Management of Labor and Delivery

Management of Labor and Delivery

EDITED BY

George A. Macones MD

Mitchell and Elaine Yanow Professor and Chair
Department of Obstetrics and Gynecology
Washington University School of Medicine
St Louis, MO, USA

SECOND EDITION

WILEY Blackwell

This edition first published 2016 © 2016, 1997 by John Wiley & Sons, Ltd

Registered Office
John Wiley & Sons, Ltd, The Atrium, Southern Gate, Chichester, West Sussex, PO19 8SQ, UK

Editorial Offices
9600 Garsington Road, Oxford, OX4 2DQ, UK
The Atrium, Southern Gate, Chichester, West Sussex, PO19 8SQ, UK
111 River Street, Hoboken, NJ 07030-5774, USA

For details of our global editorial offices, for customer services and for information about how to apply for permission to reuse the copyright material in this book please see our website at www.wiley.com/wiley-blackwell

Library of Congress Cataloging-in-Publication Data

Management of labor and delivery / [edited by] George A. Macones. – Second edition.
p. ; cm.
Preceeded by Management of labor and delivery / [edited by] Robert K. Creasy, c1997.
Includes bibliographical references and index.
ISBN 978-1-118-26864-3 (cloth)
I. Macones, George A., editor.
[DNLM: 1. Labor, Obstetric. 2. Delivery, Obstetric. WQ 300]
RG651
618.4–dc23

2015018495

A catalogue record for this book is available from the British Library.

Wiley also publishes its books in a variety of electronic formats. Some content that appears in print may not be available in electronic books.

Cover image: http://www.istockphoto.com/photo/doctor-holding-new-born-12676907
photo/doctor-holding-new-born © Reynardt

Set in 9.5/13pt Meridien by SPi Global, Pondicherry, India

Printed in Singapore by C.O.S. Printers Pte Ltd

1 2016

Contents

Contributor List

Valerie A. Arkoosh MD, MPH
Department of Anesthesiology and Critical Care, Perelman School of Medicine, University of Pennsylvania, Philadelphia, PA, USA

Emily J. Baird MD
Department of Anesthesiology and Critical Care, Perelman School of Medicine, University of Pennsylvania, Philadelphia, PA, USA

Alison Cahill MD, MSCI
Associate Professor, Director, Division of Maternal-Fetal Medicine, Department of Obstetrics and Gynecology, Washington University School of Medicine, St Louis, MO, USA

Aaron B. Caughey MD, PhD
Professor and Chair, Department of Obstetrics and Gynecology, Oregon Health and Science University, Portland, OR, USA

Yvonne W. Cheng MD, PhD
Department of Obstetrics, Gynecology, and Reproductive Sciences, University of California, San Francisco, CA, USA

Gary A. Dildy, III MD
Professor and Vice Chairman of Quality and Patient Safety, Department of Obstetrics and Gynecology, Baylor College of Medicine; Chief Quality Officer, Obstetrics and Gynecology, Texas Children's Hospital, Houston, TX, USA

Karin A. Fox MD, MEd
Assistant Professor, Division of Maternal-Fetal Medicine, Department of Obstetrics and Gynecology, Baylor College of Medicine, Houston, TX, USA

William D. Fraser MD, MSc, FRCSC
Professor, Department of Obstetrics and Gynecology, Director, Research Centre, Hospital Centre of the Université de Sherbrooke, Sherbrooke, QC, Canada

Edmund F. Funai MD
Vice President and Chief Operating Officer, USF Health, Vice Dean, Morsani College of Medicine, Professor, Department of Obstetrics and Gynecology, University of South Florida, Tampa, FL, USA

Jessica C. Garrett RN, BSN
Department of Obstetrics and Gynecology, Washington University in St Louis, St Louis, MO, USA

Katherine R. Goetzinger MD, MSCI
Assistant Professor, Division of Maternal-Fetal Medicine, Department of Obstetrics and Gynecology, Washington University School of Medicine, St Louis, MO, USA

Christopher Goodier MD
Fellow, Maternal-Fetal Medicine, Department of Obstetrics and Gynecology, Medical University of South Carolina, Charleston, SC, USA

William Grobman MD, MBA
Arthur Hale Curtis Professor, Department of Obstetrics and Gynecology, Feinberg School of Medicine, Northwestern University Medical School, Chicago, IL, USA

Christina S. Han MD
Adjunct Assistant Professor, Department of Obstetrics, Gynecology, and Reproductive Sciences, Yale University School of Medicine, New Haven, CT, USA

Laura Houston MD
Fellow, Maternal-Fetal Medicine, Medical University of South Carolina, Charleston, SC, USA

Kristina J. Hung MD
San Francisco General Hospital and Trauma Center, San Francisco, CA, USA

Megan Jones MD
Division of Maternal-Fetal Medicine, Department of Obstetrics and Gynecology, Banner Good Samaritan Medical Center, Phoenix, AZ, USA

Audrey Lyndon PhD, RN
Associate Professor, Department of Family Health Care Nursing, School of Nursing, University of California, San Francisco, CA, USA

Romy-Leigh McMaster MSc
Research Assistant, Department of Obstetrics and Gynecology, CHU Sainte-Justine, University of Montreal, Montréal, Canada

Audrey Merriam MD
Clinical Fellow, Division of Maternal-Fetal Medicine, Department of Obstetrics and Gynecology, Columbia University, New York, NY, USA

Emily Miller MD, MPH
Assistant Professor, Department of Obstetrics and Gynecology, Feinberg School of Medicine, Northwestern University Medical School, Chicago, IL, USA

Richard C. Month MD
Assistant Professor of Clinical Anesthesiology, Chief of Obstetric Anesthesiology, Department of Anesthesiology and Critical Care, University of Pennsylvania Health System, Philadelphia, PA, USA

Roger Newman MD
Professor and Maas Chair for Reproductive Sciences; Vice Chair, Academic Affairs and Women's Health Research, Medical University of South Carolina, Charleston, SC, USA

John Ozimek MD
Division of Maternal-Fetal Medicine, Department of Obstetrics and Gynecology, Banner Good Samaritan Medical Center, Phoenix, AZ, USA

Jordan H. Perlow
Division of Maternal-Fetal Medicine, Department of Obstetrics and Gynecology, Banner Good Samaritan Medical Center, Phoenix, AZ, USA

Christian M. Pettker MD
Associate Professor, Chief of Obstetrics, Department of Obstetrics, Gynecology, and Reproductive Sciences, Yale University School of Medicine, New Haven, CT, USA

Shu Qin Wei MD, PhD
Ajunct Professor, Department of Obstetrics and Gynecology, CHU Sainte-Justine, University of Montreal, Montréal, Canada

Susan M. Ramin MD
Henry and Emma Meyer Chair in Obstetrics and Gynecology, Professor and Vice Chair of Education, Department of Obstetrics and Gynecology, Baylor College of Medicine, Houston, TX, USA

Mildred M. Ramirez
Professor, Department of Obstetrics and Gynecology, Baylor College of Medicine, Houston, TX, USA

Anthony Sciscione DO
Director of Maternal-Fetal Medicine, Department of Obstetrics and Gynecology, Christiana Hospital, Newark, DE, USA

Anthony Shanks MD
Assistant Professor, Division of Maternal-Fetal Medicine, Department of Obstetrics and Gynecology, Washington University School of Medicine, St Louis, MO, USA

David M. Stamilio MD
Clinical Professor, Division of Maternal-Fetal Medicine, Department of Obstetrics and Gynecology, University of North Carolina at Chapel Hill, Chapel Hill, NC, USA

Molly J. Stout MD
Assistant Professor, Division of Maternal-Fetal Medicine, Department of Obstetrics and Gynecology, Washington University in St Louis, St Louis, MO, USA

Scott A. Sullivan MD
Associate Professor, Department of Obstetrics and Gynecology, Medical University of South Carolina, Charleston, SC, USA

Laurie S. Swaim MD
Associate Professor; Director, Division of Gynecologic and Obstetric Specialists, Department of Obstetrics and Gynecology, Baylor College of Medicine; Chief of Gynecological Services, Texas Children's Hospital, Houston, TX, USA

Methodius G. Tuuli MD, MPH
Assistant Professor, Division of Maternal-Fetal Medicine, Department of Obstetrics and Gynecology, Washington University in St Louis, St Louis, MO, USA

Kirsten Wisner MS, RNC
Salinas Valley Memorial Hospital, Seaside, CA, USA

Jun Zhang MD, PhD
Professor, Xinhua Hospital, Shanghai Jiao Tong University School of Medicine, Shanghai, China

CHAPTER 1

Antenatal preparation for labor

Molly Stout[1], Jessica C. Garrett[1], and David M. Stamilio[2]

[1] *Department of Obstetrics and Gynecology, Washington University in St Louis, St Louis, MO, USA*

[2] *Department of Obstetrics and Gynecology, University of North Carolina at Chapel Hill, Chapel Hill, NC, USA*

1.1 Introduction

Childbirth most often is viewed as a joyful event and most commonly culminates in a happy outcome. However, it is also a major life change for the pregnant woman that frequently produces anxiety, stress, and fear, and is associated with considerable pain and a need for substantial physical and emotional exertion. Women have described childbirth pain as severe, with 60% of women reporting labor pain as the most intense that they had ever experienced [1–2]. Some authors have described pregnancy and childbirth as having a crisis character, similar in some ways to the crisis character of surgery. Thus, the pregnant patient must, in some way, cope with the critical nature of childbirth [3–4]. And her ability to cope with the pain and stress of childbirth can determine whether she views it as a positive or a negative experience. Further, her perception of childbirth and how she coped with the process has the potential to shape either favorably or detrimentally her own self-image, and to affect attitudes and relationships with her newborn child, partner, and other family members. Thus, childbirth has great potential to cause long-lasting changes in a woman's adaptation to and progression through life.

Antenatal childbirth education as a formal construct was initially conceived in the 1930s and then further developed in the 1960s and 1970s to address the critical nature of childbirth and to better prepare pregnant women for the stress associated with this major life-event, in hopes of improving physical and emotional outcomes related to pregnancy [5–9]. The pregnant patient is faced with several stressors associated with childbirth. While historically pain has been the primary focus for obstetric providers, other stressors for the pregnant patient include fear of the unknown, fatigue, loss of dignity, loss of ability to

Management of Labor and Delivery, Second Edition. Edited by George A. Macones.

actively participate in the birthing process, aloneness, and health threats to mother and newborn [10]. In response to these stressors, various antenatal childbirth education programs have been developed with goals to: "influence health behavior; build women's confidence in their ability to give birth; prepare women and their partners for childbirth; prepare for parenthood; develop social support networks; promote confident parents; and contribute to reducing perinatal morbidity and mortality." Indeed, women commonly report that their primary reason for attending childbirth classes is to reduce anxiety about labor and birth [11]. Women also seek antenatal education to get information on physiologic changes of pregnancy, fetal development, the course of labor and birth, their care options in labor and birth, possible birth-related complications, and newborn care [11–12].

Antenatal childbirth education has remained popular over the last six decades, although some centers are reporting a decreased attendance, perhaps related to the expanding popularity and accessibility of internet-based information [13]. Still, medical professional organizations and providers commonly recommend antenatal childbirth education to patients, and a substantial proportion of patients, especially primiparas, seek and attend education programs [9,11,13]. Several observational and qualitative studies, many on the psychoprophylaxis of Lamaze, indicate that women who take prepared childbirth classes rate birth experiences more positively [10], and the large majority of participants report high satisfaction with their selected educational program [14]. The efficacy of antenatal childbirth classes has been a source of debate, in part, due to the variability in the outcomes assessed by investigators, but also likely a manifestation of the wide variability in the content of and approach to antenatal education. This topic will be discussed in detail later in the chapter, but there are mounting data on the efficacy, benefits, and utility of antenatal childbirth programs.

1.2 Goals of antenatal childbirth education

Various childbirth education programs have been developed to achieve multiple and often varied goals. The variability in program aims not only influences educational content but also produces controversy in the expert community regarding the purpose and effectiveness of antenatal childbirth education. In his expert commentary, Dr Enkin cautions clinicians and investigators that childbirth classes are an educational rather than obstetric intervention, and that effectiveness of childbirth classes should be evaluated by assessing outcomes that reflect their objectives, as determined by the attendees [15]. Women attend childbirth classes not just to improve pregnancy outcomes or to minimize the use of analgesic drugs, but "to be informed, to learn what to expect during labor and afterward, to learn about obstetric interventions and hospital routines, to obtain advice and answers to questions, to reduce anxiety, to meet other

Table 1.1 Goals of antenatal childbirth classes.

Patient-based	Learn about childbirth
	Learn about obstetrical interventions
	Obtain medical advice
	Reduce anxiety
	Learn about baby care
	Establish social support
Provider-based	Influence health behavior
	Potentially reduce morbidity and mortality
	Improve maternal satisfaction with childbirth

expectant parents, and to learn about baby care and feeding" [15]. Thus, he urges that the efficacy and utility of childbirth classes be assessed using the educational objectives that are important to the women attending rather than the obstetrical outcomes important to clinicians. While it is important to assure that clinical outcomes are not compromised and it would be advantageous if the educational objectives could result in improved pregnancy outcomes, the success of programs in achieving educational goals must also be prioritized and assessed directly. The goals of antenatal childbirth education should be to inform about childbirth, influence health behavior, build the woman's confidence in her ability to birth, prepare women and partners for childbirth and parenthood, develop social support networks, and, potentially, reduce perinatal morbidity and mortality [11]. Humenic reviewed the literature on childbirth preparation and pain management and identified maternal control during and satisfaction with the birthing process as important factors or steps in achieving improved psychosocial outcomes, such as less postpartum depression, improved self-esteem, and better self-perception after delivery [3]. Thus she identified improved maternal satisfaction with the labor and delivery experience and an improved perception of control or "mastery" of the birth process as the major goals of childbirth preparation (Table 1.1) [10].

1.3 Theoretical approaches to antenatal childbirth education

As antenatal childbirth education evolved in the 1970s, there was a major shift in the theoretic framework of maternal satisfaction with childbirth and the positive effects of childbirth preparation. The prevailing model for childbirth satisfaction assumed pain control to be the primary factor in achieving satisfaction in childbirth. In opposition to this "Pain Management Model" (Figure 1.1), Humenic developed the "Mastery Model" (Figure 1.2) as a more comprehensive theory to explain maternal satisfaction with the birth process and consequential improved psychosocial outcomes and mental health [10]. The Mastery Model

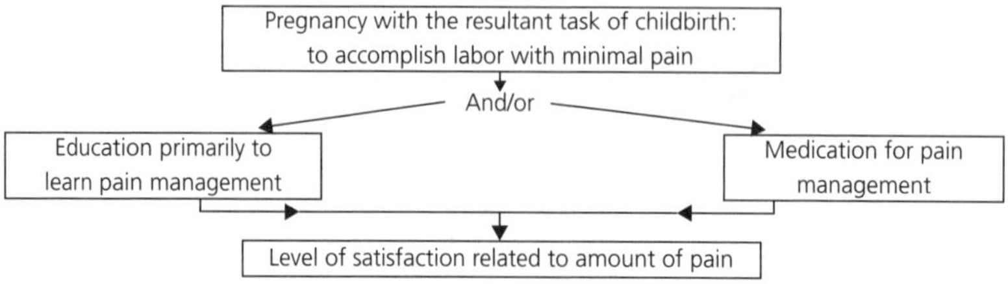

Figure 1.1 The Pain Management Model. *Source*: Humenick, 1981 [10]. Reproduced with permission from Wiley.

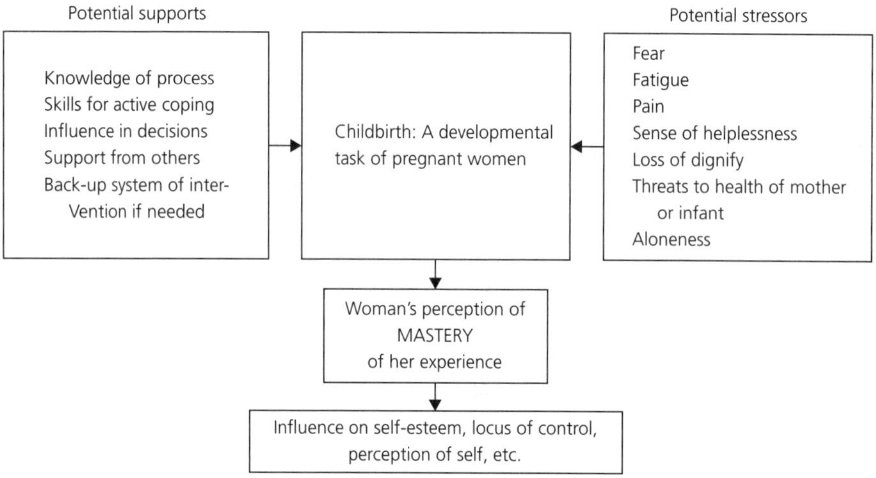

Figure 1.2 Mastery as the key to childbirth satisfaction. *Source*: Humenick, 1981 [10]. Reproduced with permission from Wiley.

was constructed from the qualitative and observational research that explored the effects of pharmaceutical pain control versus childbirth classes on maternal satisfaction with childbirth. The model was also based on qualitative research that related maternal satisfaction and improved mental health to various factors associated with control or "mastery" of the childbirth process. Control was most often identified as a key factor in satisfaction and was defined by women as the ability to influence decisions made, not surrendering all decisions and responsibilities to care providers, and maintaining a working alliance with healthcare providers [10,16]. Unlike the Pain Management Model, which identified pain as the primary important birth stressor, the Mastery Model identifies pain as one of several potential maternal stressors, such as fear, fatigue, sense of helplessness, loss of dignity, and health threats (Figure 1.2). Via childbirth classes and preparation, these stressors are minimized by providing women with mechanisms to control these stressors, such as knowledge, coping skills, and support from others. Armed with these supports, the pregnant woman has a sense of greater control in the birthing process and a perception of mastery of her childbirth experience. In turn, this mastery positively influences self-esteem, self-perception, locus of control, and sense of satisfaction, all of which influence the woman's ability to assume the task of parenthood and relate to her child and others. These positive psychosocial effects may also directly improve clinical outcomes such as postpartum depression, or indirectly improve clinical outcomes by promoting healthy behavior, as a consequence of improved mental health. The Mastery Model aims to encourage assertive, self-reliant behaviors via comprehensive childbirth preparation. Childbirth classes are designed to inform about the labor and birth process, encourage realistic maternal childbirth goals, teach coping skills for pain management, prepare the woman for active participation in decision making, and assist in developing an adequate support system [10].

There are several types or brands of childbirth preparation programs that are currently available and prevalent in the US and Europe, but most have a theoretic framework that is based on or extrapolated from the earlier work of Dr Grantly Dick-Read who developed and published the concept of "natural birth." Dick-Read's approach included childbirth preparation with education about labor and birth, as well as relaxation techniques and other forms of psychological preparation [5–6]. One of the most common methods taught in the US is the Lamaze method of childbirth preparation; however, the Bradley method, and more recently the Mongan method (a.k.a. HypnoBirthing) and Balaskas's "active birth" method, are also prevalent and popular methods for childbirth preparation, among others [7,17–19]. Although certain components of the childbirth education are emphasized variably across methods and specific coping strategies differ by the method, these childbirth preparation classes share common tenets, including education on the labor and birth process, emphasizing childbirth as a normal, healthy process rather than a disease process, decreasing fear and anxiety, instruction on relaxation techniques, and identifying a support person or multiple support people. The Lamaze psychoprophylaxis method was introduced by Dr Fernand Lamaze, a French obstetrician. The ultimate goal of the Lamaze method is to assure that women are confident in their ability to give birth, are free to find comfort in a variety of ways, and are supported by family or friends and healthcare professionals. While this method initially relied primarily on focused breathing to cope with labor pain, the method has evolved to include other techniques such as movement and massage. Although the program teaches about necessary obstetric interventions with informed consent, there is an emphasis on the woman's "right to give birth free from *routine* medical intervention" including but not specific to pain medication. Lamaze International (Position Paper 2007) has identified six care practices that promote normal birth and serve as the foundation for childbirth education:

- labor begins on its own
- freedom of movement throughout labor
- continuous labor support

- no routine interventions
- spontaneous pushing in upright or gravity-neutral positions
- no separation of mother and baby with unlimited opportunities for breastfeeding.

The Bradley method of natural (i.e. drug free) childbirth was developed by Dr Robert Bradley in the late 1940s and then gained popularity in the 1960s after his method was published widely. This method emphasizes the husband or partner as a labor coach and is therefore also known as "Husband-Coached Childbirth," the title of his book. The Bradley method also underscores labor as a normal, natural process. The primary goal is to promote healthy, "low risk" mothers and babies so as to avoid medical intervention; to that end, 12 weekly classes emphasize good nutrition and exercise, breathing and other relaxation techniques to cope with labor pain, and active participation of the husband or partner as a coach. According to the Bradley method, to achieve natural childbirth, the woman must have complete relaxation with abdominal breathing and other techniques, as well as quiet, darkness and solitude, physical comfort, and closed eyes. Similar to Lamaze and other childbirth preparation methods, the Bradley method encourages active participation by the patient in clinical decision making. The Mongan method, or HypnoBirthing, is also based on Dr Dick-Read's philosophy of natural childbirth, but, as the name indicates, with an emphasis on hypnosis techniques for relaxation as well as programming and conditioning by practicing a "few key techniques." In a series of five 2.5-hour classes, this program also encompasses education on the birthing process, labor positions, nutrition, breathing methods, and body toning exercises (www.hypnobirthing.com). The "active birth" method was founded in the late 1970s by Janet Balaskas, a childbirth educator in the UK. According to the Active Birth Centre, the method's central principle is "for the woman to move spontaneously and be led by her body, adopting upright positions during labour and birth." This method promotes women as "active birthgivers" rather than passive patients (www.activebirthcentre.com). In addition to informing patients about labor and birth, the program relies heavily on the instruction of yoga to promote free movement and good positioning during labor and delivery.

In addition to variability in class content and philosophy, there are various types of settings or venues for education. Classes are offered with a wide spectrum in length, from intensive one-day classes to a series of classes over several weeks. Educational programs can be stand-alone, which tend to be more comprehensive, "bench" classes that are offered in the clinic (often by the office nurse) while waiting for the obstetrical provider, or self-learning programs that use video (e.g. DVD) or Internet computer-based learning instead of didactic in-person instruction. Other non-traditional childbirth education programs exist, such as local "grass roots" programs or personalized programs such as "Birthing from Within," which is tailored instruction provided via telephone. Education can be provided either individually or in groups [11,13]. Group prenatal care and childbirth education have gained popularity in the last two decades and this group approach to care has recently been a focus of research to assess if it can improve pregnancy outcomes. Thus, the topic is presented in more detail later in the chapter.

1.4 Effectiveness of childbirth preparation: educational goals and pregnancy outcomes

The literature on the effectiveness of childbirth education is quite difficult to interpret as there is great variability in class content, populations studied, and outcomes assessed. By and large, childbirth classes appear to be more effective when educational or psychosocial goals are assessed as the primary outcome compared to when obstetrical outcomes are defined as the primary outcome. Except for more recent research on group prenatal care, most studies that assess the efficacy of antenatal childbirth education are observational studies that rely on convenience sampling rather than randomization. Thus, there is great potential for selection bias in most studies. For example, women who elect to participate in childbirth classes are more often primiparous, tend to smoke less frequently, have higher income and educational levels, are more knowledgeable about pregnancy at baseline, and have less "background negativity" and a "more positive self-concept" than women who do not seek childbirth education [9,14,20]. Those who do not attend classes tend to have lower socioeconomic status, are younger, and are more often single [14]. Many of these characteristics have been associated with obstetrical and/or psychological outcomes. Therefore, for most studies it is possible that observed positive effects of childbirth preparation programs may be in part or completely due to study group differences from selection bias.

1.4.1 Educational goals and psychological impact

As noted previously, most women seek childbirth education to become better informed about birth and parenting and to reduce anxiety related to the anticipation of the birthing process. Indicators that show whether or not childbirth classes achieve these goals include measurement of maternal enjoyment and satisfaction with the birth experience, assessment of maternal anxiety levels, assessment of the ability to adapt to and endure the birthing process and to assume the parenting role, and evaluation of maternal knowledge. Multiple studies have reported increased satisfaction with the birthing process among patients who take childbirth classes [9,21–23]. These studies generally used educational programs based on the natural birth methods of Dick-Read or the psychoprophylaxis methods of Lamaze. While not all studies detected a measurable reduction in labor pain with childbirth classes, most studies report that women who undergo childbirth preparation more commonly view birth as a positive experience. Underlying factors for satisfaction with the birth experience include a sense of self-reliance, self-control, and independence, as well as both the desire and the opportunity to play an active role in childbirth [10,16,21]. In a cohort study of 36 women who did or did not participate in Lamaze or natural childbirth classes, Tanzer (1968) observed that class takers perceived less pain, particularly in the late stages of labor, and they received less pain medication [25]. Further, the pregnant women's experience was improved with the husband present. Other studies have also observed that women who take childbirth classes receive less pain medication [22–26]. In a similar cohort study of 75 women, Davenport and Boylan did not observe a reduction in pain perception with participation in natural childbirth classes, but trained women behaved more calmly in labor and birth with less "body tenseness" [21]. Further, a woman's desire to be an active participant was a major factor for having a positive childbirth experience. In a cohort of 294 primiparas, Redman observed increased knowledge of childbirth among patients who took classes but did not observe a difference in use of epidural or other pain medications or in patient satisfaction with the birth [14]. Childbirth classes have also been shown to decrease the amount of maternal anxiety with labor and birth [3,20,26]. Patients who took Lamaze classes have been shown to be more prepared for labor, which leads to a higher level of awareness at delivery and consequently promotes more positive reactions to the infant and improved attitude about childbirth [4].

Summarizing these data, a sense of control experienced by laboring patients, in the form of being an active participant and decision-maker, is an important predictor of and generally a necessary step in birth satisfaction [27]. Increased prenatal control in the form of childbirth preparation has been shown to teach the mother techniques to maintain control in the delivery room and to develop healthy expectations [28]. Women who experience greater control during childbirth report increased satisfaction with their birth experience; control is commonly described by patients as the ability to play an active role in decisions such as pain control, body position, birth method, and medical interventions [29–34].

Further, there is evidence to suggest that childbirth preparation could promote improved long-term psychosocial outcomes by reducing dissatisfaction as unsatisfying birth experiences have been associated with postpartum depression and post-traumatic stress disorder [29,32–33,35]. Similarly, adverse pregnancy outcomes may be decreased as childbirth preparation can reduce maternal anxiety, and anxiety is associated with a greater number of risk behaviors, such as scant prenatal care, smoking, drugs, and poor diet, as well as increased risks of preterm birth and low birthweight [3]. Significant differences between maternal expectations and experience reduce birth satisfaction; childbirth classes may improve satisfaction by reducing the disparity between expectations and experience [28,32,36].

1.4.2 Pregnancy outcomes

Clinicians and clinical investigators have explored the possibility that childbirth preparation improves obstetrical outcomes in addition to achieving educational objectives. Findings have been mixed regarding the efficacy of childbirth classes for improving pregnancy outcomes, which is not surprising given the heterogeneity in the outcomes studied, the types of antenatal education programs used, and the population characteristics. Most studies are observational but there is one meta-analysis of nine randomized trials [11]. Study variability among those included in the meta-analysis was so marked that data could not be pooled to estimate summary effects (odds ratios). In the largest of the trials included, childbirth education did not alter the rates of maternal blood transfusion, instrumental delivery, low 5-minute Apgar score, or neonatal intensive care unit admission and did not affect the rates of vaginal birth after cesarean (VBAC) attempt or success. In smaller trials included in the meta-analysis, childbirth education did not alter the rates of preterm birth, fetal growth restriction, congenital anomalies, or cesarean. There was also no effect on the length of labor or frequency of episiotomy. Data were quite limited but no differences in outcomes were identified across different types of childbirth education, including group, individual, and expanded educational programs.

Cogan reviewed observational studies on the efficacy of childbirth education [9]. Findings were inconsistent with regard to the effect of childbirth classes on the length of labor and frequency of forceps-assisted delivery. For example, six studies indicated that labor length was shorter after childbirth education but seven studies observed similar or increased labor length. Most recent studies of childbirth education have also not identified a reduction in labor length, forceps-assisted delivery rate, oxytocin use, cesarean rate, or use of regional anesthesia or analgesia [3,37–38]. While findings are inconsistent, a few studies observed lower cesarean rates in patients who attended childbirth classes and one study revealed a lower rate of forceps delivery [3,37]. Research on the effect of childbirth on perinatal and neonatal outcomes is very limited. However, Hughey and colleagues observed a lower rate of "fetal distress" in patients who attended childbirth classes [39]. Consonni and colleagues observed a shorter mean length of newborn admission among class attendees [3]. In one moderately sized cohort study (N = 616) antenatal childbirth education was associated with increased rate of breastfeeding and decreased visits for false labor [40–41]. As discussed previously, there is great potential for selection bias in the observational studies, which may result in erroneous observations.

Antenatal childbirth education is popular with and desired by a significant proportion of pregnant patients. Attendees are generally satisfied with their choice to seek antenatal education and are most often quite satisfied with the education and preparation received.

To summarize the efficacy of antenatal childbirth education, data are quite limited in methodology and quantity, but educational programs appear to

Table 1.2 Potential effects of childbirth classes identified in research.

Obstetrical impact	Improved social interaction with newborn and family Reduced labor pain? Improved sense of control Improved knowledge about childbirth Reduced anxiety Reduced cesarean risk? Increased breastfeeding rate Decreased frequency of visits for "false labor"

improve maternal knowledge about labor and childbirth and likely have a favorable impact on the rate or severity of maternal anxiety. Childbirth classes also appear to improve the likelihood that a pregnant woman will be satisfied with the childbirth experience, which may be achieved via an improved maternal perception of control and active participation in the birthing process. The restricted amount of data from randomized clinical trials does not provide evidence that antenatal childbirth education improves perinatal or maternal pregnancy outcomes. While fraught with the great potential for selection bias, observational studies provide some evidence that childbirth education may reduce cesarean rate and increase breastfeeding rate. Education may also reduce the frequency at which patients present for evaluation of threatened or false labor (Table 1.2).

1.5 Future direction for advancing antenatal childbirth education

As several clinical and research experts have stated, there is a great need for well-designed clinical trials to assess the content and efficacy of antenatal childbirth education programs [1,11,42–43]. Evaluating the effectiveness of childbirth education is necessary and important because currently an extensive amount of healthcare resources are utilized in promoting and providing childbirth classes even though the effects of the intervention have not been rigorously studied. Designing and completing a clinical trial for this topic will be challenging since there is a large amount of variability in program content, format, and methods. Importantly, investigational outcomes selected should reflect those that are important to both the consumer and the healthcare provider. Thus, selected outcomes should include both educational goals and clinical outcomes. Additionally, effects of childbirth education should be assessed in both general and specific high-risk patient populations to improve generalizability of findings and to assess if effectiveness is differential by population type. Identifying high-risk patients most likely to benefit may allow them to be targeted for specific educational programs. Lastly, research on specific class content and best practices for childbirth education is needed to inform educators on the optimal approach for childbirth preparation. Escott, Slade, and Spiby, in a review of the psychological aspects of childbirth education, noted that there is a "limited range of coping strategies taught" in antenatal classes [1]. They recommend that, beyond controlled breathing, relaxation, and position change, other cognitive strategies (e.g. imagery, distraction, self-statements) and behavioral strategies (e.g. operant conditioning or biofeedback) be used and investigated. They suggest areas for improvement and research, including: (1) increasing the range of coping strategies taught, (2) helping identify patient coping preferences and styles, (3) using classes to help develop a unique set of strategies for an individual, (4) strengthening coping self-efficacy (i.e. confidence) by practice and reinforcement in class, (5) developing prompting and reinforcement of a set of strategies by the partner, and (6) developing implementation intentions that account for the changing environment in childbirth. In their systematic review, Lally and colleagues acknowledged a need for improved educational content and approach because they identified "a mismatch between women's expectations and their actual experiences ... there is a mismatch between how painful women expect labour to be, how long it will last, what pain relief they will need, how in control they will be and what the actual experience is like." They state that in order to improve a woman's satisfaction with childbirth experience, researchers need to investigate how education can be improved so that "expectations of women can be brought more in line with their actual experience" [43].

1.6 Who teaches childbirth education classes and where?

In the United States, family childbirth education may be offered at hospitals, birth centers, clinics, and community sites, and privately. Childbirth class educators may include nurses, nurse practitioners, midwives, doulas, or other types of experienced educators in maternal and newborn health. Class offerings range widely in terms of content, scope, and style of presentation. Types of classes may include:

- sequential series, usually starting in the second trimester and ending near term gestation
- a one-time refresher course, often offered to families with previous childbirth experience
- ongoing childbirth education that is incorporated into group prenatal care visits, occurring throughout the duration of the pregnancy, such as the CenteringPregnancy curriculum [44].

Certain childbirth education curricula, such as CenteringPregnancy, Lamaze International, Bradley Method, International Childbirth Education Association, and Prepared Childbirth Educators, have specific instructor training

Table 1.3 Prevalent models of antepartum education.

CenteringPregnancy
Lamaze International
Bradley Method
International Childbirth Education Association
Prepared Childbirth Educators
HypnoBirthing/Mongan Method
Active Birth Method

and certification unique to the particular focus and content of that program (Table 1.3). No one specific course or method is endorsed by the American College of Obstetricians and Gynecology (ACOG) or the American College of Nurse Midwives. Resource information on some of the more well-known methods are offered on the ACOG website: http://www.yourpregnancyandchildbirth.com/topics.php?page=resources

The pregnant mother may choose the type of childbirth preparation class that best fits her needs. A mother may choose any support person (father of the baby, partner, mother, sister, friend, doula, etc.) to attend childbirth education with her. It is recommended that the support person be consistently present at all classes with the mother and be available as the primary support person during the mother's actual labor and birth experience. The presence of a consistent support person is associated with clinically meaningful benefits for the mother, including shorter labor, improved maternal satisfaction, and an increased likelihood of having a vaginal birth [45]. Introduction of the support person to the obstetric provider and communication about the choice of childbirth education class may help to clarify the family's preparedness level, as well as hopes and expectations for childbirth.

1.7 Prenatal education class content

1.7.1 Signs of labor

Recognition of the signs and symptoms of labor is a key step in preparing for labor and delivery. Prenatal education classes may cover normal symptomatology of the third trimester. Women who attend antenatal childbirth classes are generally instructed on the following concepts: signs and symptoms of labor, normal symptomatology of late pregnancy (fatigue, low back pain, abdominal discomfort), and strategies to alleviate some of the discomfort of pregnancy. In addition, prenatal classes can provide guidance about what symptoms may indicate the true onset of labor and should prompt the woman to be evaluated by obstetric providers.

1.7.2 Process of labor

During labor and delivery there are many steps that without preparation may seem foreign to the laboring mother. Childbirth education can prepare a mother for what to expect during the process of labor. Certain topics that may be addressed are the typical progression of cervical change, spontaneous versus artificial rupture of membranes, internal versus external fetal heart rate monitoring, contraction monitoring, and use of medications in labor. In addition, classes may review different positions for pushing as well as techniques for effective pushing. Familiarity with these topics may decrease maternal anxiety and improve patient-provider communication during the labor process.

1.7.3 Pain coping, comfort, and relief

Both coping-centered and pharmacologic pain control approaches may be useful to the laboring mother. A trusting patient-provider relationship is integral to determining the right approach for each individual person, both prior to and with ongoing assessment during the labor process. An understanding of the breadth of available pain control options, including coping techniques, as well as pharmacologic or regional pain relief, will help the mother make informed decisions during the labor process. Familiarity with pain control options prior to the onset of labor is helpful; conversely, exploring these decisions for the first time during the acute pain associated with labor may be overwhelming for the mother. Childbirth education classes typically cover both non-pharmacologic and pharmacologic pain control options. It is important for both the patient and the provider to maintain flexibility with respect to pain control options, as a mother's wants and needs may change during the labor process.

1.7.4 Non-pharmacologic pain coping

Most women experience pain during labor, while giving birth, and/or postpartum. Healthy labor is a unique situation in which moderate to severe pain is not associated with injury or pathology but is instead part of the normal process. During normal labor, uterine contraction pain is expected. However, maternal suffering is not necessary and all efforts should be made by the medical team and support person to assist the mother with pain relief to minimize maternal suffering. Coping-centered pain management options are discussed in most kinds of childbirth classes. Selecting a class that includes pain coping strategies can help an expectant mother and her support person to be prepared for the pain typically associated with labor [46]. Excessive maternal pain and suffering can, in some cases, be associated with long-term maternal-infant bonding impairment, and more generally, with maternal symptoms of depression, anxiety, and post-traumatic stress disorder [47]. Education for the mother and her support person can focus on strategies to prevent pain-related psychological suffering, helplessness, and distress associated with the feeling of having insufficient resources for coping with labor [48].

With guidance in prenatal classes, women and their support persons are able to learn about, discuss, and practice coping strategies in preparation for labor and birth-associated pain. As perceptions of and responses to pain vary widely from person to person, each pregnant mother may prepare for childbirth by identifying and understanding the nature of her own coping styles and preferences, including any dysfunctional coping patterns [1]. Non-pharmacologic coping-centered pain control may include methods such as physical movement, hydrotherapy, meditation, focused breathing, and listening to music. Many childbirth curricula include information specifically for the support person to become familiar with techniques to help the laboring mother cope with pain. Massage, acupressure, guided imagery, and partnered breathing are just of few of many practices that, with training, a support person may use to help a laboring mother manage pain and prevent suffering. Information about useful labor tools like the birthing ball, chair, and bar, wireless fetal monitoring equipment, and tubs designed specifically for hydrotherapy in labor, are also often included in childbirth education.

1.7.5 Pharmacologic pain control options

Certain types of intravenous analgesia and regional anesthesia are considered safe medical interventions for decreasing labor pain. According to an ACOG committee opinion on pain control during labor, "There is no other circumstance where it is considered acceptable for an individual to experience untreated severe pain, amenable to safe intervention, while under a physician's care" [49]. The medical approach to labor pain management places emphasis on the elimination of the physical sensation of labor pain. ACOG recommends that regional anesthesia be provided to any woman in labor who requests it, regardless of insurance. The only exception to this statement is the rare circumstance of a coexisting medical condition which is a contraindication to regional anesthesia [49].

Most childbirth education programs provide information on pharmaceutical-based approaches for pain control during labor. Albeit the description of risks and benefits of therapy and the extent that pharmaceutical therapy is encouraged or discouraged varies by the specific educational program. Common medical pain control topics discussed in childbirth education are summarized below. Medical options for pain control during labor include intravenous opioids, sedatives, regional neuraxial anesthesia (epidural), paracervical or pudendal local nerve blocks, and local anesthetic injections. Systemic opioids or sedatives may be used for pain control during labor but have associated risks of neonatal respiratory depression and therefore may be used predominantly during the early stages of labor. Regional anesthesia such as spinal block or epidural anesthesia is the most commonly used form of pain relief during labor in the United States [50] and is administered and monitored by trained anesthesiologists and advanced nurse practitioners. A secondary benefit of epidural catheters is the ability to rapidly dose the epidural if an emergency indication for cesarean arises.

Table 1.4 Common methods of non-pharmacologic and pharmacologic pain control for labor and delivery.

Non-pharmacologic	Pharmacologic
Physical movement (walking, birthing ball, changing positions, yoga)	Regional anesthesia
Hydrotherapy	Intravenous analgesia/sedative medication
Meditation	Pudendal block
Focused breathing	Local anesthesia
Listening to music	
Massage	
Acupressure	

Common side effects associated with regional anesthesia include hypotension, spinal headache, and back pain at the injection site. Anesthetic toxicity, high spinal block, and paralysis or nerve injury are extremely rare complications of epidural anesthesia. Paracervical block may decrease pain associated with cervical dilation. However, its use for obstetric analgesia has fallen out of favor. Pudendal nerve blockade introduces local anesthetic into the pudendal nerve as it traverses just below the ischial spine and provides pain control for the perineal region only. Thus, the utility of pudendal nerve blockade is primarily for vaginal laceration repair, episiotomy, or operative vaginal deliveries where regional anesthesia is not present or is inadequate.

Obstetric anesthesiologists provide expertise in the safe use of regional and general anesthesia, as well as prevention and management of any complications related to neuraxial anesthesia. Collaboration with anesthesia colleagues for pain management strategies for women with or without epidurals, and with medical and obstetric complications, can be extremely useful and beneficial to the patient to maximize pain control while minimizing medical risks. Effective and thorough patient education is the foundation of informed decision making on pain control options. Education best begins during pregnancy, before the stress of labor or hospitalization occurs. Education on pharmacologic pain relief methods is typically emphasized in childbirth education classes in settings where a medical approach may be used, as with hospital-based childbirth education classes (Table 1.4).

1.7.6 Immediate post-delivery events

Childbirth classes may reduce anxiety surrounding the anticipated birth by informing the pregnant woman about typical birth scenarios and hospital-specific standard approaches and facilities, as well as informing her about available emergency maternal and pediatric care resources. Both obstetric and pediatric providers may be present at delivery; information about the roles of each, as well as about the immediate post-birth assessment of the newborn, is typically offered during class. Separation of infant from mother immediately after birth has been common in the United States, both for high- and low-risk deliveries. Because of increasing evidence supporting the benefits of early maternal-newborn skin-to-skin contact, many classes currently offer information on these benefits. For example, early continuous skin-to-skin contact improves neonatal cardio-respiratory stability, breastfeeding outcomes, and maternal-newborn bonding, and is associated with decreased infant crying, with no apparent short- or long-term negative effects [51]. Prenatal educators should address circumstances that may necessitate more immediate examination and intervention for the newborn. For example, newborns that underwent operative delivery, have anomalies, or demonstrate difficulty transitioning to extrauterine life should be assessed by pediatric providers at delivery. The assessment may sometimes be accomplished while the newborn is being held by his or her mother; at other times the support devices and accessibility available via an infant warmer are required for safe newborn assessment and resuscitation.

1.7.7 Cesarean and operative delivery

Most women who enter labor anticipate a vaginal delivery. However, circumstances may arise that necessitate an operative vaginal delivery or cesarean delivery. Childbirth education classes may address some of the indications for these interventions. It may help mothers to be familiar with what obstetric physicians are assessing during the labor progress and which conditions (such as non-reassuring fetal status or labor dystocia) might necessitate operative interventions. Although these topics may be discussed briefly during antenatal education classes, communication between the mother and the obstetric providers during the course of labor is of utmost importance. Certain signs may portend the need for an operative intervention and the obstetric providers should communicate findings to the mother during labor. However, non-reassuring fetal status may occur abruptly without warning and may necessitate urgent or emergency cesarean or operative vaginal delivery. Especially for circumstances where rapid clinical interventions are indicated, some familiarity with these procedures may be helpful for the mother. In addition, informed consent for cesarean and operative vaginal delivery is best sought prior to or early in the labor process where appropriate time for explanation, questions, and answers can be allotted in the event that a rapid intervention is needed during labor.

1.7.8 Postpartum care, breastfeeding challenges, bonding, sleep, community support

Childbirth classes typically include information about postpartum care of the mother, newborn care, common breastfeeding challenges, parent-newborn bonding, and community support resources. The amount of detail discussed on these topics varies widely and depends on the type and duration of the class. As with symptoms during late pregnancy, women may be helped by education regarding normal symptoms during the postpartum period. Physical fatigue, both from the labor process and from decreased sleep, is a challenge in the immediate postpartum period. Follow-up with obstetric providers is important to address contraception and uterine and vaginal healing, and to assess mood symptoms. Emotional challenges such as postpartum blues may be present, and both the mother and her support person should be educated regarding signs and symptoms of postpartum depression or psychosis that would warrant immediate medical attention. Many resources are available to women for breastfeeding support. Breastfeeding technique may be addressed in antenatal education classes, but are best addressed by nurses and lactation consultants during the postpartum period where bedside assessment of both the newborn and the mother can be performed to optimize breastfeeding success.

1.8 Group prenatal care

The typical model for medical care consists of one-on-one patient-provider (e.g. physician, nurse practitioner, midwife) interaction. However, starting in the late 1990s, group prenatal care, commonly called CenteringPregnancy, was introduced as a new model of prenatal care for pregnant women in which a group of 8–12 pregnant women meet for 10 sessions with an obstetric provider. The goal of CenteringPregnancy is the integration of three main components of prenatal care: health assessment, education, and support [44]. Women participate in their own assessment by measuring their own weight and blood pressure and contributing to documentation on their own medical chart. In addition, educational topics such as nutrition, exercise, newborn care, substance abuse, relaxation techniques, parenting technique, and social support are discussed in 10 2-hour sessions. Group participation allows women to discuss questions and concerns together, facilitating both a sense of self-responsibility and support within the group. Many women report that their experience with CenteringPregnancy was positive, resulting in more active participation in their own health care and facilitating a sense of camaraderie with other women alleviating anxiety and loneliness in pregnancy [52].

A recent study reported positive opinions of attendees after women participated in group prenatal care; participants reported that they learned information they may not otherwise have learned without group participation. Furthermore, women reported satisfaction with efficiency of medical care (e.g. less waiting for doctor appointments, improved sense of social support, decreased loneliness, and improved awareness of their own health) [53]. Another study, of more than 4000 patients, suggested an improvement in adequacy of prenatal care evidenced by improved prenatal visit attendance in women participating in group prenatal care. In addition, there appeared to be a decreased risk for preterm birth

Table 1.5 Possible benefits of group prenatal care.

Active participation in care
Improved awareness of self-health
Sense of support from other participants in group
Combination of prenatal care and antenatal education
Decreased loneliness
Increased compliance with attendance to prenatal visits

among the women in group prenatal care compared to those in regular obstetric care. A systematic review and meta-analysis of eight randomized control trials and cohort studies evaluated both clinical outcomes and maternal satisfaction outcomes associated with group prenatal care. The investigators reported a slight decrease in the risk for preterm birth in the randomized control trials, a slight decrease in the risk for low birthweight in the cohort studies, and no evidence for improvements in any other clinical outcomes associated with group prenatal care. However, breastfeeding rate, maternal knowledge, and maternal satisfaction with prenatal care were improved in group prenatal care models. Importantly, the authors report that the available studies on group prenatal care are of poor quality with only two high-quality randomized studies and several cohort studies with potential for significant biases of the observed results [42]. A Cochrane systematic review included nine randomized clinical trials of the effects of group or individual antenatal childbirth classes. Meta-analytic methods were not applied due to the large amount of variability and heterogeneity across studies. The investigators found no consistent results with regard to the influence of group or individual childbirth classes on knowledge acquisition, anxiety, sense of control, labor pain, factors related to infant-care competencies, or labor and birth outcomes (Table 1.5) [11]. Thus, the effects of group or individual childbirth education are largely unknown. Further studies are needed to determine whether group prenatal care for women in specific high-risk groups, such as those with a risk for preterm birth, those with diabetes or chronic pain, or those for whom substance abuse is a consideration, may improve obstetric and neonatal outcomes [54]. In addition to CenteringPregnancy, the Centering program also offers education programs in parenting (CenteringParenting) and aging/chronic disease (CenteringLifeCycle).

1.9 Self-prepared birth plans

A birth plan is a written document prepared prior to labor in which a woman outlines her hopes and expectations for her birth experience. The preparation of a birth plan often takes place in the context of childbirth education class. Written birth plans are intended to encourage informed decision making and provider-patient communication and have been in use in the US since the 1980s [55]. The original intent of formulating a birth plan was as a "vehicle for trust and communication" between pregnant women and the providers who care for them during labor and birth. Their effectiveness has been a source of controversy since inception. While some disagreement remains, the majority of providers and patients view birth plans as an effective means for communication and education. Vocal minorities remain adversarial, with some suggesting that birth plans are necessary to protect the patient from unneeded intervention while others insist that birth plans obstruct the delivery of health care. On the contrary, a carefully crafted birth plan can stimulate conversation between patient and provider, inform both patient and provider on needs and expectations, and foster a collaborative, safe approach to childbirth.

Proponents of birth plans highlight that a properly used birth plan improves communication, increases a woman's sense of control, and makes women more aware of the choices they may have during the birthing process. Critics of birth plans claim that they may foster a sense of distrust in the doctor-patient relationship [56]. There are concerns that conflict can arise when a mismatch occurs between the physician's opinion regarding medical safety and the patient's desires for birth [57]. Birth plans may cover topics such as maternal desire to walk and move during labor, requests for pain control, whether a woman wishes to be offered an epidural or not, who she desires to be present at the time of birth, whether the baby will go immediately to the mother's chest or to be warmed and assessed by the pediatric team, and who will cut the umbilical cord. The emphasis of a birth plan should be to communicate a woman's desires for the birth experience. However, satisfaction with the birth experience will be maximized if there is a strong sense of trust between the obstetric provider and the patient. The goal of a birth plan should not be, therefore, to protect a woman from bad intentions of medical intervention, but instead to allow for a satisfying and medically safe birthing experience for both the mother and the infant. Like a living will, a birth plan can communicate preferences for care during a major life-event [58]. It is generally advised to share the birth plan with the provider during a prenatal visit prior to admission for labor. A discussion between the provider and the patient is important to communicate the patient's wishes and to discuss any aspect of the birth plan that cannot or should not be accommodated, and to allow for the development of a mutually agreeable plan [58].

A recent study evaluated obstetric outcomes in women who prepared an antepartum birth plan compared to those who did not. There was no significant difference in rate of cesarean, spontaneous vaginal delivery, or operative vaginal delivery between women who prepared birth plans and those who did not. Women who prepared birth plans were significantly less likely to receive epidural or intravenous analgesia. There was no difference in third- to fourth-degree perineal lacerations in women who prepared a birth plan compared to those who did not [59]. In a questionnaire-based cross-sectional study of women who had prepared birth plans, 60% of women reported that labor did not progress according to the birth plan or that the plan was only partly followed. However, most of those women reported that they were satisfied with their birth experience nonetheless. When asked how the birth plan contributed to their sense of control, 50% of women reported that it did not make any difference in their sense of control while 33% reported that it helped their sense of control during labor and delivery [60].

Creation of a birth plan may be an important exercise for some women to think through their wishes for the birthing experience. However, during creation of a birth plan it must be emphasized that progress through labor is often unpredictable, as evidenced by the large percentage of women who report that their birth plan was only partly followed. Emphasizing the importance of flexibility during the labor process may help mothers be comfortable in assessing and reassessing their desires in the context of changes during labor. In summary, whether or not a woman prepares a birth plan, the goal is to form a trusting and safe relationship with shared decision making between the patient and the treating obstetric provider with the ultimate goal of maximizing maternal and fetal safety and satisfaction with the labor and birthing experience.

References

1 Escott D, Slade P, and Spiby H. Preparation for pain management during childbirth: the psychological aspects of coping strategy development in antenatal education. *Clinical Psycholology Revue* 2009;**29**(7):617–622.

2 Niven C and Gijsbers K. A study of labour pain using the McGill Pain Questionnaire. *Social Science & Medicine* 1984;**19**(12):1347–1351.

3 Consonni EB *et al.* A multidisciplinary program of preparation for childbirth and motherhood: maternal anxiety and perinatal outcomes. *Reproductive Health* 2010;**7**:28.

4 Doering SG and Entwisle DR. Preparation during pregnancy and ability to cope with labor and delivery. *American Journal of Orthopsychiatry,* 1975;**45**(5):825–837.

5 Dick-Read G. *Childbirth Without Fear.* New York: Harper & Row. 1944.

6 Dick-Read G. [Natural childbirth]. *Medizinische Klinik* (Munich) 1957;**52**(33):1395–1398.

7 Lamaze F. *Painless Childbirth. Psychoprophylactic Method.* 1958. London: Burke.

8 Lamaze F and Vellay P. [Psychoprophylaxis and guided labor]. *Gynaecologia* 1957; **144**(Suppl.):125–128.

9 Cogan R. Effects of childbirth preparation. *Clinical Obstetrics and Gynecology* 1980; **23**(1):1–14.

10 Humenick S. Mastery: The key to childbirth satisfaction? A review. *Birth and the Family Journal* 1981;**8**(2):79–83.

11 Gagnon AJ and Sandall J. Individual or group antenatal education for childbirth or parenthood, or both. *Cochrane Database of Systematic Reviews* 2007;(**3**):CD002869.

12 Sullivan PL. Felt learning needs of pregnant women. *Canadian Nurse* 1993;**89**(1):42–45.

13 Bailey JM, Crane P and Nugent CE. Childbirth education and birth plans. *Obstetrics and Gynecology Clinics of North America* 2008;**35**(3):497–509, ix.

14 Redman S *et al.* Evaluation of an antenatal education programme: characteristics of attenders, changes in knowledge and satisfaction of participants. *Australian and New Zealand Journal of Obstetrics and Gynaecology* 1991;**31**(4):310–316.

15 Enkin MW. Commentary: are the correct outcomes of prenatal education being measured? *Birth* 1990;**17**(2):90–91.
16 Willmuth LR. Prepared childbirth and the concept of control. *Journal of Obstetric, Gynecologic, & Neonatal Nursing* 1975;**4**(5):38–41.
17 Balaskas J. *Active Birth: The New Approach to Giving Birth Naturally*. Boston: Harvard Common Press. 1992.
18 Bradley R. *Husband-Coached Childbirth*. 4th edn. New York: Bantam Books. 1996.
19 Mongan M., *HypnoBirthing: The Mongan Method: a Natural Approach to a Safe, Easier, More Comfortable Birthing*. 3rd edn. Deerfield Beach, FL: Health Communications Inc. 2005.
20 Davis CD and Morrone FA. An objective evaluation of a prepared childbirth program. *American Journal of Obstetrics & Gynecology* 1962;**84**:1196–1206.
21 Davenport-Slack B and Boylan CH. Psychological correlates of childbirth pain. *Psychosomatic Medicine* 1974;**36**(3):215–223.
22 Huttel FA *et al.* A quantitative evaluation of psycho-prophylaxis in childbirth. *Journal of Psychosomatic Research* 1972;**16**(2):81–92.
23 Enkin MW *et al. Psychosomatic Medicine in Obstetrics and Gynaecology, 3rd International Congress*, Morris N (ed.). 1972. Steiner & Co.: Basel.
24 Hogan M and Laird MD. An elective program on preparation for childbirth at the Sloane Hospital for Women, May, 1951, to June, 1953. *American Journal of Obstetrics & Gynecology* 1956;**72**(3):641–647.
25 Tanzer D. Natural childbirth: pain or peak experience? *Psychology Today* 1968;**2**(5):17–21.
26 Bergstrom-Walan J. Efficacy of education for childbirth. *Journal of Psychosomatic Research* 1963;**7**:131.
27 Fair CD and Morrison TE. The relationship between prenatal control, expectations, experienced control, and birth satisfaction among primiparous women. *Midwifery* 2012; **28**(1):39–44.
28 Goodman P, Mackey MC and Tavakoli AS. Factors related to childbirth satisfaction. *Journal of Advanced Nursing* 2004;**46**(2):212–219.
29 Ford E, Ayers S, and Wright DB. Measurement of maternal perceptions of support and control in birth (SCIB). *Journal of Women's Health* (Larchmt), 2009;**18**(2):245–252.
30 Harriott EM, Williams TV, and Peterson MR. Childbearing in U.S. military hospitals: dimensions of care affecting women's perceptions of quality and satisfaction. *Birth* 2005; **32**(1):4–10.
31 Lavender T, Walkinshaw SA, and Walton I. A prospective study of women's views of factors contributing to a positive birth experience. *Midwifery* 1999;**15**(1):40–46.
32 Maggioni C, Margola D, and Filippi F. PTSD, risk factors, and expectations among women having a baby: a two-wave longitudinal study. *Journal of Psychosomatic Obstetrics and Gynecology* 2006;**27**(2):81–90.
33 Rudman A, El-Khouri B, and Waldenstrom U. Women's satisfaction with intrapartum care – a pattern approach. *Journal of Advanced Nursing* 2007;**59**(5):474–487.
34 Waldenstrom U et al. A negative birth experience: prevalence and risk factors in a national sample. *Birth* 2004;**31**(1):17–27.
35 Soet JE, Brack GA, and DiIorio C. Prevalence and predictors of women's experience of psychological trauma during childbirth. *Birth* 2003;**30**(1):36–46.
36 Hauck Y *et al.* The influence of childbirth expectations on Western Australian women's perceptions of their birth experience. *Midwifery* 2007;**23**(3):235–247.
37 Hetherington SE. A controlled study of the effect of prepared childbirth classes on obstetric outcomes. *Birth* 1990;**17**(2):86–90.
38 Sturrock WA and Johnson JA. The relationship between childbirth education classes and obstetric outcome. *Birth* 1990;**17**(2):82–85.

39 Hughey MJ, McElin TW, and Young T. Maternal and fetal outcome of Lamaze-prepared patients. *Obstetrics & Gynecology* 1978;**51**(6):643–647.

40 Artieta-Pinedo I *et al.* The benefits of antenatal education for the childbirth process in Spain. *Nursing Research* 2010;**59**(3):194–202.

41 Paz-Pascual C *et al.* Design and process of the EMA Cohort Study: the value of antenatal education in childbirth and breastfeeding. *BMC Nursing* 2008;**7**:5.

42 Ruiz-Mirazo E, Lopez-Yarto M, and McDonald SD. Group prenatal care versus individual prenatal care: a systematic review and meta-analyses. *Journal of Obstetrics and Gynaecology Canada* 2012;**34**(3):223–229.

43 Lally JE *et al.* More in hope than expectation: a systematic review of women's expectations and experience of pain relief in labour. *BMC Medicine* 2008;**6**:7.

44 *Centering Pregnancy: Healthcare in a Group Setting.* 2012. Available from: https://www.centeringhealthcare.org/pages/centering-model/pregnancy-overview.php (accessed May 15, 2015).

45 Hodnett ED *et al.* Continuous support for women during childbirth. *Cochrane Database of Systematic Reviews* 2011;(**2**):CD003766.

46 Simpkin P. Update on nonpharmacologic approaches to relieve labor pain and prevent suffering. *Journal of Midwifery & Womens Health* 2004;**49**:489–504.

47 Beck CT *et al.* Posttraumatic stress disorder in new mothers: results from a two-stage U.S. national survey. *Birth* 2011;**38**(3):216–227.

48 Lowe NK. The nature of labor pain. *American Journal of Obstetrics & Gynecology* 2002; **186**(5 Suppl Nature):S16–24.

49 American College of Obstetricians and Gynecologists Committee Opinion No. 295: pain relief during labor. *Obstetrics & Gynecology* 2004;**104**(1):213.

50 American College of Obstetricians and Gynecologists Practice Bulletin No. 36: Obstetric analgesia and anesthesia. *International Journal of Gynecology & Obstetrics* 2002;**78**(3): 321–335.

51 Moore ER *et al.* Early skin-to-skin contact for mothers and their healthy newborn infants. *Cochrane Database of Systematic Reviews* 2012;(**5**):CD003519.

52 Rising SS. Centering pregnancy. An interdisciplinary model of empowerment. *Journal of Nurse-Midwifery* 1998;**43**(1):46–54.

53 McNeil DA *et al.* Getting more than they realized they needed: a qualitative study of women's experience of group prenatal care. *BMC Pregnancy and Childbirth* 2012;**12**(1):17.

54 Picklesimer AH *et al.* The effect of CenteringPregnancy group prenatal care on preterm birth in a low-income population. *American Journal of Obstetrics & Gynecology* 2012;**206**(5): 415 e1–7.

55 Simpkin P. Birth plans: after 25 years, women still want to be heard. *Birth* 2007;**34**:49–51.

56 Too SK. Do birthplans empower women? A study of midwives' views. *Nursing Standard* 1996;**10**(32):44–48.

57 Lothian J. Birth plans: the good, the bad, and the future. *Journal of Obstetric, Gynecologic, and Neonatal Nursing* 2006;**35**:295–303.

58 Philipsen NaHD. The similarities between birth plans and living wills. *Journal of Perinatal Education* 2005;**14**(4):46–48.

59 Hadar E *et al.* Obstetrical outcome in women with self-prepared birth plan. *Journal of Maternal-Fetal and Neonatal Medicine* 2012.

60 Whitford HM and Hillan EM. Women's perceptions of birth plans. *Midwifery* 1998; **14**(4):248–253.

CHAPTER 2
Normal labor and delivery

Shu Qin Wei[1], Jun Zhang[2], Romy-Leigh McMaster[1], and William D. Fraser[3]

[1] *Department of Obstetrics Gynecology, CHU Sainte-Justine, University of Montreal, Montréal, Canada*
[2] *Xinhua Hospital, Shanghai Jiao Tong University School of Medicine, Shanghai, China*
[3] *Department of Obstetrics and Gynecology, Université de Sherbrooke, Sherbrooke, QC, Canada*

2.1 Introduction

Labor and delivery are physiological processes that begin with the onset of regular uterine contractions and end with the expulsion of the products of conception from the uterus [1]. Labor is characterized by the presence of uterine contractions of sufficient intensity, frequency, and duration to bring about demonstrable effacement and dilation of the cervix. The progress of labor is measured by changes in cervical dilatation and fetal descent. Detection of deviations from normal progress in labor allows for timely and appropriate intervention to optimize maternal and fetal well-being [2]. However, defining normal labor progression has been a long-standing challenge [3]. Friedman was the first to depict a labor curve and divide the labor process into three stages (first, second, and third) in a continuous process [4,5]. The first stage of labor, from the onset of uterine contractions to full cervical dilation, is further divided into the latent phase (the presence of uterine contractions resulting in progressive effacement and dilatation of the cervix to 4 cm) and the active phase (regular uterine contractions accompanied by cervical dilatation and effacement from 4 cm until full dilatation and effacement of the cervix). The second stage of labor is from full dilatation and effacement of the cervix to birth of the neonate. The third stage of labor refers to the period following the completed delivery of the newborn until the completed delivery of the placenta [4,5].

According to Friedman, normal labor progress in the active phase is defined as cervical dilation of at least 1.2 cm/h in nulliparous women and 1.5 cm/h in multiparous women [4,5]. In the past half century, these measures have come to govern labor management. However, these criteria may no longer be applicable to contemporary obstetric populations and may not be appropriate for

---

Management of Labor and Delivery, Second Edition. Edited by George A. Macones.

current obstetric management [6]. Increasing maternal age and maternal and fetal body sizes have made labor a more challenging process. Large increases in the rate of cesarean section deliveries in the US during the 1990s and 2000s, particularly those with indications of labor arrest or dystocia, without evidence of concurrent decreases in rates of maternal or neonatal morbidity and mortality, have highlighted a concern for the frequent use of this obstetric intervention [7,8]. Most recently, the American College of Obstetrics and Gynecology (ACOG) released a consensus statement regarding the safe prevention of the primary cesarean section that recognized that labor progresses at a rate much slower than previously thought, and included, among others, a recommendation to reexamine definitions of labor dystocia and failure to progress based on the results from recent data [9]. In addition, improved and standardized fetal heart rate monitors may have an effect on obstetric intervention such as induction and oxytocin use [9], which may have altered the labor process.

This chapter evaluates the classic definitions of labor progress in a modern context through review of the current scientific literature, outlines patient and care characteristics that have been shown to have an effect on labor progress, and discusses outcomes associated with prolonged or abnormal progression of labor. Finally, this chapter discusses trends in normal labor onset and outcomes from an epidemiologic perspective.

2.1.1 Definitions of normal labor and normal delivery

According to a joint policy statement on normal childbirth [10], normal labor is defined as spontaneous onset and progress of labor to a spontaneous delivery at 37–42 weeks of gestation with a normal third stage. A normal delivery is defined as spontaneous in onset, is low-risk at the start of labor, and remains so throughout labor and birth. The infant is born spontaneously in vertex position between 37 and 42 completed weeks of pregnancy [10].

2.2 Labor onset

The prospective diagnosis of labor of spontaneous onset relies on the presence of regular uterine contractions, progressive cervical effacement and dilation, and "show" (discharge of cervical mucus). Cervical insufficiency may be indicated when there is cervical dilation without regular uterine contraction. Conversely, uterine contractions without cervical change may be due to "false labor" or uterine irritability [11]. Neither of these two latter scenarios meets the clinical criteria for true labor.

Labor onset may be either spontaneous or induced. The latter may be further classified as induced labor with or without medical indication [12]. This chapter focuses primarily on spontaneous labor onset. Labor induction is discussed in Chapter 4.

Oxytocin plays a key role in the spontaneous onset of labor, primarily through initiating, strengthening, and regulating uterine contractions. Produced in the hypothalamus and stored in the posterior pituitary, the release of oxytocin in turn causes the release of previously bound calcium from the sarcoplasmic reticulum, thus activating the contractile system and directly initiating labor [13].

The approach to assessment and care in early labor can have a sizable impact on outcomes [14]. For women with healthy pregnancies who plan to birth in a hospital setting, it is recommended that they not be admitted to the labor and birth area until active labor is confirmed. The criteria for the admission to the labor unit have been proposed by The Society of Obstetricians and Gynaecologists of Canada as follows: cervical dilation of 3–4 cm and 80–90% effacement for nulliparity; or cervical dilation of 3–4 cm and 70–80% effacement in multiparous women [15].

The goal of this recommendation is to minimize the risk of unnecessary interventions and to shorten length of stay in hospital [13]. Holmes *et al.* [16] examined the association between cervical dilation at admission and the likelihood of delivery by cesarean section and found that women who presented to hospital in earlier stages of labor (0- to 3-cm cervical dilation) were more likely to have obstetric intervention than those who presented in more active phases of labor. Janssen *et al.* conducted a clinical trial comparing early labor assessment and support at home to telephone triage on labor outcomes [17]. Significantly fewer women in the home care group arrived at the hospital in latent phase labor, although there was no statistically significant difference between the two groups with respect to cesarean delivery and use of epidural analgesia in labor. Adverse neonatal outcomes were rare and did not differ between the study groups. Hodnett *et al.*, in a randomized controlled trial, evaluated an intervention consisting of early labor assessment by a nursing team, the provision to women of strategies to deal with the discomfort of early labor, and advice on avoiding early admission to the labor suite. The study intervention did not result in a reduction in cesarean deliveries [18].

2.3 First stage of labor

The first stage of labor begins with the onset of labor contractions and ends when the cervix is 100% effaced and completely dilated (10 cm) [1]. Friedman, in his landmark study of 500 nulliparous women [4], subdivided the first stage into an early "latent phase" and an ensuing "active phase." According to Freidman, the latent phase refers to the interval from the time of onset of labor to cervical dilatation of 4 cm and has an expected duration of less than 20 hours for primiparas and less than 14 hours for multiparas. Friedman's latent phase is followed by an active phase of labor, which was considered to begin at about 4 cm of cervical dilatation and end with complete cervical dilatation at 10 cm. It is characterized by cervical dilation at an accelerated rate, as well as descent of the presenting fetal part [1]. According to Friedman, the active phase is further divided into an acceleration phase, a phase of maximum slope, and a deceleration phase.

2.3.1 Measuring progress in labor: labor curves

Labor curves display progress in labor (i.e. cervical dilation) as a function of time and are commonly used to diagnose delays in progress. Friedman was first to describe the relationship between cervical dilation and duration of labor using a graphic format [5].

Friedman considered normal labor progress in the active phase as cervical dilation of at least 1.2 cm/h in nulliparous women and of at least 1.5 cm/h in multiparous women. However, some studies suggest that the Friedman curve might no longer be appropriate for the management of labor [19,6]. Friedman's study population, which included only nulliparous women delivering at term, had low rates of epidural analgesia use (8%) and oxytocin augmentation (9%), and had a high rate of instrumental or cesarean section delivery (Table 2.1). Data from recent studies have suggested that normal labor can progress without intervention at a rate much slower than that described by Friedman [20,21].

One such study, conducted by Zhang *et al.* [6], assessed progression of spontaneous labor in 1162 nulliparous women. He observed that the average time interval from 4- to 10-cm cervical dilation was 5.5 hours (compared to 2.5 hours using the Friedman curve) (Figure 2.1). Zhang did not observe any deceleration phase of active labor. Figure 2.2 displays average labor curves for cervical dilation and fetal decent.

Kilpatrick *et al.* [22] reported that the mean length for the first stage of labor is 8.1 hours, and Albers *et al.* [23] also reported that the median lengths of first and second stages of labor were longer than those that Friedman suggested.

More recently, Neal *et al.* [24] published a meta-analysis assessing studies from 1990–2008 and concluded that modern labor is, on average, slower than

Table 2.1 Comparison of study populations between Friedman's study and the current study.

	Friedman study (n = 500)	Current study (n = 1162)
Year of data collection	Early 1950s	1992–1996
Birthweight between 2500–4000 g (%)	85	100
Labor induction (%)	4	0
Caudal/epidural anesthesia (%)	8	48
Oxytocin augmentation (%)	9	50
Breech delivery and twin gestation (%)	4	0
Low forceps/vacuum (%)	51	13
Mid forceps of cesarean delivery (%)	6	0

Source: Zhang *et al.*, 2002 [6]. Reproduced with permission of Elsevier.

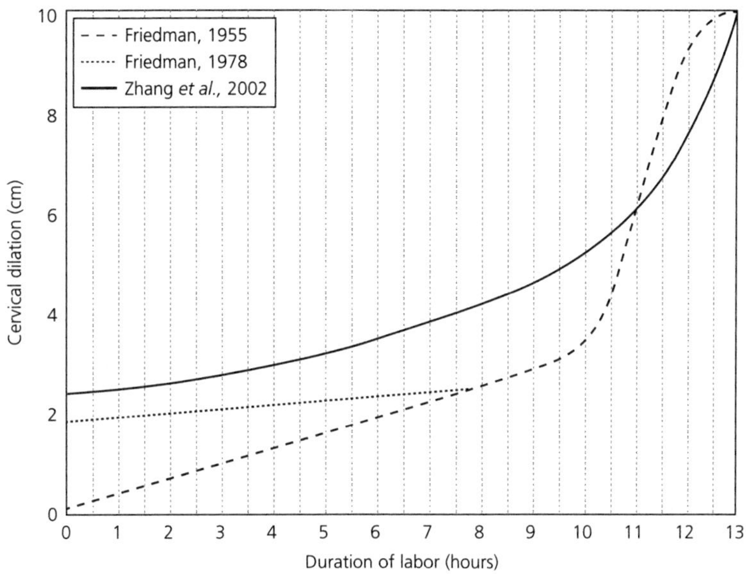

Figure 2.1 Comparison between the Friedman curve and the pattern of cervical dilation based on the current data. *Source*: Zhang *et al.*, 2002 [27]. Reproduced with permission of Elsevier.

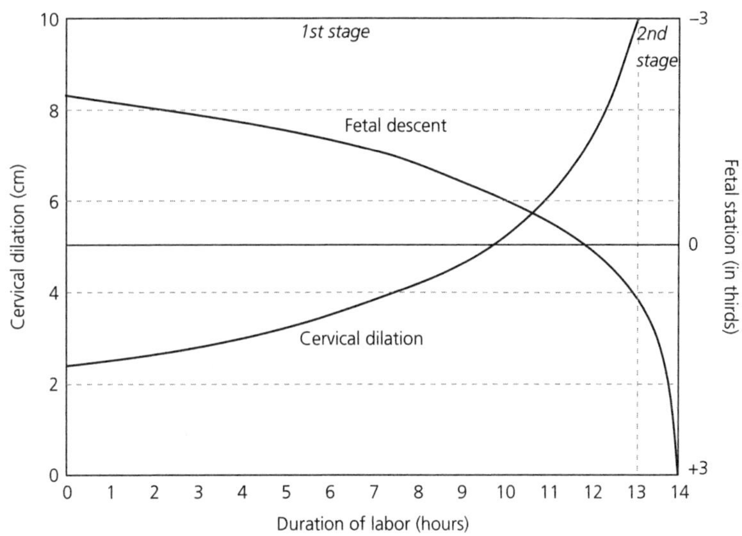

Figure 2.2 Patterns of cervical dilation (left) and fetal descent (right) in nulliparous women. *Source*: Zhang *et al.*, 2002 [27]. Reproduced with permission of Elsevier.

labor among the women who contributed to the construction of Friedman's curve. In fact, they found that the *average* cervical dilation rate per hour among first-time laboring women was the same as Friedman's *lowest* acceptable rate of 1.2 cm/h.

The Consortium on Safe Labor (CSL) was a multicenter, retrospective, observational study that abstracted detailed labor and delivery information for 228,562 deliveries from electronic medical records in 12 clinical centers (with 19 hospitals) across nine ACOG districts from the period 2002–2008; 87% of births occurred in 2005–2007 [25,26]. Zhang *et al.* [27] examined the contemporary labor patterns of spontaneous labor with normal neonatal outcomes using CSL data. The characteristics of the parturients by parity (weighted) in CSL are shown in Table 2.2. With increasing parity, both maternal age and body mass increased. In this large, modern obstetric population of pregnant women who had a vaginal delivery of a singleton term gestation with a normal perinatal outcome after spontaneous onset of labor, cervical dilation from 4 to 5 cm sometimes took longer than 6 hours and dilation from 5 to 6 cm sometimes took longer than 3 hours (Table 2.3). Regardless of parity, women appeared to progress at similar rates before 6 cm dilation. Only after reaching a cervical dilation of 6 cm did differences in parity become apparent, with multiparous women progressing to full

Table 2.2 Characteristics of the parturients by parity (weighted), Consortium on Safe Labor, 2002–2008.

	Parity 0	Parity 1	Parity 2+
Unweighted cohort (n)	27,170	17,850	17,395
Weighted cohort (n)	453,693	368,131	311,248
Maternal race			
White	60	55	51
African American	12	12	15
Hispanic	20	26	29
Asian or Pacific Islanders	4	4	2
Others	4	3	3
Maternal age (y)	24.6±5.8	27.7±5.7	30.0±5.4
Body mass index before pregnancy (kg/m^2)	23.4±4.6	24.2±5.1	25.5±5.6
Body mass index at delivery (kg/m^2)	29.1±5.0	29.6±5.2	30.5±5.5
Cervical dilation at admission (cm)	4(1, 7)	4.5 (2, 8)	5 (2, 8)
Effacement at admission (%)	90 (60, 100)	90(50, 100)	80 (50, 100)
Station at admission	−1 (−3, 0)	−1 (−3, 0)	−2 (−3, 0)
Oxytocin use in spontaneous labor	47	45	45
Epidural analgesia	84	77	71
Total number of vaginal examinations in first stage	5(1, 9)	4 (1, 7)	4(1, 7)
Instrumental delivery	12	3	2
Gestational age at delivery (wk)	39.3±1.2	39.2±1.2	39.1±1.1
Birth weight (g)	3,296±406	3,384±421	3,410±428

Data are %, mean ± standard deviation, or median (10th, 90th percentile) unless otherwise specified.

Source: Cheng *et al.*, 2010 [37]. Reproduced with permission of Lippincott Williams & Wilkins.

Table 2.3 Duration of labor in hours by parity in spontaneous onset of labor.

Cervical dilation (cm)	Parity 0 (n = 25,624)	Parity 1 (n = 16,755)	Parity 2+ (n = 16,219)
3–4	1.8 (8.1)	—	—
4–5	1.3 (6.4)	1.4 (7.3)	1.4 (7.0)
5–6	0.8 (3.2)	0.8 (3.4)	0.8 (3.4)
6–7	0.6 (2.2)	0.5 (1.9)	0.5 (1.8)
7–8	0.5 (1.6)	0.4 (1.3)	0.4 (1.2)
8–9	0.5 (1.4)	0.3 (1.0)	0.3 (0.9)
9–10	0.5 (1.8)	0.3 (0.9)	0.3 (0.8)
Second stage with epidural analgesia	1.1 (3.6)	0.4 (2.0)	0.3 (1.6)
Second stage without epidural analgesia	0.6 (2.8)	0.2 (1.3)	0.1 (1.1)

Data are median (95th percentile).

Source: Zhang *et al.*, 2010 [6]. Reproduced with permission of Lippincott Williams & Wilkins.

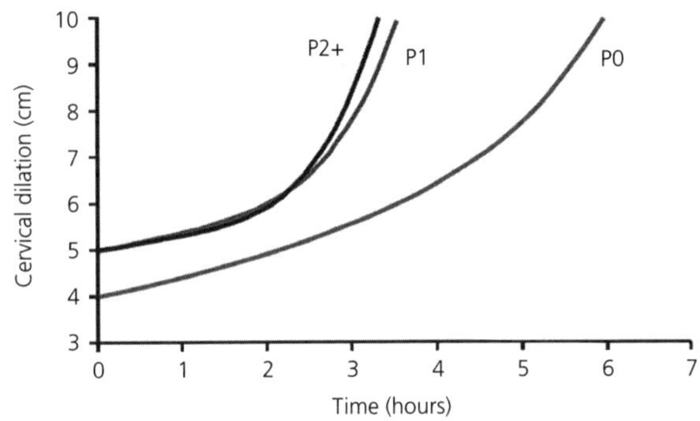

Figure 2.3 Average labor curves by parity in singleton term pregnancies with spontaneous onset of labor, vaginal delivery, and normal neonatal outcomes. P0, nulliparous women; P1, women of parity 1; P2, women of parity 2 or higher. The Consortium on Safe Labor, 2002–2008. *Source*: Zhang *et al.*, 2010 [6]. Reproduced with permission of Lippincott Williams & Wilkins.

dilation more quickly than nulliparous women (Figure 2.3). The authors found that the transition point between the latent and the active phase of labor occurred at a point further along in cervical dilation than previously explained by Friedman [27].

Laughon *et al.* [28] examined the differences in labor patterns between the Collaborative Perinatal Project (CPP), which was comprised of data from 39,491 deliveries between 1959 and 1966, and the CSL. Women in the latter (modern) cohort were more likely to be older and have a higher body mass index, and had more frequent use of epidural analgesia and oxytocin in labor as well as cesarean delivery (Table 2.4). These women had a longer first stage of labor, by a median of 2.6 hours in nulliparas and 2.0 hours in multiparas (Figure 2.4 and Figure 2.5).

Table 2.4 Comparison between CPP and CSL in nulliparous women.

Parameter	CPP (n = 14,791)	CSL (n = 43,576)	Adjusted median difference[a]	Adjusted *p* value
Maternal age, y (mean ± SD)	20.4 ± 4.0	24,4 ± 5.7		< .001
Delivery BMI, kg/m^2	25.5 ± 3.4	29.6 ± 4.9		< .001
Admission characteristics				
Gestational age at delivery, wks	39.3 ±3.4	38.6 ± 2.4		< .001
Dilation on admission				
Median (10th, 90th percentiles)	3 (1, 6.5)	3.5 (1,7)		
Mean ± SD	3.5 ± 2.2	3.8 ± 2.3	0.6[b]	< .001
Effacement on admission				
Median (10th, 90th percentiles)	85 (40, 100)	90 (60, 100)		
Mean ± SD	77 ± 25	84 ± 18	7.3[b]	< .001
Spontaneous ROM prior to admission, %	16	41	18	< .001
Lahor characteristics				
Epidural, %	5	60	37	< .001
Oxytocin augmentation, %	16	37	8	< .001
First-stage durations, h (median, 95th percentiles)				
From 4 cm to C/C	3.9 (18.5)	6.5 (24.0)	2.6	< .001
From 5 cm to C/C	2.1 (11.8)	3.6 (15.1)	1.3	< .001
From 6 cm to C/C	1.2 (8.2)	2.2 (10.0)	0.7	< .001
Second-stage durations, h				
With spontaneous delivery (median, 95th percentiles)	0.45 (2.0)	0.90 (3.1)	0.22	< .001
With assisted delivery (median, 95th percentiles)	0.75(3.1)	1.65 (4.25)	0.49	< .001
Forceps, %	66	3	−51	< .001
Vacuum. %	0.2	6	4	< .001
Forceps or vacuum. %	66	10	−47	< .001
Episiotomy. %	92	27	−51	< .001
Third- or fourth-degree laceration, %	8	5	−4	< .001
Intrapartum cesarean delivery, %	3	16	5	< .001
Neonatal characteristics				
Birthweight, g (mean ± SD)	3077 ± 571	3190 ± 573		

Table 2.4 *(continued)*

Parameter	CPP (n = 14,791)	CSL (n = 43,576)	Adjusted median difference[a]	Adjusted *p* value
Apgar score at 1 min (mean)	7.5 ± 2.1	7.9 ± 1.4		
<4, %	7	3		
4-6	17	6		
≥7	76	91		
Apgar score at 1 min <7, %	24	9	−13	< .001
Apgar score at 5 min (mean)	8.9 ± 1.4	8.8 ± 0.3		
<4, %	1.8	0.5		
4-6	3.9	1.3		
≥7	94.4	98.2		
Apgar score at 5 min <7, %	6	2	−4	< .001

BMI, body mass index; C/C, completely dilated and completely effaced (end of first stage of labor); CSL, Consortium on Safe Labor; CPP, Collaborative Perinatal Project; ROM, rupture of membranes.
[a] Median difference (except where noted) for parameter in the CSL minus the CPP, adjusted for maternal age, race, gestational age at delivery, BMI at delivery, spontaneous rupture of membranes, and birth weight;
[b] Adjusted mean difference.
Source: Laughon *et al*., 2012 [26]. Reproduced with permission of Elsevier.

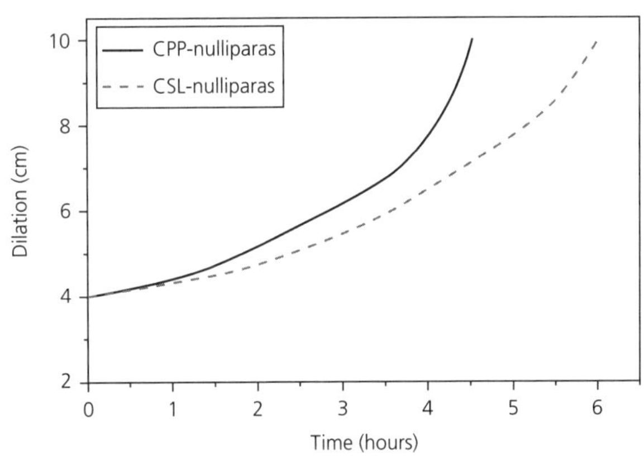

Figure 2.4 The average labor curves for nulliparas in the CPP and CSL cohorts. Average labor curves for women by study with singleton term pregnancies presenting in spontaneous labor with vaginal delivery for nulliparas. Curves were evaluated at the average values of the combined population for maternal age, maternal race, body mass index at delivery, spontaneous rupture of membranes, gestational age, and birthweight. Collaborative Perinatal Project (CPP) was conducted from 1959 to 1966; Consortium on Safe Labor (CSL) was conducted from 2002 to 2008. *Source*: Laughon *et al.*, 2012 [26]. Reproduced with permission of Elsevier.

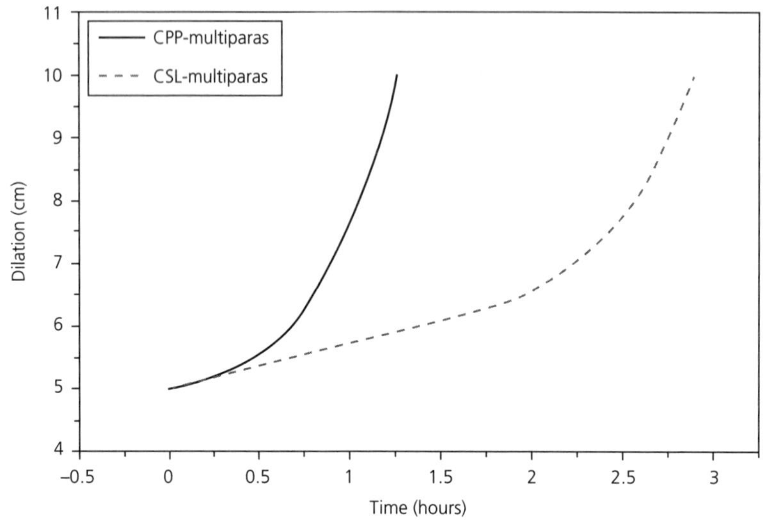

Figure 2.5 The average labor curves for multiparas in the CPP and CSL cohorts. Average labor curves for women by study with singleton term pregnancies presenting in spontaneous labor with vaginal delivery for nulliparas. Curves were evaluated at the average values of the combined population for maternal age, maternal race, body mass index at delivery, spontaneous rupture of membranes, gestational age, and birthweight. Collaborative Perinatal Project (CPP) was conducted from 1959 to 1966; Consortium on Safe Labor (CSL) was conducted from 2002 to 2008. *Source*: *Laughon et al.*, 2012 [26]. Reproduced with permission of Elsevier.

The increased duration of the first stage of labor remained even after adjustment for patient characteristics.

Zhang *et al.* [27] studied the natural history of the normal first stage of labor in 26,838 pregnant women who had a singleton term gestation with spontaneous onset of labor, vertex presentation, and a normal perinatal outcome. They conducted a detailed analysis on labor progression, which showed that rates of cervical dilation increased as labor progressed, and that these rates varied by parity. For example, among nulliparous women, who had the longest durations of labor, progression of cervical dilation from 3 to 4 cm took 1.2 hours (median), but from 7 to 8 cm took only 0.4 hours (median) (Table 2.5). The authors also presented an alternate approach to the diagnosis of labor arrest, based on graduated levels of cervical dilation, given their findings that a 2-hour limit may be too short when cervical dilation has not reached 6 cm, but that a 4-hour limit may be too long after 6 cm dilation has been reached (Figure 2.6).

"Failure to progress" is a common indication for cesarean section in the US and the cesarean section rate has also been increasing in recent years. In 2010, *Zhang et al.*, in a study spanning 6 years and 233,844 newborns, found that 53% of all induced women having a cesarean section for an indication of failure to progress had not reached 6 cm dilation. Similarly, Boyle *et al.* [28] found that

Table 2.5 Duration of labor (in hours) in nulliparas based on cervical dilation at admission, National Collaborative Perinatal Project (CPP), 1959–1966.

Cervical dilation (cm)	Admitted at 2 or 2.5 cm	Admitted at 3 or 3.5 cm	Admitted at 4 or 4.5 cm	Admitted at 5 or 5.5 cm
Adm. to 3	1.0 (8.5)			
Adm. to 4	2.3 (12.6)	0.7 (6.5)		
Adm. to 5	3.6 (15.3)	1.9 (10.5)	0.5 (5.4)	
Adm. to 6	4.5 (1 7.0)	2.7 (12.4)	1.3 (8.4)	0.4 (3.4)
Adm. to 7	5.1 (18.0)	3.3 (13.3)	2.0 (10.1)	0.9 (5.5)
Adm. to 8	5.5 (18.8)	3.7 (14.1)	2.4 (11.4)	1.3 (6.6)
Adm. to 9	5.9 (19.8)	4.1 (15.2)	2.8 (12.7)	1.7 (8.2)
Adm. to 10	6.3 (20.7)	4.5 (16.2)	3.2 (1 4.1)	2.1 (9.3)

Source: Zhang *et al.*, 2010 [27]. Reproduced with permission of Lippincott Williams & Wilkins.

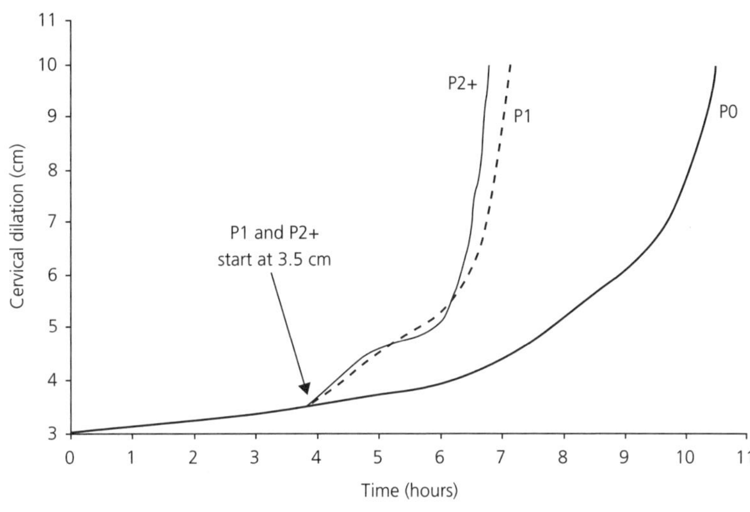

Figure 2.6 The average labor curves by parity in women with singleton term pregnancies with spontaneous onset of labor and vertex presentation who completed the first stage of labor and whose newborns had 5-minute Apgar scores of at least 7. The National Collaborative Perinatal Project, 1959–966. P0, nulliparas; P1, parity 1; P2_, parity 2 or higher. *Source: Zhang et al.*, 2010 [29]. Reproduced with permission of Lippincott Williams & Wilkins.

more than 40% of women having a cesarean section for failure to progress had not reached 5 cm dilation.

Although many patient characteristics have been associated with an increased likelihood for cesarean section, Hamilton has identified a modifiable clinical factor as a significant contributor: variation in the identification of dystocia or labor progressing too slowly. Hamilton has developed a mathematical model to help care providers answer the question "How slow is too slow?" and that can be used to safely lower the risk of cesarean section for the indication of dystocia. The model compares an individual's progress in cervical dilation to an appropriate reference group and differs from the Friedman curve in that it incorporates ranges of normal responses and is dynamic (it is updated as factors change in labor). Although a prospective randomized clinical trial evaluating the effectiveness of the model showed no significant impact on the risk of cesarean section, a pretest-posttest analysis showed a reduction in rates from 19.54% (pretest) to 16.62% at 12 months [29].

2.3.2 Factors that affect duration of first stage of labor

Several factors are associated with the duration of the first stage of labor. Friedman noted that early or excessive sedation, early administration of epidural analgesia, and unfavorable cervix at the onset of labor were associated with prolonged first stage of labor [20]. Nulliparity is associated with a longer labor compared to multiparity, although increasing parity does not further shorten the first stage of labor [30]. Some researchers have observed that the length of labor differs among racial/ethnic groups. Tuck *et al.* reported Asian women to have the longest first and second stages of labor compared to Caucasian or African American women [31]. However, others report conflicting findings [32,33]. Differences in findings may be due to variations in study designs, study populations, labor management, or statistical power. Finally, a large, retrospective study (n = 2373) assessed the impact of fetal gender on duration of labor and found an association between male gender and longer active phase of the first stage of labor [34].

A study by Kominiarek *et al.* in 2011 [35] using data from the CSL compared labor patterns by maternal body mass index (BMI) and found that the first stage of labor progressed significantly more slowly with increasing maternal BMI. For example, among nulliparas, the median time to reach 10-cm cervical dilation (from 4 cm) was 7.7 hours (95th percentile 25.6 hours) among women with a BMI >= 40.0 as compared to 5.7 hours (95th percentile 18.8 hours) among women with a BMI between 25.0 and 29.9. This effect was observed among multiparas as well.

Sheiner *et al.* [36] conducted a population-based study of 92,918 singleton vertex term deliveries between the years 1988 and 1999, comparing patients who underwent cesarean for delay in progress during the first stage with those whose labors progressed normally. Independent risk factors for longer first stage, using a multivariable analysis, were premature rupture of membranes (OR 3.8, 95% CI 3.2–4.5), nulliparity (OR 3.8, 95% CI 3.3–4.3), labor induction (OR 3.3, 95% CI 2.9–3.7), maternal age > 35 years (OR 3.0, 95% CI 2.6–3.6), birthweight > 4 kg (OR 2.2, 95% CI 1.8–2.7), hypertensive disorders (OR 2.1, 95% CI 1.8–2.6), hydramnios (OR 1.9, 95% CI 1.5–2.3), fertility treatment (OR 1.8, 95% CI 1.4–2.4), epidural analgesia (OR 1.6, 95% CI 1.4–1.8), and gestational diabetes (OR 1.4, 95% CI 1.1–1.7) [38].

Cheng *et al.* [37] conducted a retrospective cohort study of 10,661 nulliparous women with term singleton gestations between 1990 and 2008. Maternal characteristics associated with a length of first stage of more than 30 hours included: maternal age, gestational age at delivery greater than 41 weeks,

Table 2.6 Maternal and labor characteristics of nulliparous women stratified by length of the first stage of labor.*

Length of the first stage	Less than the 5th percentile (0–2.8 h) (n = 525)	5th to 95th percentile (2.8–30 h) (n = 9611)	Greater than the 95th percentile (more than 30 h) (n = 525)	*p*
Maternal age (y)				
Younger than 35 (n = 9,006)	5.1	90.4	4.5	< .001
35 or older (n = 1,640)	4.0	88.9	7.1	
Rice/Ethnicity				
White (n = 4,714)	4.5	90.0	5.8	
African American (n = 1,196)	6.4	90.0	3.7	.04
Latina (n = 1,056)	5.4	89.7	4.9	
Asian (n = 2,996)	4.6	90.6	4.8	
Gestational age (wk)				
Less than 41 (n = 8,582)	5.4	90.2	4.4	< .001
41 or more (n = 2,072)	2.9	90.3	6.7	
Maternal body mass index (kg/m^2)				
Low [less than 19.5) (n = 1,254)	6.1	91.6	2.4	
Normal (19.5–25) (n = 4,234)	4.6	91.2	4.3	< .001
High (26–28} (n = 684)	4.5	89.0	6.4	
Obese (29 or greater) (n = 628)	4.1	89.3	6.5	
Marital status				
Married (n = 6,648)	4.5	90.3	5.2	.02
Not married (n = 3,805)	5.4	90.3	4.3	
Oxytocin augmentation of labor				
No oxytocin (n = 5,690)	6.1	91 0	2.9	< .001
Had Oxytocin) (n = 4,943)	3.5	89.4	7.1	
Epidural use				
No epidural use) (n = 3,897)	9.6	88.3	2.1	< .001
Epidural use (n = 7,211)	2.7	91.1	6.2	
Fetal occiput position				
OA position (n = 9,088)	5.3	90.5	4.2	< .001
OP position (n = 911)	1.2	89.1	9.7	
Birth weight (g)				
4,000 or less (n = 9,736)	5.1	90.2	4.7	< .001
More than 4,000 (n = 914)	2.9	90.0	7.0	

OA, occiput anterior; OP, occiput posterior.
Data are % Unless Otherwise Specified.
*The length of the first stage of labor was examined as a categorical variable using Pearson's χ^2 test.
Source: Cheng *et al.*, 2010 [37]. Reproduced with permission of Lippincott Williams & Wilkins.

high prepregnancy maternal body mass index, and being married. Oxytocin augmentation of labor was more frequent with longer first stage as was epidural analgesia use, persistent occiput posterior position at delivery, and birthweight greater than 4000 g (Table 2.6).

2.3.3 The length of the first stage of labor and maternal and perinatal outcomes

A number of researchers have reported associations between the length of the first stage of labor and maternal and perinatal outcomes. In a study by Cheng *et al.* [39], women with a first stage of labor longer than 30 hours (when compared to women with a first stage of labor between 2.8 and 30 hours) had a higher risk of cesarean delivery (aOR 2.28, 95% CI 1.92–2.72) and higher odds of chorioamnionitis (aOR 1.58, 95% CI 1.25–1.98), as well as increased risk of admission to the neonatal intensive care unit (aOR 1.53, 95% CI 1.18–1.97) (Table 2.7).

Table 2.7 Adjusted odds ratios of perinatal outcomes in multivariate logistic regression analyses stratified by length of the first stage of labor.

Length of the first stage	Less than the 5th percentile (less than 2.8 h)		Greater than the 95th percentile (more than 30 h)	
	aOR	95% CI	aOR	95% CI
Mode of delivery				
Cesarean (first and second stages)	0.62	0.45–0.84	2.28	1.92–2.72
Cesarean (second stage only)	0.58	0.39–0.89	1.70	1.35–2.14
Operative vaginal†	1.12	0.94–1.34	0.80	0.68–0.96
Maternal outcomes				
3rd- or 4th-degree perineal laceration†	1.08	0.86–1.35	1.10	0.86–1.39
Postpartum hemorrhage	0.95	0.74–1.22	1.18	0.95–1.45
Chorioamnionitis	0.31	0.17–0.56	1.58	1.25–1.98
Endomyometritis	0.72	0.39–1.32	0.94	0.62–1.43
Neonatal outcomes				
5-min Apgar score less than 7	0.73	0.44–1.22	1.27	0.88–1.85
UA pH less than 7.0	0.37	0.29–2.51	0.73	0.22–2.42
Meconium aspiration	0.64	0.20–2.13	1.36	0.52–3.51
Neonatal sepsis	–	–	1.07	0.13–8.87
Shoulder dystocia	0.71	0.33–1.48	1.00	0.51–1.95
Birth trauma‡	0.96	0.23–4.08	–	–
Neonatal intensive care unit admission	0.91	0.67–1.25	1.53	1.18–1.97

aOR, adjusted odds ratio; CI, confidence interval; UA, cord umbilical artery.

Reference comparison group; white, length of first stage of labor in the 5th to 95th percentile.

*Adjusted for maternal age, gestational age at delivery, ethnicity, gestational diabetes, preeclampsia, placenta abruption, year of delivery, delivery attendant, and epidural anesthesia (episiotomy and operative vaginal delivery additionally included for perineal lacerations, and shoulder dystocia; oxytocin augmentation additionally included for chorioamnionitis; mode of delivery and chorioamnionitis additionally adjusted for postpartum hemorrhage and neonatal intensive care unit admission).

†For vaginal deliveries only.

‡Birth trauma: composite variable of skull fracture, clavicle fracture, brachial plexus palsy, facial nerve palsy, and other nonspecified trauma.

Source: Cheng *et al.*, 2010 [37]. Reproduced with permission of Lippincott Williams & Wilkins.

Rouse *et al.* [38] prospectively evaluated a labor management protocol for spontaneous labor with active phase labor arrest (cervix at least 4 cm dilated and 1 cm or less of cervical progress in 2 hours) in the first stage of labor that mandated at least 4 hours of oxytocin augmentation before cesarean delivery. They found that this protocol was effective, resulting in a high rate of vaginal delivery (92%), and safe, with no severe adverse maternal and fetal or neonatal outcomes.

Sheiner *et al.* [37] studied the outcome of failure to progress during the first stage of labor. Maternal anemia (defined as hemoglobin level less than 10 mg/dL) and the rate of packed cell transfusion were higher among pregnancies complicated with failure of labor to progress during the first stage as compared to controls. Deliveries that failed to progress during the first stage were significantly associated with non-reassuring fetal heart rate patterns. The women with the prolonged first stage labor had significantly higher rates of intrauterine growth restriction and Apgar scores lower than 7 at 5 min.

2.4 Second stage of labor

The second stage of labor has traditionally been defined as the period from full cervical dilation to the birth of the baby. The ACOG has suggested that second stage nulliparous labor should be considered as normal when its duration does not exceed 3 hours in the presence of regional anesthesia or 2 hours in its absence. In multiparous women, such a diagnosis can be made if the second stage of labor does not exceed 2 hours with regional anesthesia or 1 hour without it [1]. The adoption in some centers of "delayed pushing" or "laboring down" has raised new questions about the duration of the second stage of labor.

2.4.1 Factors that affect duration of second stage of labor

Maternal position during labor is an important consideration in the care of women in labor. Two systematic reviews [39,40] of clinical trials assessing the effect of the maternal position on the duration of the second stage of labor both concluded that women delivering in upright positions had a reduction in second stage duration. Despite this evidence, most women continue to labor and deliver in a reclined or lithotomy position.

Fetal position also has been shown to have an effect on second-stage duration. Senécal *et al.* [41] showed that the following factors are significant determinants of prolonged second stage of labor (>3 hours): fetal malposition at the beginning of the second stage (aOR 2.37, 95% CI 1.69–3.32, $p < .001$ for occiput posterior and aOR 1.57, 95% CI 1.13–2.18, $p = .008$ for occiput transverse); station of the fetal head at 0 at the beginning of the second stage (aOR 1.45, 95% CI 1.15–1.84, $p = .002$); advanced maternal age (aOR 2.83, 95% CI 1.91–4.20, $p < .001$ for women aged 35 years or older); birthweight of 4000 g or higher (aOR 1.85, 95% CI 1.32–2.61, $p < .001$); and second-stage oxytocin administration (aOR 1.45,

95% CI 1.18–1.78, $p < .001$). A policy of early pushing during the second stage had a protective effect on a prolonged second stage of labor (aOR 0.26, 95% CI 0.22–0.32, $p < .001$). Conversely, delayed pushing shortened the duration of expulsive efforts.

Schiessl *et al.* [42] conducted a univariate analysis of a range of potential determinants of second stage duration among 1200 consecutive vaginal deliveries and found that occipito-posterior presentation was a significant parameter associated with a prolonged second stage of labor. They also observed that nulliparity and epidural analgesia use were risk factors for the prolonged second stage of labor.

Paterson *et al.* [43] conducted a retrospective analysis of 25,069 women delivered of an infant of at least 37 weeks of gestation with a cephalic presentation following the spontaneous onset of labor. They found that the duration of the second stage was strongly negatively associated with parity and positively associated with the use of epidural analgesia. Maternal age, baby birthweight, and maternal height were also independently associated with the duration of the second stage. There were longer durations of the second stage of labor in the women with epidural analgesia and those using alternate methods of pain relief.

In a large retrospective study on determinants of the length of labor, specifically focusing on race and/or ethnicity, the authors observed that the second stage was shorter in African American women than in Caucasian women, both for nulliparas (−22 min) and multiparas (−7.5 min). Compared with their Caucasian counterparts, Hispanic nulliparas also had a shortened second stage, whereas no differences were seen for multiparas. In contrast, Asian nulliparas had a significantly prolonged second stage compared with their Caucasian counterparts, and no differences were seen for multiparas [44].

As compared to the obstetric population when Friedman's curve was developed, the use of epidural analgesia as a method of pain relief in labor is now much more common. In 2005/2006, it was estimated that epidural analgesia was administered to 47.9% of all women delivering in Canada [45]. A recent (2011) meta-analysis assessed the effects of epidural analgesia on labor and delivery outcomes as compared to other forms of pain relief and to no pain relief modalities. The meta-analysis found that the use of epidural analgesia as compared to non-epidural or no pain relief in labor is associated with an increase in the duration of second stage of labor only (mean difference 13.66 minutes, 95% CI 6.67–20.66) (n = 4233) and may also increase the need to strengthen contractions through the use of augmentation with oxytocin [46].

2.4.2 The length of the second stage of labor and maternal and perinatal outcomes

Cohen was the first to evaluate the influence of the duration of second stage labor on perinatal outcome and postpartum morbidity [47]. He observed that certain maternal morbidities, specifically postpartum hemorrhage and fever, were increased when the second stage of labor was prolonged, although neither 5-minute Apgar scores nor perinatal mortality were related to second stage duration.

Saunders *et al.* [48] conducted a retrospective analysis of 25,069 women delivered of an infant of at least 37 weeks of gestation with a cephalic presentation following the spontaneous onset of labor to investigate the relation between the duration of the second stage of labor and subsequent early neonatal and maternal morbidity. The authors found a statistically significant association between prolonged duration of second stage of labor and risk of both postpartum hemorrhage and maternal infection, although risk of low Apgar score and admission to a special care baby unit were not found to be statistically significant. Presumably because relatively few women in their cohort had second stage durations that exceeded 3 hours, they limited their conclusions to durations that did not exceed this threshold.

In a study of 5158 multiparous women, Cheng *et al.* [49] compared women who delivered after a second stage of labor lasting between 0 and 2 hours with women with a second stage lasting more than 3 hours, and found several significant adverse outcomes. Women with longer second stages had higher risks of operative vaginal deliveries, cesarean deliveries, and maternal morbidity including third- or fourth-degree perineal lacerations, postpartum hemorrhage, and chorioamnionitis. Additional adverse neonatal outcomes associated with longer second stages of labor included higher risks of a 5-minute Apgar score of less than 7, admission to an intensive care nursery (OR 2.08; 95% CI 1.15–3.77), and longer neonatal stay in hospital [51].

Similarly, Allen *et al.* [50] conducted a population-based cohort study of 121,517 women with low-risk singleton vertex nonanomalous deliveries at or after 37 weeks of gestation and estimated maternal and perinatal outcomes among women, where duration of the second stage of labor was the exposure variable. They found several adverse outcomes associated with increased second stage labor duration. These included an increased risk in both maternal (obstetric trauma, postpartum hemorrhage, puerperal febrile motility) and neonatal (low 5-minute Apgar score, admission to neonatal intensive care units, composite neonatal morbidity) outcomes.

Rouse *et al.* [51] analyzed data that were collected prospectively from 14 centers and reaffirmed that the duration of the second stage of labor was associated principally with adverse maternal as opposed to adverse neonatal outcomes. For example, they found significantly increased risks in adjusted rates of chorioamnionitis and third- or fourth-degree perinatal laceration when second stage duration was 3 hours or longer, but found no significant differences in risk of adjusted rates of sepsis, admission to neonatal intensive care, 5-minute Apgar < 4, umbilical artery pH < 7, or intubation in delivery room. The authors concluded that intervention during second stage should not be determined by duration alone [53].

2.4.3 Delayed pushing with epidural analgesia

After complete dilation of the cervix and a labor transition to the second stage, some women may feel an involuntary urge to beginning pushing. However, not all women experience this urge at the same time, particularly in the presence of epidural analgesia. The urge to push can occur before or after complete dilation of the cervix, when the presenting part of the fetus is also at an advanced station [52]. Allowing passive decent of the fetal head (laboring down) was first suggested by Maresh [53] as a means of protecting the pelvic floor in women who were experiencing the second stage of labor with epidural analgesia. With delayed pushing, women are advised to avoid pushing either until there is an irresistible urge to push or until the presenting part has descended to the perineum [54].

In the multicenter Pushing Early or Pushing Late with Epidural clinical trial (PEOPLE), Fraser *et al.* [56] evaluated whether a policy of delayed pushing for nulliparous women with continuous-infusion epidural analgesia reduces the risk of difficult delivery, with objectives to assess the effects of delayed pushing on spontaneous vaginal delivery, on indicators of maternal, fetal, and neonatal morbidity, and on women's experience of delivery. Their results showed that delayed pushing was associated with a reduction in difficult deliveries (RR 0.79, 95% CI 0.66–0.95), with the greatest effect on midpelvic procedures (RR 0.72, 95% CI 0.55–0.93). The delayed pushing group also demonstrated a higher frequency of spontaneous vaginal delivery (RR 1.09, 95% CI 1.00–1.18) but an increase in abnormal umbilical cord blood pH (RR 2.45, 95% CI 1.35–4.43). A summary neonatal morbidity index did not differ significantly between the two groups.

Petrou *et al.* [55] evaluated the cost-effectiveness of delayed pushing and found that although the laboring down approach significantly reduced the incidence of difficult delivery, it was also associated with an increase in intrapartum and postnatal costs. The delayed pushing group required more clinical resources, such as nursing care, epidural boluses, oxytocin infusion, and other consumables. The cesarean deliveries and difficult deliveries required by the early pushing group required a different kind of resources, such as a pediatrician in the operating room, but the overall costs of extended labor care for the delayed pushing group increased the cost by $68.

Tuuli *et al.* [56] recently conducted a systematic review and meta-analysis of 12 randomized controlled trials and they found that there were few clinical differences in outcomes with immediate compared with delayed pushing in the second stage of labor. When compared to immediate pushing, delayed pushing was associated with an increased rate of spontaneous vaginal delivery (RR 1.09, 95% CI 1.03–1.15), an increase in total second stage duration (weighted mean difference 57 minutes, 95% CI 42–72), but a shortened duration of active pushing (weighted mean difference of −22 minutes, 95% CI −31 to −13). Operative vaginal delivery rates did not differ significantly between the immediate and the delayed pushing groups.

2.5 Third stage of labor

The third stage of labor is defined as the time between the delivery of the fetus and the delivery of the placenta and fetal membranes. During this period, uterine contractions decrease basal blood flow, resulting in thickening and reduction in the surface area of the myometrium underlying the placenta with subsequent detachment of the placenta [57]. Placental separation during the third stage of labor is an important part of normal delivery. Herman *et al.* [58] were the first to describe spontaneous separation of the placenta by using real-time ultrasound. They were able to divide the separation process into four phases: latent (placenta-site wall remains thin while placenta-free wall is thick), contraction (thickening of placenta-site wall), detachment (actual separation of the placenta from the adjacent uterine wall), and expulsion (sliding of the placenta out of the uterine cavity). The normal duration of the third stage of labor is less than 30 minutes, and most often lasts 5–15 minutes. Third stages of labor lasting longer than 30 minutes may require intervention to minimize adverse outcomes.

2.5.1 Factors that affect duration of third stage of labor

The location of the placenta has been indicated to affect the duration of the third stage of labor. Lurie *et al.* [59] evaluated the association between placental location and length of the third stage of labor in term singleton pregnancies. Anterior location of the placenta was noted in 96 women (48%), posterior in 66 (33%), fundal in 26 (13%), and lateral in 12 (6%). The duration of the third stage of labor was statistically significantly longer when the placenta was located in the fundal area of the uterus (12.8 +/− 9.5 min, $p < 0.05$) when compared to other locations, such as anterior (9.5 +/− 5.5 min), posterior (9.4 +/− 5.3 min), and lateral (7.6 +/− 3.5 min). In contrast, Altay *et al.* [60] conducted a prospective study examining the association between location of the placenta and the duration of the third stage of labor and they observed a significantly shorter length of third stage of labor when the placenta was in the fundal location.

Grinsted *et al.* [61] studied the duration of the third stage of labor retrospectively by comparing the third stage of labor of women with previously induced abortions and that of women with previously uncomplicated pregnancies. They found that the third stage of labor lasted significantly longer among women with previously induced abortions than among the other group included in the study.

2.5.2 Active management of the third stage of labor

Postpartum hemorrhage is a common complication during the third stage of labor and is the leading cause of maternal death in many countries worldwide. According to the World Health Organization, normal blood loss during the third stage of labor is ≤500 ml [62]. Uterine atony, prolonged third stage (>30 min), and retained placenta are the most common causes of severe postpartum hemorrhage, and these deviations from normal third stage of labor often necessitate active management [63,64]. Major risk factors associated with postpartum hemorrhage include primiparity, retained placenta, placenta previa, failure to progress in the second stage, and multiparity [65,66]. Despite the known predisposing factors, postpartum haemorrhage can also occur in women without any apparent risk factors.

Magann *et al.* [66] conducted a prospective observational study to estimate the relationship between the length of the third stage of labor and the risk of postpartum hemorrhage. Postpartum hemorrhage was defined as more than 1000 mL blood loss or hemodynamic instability related to blood loss requiring a blood transfusion. The study found a significantly associated risk of postpartum haemorrhage when the third stage of labor was longer than 18 minutes. An additional sixfold risk of postpartum hemorrhage was found when the third stage of labor had a duration of at least 30 minutes.

Active management of the third stage of labor, which includes administration of an oxytocin agent after birth of the baby, early cord clamping, and controlled umbilical cord traction, has been shown to reduce the risk of postpartum hemorrhage. Jangsten *et al.* [67] conducted a randomized clinical trial to compare blood loss in women actively and expectantly managed in the third stage of labor. Both prolonged duration of the third stage of labor and increased placenta weight were associated with increased blood loss (> 1000 mL). Active management of the third stage of labor was associated with a significant reduction in blood loss compared with expectant management (10% vs 16.8%, $p < 0.001$) [69].

As part of the active management of the third stage of labor, early cord clamping is understood to occur immediately (or before 30 seconds) after birth. However, recent systematic reviews [68–70] have demonstrated an association between delayed cord clamping (30–60 seconds after birth) and a number of neonatal benefits, including increased blood volume, reduced need for blood transfusions, and decreased frequency of iron deficiency anemia in term infants. Although the effects of delayed cord clamping on maternal postpartum hemorrhage have not been thoroughly studied, a 2008 systematic review of term infants found no significant differences in postpartum hemorrhage between early and delayed cord clamping [71]. The ideal timing for umbilical cord clamping that maximizes neonatal benefit while minimizing the risk of postpartum hemorrhage has yet to be established.

2.6 Intrapartum care during normal labor and delivery

2.6.1 Self-care

Restricting fluid and food intake in labor is a historical practice done to minimize the risk of aspiration pneumonitis and anaesthia-related complications, but may decrease maternal satisfaction and is not grounded in strong evidence for low-risk women. A review conducted by Singata *et al.* [72] assessed the effects of restriction versus no restriction of food and/or fluids in labor. All five reviewed studies (3130 women) included women in active labor with low risk of requiring general anesthetic. The authors concluded that there were no statistically significant differences in any of the assessed outcomes, including cesarean section, operative vaginal birth, and low 5-minute Apgar score. They found no justification for fluid or food restrictions in labor for low-risk women in normally progressing labor.

The majority of women in developed countries labor in bed. However, current findings have shown that walking and upright positions reduce the duration of first stage of labor as well as the risk for use of epidural analgesia and cesarean birth. Low-risk women in active labor should be encouraged to labor in positions that are most comfortable to them [73].

2.6.2 Care from non-medical person (continuous support)

Historically, women in labor have been supported by other women in non-hospital settings. However, modern obstetrics, with increasing numbers of births in hospital, has had the unintended effect of isolating women from these informal support systems, and continuous support during labor and birth has become less routine, increasing the risk of interference with the normal and natural progression of labor. Continuous support in labor may include emotional support and the provision of comfort measures for both the woman and her partner, as well as playing a role in advocacy. A recent Cochrane systematic review [74] analyzed 23 trials from 16 countries and included 15,288 women in an analysis of the effects of continuous support in labor and birth. The authors concluded that continuous support in labor from someone who was neither part of the hospital staff nor of the women's social network or family was of significant clinical benefit and demonstrated no harm. Specifically, they found an increased chance of vaginal birth (RR 1.08, 95% CI 1.04–1.12) and decreased rates of reported maternal dissatisfaction (RR 0.69, 95% CI 0.59–0.79). The authors recommended that all women in labor should receive continuous, one-on-one support throughout labor and birth.

2.6.3 Choice of care provider

For women with healthy pregnancies who expect a normal labor and who have a choice of care provider, the question arises as to the optimal care model to select. A recently updated Cochrane review by Sandall *et al.* compared midwife-led care to other forms of care, including doctor-led care [75]. Women who had midwife-led continuity models of care were less likely to experience regional analgesia (RR 0.83, 95% CI 0.76–0.90), episiotomy (RR 0.84, 95% CI 0.76–0.92), and instrumental birth (average RR 0.88, 95% CI 0.81–0.96), and were more likely to experience no intrapartum analgesia/anaesthesia (average RR 1.16, 95% CI 1.04–1.31), spontaneous vaginal birth (average RR 1.05, 95%

CI 1.03–1.08), attendance at birth by a known midwife (average RR 7.83, 95% CI 4.15–14.80), and a longer mean length of labor (hrs) (mean difference (hrs) 0.50, 95% CI 0.27–0.74). There were no differences between groups in cesarean births (average RR 0.93, 95% CI 0.84–1.02). Maternal satisfaction tended to be high in the midwife-led care groups.

2.7 Conclusion

The term "obstetrician" is derived from the Latin *obstare*, or "to stand by." This is to be distinguished from the "surgeon," a term derived from the Greek *kheirourgos*, "working or done by hand." The "one who stands by" must know when it is timely to intervene, to perform the "work done by hand." This ability to judge the timeliness of intervention is the essence of the profession of obstetrics. For women in labor with a healthy, normally grown baby, clinical care should be based on: (1) criteria for normal labor progress that are based on norms derived from recent, relevant obstetrical data and adapted to the specific characteristics of the patient; and (2) the premise that obstetrical interventions should be reserved for diagnoses where there are proven benefits from intervention. Patterns of labor progress appear to have changed since the 1950s, and it is no longer appropriate to apply outdated standards of progress that are not based on observations taken from current populations. Clinical practice guidelines for the care of normal women with a healthy fetus should be designed to minimize the obstetrical risk to the fetus associated with labor and delivery but, importantly, to avoid obstetrical interventions that are not evidence based, and that can potentially lead to iatrogenic morbidity. Obstetrics has a long and proud history of practice audit. The application of improved reference standards to assess labor progress will provide a rational basis for clinical care, facilitate audit, and ultimately lead to both a reduction in perinatal and maternal morbidity and mortality, and an improvement in the quality of the birthing experience for mothers and families.

References

1 American College of Obstetricians and Gynecologists Practice Bulletin No. 49: Dystocia and augmentation of labor. Clinical management guidelines for obstetricians-gynecologists. ACOG: Washington, DC, 2003.

2 Vause S. *Labor and delivery. Obstetrics: Normal Labor.* Cambridge University Press. 2008.

3 Zhang J, Landy HJ, Branch DW *et al.* Consortium on safe labor. Contemporary patterns of spontaneous labor with normal neonatal outcomes. *Obstetrics & Gynecology* 2010;**116**: 1281–1287.

4 Friedman EA. The graphic analysis of labor. *American Journal of Obstetrics & Gynecology* 1954;**68**:1568–1575.

5 Friedman EA. Primigravid labor: a graphicostastistical analysis. *Obstetrics & Gynecology* 1955;**6**:567–589.
6 Zhang J, Troendle JF, and Yancey MK. Reassessing the labor curve in nulliparous women. *American Journal of Obstetrics & Gynecology* 2002;**187**:824–828.
7 Martin JA, Hamilton BE, Ventura SJ, Osterman MJ, and Mathews TJ. Births: final data for 2011. *National Vital Statistics Reports* 2013;**62**:1–90.
8 Barber EL, Lundsberg LS, Belanger K, Pettker CM, Funai EF, Illuzzi JL. Indications contributing to the increasing cesarean delivery rate. *Obstetrics & Gynecology* 2011;**118**:29–38.
9 American College of Obstetricians and Gynecologists. Safe prevention of the primary cesarean delivery. Obstetric Care Consensus No. 1. American College of Obstetricians and Gynecologists. *Obstetrics & Gynecology* 2014;**123**:693–711.
10 SOGC. Joint policy statement on normal childbirth. *Journal of Obstetrics and Gynaecology Canada* 2009;**30**(12):1163–1165.
11 Steer P and Flint C. Physiology and management of normal labour. *BMJ* 1999 Mar 20;**318**(7186):793–796.
12 Bailit JL, Gregory KD, Reddy UM, Gonzalez-Quintero VH, Hibbard JU, Ramirez MM *et al.* Maternal and neonatal outcomes by labor onset type and gestational age. *American Journal of Obstetrics & Gynecology* 2010;**202**(3): 245.e1–245.e12.
13 McNiven PS, Williams JI, Hodnett E, Kaufman K, and Hannah ME. An early labor assessment program: a randomized, controlled trial. *Birth* 1998;**25**:5–10.
14 Morris H, Ruderman J, and Lacy J. The development and evaluation of an obstetrical triage programme. *Journal of Obstetrics and Gynaecology Canada* 1996;**18**:337–346.
15 SOGC Policy Statement No. 40 "Dystocia." October 1995.
16 Holmes P, Oppenheimer LW, and Wen SW. The relationship between cervical dilatation at initial presentation in labour and subsequent intervention. *BJOG: An International Journal of Obstetrics and Gynaecology* 2001;**108**(11):1120–1124.
17 Janssen PA, Still DK, Klein MC, Singer J, Carty EA, Liston RM *et al.* Early labor assessment and support at home versus telephone triage: a randomized controlled trial. *Obstetrics & Gynecology* 2006;**108**:1463–1469.
18 Hodnett ED, Stremler R, Willan AR, Weston JA, Lowe NK, Simpson KR *et al.* SELAN (structured early labour assessment and care by nurses) trial group. *BMJ* 2008;**337**:a1021.
19 Friedman E. *Labor: Clinical Evaluation and Management.* 2nd edn. New York: Appleton-century-Crofts. 1978.
20 Friedman EA and Sachtleben MR. Dysfunctional labor. I. Prolonged latent phase in the nullipara. *Obstetrics & Gynecology* 1961;**17**:135–148.
21 Friedman EA and Sachtleben MR. Dysfunctional labor. II. Protracted active-phase dilatation in the nullipara. *Obstetrics & Gynecology* 1961;**17**:566–578.
22 Kilpatrick SJ and Laros RK Jr. Characteristics of normal labor. *Obstetrics & Gynecology* 1989;**74**:85–87.
23 Albers LL. The duration of labor in healthy women. *Journal of Perinatology* 1999; **19**:114–119.
24 Neal JL, Lowe NK, Patrick TE, Cabbage LA, and Corwin EJ. What is the slowest-yet-normal cervical dilation rate among nulliparous women with spontaneous labor onset? *Journal of Obstetric, Gynecologic, & Neonatal Nursing* 2010;**39**(4):361–369.
25 Zhang J, Landy HJ, Branch DW *et al.* Contemporary patterns of spontaneous labor with normal neonatal outcomes. *Obstetrics & Gynecology* 2010;**116**:1281–1287.
26 Laughon SK, Branch DW, Beaver J *et al.* Changes in labor patterns over 50 years. *American Journal of Obstetrics & Gynecology* 2012;**206**:419.e1–9.
27 Zhang J, Troendle J, Mikolajczyk R, Sundaram R, Beaver J, and Fraser W. The natural history of the normal first stage of labor. *Obstetrics & Gynecology* 2010;**115**:705–710.

28 Boyle A, Reddy UM, Landy HJ, Huang CC, Driggers RQ, and Laughon SK. Primary cesarean delivery in the United States. *Obstetrics & Gynecology* 2013;**122**(1):33–40.

29 Hamilton E, Platt R, Gauthier R, McNamara H, Miner L, Rothenberg S *et al.* The effect of computer-assisted evaluation of labor on cesarean rates. *Journal for Healthcare Quality* Jan–Feb 2004;**26**(1):37–44.

30 Vahratian A, Hoffman MK, Troendle JF, and Zhang J. The impact of parity on course of labor in a contemporary population. *Birth* 2006;**33**:12–7.

31 Tuck SM, Cardozo LD, Studd JW *et al.* Obstetric characteristics in different racial groups. *BJOG: An International Journal of Obstetrics and Gynaecology* 1983;**90**(10):892–897.

32 Duignan NM, Studd JW, and Hughes AO. Characteristics of normal labour in different racial groups. *BJOG: An International Journal of Obstetrics and Gynaecology* 1975;**82**(8):593–601.

33 Sills ES, Baum JD, Ling X *et al.* [Average length of spontaneous labor in Chinese primigravidas]. *Journal de Gynécologie Obstétrique et Biologie de la Reproduction* (Paris) 1997;**26**:704–710.

34 Cahill AG, Roehl KA, Odibo AO, Zhao Q, and Macones GA. Impact of fetal gender on the labor curve. *American Journal of Obstetrics & Gynecology* 2012;**206**:335.e1–5.

35 Kominiarek MA, Zhang J, Vanvaldhuisen P, Troendle J, Beaver J, and Hibbard JU. Contemporary labor patterns: the impact of maternal body mass index. *American Journal of Obstetrics & Gynecology* 2011;**205**(3):244:e1–8.

36 Sheiner E, Levy A, Feinstein U, Hallak M, and Mazor M. Risk factors and outcome of failure to progress during the first stage of labor: a population-based study. *Acta Obstetricia et Gynecologica Scandinavica* 2002;**81**:222–226.

37 Cheng YW, Shaffer BL, Bryant AS, and Caughey AB. Length of the first stage of labor and associated perinatal outcomes in nulliparous women. *Obstetrics & Gynecology* 2010; **116**:1127–1135.

38 Rouse DJ, Owen J, and Hauth JC. Active-phase labor arrest: oxytocin augmentation for at least 4 hours. *Obstetrics & Gynecology* 1999;**93**(3):323–328.

39 Gupta JK, Hofmeyr GJ, and Smyth R. Position in the second stage of labour for women without epidural anaesthesia. *Cochrane Database of Systematic Reviews* 2004;(**1**):CD002006. DOI: 10.1002/14651858.CD002006.

40 Roberts CL, Algert CS, Cameron CA, and Torvaldsen S. A meta-analysis of upright positions in the second stage to reduce instrumental deliveries in women with epidural anesthesia. *Acta Obstetricia et Gynecologica Scandinavica* 2005;**84**:794–798.

41 Senécal J, Xiong X, and Fraser WD. Pushing early or pushing late with epidural study group. Effect of fetal position on second-stage duration and labor outcome. *Obstetrics & Gynecology* 2005;**105**:763–772.

42 Schiessl B, Janni W, Jundt K, Rammel G, Peschers U, and Kainer F. Obstetrical parameters influencing the duration of the second stage of labor. *European Journal of Obstetrics & Gynecology and Reproductive Biology* 2005;**118**:17–20.

43 Paterson CM, Saunders NS, and Wadsworth J. The characteristics of the second stage of labour in 25,069 singleton deliveries in the North West Thames Health Region, 1988. *BJOG: An International Journal of Obstetrics and Gynaecology* 1992;**99**:377–380.

44 Greenberg MB, Cheng YW, Hopkins LM *et al.* Are there ethnic differences in the length of labor? *American Journal of Obstetrics & Gynecology* 2006;**195**:743–748.

45 Canadian Institute for Health Information. *Giving Birth in Canada: Providers of Maternity and Infant Care*. Ottawa: CIHI. 2004.

46 Anim-Somuah M, Smyth RMD, and Jones L. Epidural versus non-epidural or no analgesia in labour. *Cochrane Database of Systematic Reviews* 2011;(12):CD000331. DOI: 10.1002/14651858.CD000331.pub3.

47 Cohen WR. Influence of the duration of second stage labor on perinatal outcome and puerperal morbidity. *Obstetrics & Gynecology* 1977;**49**:266–269.

48 Saunders NS, Paterson CM, and Wadsworth J. Neonatal and maternal morbidity in relation to the length of the second stage of labour. *BJOG: An International Journal of Obstetrics and Gynaecology* 1992;**99**:381–385.

49 Cheng YW, Hopkins LM, Laros RK Jr, and Caughey AB. Duration of the second stage of labor in multiparous women: maternal and neonatal outcomes. *American Journal of Obstetrics & Gynecology* 2007;**196**:585.e1–6.

50 Allen VM, Baskett TF, O'Connell CM, McKeen D, and Allen AC. Maternal and perinatal outcomes with increasing duration of the second stage of labor. *Obstetrics & Gynecology* 2009;**113**:1248–1258.

51 Rouse DJ, Weiner SJ, Bloom SL, Varner MW, Spong CY, Ramin SM *et al.* Eunice Kennedy Shriver National Institute of Child Health and Human Development Maternal-Fetal Medicine Units Network. Second-stage labor duration in nulliparous women: relationship to maternal and perinatal outcomes. *American Journal of Obstetrics & Gynecology* 2009;**201**:357.e1–7.

52 Roberts J, Goldstein S, Gruener J, Maggio M, and Mendez-Bauer C. A descriptive analysis of involuntary bearing-down efforts during the expulsive phase of labor. *Journal of Obstetric, Gynecologic, & Neonatal Nursing* 1987;**16**:48–55.

53 Maresh M, Choong KH, and Beard RW. Delayed pushing with lumbar epidural analgesia in labour. *BJOG: An International Journal of Obstetrics and Gynaecology* 1983;**90**:623–627.

54 Fraser WD, Marcoux S, Krauss I, Douglas J, Goulet C, Boulvain M. Multicenter, randomized, controlled trial of delayed pushing for nulliparous women in the second stage of labor with continuous epidural analgesia. The PEOPLE (pushing early or pushing late with epidural) study group. *American Journal of Obstetrics & Gynecology* 2000;**182**:1165–1172.

55 Petrou S, Coyle D, and Fraser WD. Cost-effectiveness of a delayed pushing policy for patients with epidural anesthesia. The PEOPLE (pushing early or pushing late with epidural) study group. *American Journal of Obstetrics & Gynecology* 2000;**182**:1158–1156.

56 Tuuli MG, Frey HA, Odibo AO, Macones GA, and Cahill AG. Immediate compared with delayed pushing in the second stage of labor: a systematic review and meta-analysis. *Obstetrics & Gynecology* 2012;**120**:660–668.

57 Herman A, Zimerman A, Arieli S *et al.* Down-up sequential separation of the placenta. *Ultrasound in Obstetrics & Gynecology* 2002;**19**:278–281.

58 Herman A, Weinraub Z, Bukovsky I, Ariely S, Zabow P, Caspi E *et al.* Dynamic ultrasonographic imaging of the third stage of labor: New perspective into third stage mechanism. *American Journal of Obstetrics & Gynecology* 1993;**168**:1496–1499.

59 Lurie S, Gomel A, Sadan O, Ginath S, Rotmensch S, and Glezerman M. The duration of the third stage of labor is subject to the location of placental implantation. *Gynecologic and Obstetric Investigation* 2003;**56**:14–16.

60 Altay MM, Ilhan AK, and Haberal A. Length of the third stage of labor at term pregnancies is shorter if placenta is located at fundus: prospective study. *Journal of Obstetrics and Gynaecology Research* 2007;**33**:641–644.

61 Grinsted L and Grinsted J. Effects of induced abortion on the third stage of labor in subsequent pregnancy. *Acta Obstetricia et Gynecologica Scandinavica* 1987;**66**:685–688.

62 WHO/MCH. *Prevention and Management of Postpartum Haemorrhage.* Report of technical working group, July 1989. WHO/MCH/90.7. Geneva.1990.

63 Stones RW, Paterson CM, and Saunders NJ. Risk factors for major obstetric haemorrhage. *European Journal of Obstetrics & Gynecology and Reproductive Biology* 1993;**48**:15–18.

64 Magann EF, Evans S, Chauhan SP, Lanneau G, Fisk AD, and Morrison JC. The length of the third stage of labor and the risk of postpartum hemorrhage. *Obstetrics & Gynecology* 2005;**105**:290–293.

65 Kramer MS, Dahhou M, Vallerand D, Liston R, and Joseph KS. Risk factors for postpartum hemorrhage: can we explain the recent temporal increase? *Journal of Obstetrics and Gynaecology Canada* 2011;**33**(8):810–819.

66 Sheiner E, Sarid L, Levy A, Seidman DS, and Hallak M. Obstetric risk factors and outcome of pregnancies complicated with early postpartum hemorrhage: a population-based study. *Journal of Maternal-Fetal and Neonatal Medicine* 2005;**18**(3):149–154.

67 Jangsten E, Mattsson LÅ, Lyckestam I, Hellström AL, and Berg M. A comparison of active management and expectant management of the third stage of labour: a Swedish randomised controlled trial. *BJOG: An International Journal of Obstetrics and Gynaecology* 2011;**118**:362–369.

68 Rabe H, Diaz-Rossello JL, Duley L, and Dowswell T. Effect of timing of umbilical cord clamping and other strategies to influence placental transfusion at preterm birth on maternal and infant outcomes. *Cochrane Database of Systematic Reviews* 2012;(8): CD003248. DOI: 10.1002/14651858.CD003248.pub3.

69 Rabe H, Reynolds G, and Diaz-Rossello J. A systematic review and meta-analysis of a brief delay in clamping the umbilical cord of preterm infants. *Neonatology* 2008;**93**:138–144.

70 Hutton EK and Hassan ES. Late vs early clamping of the umbilical cord in full-term neonates: systematic review and meta-analysis of controlled trials. *Journal of the American Medical Association* 2007;**297**:1241–1252.

71 McDonald SJ and Middleton P. Effect of timing of umbilical cord clamping of term infants on maternal and neonatal outcomes. *Cochrane Database of Systematic Reviews* 2008;(2):CD004074. DOI: 10.1002/14651858.CD004074.pub2.

72 Singata M, Tranmer J, and Gyte GM. Restricting oral fluid and food intake during labour. *Cochrane Database of Systematic Reviews* 2013;(8):CD003930.

73 Lawrence A, Lewis L, Hofmeyr GJ, and Styles C. Maternal positions and mobility during first stage labour. *Cochrane Database of Systematic Reviews* 2013;(10):CD003934.

74 Hodnett ED, Gates S, Hofmeyr GJ, and Sakala C. Continuous support for women during childbirth. *Cochrane Database of Systematic Reviews* 2013;(7):CD003766.

75 Sandall J, Soltani H, Gates S, Shennan A, and Devane D. Midwife-led continuity models versus other models of care for childbearing women. *Cochrane Database of Systematic Reviews* 2013;(8):CD004667.

CHAPTER 3

Management of labor and delivery in low-risk subjects

Anthony Shanks and Alison Cahill*

Division of Maternal-Fetal Medicine, Department of Obstetrics and Gynecology, Washington University School of Medicine, St Louis, MO, USA

3.1 Introduction

The cesarean delivery rate continues to rise to historic proportions [1]. Given the increased morbidity associated with the procedure as compared to spontaneous delivery, it is imperative that women who are candidates to deliver vaginally continue to have the opportunity. Identifying and encouraging trial of labor after cesarean (TOLAC) is one method to combat the rising rate. An equally important method is to decrease the primary cesarean rate. The abnormal progression of labor, termed dystocia, is the leading indication for primary cesarean delivery in the United States [2]. Clearly, the optimal labor management of the low-risk patient could have far-reaching effects.

Our understanding of labor dystocia was initially presented over half a century ago. Dr. Emanuel Friedman in the 1950s laid down the groundwork for our understanding of the labor process [3,4]. He used a prospective cohort study to identify 200 women in order to characterize ideal labor. Data in the 1980s yielded similar results [5]. The result of these works is the labor curve that is ubiquitous in labor and delivery units and medical schools across the country. Though the mean latent phase of labor was 8.6 hours, the 95th percentile was noted to be significantly longer at 20.6 hours. Rates of dilation of 1.5 cm/h in multiparous and 1.2 cm/h in nulliparous patients in the active phase of labor represented the 95th percentile for rates of dilation and led to the thinking that dilation of 1 cm/h should be the minimum acceptable rate before noting a labor dystocia [4]. This became an important distinction because currently an estimated 60% of all cesarean deliveries are performed for the diagnosis of dystocia [6].

*Dr Cahill is a Robert Wood Johnson Faculty Physician Scholar

Management of Labor and Delivery, Second Edition. Edited by George A. Macones.

Labor dystocia is the leading cause of operative vaginal and cesarean delivery and their potential complications and, despite the high prevalence of labor dystocia disorders, considerable variability exists in the management of dystocia [2]. One attempt to decrease the rate of cesarean delivery due to dystocia was the concept of active management. Active management of labor was popularized in the 1980s based on findings in Ireland [7]. Protocols included admission only when labor was established (painful contractions and spontaneous rupture of membranes, 100% effacement, or passage of bloodstained mucus); artificial rupture of membranes on diagnosis of labor; aggressive oxytocin augmentation for labor progress of less than 1 cm/h with high dose oxytocin (6 mIU/min initial dose, increased by 6 mIU/min every 15 minutes to a maximum of 40 mIU/min); and patient education [7]. Results of this initial study yielded a reported cesarean delivery rate of 5.5% and delivery within 12 hours in 98% of women. Unfortunately, these results were not routinely reproducible in US populations [8,9]. A meta-analysis of four randomized trials did not demonstrate a decrease in cesarean deliveries related to active management of labor (RR 0.93, 95% CI 0.8–1.08) [10]. Applicability of these results leads one to question whether standards are different across differing populations and also if the initial results of Friedman are applicable today.

New studies challenge those initial works and lead us to potentially reevaluate what is a "normal" labor curve. Doing so would lead us to reconsider our interventions for dystocia – including cesarean delivery – as well as other measures in the management of labor and delivery in the low-risk subject.

3.2 First stage

Labor is divided into three stages – first, second, and third [11]. The first stage marks the time from the onset of contractions to complete cervical dilation. The second stage is the time from complete cervical dilation to expulsion of the fetus. The third stage is the time from delivery of the fetus to expulsion of the placenta. The first stage can be further subdivided into a latent phase and an active phase based on the work initially described by Friedman on labors in women managed at a single institution [12]. Since that time, practice patterns and even maternal demographics have changed.

To evaluate these differences, attention has been paid to two large cohorts. The historical comparison often used is the Collaborative Perinatal Project, which consisted of 48,197 women and 54,390 births delivered between 1959 and 1966 [13]. The second, more modern cohort is the Consortium on Safe Labor (CSL). This was a retrospective cohort study by the Eunice Kennedy Shriver National Institute of Child Health and Human Development and National Health and consisted of 228,668 deliveries in 12 clinical centers and 19 hospitals representing nine American College of Obstetrics and Gynecology districts between 2002 and 2008 [14]. In a comparison of labor patterns in these two cohorts, the more modern cohort consisted of older women (26.8 + 6.0 vs 24.1 + 6.0 years), were heavier (body mass index 29.9 + 5.0 vs 26.3 + 4.1 kg/m^2), had higher epidural (55% vs 4%) and oxytocin use (31% vs 12%), and higher cesarean delivery rates (12% vs 3%) [13]. The first stage of labor was also significantly longer in the modern cohort by a median of 2.6 hours in nulliparas and 2.0 hours in multiparas. Even after adjusting for maternal and pregnancy characteristics, the prolonged labor persisted, suggesting changes in practice patterns.

In addition to the total duration of the first stage of labor, the rate of cervical change has also been investigated in modern cohorts. In 2002, Zhang *et al.* evaluated 1329 nulliparous term singletons and documented the rate of cervical change [15]. They discovered that the fifth percentile rate of cervical dilation was less than 1 cm/h and no perceivable change for 2 hours prior to 7 cm was not uncommon. A more recent analysis by the same group extrapolated on these findings. In it, data from the CSL evaluated 62,415 women with singleton gestations, spontaneous labor, vaginal deliveries, and normal perinatal outcomes [14]. In this population, the rate of cervical dilation accelerated after 6 cm, and progress from 4 cm to 6 cm was far slower than previously described. When contrasted to prior work by Friedman, there is faster progress toward the point of complete dilation and no deceleration phase was noted. These data suggest that interventions – such as cesarean delivery – prior to 6 cm may be hasty.

The active phase of labor has previously been thought to occur at 4 cm [12]. If current cohorts demonstrate that this occurs at 6 cm, many cesarean sections for dystocia could potentially be avoided. Research into the contemporary delivery practice in the US has been further investigated to highlight the impact of this 6-cm cutoff. Zhang *et al.* in 2010 used the CSL cohort to discover that 31.2% of nulliparous women were delivered by cesarean delivery [1]. Pre-labor repeat cesarean delivery due to previous uterine scar contributed to 30.9% of all cesarean sections. For women who attempted TOLAC, the success rate for vaginal birth after caesarean was 57.1% for the 28.8% of women with a uterine scar. Interestingly, half of cesarean deliveries for dystocia were performed prior to 6 cm of dilation. The results of this study highlight the potential impact of avoiding cesarean section for dystocia prior to 6 cm.

The question of whether this rule regarding dystocia applies to induced versus spontaneous labor has recently been investigated. Harper *et al.* used a retrospective cohort of 5388 women presenting for labor between 2004 and 2008 [16]. In this cohort, 2021 women spontaneously labored, 1720 were augmented, and 1647 were induced. The authors adjusted for race, obesity, macrosomia, and Bishop score and discovered that the median time to progress 1 cm dilation in active labor (6 cm or greater) was similar in induced and spontaneous labor. However, the time to progress 1 cm dilation in latent labor (less than 6 cm) was significantly longer in women who were induced compared to those who had a spontaneous labor. The authors conclude that arrest disorders diagnosed prior to 6 cm in labor inductions should be made cautiously.

Further research has continued to focus on different subgroups and analyzing whether differences exist in their first stage of labor. Graseck *et al.* recently used a retrospective cohort to evaluate the first stage of labor in women undergoing TOLAC [17]. In this study, 1881 laboring women with no previous cesarean delivery were compared with 140 women undergoing TOLAC. Adjustments for race, obesity, macrosomia, and previous vaginal delivery were performed. They reported that there was no significant difference in rates of cervical dilation between the two groups. The median time for dilation from 4 to 10 cm was 3.0 hours for TOLAC and 2.8 hours for the subjects without a previous cesarean delivery ($p = 0.52$). The authors conclude that there was no difference in first-stage labor groups in women undergoing TOLAC and those without a previous cesarean. Certainly women that elect to undergo TOLAC deserve special consideration. However, labor disorders should be diagnosed using similar standards to those used for patients without a prior uterine scar.

The obese population deserves special attention as well. Maternal obesity has been identified as an independent risk factor for cesarean delivery [18,19] and obese women have higher rates of wound complications, wound infections, dehiscence, and surgical tissue injury associated with cesarean delivery [20–23]. Given that dystocia and arrest disorders are cited as leading indications for cesarean delivery [24], it would certainly be worthwhile to note if historically accepted norms apply to this group. Norman *et al.* used a retrospective cohort study of 5204 consecutive term parturients with singleton term pregnancies greater than 37 weeks [25]. Two comparison groups were defined by body mass index (BMI). There were 2413 women with BMI < 30 and 2791 with BMI > 30. Multivariable regression analysis revealed that a BMI of > 30 resulted in longer duration and slower progression of the first stage of labor for both nulliparous and multiparous women (4–10 cm: 4.7 compared with 4.1 hrs, $p < 0.01$). There was also a slower progression from 4 to 6 cm dilation (2.2 compared with 1.9 hrs, $p < 0.01$ with a range of 0.5–10.0 hrs) in this group of patients. The authors conclude that obesity should be considered when defining norms for the management of labor, particularly in the first stage [21].

Given the impact of dystocia diagnosis, an important consideration is how often to check the laboring patient. Though each institution has their own protocol, many will perform cervical exams every 2–4 hours in the laboring patient. The concern of increased febrile morbidity exists for the laboring patient receiving multiple cervical exams. Cahill *et al.* used a 4-year retrospective cohort of term (≥37 weeks of gestation) singleton deliveries reaching the second stage of labor. They identified women who developed an intrapartum fever and compared them with women who remained afebrile through 6 hours postpartum. Of the 2395 women who were afebrile at admission, 174 (7.2%) developed an intrapartum fever. There was no significant association between increasing number of examinations and risk of fever – even for women with seven or more examinations during the second stage. Their conclusion was that the number of examinations does not increase the risk of maternal fever. Therefore, checking women for dystocia can be done without fear of maternal febrile morbidity so allowing for an accurate diagnosis.

It appears that the maternal demographics have changed over the past century and our understanding of the labor process with it. The active phase does not start until 6 cm so cesarean delivery for the diagnosis of dystocia prior to 6 cm may be premature. The rate of cervical dilation appears to be the same whether the patient is induced or labors spontaneously and patients undergoing TOLAC witness similar progression rates in the first stage to those without a prior uterine scar. Importantly, the risk of febrile morbidity does not appear to be related to the number of cervical exams. In practical terms, laboring patients may not need to be checked as often prior to 6 cm and perhaps need to be evaluated more frequently afterward when true dystocia can be diagnosed. In the near future, customized labor curves including factors such as BMI may be used to optimize labor management.

3.3 Amniotomy

There are other interventions that are commonly performed in the low-risk obstetrical patient in order to augment their labor. Some providers routinely perform amniotomy to accelerate labor but its effect is unclear. A systematic review of 14 randomized trials involving 4893 women compared women with routine amniotomy versus those in whom preservation of intact membranes was planned [26]. There was no statistically significant difference in length of the first stage of labor (WMD −20.43, 95% CI −95.93–55.06) or low Apgar score less than 7 at 5 minutes (RR 0.55, 95% CI 0.29–1.05). Amniotomy was associated with an increased risk of cesarean section but this difference was not statistically significant (RR 1.26, 95% CI 0.98–1.62). Amniotomy is recommended when monitoring of fetal status (fetal scalp electrode [FSE]) is needed though it is does not appear to be beneficial for augmenting labor by itself.

The addition of oxytocin to amniotomy, however, may provide more benefits. A meta-analysis evaluated the effects of amniotomy with oxytocin [27]. Twelve trials with 7792 women were included. A policy of early amniotomy and early oxytocin was associated with a shortened duration of labor (mean difference −1.11 hr). There were no significant effects in regards to maternal or neonatal morbidity. It appears that the performance of amniotomy by itself does not hasten labor progression. Its use should be considered if an FSE is needed or if oxytocin is planned.

3.4 Second stage

As maternal demographics change, the rate of progress in the first stage has been reevaluated. Investigation into the second stage of labor, however, has showed more similarities to historical cohorts. In one classic review of nearly 7000 women with minimal intervention, the mean length of the second stage of labor was 19 minutes in multiparous women and 54 minutes in nulliparous women [5]. The use of conduction anesthesia increased the rates by approximately 30 minutes and gave way to the diagnosis of prolonged second stage when it exceeded 3 hours if regional anesthesia was used and 2 hours if none was administered in the nulliparous patient [2]. Prolonged second stage for multiparous patients had definitions of 2 hours with regional anesthesia and 1 hour without regional anesthesia [2]. Recently, Zhang *et al.* used the CSL to evaluate second stage characteristics. In this study, the 95th percentiles of the second stage of labor in nulliparous women with and without epidural anesthesia were 3.6 and 2.8 hours, respectively [14]. These time frames are remarkably similar to the results reported by Friedman *et al.*

More important than a historical comparison is the issue of whether the amount of time spent in the second stage has an impact on maternal and neonatal outcomes. One study that attempted to answer this question was performed by Rouse *et al.* where the authors evaluated 5341 women, 4126 of whom reached the second stage of labor [28]. As the duration of the second stage increased, spontaneous vaginal delivery rates declined from 85% when the duration was < 1 hour to 9% when it was ≥ 5 hours. Rates of chorioamnionitis (overall rate 3.9%), third- or fourth-degree perineal laceration (overall rate, 8.7%), and uterine atony (overall rate, 3.9%) were associated significantly with the duration of the second stage of labor. In terms of neonatal outcomes, only admission to neonatal intensive care units was significantly associated with second stage duration (OR 1.4). The results of this study show that increasing the amount of time in the second stage has increased rates of adverse outcomes for both the mother and the baby.

Another study looked at vaginal delivery success and outcomes based on the amount of time spent in the second stage of labor. Le Ray *et al.* performed a secondary analysis of 1862 nulliparous women with epidural anesthesia who were in the second stage of labor [29]. They found that relative to the first hour of expulsive efforts, the chances of a spontaneous vaginal delivery of a newborn infant without signs of asphyxia decreased significantly every hour (1- to 2-hr aOR 0.4, 95% CI 0.3–0.6; 2- to 3-hr aOR 0.1, 95% CI 0.09–0.2; > 3-hr aOR 0.03; 95% CI 0.02–0.05). The risk of postpartum hemorrhage and intrapartum fever increased significantly after 2 hours of pushing. The authors concluded that with increased maternal risk of morbidity after 2 hours and a decreasing probability of vaginal delivery, the concept of continued expulsive efforts after 2 hours should be reevaluated.

There is also the potential concern for adverse outcomes the longer a patient is subjecting to maternal expulsive efforts. To address this, some practitioners have adopted the practice of laboring down in order to improve outcomes. This practice involves allowing the patient to wait to push until she has the urge once complete. This technique has been evaluated multiple times with conflicting results. Fraser *et al.* in 2000 performed a large, multicenter trial randomizing nulliparous women with continuous epidural anesthesia to early pushing versus delayed pushing (waiting ≥ 2 hrs from reaching complete dilation) [30]. Their primary outcome was difficult delivery defined as cesarean delivery, operative delivery from a mid-pelvic position, or low-pelvic procedures with rotation > 45 degrees. In the study, the authors concluded that difficult delivery was reduced with delayed pushing (RR 0.79; 95% CI 0.66–0.95); however, abnormal umbilical cord pH (< 7.15 venous value or < 7.10 arterial value) was more frequent with delayed pushing. Another recent retrospective cohort study found a similar finding with decreased umbilical cord pH in patients selected to labor down [31]. Frey *et al.* evaluated 57,290 women, 91.1% pushed immediately after complete dilation and 8.9% delayed pushing for > 60 minutes after complete dilation. The group that delayed pushing was found to be associated with an increased rate of cesarean delivery, operative vaginal delivery, and maternal fever, in addition to decreased cord pH.

Conversely, there is data to suggest that passive descent may have benefit. Brancato *et al.* in 2008 performed a meta-analysis evaluating passive descent versus immediate pushing in nulliparous women with epidural anesthesia in the second stage of labor [32]. Seven studies including 2827 women were evaluated. Their study revealed that passive descent increased a woman's chance of having a spontaneous vaginal birth (RR 1.08, 95% CI 1.01–1.15), deceased the risk of having an instrument-assisted delivery (RR 0.77, 95% CI 0.77–0.85), and decreased pushing time (mean difference −0.19 hrs, 95% CI −0.27–0.12). No differences were found in the rates of cesarean births (RR 0.80, 95% CI 0.57–1.12), lacerations (RR 0.88, 95% CI 0.72–1.07), or episiotomies (RR 0.97, 95% CI 0.88–1.06). The authors conclude that significant positive effects can be gained by passive descent in the second stage of labor.

The question of immediate pushing versus delayed pushing has yielded conflicting data – especially in terms of neonatal outcomes. Tuuli *et al.* performed a meta-analysis of 12 randomized controlled trials with 1584 patients employing immediate pushing and 1531 performing delayed pushing [33]. Overall, delayed pushing was associated with an increased rate of vaginal delivery (61.5% vs 56.9%, RR 1.09, 95% CI 1.03–1.15) but the findings were only statistically significant in lower quality studies. Delayed pushing may lead to an increased chance of spontaneous vaginal delivery; however, there is an increased risk of prolongation of the second stage in addition to potentially decreased pH cord gases in delivered fetuses when delayed pushing is employed. Given these findings, the decision for delayed pushing should be individualized.

3.5 Perineal massage

Whether a patient has a cesarean delivery is not the only outcome worth evaluating in the low-risk obstetrical patient. There is also the issue of perineal trauma and methods to decrease this risk. A Cochrane review in 2006 evaluated antenatal perinatal massage for reducing perineal trauma [34]. The authors posited that perineal massage may increase the flexibility of the perineal muscles and therefore decrease muscular resistance leading to decreased genital trauma with vaginal delivery. Three trials with 2434 women were included. Antenatal perineal massage was associated with an overall reduction in the incidence of trauma requiring suturing (RR 0.91, 95% CI 0.86–0.96) though this was only statistically significant for women without a previous vaginal birth (three trials, 1925 women, RR 0.90, 95% CI 0.84–0.96). These women were also at a decreased risk for episiotomy (three trials, 2417 women, RR 0.85, 95% CI 0.74–0.97). No differences were seen in the incidence of first- or second-degree perineal tears or third- or fourth-degree perineal trauma. Only women with a previous delivery reported a significant reduction in the incidence of pain 3 months postpartum (one trial, 376 women, RR 0.68, 95% CI 0.50–0.91). Interestingly, the reduction in the incidence of episiotomy and of perineal trauma requiring suturing was not more pronounced in the women who massaged the most frequently. It was also found that the women who massaged the most frequently had the longest second stage of labor. The authors conclude that antenatal perineal massage reduces the likelihood of perineal trauma and that women should be provided with information and instructions on its performance. More recently, Aasheim *et al.* performed a meta-analysis of eight trials involving 11,651 randomized women [35]. The authors reported that the use of warm compresses on the perineum during the second stage of labor reduced third- and fourth-degree tears (RR 0.48, 95% CI 0.28–0.84). Given the relative ease and safety of this maneuver, its use can be considered in the low-risk laboring patient.

Pelvic floor muscle training to decrease the rate of perineal trauma has also been evaluated [36]. Bo *et al.* evaluated 18,865 primiparous women via questionnaire to assess the impact of antenatal pelvic muscle floor training. Women who performed pelvic muscle floor training at least three times per week had similar rates of episiotomy (29.1% vs 24.9%), vacuum/forceps delivery (15.9% vs 15.0%), and acute cesarean delivery (9.5% vs 7.5%) compared to women who trained less than once per week. Additionally, third- and fourth-degree lacerations were similar between the groups (aOR 0.86, 95% CI 0.60–1.24). The authors conclude that pelvic muscle floor training during pregnancy does not affect birth complication rates.

3.6 Episiotomy

The Cochrane Database reviewed the evidence for episiotomy for vaginal birth in 2000 [37]. Six studies including over 4000 women were evaluated. Compared with routine use, restrictive episiotomy involved less posterior perineal trauma (RR 0.88, 95% CI 0.84–0.92), less suturing (RR 0.74, 95% CI 0.71–0.77), and fewer healing complications (RR 0.69, 95% CI 0.56–0.85). There was an increased risk for anterior perineal trauma (RR 1.79, 95% CI 1.55–2.07) but pain measures were similar between groups. Based on this, the authors concluded that there were a number of benefits of restrictive episiotomies as compared to routine use.

More recent studies further investigated risk factors for perineal trauma and cervical lacerations. Landy *et al.* in 2011 and the CSL evaluated their robust data set to elucidate risk factors – including episiotomy – for severe perineal and cervical lacerations during labor [38]. Medical records from 19 hospitals within 12 institutions (228,668 deliveries from 2002 to 2008) were used. Third- or fourth-degree lacerations occurred in 2516 women (2223 nulliparous [5.8%], 293 multiparous [0.6%]). Risks for third- or fourth-degree lacerations included nulliparity (7.2-fold risk), being Asian or a Pacific Islander, increasing birth-weight, operative vaginal delivery, episiotomy, and longer second stage of labor. Increasing BMI was associated with fewer lacerations. Risk factors for cervical lacerations included young maternal age, vacuum vaginal delivery, oxytocin use among multiparous women, and cerclage regardless of parity. The use of episiotomy appears to be associated with significant perineal injury and its routine use should be discouraged.

3.7 Cord clamping

Many studies have tried to determine if there is any benefit to immediate versus delayed cord clamping. Rabe *et al.* in 2004 performed a Cochrane Database review in which they evaluated early versus delayed umbilical cord clamping in preterm birth [39]. Seven studies with 297 infants were included in the analysis. They discovered that delayed cord clamping was associated with a higher hematocrit 4 hours after birth (weighted mean difference 5.31, 95% CI 3.42–7.19), fewer transfusions for anemia (RR 2.01, 95% CI 1.17–5.67), and less intraventricular hemorrhage than early clamping (RR 2.58, 95% CI 1.08–2.81). They concluded that delaying cord clamping by 30–120 seconds may be associated with tangible benefits in the preterm fetus. There were no clear differences in other outcomes.

A more recent systematic review by Rabe *et al.* confirmed these findings in the preterm infant [40]. Ten studies with a total of 454 preterm infants were evaluated. The authors discovered that benefits of delayed cord clamping (30 seconds or more) included higher circulating blood volume during the first 24 hours of life, less need for blood transfusions ($p = 0.004$), and less incidence of intraventricular hemorrhage ($p = 0.002$). They conclude that delayed clamping is safe with benefits to the preterm infant in the postpartum adaptation phase.

Milking the umbilical cord has also been compared to delayed cord clamping. In a randomized controlled trial of preterm deliveries before 33 weeks, milking of the umbilical cord yielded similar mean hemoglobin values at 1 hour after birth compared to delayed clamping (17.5 vs 17.3 g/L, $p = 0.71$). There was no significant difference in the number of neonates undergoing transfusion (clamping group 15, milking group 17, $p = 0.4$) or the median number of transfusions within the first 42 days of life (median 0, range 0–7 with clamping, median 0, range 0–20 with milking). The authors conclude that milking the cord four times achieved a similar amount of placento-fetal blood transfusion to delaying cord clamping for 30 seconds.

More recent studies have evaluated term infants. Hutton *et al.* in 2007 performed a meta-analysis of 15 controlled trials and over 1912 newborns [41]. Late cord clamping was defined as delaying clamping for at least 2 minutes after birth. Early clamping was performed immediately after birth. Benefits at 2–6 months after delivery included increased hematocrit (weighted mean difference 3.7%, 95% CI 2.0–5.4%), increased ferritin concentration (WMD 17.89, 95% CI 16.58–19.21), and a clinically important reduction in the risk of anemia (RR 0.52, 95% CI 0.40–0.70). There was an increased risk of asymptomatic polycythemia (RR 3.82, 95% CI 1.11–13.21) though the results of that aspect may be benign. The authors concluded that delayed clamping by 2 minutes is beneficial and the benefits extend into infancy.

The concept of delayed cord clamping has clear benefits to the preterm neonate. There may be potential benefits to term babies in the form of increased ferritin and hematocrit but the clinical significance of this is unclear. Its use can be individualized to the patient.

3.8 Third stage

Expectant management of the third stage involves allowing the placenta to deliver spontaneously without exogenous medications. Active management involves administration of oxytocin before delivery of the placenta with usually early cord clamping and controlled cord traction of the umbilical cord. Prendiville *et al.* issued a Cochrane review on active versus expectant management in the third stage of labor [42]. Compared to expectant management, active management was associated with reduced risk of maternal blood loss (WMD −79.22 mL, 95% CI −94.29 to −64.37); postpartum hemorrhage of more than 500 mL (RR 0.38, 95% CI 0.32–0.46); and prolonged third stage of labor (WMD −9.7 minutes, 95% CI 10.0 to −9.53). Active management was associated with increased risk of maternal nausea (RR 1.95, 95% CI 1.58–2.42), vomiting, and raised blood pressure. No significant differences were observed in neonatal outcomes. The authors recommend active management to decrease the adverse hematological outcomes in the third stage of labor.

The utility of cord traction has also been assessed. Gulmezoglu *et al.* performed a randomized controlled trial evaluating placental delivery with gravity and maternal expulsive efforts compared to controlled traction of the umbilical cord [43]. Uterine massage was done after placental delivery per local policy and oxytocin 10 IU was administered immediately after birth with cord clamping after 1–3 min. Over 24,000 women were included in their study and the authors found that omission of cord traction had very little effect on the risk of severe hemorrhage (blood loss of 1000 mL, RR 1.09, 95% CI 0.91–1.31). The conclusion of this study was that cord traction had little impact on hemorrhage risk and efforts should be focused on oxytocin protocols.

3.9 Conclusion

An uncomplicated vaginal delivery is the goal of every laboring low-risk patient. Efforts by the medical community should accentuate this, which in turn would help decrease the cesarean delivery rate and its inherent increased morbidity. The most significant recent development is the concept of the active phase of labor not occurring until 6 cm. The diagnosis of dystocia as a cause for cesarean delivery is an important one and therefore should be diagnosed cautiously prior to 6 cm. Additionally, there is evidence to support – or refute – the use of certain ancillary procedures. The routine use of amniotomy has not been shown to be beneficial in accelerating labor. There may be some benefit to perineal massage and warm compresses during the second stage of labor to decrease perineal injury. The routine use of episiotomy should be avoided and active management of the third stage of delivery has been associated with decreased blood loss. The use of evidence-based medicine has informed us and allowed us to use the best available evidence to provide the best care to our obstetrical patients.

References

1 Zhang J, Troendle J, Reddy UM, Laughon SK, Branch DW, Burkman R *et al.* Contemporary cesarean delivery practice in the United States. *American Journal of Obstetrics & Gynecology* 2010;**203**(4):326 e1– e10. Epub 2010/08/17.

2 American College of Obstetricians and Gynecologists, Gynecology Committee on Practice B-O Practice Bulletin No. 49, December 2003: Dystocia and augmentation of labor. *Obstetrics & Gynecology* 2003;**102**(6):1445–1454. Epub 2003/12/10.

3 Friedman EA. Primigravid labor: a graphicostatistical analysis. *Obstetrics & Gynecology* 1955;**6**(6):567–589. Epub 1955/12/01.

4 Friedman EA. Labor in multiparas: a graphicostatistical analysis. *Obstetrics & Gynecology* 1956;**8**(6):691–703. Epub 1956/12/01.

5 Kilpatrick SJ, Laros RK Jr. Characteristics of normal labor. *Obstetrics & Gynecology* 1989;**74**(1):85–87. Epub 1989/07/01.

6 Gifford DS, Morton SC, Fiske M, Keesey J, Keeler E, and Kahn KL. Lack of progress in labor as a reason for cesarean. *Obstetrics & Gynecology* 2000;**95**(4):589–595. Epub 2000/03/22.

7 O'Driscoll K, Foley M, and MacDonald D. Active management of labor as an alternative to cesarean section for dystocia. *Obstetrics & Gynecology* 1984;**63**(4):485–490. Epub 1984/04/01.

8 Rogers R, Gilson GJ, Miller AC, Izquierdo LE, Curet LB, and Qualls CR. Active management of labor: does it make a difference? *American Journal of Obstetrics & Gynecology* 1997;**177**(3):599–605. Epub 1997/10/10.

9 Frigoletto FD Jr., Lieberman E, Lang JM, Cohen A, Barss V, Ringer S *et al.* A clinical trial of active management of labor. *New England Journal of Medicine* 1995;**333**(12):745–750. Epub 1995/09/21.

10 Sadler LC, Davison T, and McCowan LM. A randomised controlled trial and meta-analysis of active management of labour. *BJOG: An International Journal of Obstetrics and Gynaecology* 2000;**107**(7):909–915. Epub 2000/07/20.

11 Liao JB, Buhimschi CS, and Norwitz ER. Normal labor: mechanism and duration. *Obstetrics and Gynecology Clinics of North America* 2005;**32**(2):145–164, vii. Epub 2005/05/19.

12 Friedman E. The graphic analysis of labor. *American Journal of Obstetrics & Gynecology* 1954;**68**(6):1568–1575. Epub 1954/12/01.

13 Laughon SK, Branch DW, Beaver J, and Zhang J. Changes in labor patterns over 50 years. *American Journal of Obstetrics & Gynecology* 2012;**206**(5):419 e1–9. Epub 2012/05/01.

14 Zhang J, Landy HJ, Branch DW, Burkman R, Haberman S, Gregory KD *et al.* Contemporary patterns of spontaneous labor with normal neonatal outcomes. *Obstetrics & Gynecology* 2010;**116**(6):1281–1287. Epub 2010/11/26.

15 Zhang J, Troendle JF, and Yancey MK. Reassessing the labor curve in nulliparous women. *American Journal of Obstetrics & Gynecology* 2002;**187**(4):824–828. Epub 2002/10/22.

16 Harper LM, Caughey AB, Odibo AO, Roehl KA, Zhao Q, and Cahill AG. Normal progress of induced labor. *Obstetrics & Gynecology* 2012;**119**(6):1113–1118. Epub 2012/05/10.

17 Graseck AS, Odibo AO, Tuuli M, Roehl KA, Macones GA, and Cahill AG. Normal first stage of labor in women undergoing trial of labor after cesarean delivery. *Obstetrics & Gynecology* 2012;**119**(4):732–726. Epub 2012/03/22.

18 Fyfe EM, Anderson NH, North RA, Chan EH, Taylor RS, Dekker GA *et al.* Risk of first-stage and second-stage cesarean delivery by maternal body mass index among nulliparous women in labor at term. *Obstetrics & Gynecology* 2011;**117**(6):1315–1322. Epub 2011/05/25.

19 Kominiarek MA, Vanveldhuisen P, Hibbard J, Landy H, Haberman S, Learman L *et al.* The maternal body mass index: a strong association with delivery route. *American Journal of Obstetrics & Gynecology* 2010;**203**(3):264 e1–7. Epub 2010/08/03.

20 Usha Kiran TS, Hemmadi S, Bethel J, and Evans J. Outcome of pregnancy in a woman with an increased body mass index. *BJOG : An International Journal of Obstetrics and Gynaecology.* 2005;**112**(6):768–772. Epub 2005/06/01.

21 Ovesen P, Rasmussen S, and Kesmodel U. Effect of prepregnancy maternal overweight and obesity on pregnancy outcome. *Obstetrics & Gynecology* 2011;**118**(2 Pt 1):305–312. Epub 2011/07/22.

22 Alanis MC, Villers MS, Law TL, Steadman EM, and Robinson CJ. Complications of cesarean delivery in the massively obese parturient. *American Journal of Obstetrics & Gynecology* 2010;**203**(3):271 e1–7. Epub 2010/08/04.

23 Robinson HE, O'Connell CM, Joseph KS, and McLeod NL. Maternal outcomes in pregnancies complicated by obesity. *Obstetrics & Gynecology* 2005;**106**(6):1357–1364. Epub 2005/12/02.

24 Barber EL, Lundsberg LS, Belanger K, Pettker CM, Funai EF, and Illuzzi JL. Indications contributing to the increasing cesarean delivery rate. *Obstetrics & Gynecology* 2011;**118**(1):29–38. Epub 2011/06/08.

25 Norman SM, Tuuli MG, Odibo AO, Caughey AB, Roehl KA, and Cahill AG. The Effects of obesity on the first stage of labor. *Obstetrics & Gynecology* 2012;**120**(1):6.

26 Smyth RM, Alldred SK, and Markham C. Amniotomy for shortening spontaneous labour. *Cochrane Database of Systematic Reviews* 2007(4):CD006167. Epub 2007/10/19.

27 Wei S, Wo BL, Xu H, Luo ZC, Roy C, and Fraser WD. Early amniotomy and early oxytocin for prevention of, or therapy for, delay in first stage spontaneous labour compared with routine care. *Cochrane Database of Systematic Reviews* 2009(2):CD006794. Epub 2009/04/17.

28 Rouse DJ, Weiner SJ, Bloom SL, Varner MW, Spong CY, Ramin SM *et al.* Second-stage labor duration in nulliparous women: relationship to maternal and perinatal outcomes. *American Journal of Obstetrics & Gynecology* 2009;**201**(4):357 e1–7. Epub 2009/10/01.

29 Le Ray C, Audibert F, Goffinet F, and Fraser W. When to stop pushing: effects of duration of second-stage expulsion efforts on maternal and neonatal outcomes in nulliparous women with epidural analgesia. *American Journal of Obstetrics & Gynecology* 2009;**201**(4):361 e1–7. Epub 2009/10/01.
30 Fraser WD, Marcoux S, Krauss I, Douglas J, Goulet C, and Boulvain M. Multicenter, randomized, controlled trial of delayed pushing for nulliparous women in the second stage of labor with continuous epidural analgesia. The PEOPLE (pushing early or pushing late with epidural) study group. *American Journal of Obstetrics & Gynecology* 2000;**182**(5):1165–1172. Epub 2000/05/20.
31 Frey HA, Tuuli MG, Cortez S, Odibo AO, Roehl KA, Shanks AL *et al.* Does delayed pushing in the second stage of labor impact perinatal outcomes? *American Journal of Perinatology* 2012. Epub 2012/07/10.
32 Brancato RM, Church S, and Stone PW. A meta-analysis of passive descent versus immediate pushing in nulliparous women with epidural analgesia in the second stage of labor. *Journal of Obstetric, Gynecologic, and Neonatal Nursing* 2008;**37**(1):4–12. Epub 2008/01/30.
33 Tuuli MG, Frey HA, Odibo AO, Macones GA, and Cahill AG. Immediate compared with delayed pushing in the second stage of labor: a systematic review and meta-analysis. *Obstetrics & Gynecology* 2012. Epub 2012/08/09.
34 Beckmann MM and Garrett AJ. Antenatal perineal massage for reducing perineal trauma. *Cochrane Database of Systematic Reviews* 2006(1):CD005123. Epub 2006/01/27.
35 Aasheim V, Nilsen AB, Lukasse M, and Reinar LM. Perineal techniques during the second stage of labour for reducing perineal trauma. *Cochrane Database of Systematic Reviews* 2011(12):CD006672. Epub 2011/12/14.
36 Bo K, Fleten C, and Nystad W. Effect of antenatal pelvic floor muscle training on labor and birth. *Obstetrics & Gynecology* 2009;**113**(6):1279–1284. Epub 2009/05/23.
37 Carroli G and Belizan J. Episiotomy for vaginal birth. *Cochrane Database of Systematic Reviews* 2000(2):CD000081. Epub 2000/05/05.
38 Landy HJ, Laughon SK, Bailit JL, Kominiarek MA, Gonzalez-Quintero VH, Ramirez M *et al.* Characteristics associated with severe perineal and cervical lacerations during vaginal delivery. *Obstetrics & Gynecology* 2011;**117**(3):627–635. Epub 2011/02/24.
39 Rabe H, Reynolds G, and Diaz-Rossello J. Early versus delayed umbilical cord clamping in preterm infants. *Cochrane Database of Systematic Reviews* 2004(4):CD003248. Epub 2004/10/21.
40 Rabe H, Reynolds G, and Diaz-Rossello J. A systematic review and meta-analysis of a brief delay in clamping the umbilical cord of preterm infants. *Neonatology* 2008;**93**(2):138–144. Epub 2007/09/25.
41 Hutton EK and Hassan ES. Late vs early clamping of the umbilical cord in full-term neonates: systematic review and meta-analysis of controlled trials. *Journal of the American Medical Association* 2007;**297**(11):1241–1252. Epub 2007/03/22.
42 Prendiville WJ, Elbourne D, and McDonald S. Active versus expectant management in the third stage of labour. *Cochrane Database of Systematic Reviews* 2000(**3**):CD000007. Epub 2000/07/25.
43 Gulmezoglu AM, Lumbiganon P, Landoulsi S, Widmer M, Abdel-Aleem H, Festin M *et al.* Active management of the third stage of labour with and without controlled cord traction: a randomised, controlled, non-inferiority trial. *Lancet* 2012;**379**(9827):1721–1727. Epub 2012/03/09.

CHAPTER 4

Induction and augmentation of labor

Karin A. Fox, Mildred M. Ramirez, and Susan M. Ramin*
Department of Obstetrics and Gynecology, Baylor College of Medicine, Houston, TX, USA

4.1 Introduction

Labor resembles a "Rube Goldberg" machine – a complex system that once set into motion, causes a chain reaction that ultimately results in the accomplishment of a basic task. One might imagine a contraption in which an old-fashioned alarm clock rings. As the bells vibrate, a marble falls off of a carefully balanced stand into a bucket that causes a lever to fall. Attached to the far end of the lever is a match that strikes sandpaper as the lever moves and ignites a fuse. Upon burning out, a window blind springs open, letting in sufficient sunlight to awaken the inventor. In the case of natural labor, we now know there is an intricate interplay between hormonal and biochemical crosstalk between the fetal, placental, and maternal compartments [4], alterations in gene expression regulating hormone receptors, inflammatory responses and gap junctions in the myometrium [5–7], and cervical remodeling, including alterations of cervical collagen, glycogen, and glycosaminoglycans [8–10]. The interconnected roles of the immune system, complement cascade, placental tissues, and fetal endocrine signaling on the initiation and propagation of labor, and ultimately the bioelectric signaling and mechanical forces of the uterus are all thought to play a part to expel a fetus from the womb into the world. Although the complex mechanisms behind natural labor are becoming better elucidated, the precise cascade of events that occurs in the labor process remains elusive.

From a teleological perspective, having multiple, redundant pathways to promote parturition is beneficial. Should conditions such as infection, stress, famine, or maternal illness threaten either the mother or her fetus, delivery may

*The authors report no proprietary or commercial interest in any product mentioned or concept discussed in this chapter.

Management of Labor and Delivery, Second Edition. Edited by George A. Macones.

mean survival for either one or both. Induction of labor is a medical intervention in pregnancy designed to effect parturition by inciting cervical change and uterine contractions prior to the onset of spontaneous labor.

Historically, efforts to "jump-start" uterine contractility using nipple stimulation and mechanical cervical dilatation date back to Hippocrates, with numerous later reports of cervical dilatation and the use of herbal or folk remedies [11]. In 1906, Sir Henry Dale reported that bovine pituitary extract could induce uterine contractions in a pregnant cat [12]. In 1948, Theobald and colleagues reported intravenous human administration of this pituitary extract, to induce labor [13]. Five years later, du Vignaud and colleagues successfully synthesized the endocrine polypeptide oxytocin [14,15], which has since been a mainstay of labor augmentation and induction. This led to increasing acceptance of intervention in the form of labor induction as a means to prevent fetal death or morbidity. There is clear evidence that for each week a pregnancy continues past 40 weeks of gestation, the relative risk for intrauterine and perinatal death increases [16,17]. In developing regions, such as Africa, the rates of maternal mortality, stillbirth, and perinatal mortality are among the highest in the world, yet the induction rate is as low as approximately 3–6%, and experts call for improved access to safe and effective induction of labor to reduce the burden of maternal and perinatal death in these regions [18].

With widespread acceptance of labor induction came an increase in the total number of women undergoing the procedure, and a broadening in the reasons used to justify the intervention. Between 1989 and 2011 the rate of induction had more than doubled, from a rate of approximately 9.0% to a rate of 23.2% of all deliveries in the United States [1,19,20]. Not only were labor inductions for medical indications on the rise, but inductions for more psychosocial reasons such as distance from the hospital and practitioner or maternal convenience have been cited as justifications for induction of labor [21]. The rate of late preterm inductions rose concomitantly, by more than one-third from the 1980s through 2006 [20]. In the early 2000s, experts began to recognize the public health burden due to the increase in late preterm births [22], and the role of labor inductions without clear medical indications have since been implicated in this rise [23,24].

4.2 Indications and contraindications for induction or augmentation of labor

Despite the increase in late preterm deliveries there has been a decline in the number of stillbirths and in perinatal mortality [25]. The need to balance the benefits of induction of labor when medically necessary with potential risks of continuing pregnancy are the focus of recent educational efforts and clinical recommendations, such as those published by the March of Dimes, the

Society for Maternal-Fetal Medicine, and the American College of Obstetricians and Gynecologists (ACOG) [2,3,26,27]. Included in these initiatives are recommendations to classify scheduled inductions as "medically indicated," and to note the precise indications in the medical record, versus "non-medically indicated," or inductions scheduled without clear medical indications [28]. Clear recommendations against non-medically indicated inductions prior to 39 weeks of gestation were proposed, and implementation of local policies that discourage such inductions has been shown to reduce the number of early term and late preterm deliveries and improve neonatal outcomes [29–32]. The term "elective" induction of labor persists in older studies describing any labor induction in the absence of medical indications. However, we will primarily refer to these as non-medically indicated inductions in this text. It is important to note that the term "elective" suggests some permissibility of choice between treatment options, without implication about increased benefit or risk of one option over the other, and due to its inherent ambiguity, its use is no longer in favor [28].

The most common indication for induction of labor remains "postterm," however the average gestational age of delivery has decreased to 39 weeks of gestation in the United States coincident with a shift from the use of the strict definition of postterm as a gestational age > 42 weeks to induction after 40 to 41 weeks of gestation due to the perceived increased relative risk of intrauterine death at these gestational ages and associated additional co-morbidities such as oligohydramnios or isolated decreased fetal movements. Medical indications for induction of labor are generally those conditions that increase the risk of fetal death. Such conditions include, but are not limited to, uncontrolled hypertension or preeclampsia, uncontrolled diabetes, oligohydramnios at term, or fetal growth restriction, especially when uteroplacental insufficiency is suggested by abnormal Doppler flow in the umbilical artery.

Generally, the contraindications to induction and augmentation of labor are similar to the contraindications to spontaneous vaginal delivery. These include, but are not limited to: vasa previa or complete placenta previa; transverse fetal lie; previous classical cesarean delivery or other uterine surgery, such as myomectomy that traverses the uterine wall; umbilical cord prolapse; or active genital herpes lesions [33]. Other conditions may preclude vaginal delivery, such as history of pelvic fracture resulting in deformity or neurovascular disorders, large arteriovenous malformations or aneurysms, or maternal cardiac conditions that preclude safe Valsalva maneuver. Pregnant women with the aforementioned conditions must be considered on an individual basis, as some gravida may safely undergo induction of labor with second-stage assisted vaginal delivery. It is our opinion that such cases are preferably planned in consultation with a Maternal-Fetal Medicine specialist and appropriate multidisciplinary consultants, such as anesthesiologists, neurologists, or cardiologists.

4.3 Risks associated with labor induction

Induction of labor has been associated with increased risk of uterine tachysystole, operative delivery, lower Apgar scores, postpartum hemorrhage, prolonged hospital stay [34,35], and decreased maternal satisfaction [36] when compared to delivery after spontaneous onset of labor. Decreased satisfaction is linked to longer duration from admission to delivery, and maternal expectations of delivering within 12 hours after the start of induction, which may be linked to inadequate counseling about expectations [36]. Several studies indicate an almost twofold increased risk of cesarean delivery with non-medically indicated inductions of labor [37]; however, more recent data is conflicting, suggesting that other factors, such as maternal age, nulliparity, and cervical length at the time of induction, may contribute more to the risk of delivery by cesarean than induction alone. A major criticism of studies looking at non-medically indicated inductions of labor is that often, the control group is women in spontaneous labor, rather than women who are expectantly managed, who may require induction for medical indications, or cesarean delivery due to pregnancy complications if expectantly managed, leading to a potential bias in results. This argument was made by the authors of a large meta-analysis who compared induction of labor to expectant management at or beyond 37 weeks of gestation [38]. Whereas data was insufficient to draw conclusions about induction of labor prior to 41 weeks of gestation, at or beyond 41 weeks of gestation, induction of labor reduced the risk of cesarean delivery and meconium staining [39]. In a 2012 Cochrane review on labor induction of women at or beyond term gestation, the number needed to treat with labor induction in order to reduce one perinatal death was 410 women. Induction was associated with a reduced risk of cesarean delivery, meconium aspiration syndrome, and macrosomia, even in the stratified gestational ages of 37–39 weeks and 39–40 weeks [39]. Although the role of individual providers and physician group practices has been found to contribute to the risk of cesarean delivery with induction of labor, it is less clear how the individual physician practices contribute to this risk [37].

4.4 Predicting success of labor

Classically, a high pelvic score, as initially developed in 1964 by E.H. Bishop, has been regarded as an indicator of cervical "readiness," based on "pelvic factors that presage spontaneous labor" [40], and is one of the most commonly used predictors of labor induction success [41,42]. Cervical dilatation, effacement, consistency, position, and fetal station are the five parameters assessed in determining the Bishop score. A score of 0 to 3 is assigned to each parameter. The Bishop pelvic scoring system is summarized in Table 4.1. In general, the higher the Bishop score, the greater the success of labor induction. For example, a

Table 4.1 Bishop scoring system.

Score	Dilation (cm)	Cervical Position	Effacement (%)	Station (−3 to +3)	Consistency
0	Closed	Posterior	0–30	−3	Firm
1	1–2	Midposition	40–50	−2	Medium
2	3–4	Anterior	60–70	−1,0	Soft
3	5–6	–	80	+1,+2	–

Source: *Bishop*, 1964 [40]. Adapted with permission of Lippencott Williams, & Wilkins.

woman with a Bishop score of 9 would be considered to have a high likelihood for successful induction of labor and similar to that of a woman who spontaneously labors. Preinduction cervical ripening may be used in women with an unfavorable cervix usually defined as a Bishop score of 6 or less [33]. In one meta-analysis including 40 primary studies and a total of 13,757 women, the sensitivity of a Bishop score of 6 to predict mode of delivery was found to be only 78%, and the specificity was 44%. At lower Bishop scores, sensitivity was considerably lower, and for any Bishop score lower than 9, the sensitivity was 95%, but the specificity was only 30% [43]. In another prospective study, comparing the transvaginal sonographic cervical length measurement with Bishop scoring in 249 women, not only did cervical length measurement have better sensitivity (80% vs 64%) and marginally better positive (30% vs 27%) and negative predictive values (89 vs 83%) of need for cesarean delivery than the Bishop score, but it was also found to be better tolerated and less painful when rated on a 10-point visual analog pain scale by patients [44].

Similarly, fetal fibronectin (FFN) has been evaluated as an alternate predictor of either failure or success and duration of induction of labor. In a 1996 study of 160 women, a lower rate of cesarean delivery and shorter time from start of induction to delivery was found in women in whom cervical FFN testing was positive compared to those who had negative FFN [45]. The actual management of induction in this study was not standardized, however, and in women with a negative FFN test, fewer women had assisted rupture of membranes, an accepted method of induction. Additionally, the authors grouped women who required cervical ripening with those who did not based on cervical exam and provider preference, and a number of women with a positive FFN test were given prostaglandin, an agent commonly used for cervical ripening.

Each agent used for cervical ripening or induction carries with it a unique risk profile. Results of some comparative effectiveness studies are limited in that only one or two agents are evaluated, and it is difficult to ascertain whether or not treatment is individualized to the risks of the individual patient. In contrast to most trials that compare two agents, in practice it is far more common to employ various combinations of agents sequentially, and no single study to date adequately addresses variations in practice. Despite these limitations, there is evidence that cervical ripening prior to the use of oxytocin or assisted rupture of membranes may decrease time to delivery and increase the chances of vaginal delivery.

4.5 Mechanical cervical ripening

Cervical remodeling is an essential component of normal parturition. The cervix undergoes changes in collagen structure and arrangement, water content, and makeup of glycosaminoglycans. Additionally, cytokine and prostaglandin production is increased, and there is an influx of leukocytes into the cervical stroma. All of these biochemical processes aid in the change in physical properties in the cervix. The cervix changes from a firm, elongated column of tissue into a soft, thin, pliable one, much like a child's piece of bubblegum changes with the addition of sufficient salivary enzymes and mastication from a hard, pink wrapped chunk of gum into a chewy, stretchy blob capable of being molded into a bubble the size of the child's face.

One of the simplest and oldest methods of cervical ripening is the use of a mechanical device [46,47] to initiate cervical dilatation. Mechanical dilators include devices ranging from hydroscopic osmotic dilators, such as laminaria (*Laminaria japonicum*) or synthetic dilators such as Lamicel or Dilapan S® (Medicem, Amsterdam, Netherlands) (Figure 4.1), to balloon catheters (14–26 F, with balloon volumes ranging from 30 to 80 mL), double balloon devices (Cook® Balloon, Cook Medical, Bloomington, IN), and extra-amniotic saline infusion sets (Figure 4.2). Each type of mechanical dilator works by exerting gradual

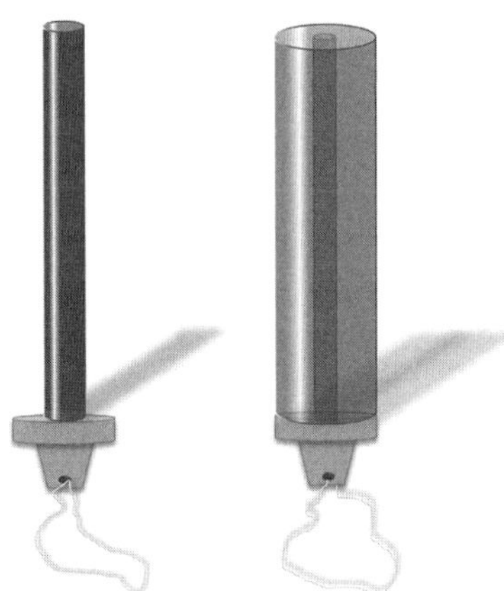

Figure 4.1 Illustration of Dilapan®. (a) Dilapan prior to insertion; (b) Dilapan after fluid absorption and expansion.

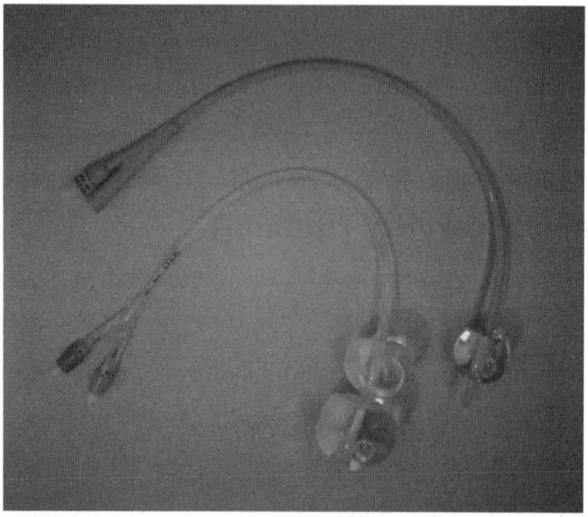

Figure 4.2 Image of balloon catheters. Top: Foley catheter inflated with 30 mL sterile saline. Bottom: Cook® Balloon catheter with 60 mL inflated in the cervical balloon and 40 mL inflated in the vaginal balloon.

pressure along the cervical canal, thereby gradually providing dilatation, while the mechanical distention is thought to cause some endogenous prostaglandin release. Still other types of mechanical dilators confer some biochemical activity. It is important to consider that mechanical dilators primarily ripen the cervix, or increase the Bishop score. When used alone, mechanical dilators are largely ineffective compared to chemical agents in causing the regular, sustained uterine contractions required to effect labor, as defined by further cervical change [46].

4.5.1 Osmotic dilators

Single or multiple osmotic dilators may be placed within the cervical canal. The dilator absorbs water from the endocervix and surrounding tissue, swells, and then slowly dilates the cervix. Laminaria are derived from dried, compressed seaweed, and are effective for cervical ripening. Complications that have been reported with the use of laminaria include infection and non-fatal anaphylaxis [47–49]. Additionally, laminaria require 24 hours to confer maximum effect. Conversely, synthetic hygroscopic dilators are thought to have improved sterility, uniformity, and predictability. Lamicel consists of a sponge impregnated with magnesium sulfate and does not exert force against the intracervical walls, but rather expands lengthwise and functions more through chemical mechanisms, whereas Dilapan S is a polyacrylonitrile, rod-shaped dilator available in 3 and 4-mm dry diameters, which exerts mechanical pressure within the endocervical canal. Both of the synthetic dilators are effective within 6 hours [50].

In one study, investigators compared the safety and efficacy of osmotic dilators in 36 women to prostaglandin E2 gel (PGE2) in 38 women for cervical ripening.

The overall change in the Bishop score, time to amniotomy, rate of cesarean delivery, maternal morbidity, and neonatal Apgar scores were similar between groups. A theoretical cost difference was found, as the group that received PGE2 gel required prolonged monitoring in the labor and delivery unit [11].

4.5.2 Balloon catheters

Balloon catheters are inserted into the cervical canal, and either one or two balloons are inflated to allow pressure to be applied to the cervix from within. Balloon catheters, particularly single-balloon bladder catheters, are readily available, inexpensive, and easy to place. One of the first descriptions of the use of a balloon catheter was by Embrey *et al.* in 1967, where they described using a 26-gauge Foley catheter with removal of the tip beyond the balloon that had been inflated with 50 mL of sterile water [51]. Catheter placement has been most often described as under direct visualization with use of a sterile speculum, after the cervix is swabbed with iodine. Grasping forceps may be used to place the catheter within the cervical os. Alternatively, a urethral stent, large sterile swab, or stylet may be used inside the catheter to guide the catheter into the cervical os. Finally, some practitioners place the catheter blindly, during digital exam, which has been reported to be less painful when compared to the use of a speculum in one randomized trial including 42 women [52].

There is a paucity of literature specifically studying infectious morbidity with catheter use or comparing the risk of infection based upon method of placement, which may be due to publication bias. As a foreign body, balloon catheters and other mechanical devices carry an increased risk of neonatal or intrauterine infection [53], especially if placed blindly upon digital exam. Other associated risks with their use include inadvertent rupture of membranes, maternal discomfort [47,54,55], transient fever, and bleeding [47]. Conversely, numerous studies cite potential benefits, including a lower risk of uterine tachysystole with balloon catheters compared to chemical ripening agents [56–59], decreased time to delivery compared to no intervention [60], and greater degree of cervical dilatation prior to initiation of oxytocin or other method of labor augmentation [60].

Balloon catheters come in various sizes, and can be inflated with differing volumes of sterile saline. Numerous randomized controlled trials have been conducted comparing catheter efficacy based on the volume of filled balloons. In one study, Levy and colleagues used either 30 or 80 mL of sterile saline for balloon inflation in 203 women [60]. The catheters were placed using aseptic technique under direct visualization using a sterile speculum, and the catheters were taped to the patient's thigh. Catheters were removed after 12 hours, or earlier if there were abnormal fetal heart tracings, and augmentation with oxytocin or amniotomy followed expulsion or removal of the balloon. The authors demonstrated that the use of larger balloon volumes resulted in less failure to achieve cervical dilatation at or beyond 3 cm by the time of balloon expulsion or removal, more frequent successful vaginal deliveries within 24 hours among both multiparous and nulliparous women, and a reduction in the mean induction-to-delivery time interval of approximately 3 hours for nulliparous women and 1 hour for multiparas. Additionally, fewer women randomized to 80 mL compared to 30 mL inflation volumes required oxytocin augmentation or epidural analgesia.

Delaney and colleagues randomized 192 women to receive a Foley catheter for cervical ripening with either 30 mL or 60 mL sterile saline [55]. In contrast to the study by Levy *et al.*, oxytocin was started within 30 minutes of balloon placement rather than at expulsion or removal. Additionally, there was no difference in the rate of delivery at 24 hours; however, the authors found a twofold higher rate of vaginal delivery by 12 hours in the group randomized to 60-mL inflation volume. On multivariate analysis, this difference was no longer found for multiparous women.

To provide additional mechanical force to the cervix, above and beyond simple inflation of the balloon, practitioners may secure the catheter tube to a weight, such as a 500- to 1000-mL bag of intravenous fluid, or tape the catheter tube to the patient's thigh. In a recent study, 191 women were randomized to either inner thigh taping or traction using a 500-mL saline bag [61]. Only a shorter time to balloon expulsion was found in the traction group. No differences were found between groups with regard to time to vaginal delivery, rate of delivery within 24 hours, patient pain score, use of epidural analgesia, or rate of cesarean delivery. This study suggests no added benefit to use of weighted traction [61]. It is our opinion that the use of a traction weight renders the patient rather immobile, as the weight is often bulky, making ambulation cumbersome, or is hung off the end of the bed. The ability for a woman undergoing cervical ripening to move about *ad libitum* is an additional hypothetical benefit of thigh taping.

4.5.3 Extra-amniotic saline infusion

Instillation of sterile saline into the extra-amniotic space via a balloon catheter has been assessed as an adjunctive method for expediting cervical ripening and the onset of labor. While some studies report a shorter time to delivery with extra-amniotic saline infusion (EASI), results are modest at best, and others show no added benefit with the addition of saline infusion to a balloon catheter [62,63]. Finally, other investigators have reported a non-significant trend toward an increased risk of cesarean delivery in women randomized to EASI [63,64].

4.5.4 Membrane sweeping

Perhaps one of the simplest and most commonly practiced methods of mechanical dilatation is membrane sweeping or stripping, whereby an examiner inserts a finger into the cervical os and gently separates the cervix from the amniotic sac. While this is technically a form of mechanical manipulation of the cervix, it is thought that membrane sweeping prompts release of endogenous prostaglandins.

In one analysis by Tan *et al.*, of 160 women undergoing membrane sweeping at 40 weeks of gestation prior to planned induction at 41 weeks of gestation, women underwent serial transvaginal cervical length measurements. The cervical length was measured immediately before and after membrane sweeping, and again before labor induction. The mean cervical length actually appeared to lengthen immediately after the procedure in a majority of the women. Cervical shortening after membrane sweeping was found in 33% of study participants, and was associated with a reduction in all-cause cesarean delivery in this study [65]. The authors did not find a reduction in the need for induction of labor. The authors postulated that cervical shortening may reflect cervical pliability, which is the actual predictor of vaginal birth, and that cervical lengthening may reflect a sonographic appearance of lengthening that occurs with brief alleviation of pressure of the fetal head on the cervix. In a similar study by Wong *et al.* [66], the mean recruitment-to-delivery interval was shorter for women who underwent membrane sweeping, but there was no difference between the groups with regard to need for induction of labor by 42 weeks of gestation or cesarean delivery. Although membrane sweeping has been associated with an increase in the release of oxytocin, and local endogenous prostaglandin release, it may not be effective in all women [67]. It remains a low-cost, simple option that can be performed in the office at term gestation, with modest, temporary discomfort to the patient and relatively low risk. The estimated number of women needed to treat with membrane sweeping to reduce the use of other methods of labor induction is eight [67].

4.6 Biochemical agents for cervical ripening

4.6.1 Prostaglandins

Prostaglandins are endogenous biochemical substances that result in changes in the collagen bundles and increase in water content of the cervix, which is associated with an increase in the softening of the cervix that leads to increased success of vaginal birth. In addition, prostaglandins trigger a cascade that results in uterine contractions and progresses to labor [68–70]. Placebo-controlled randomized trials have supported the safety and efficacy of the use of prostaglandins in women with an unscarred uterus at any gestational age. The use of prostaglandins for preinduction cervical ripening reduces the requirements for oxytocin usage for either induction or augmentation of labor [71]. Side effects of prostaglandin use include fever, chills, nausea, vomiting, diarrhea, and uterine tachysystole. The uterine tachysystole that occurs is not always, but may be, associated with fetal heart rate changes, including decelerations that may prompt maternal oxygen administration, intravenous fluid bolus, and maternal positional changes and medication discontinuation or changes. The ability to immediately ameliorate the side effect(s) of the prostaglandin varies depending upon the specific agent and the route of administration used.

Generally, whenever prostaglandins are administered intravaginally, the woman should remain recumbent for 2 to 3 hours after placement. A small amount of lubricant gel may be used to ease insertion without compromising absorption. The timing of repeat dosing or of oxytocin initiation after use of prostaglandins depends upon the type of agent used, cervical change, rate of uterine contractions, and the status of the fetal heart tracing.

Prostaglandins generally are contraindicated in women with severe asthma, glaucoma, and increased intraocular pressure.

4.6.2 Prostaglandin E1 analogues

The prostaglandin E1 (PGE1) analogue misoprostol (brand name Cytotec®, Pfizer, New York) is an FDA-approved medication for the prevention of gastric ulcers and comes in 100 or 200 mcg tablets. Although there are no large randomized clinical trials upon which to base recommendations on its use alone or in conjunction with other cervical ripening and labor inducing agents, it has been used off-label since the 1987 for these purposes [70,72,73]. The ACOG reaffirmed the recommendation for the use of PGE1 in 2009 due to its safety and efficacy in appropriately selected patients [33]. Women with a prior cesarean delivery or other hysterotomy such as transmural myomectomy are at increased risk for uterine rupture with PGE1 use [74]. However, the use of PGE1 has been shown to be safe and effective for cervical ripening and labor induction in the midtrimester even in women with a prior hysterotomy in cases of fetal death or termination of pregnancy [75,76]. PGE1 may be administered orally in doses of 50 to 100 mcg or intravaginally in doses of 25 to 50 mcg every 4–6 hours at term. Initiation of oxytocin may be as early as 4 hours after the last dose of PGE1, provided the fetal heart tracing remains Category I. The active drug is evenly distributed within the 100-mcg tablets; therefore, a 100-mcg tablet must be scored and cut prior to use. For midtrimester inductions, higher doses are typically used (ranging from 200 to 600 mcg intravaginally per dose). Route of administration for PGE1 does not change efficacy, and data regarding side effects such as the incidence of fever, abdominal pain, and uterine tachysystole are mixed [77,78]. There is a PGE1 dose-dependent risk of uterine tachysystole, meconium passage [79,80], meconium aspiration, and uterine rupture [73]. PGE1 is more frequently associated with uterine tachysystole compared to balloon catheter, oxytocin, and PGE2 [56].

The ACOG therefore recommends the 25-mcg intravaginal dose [33]. Although the toxic dose of misoprostol is unknown, serious adverse effects have been reported at cumulative daily doses above 1600 mcg.

Misoprostol is also available in 200-mcg time-released insert; although approved in other countries, it is currently not available in the United States. When compared to dinoprostone insert, misoprostol vaginal insert is associated with a significantly shorter time to vaginal delivery (21.5 hours compared to 32.8 hours). This shorter duration of labor was associated with a significant increase in uterine tachysystole (13.3% vs 4%) and no overall reduction in cesarean delivery rates [81].

4.6.3 Prostaglandin E2 analogues

Prostaglandin E2 (also known as dinoprostone) is available as a gel formulation (Prepidil 0.5 mg dinoprostone in 2.5 mL gel) that is placed via a syringe intracervically, and as a time-released insert (Cervidil®, Forest Laboratories, Inc., New York), permeated with 10 mg of dinoprostone, that is placed in the posterior vaginal fornix. Both PGE2 preparations are FDA approved for cervical ripening in women at or near term. Vaginal PGE2 analogues used for cervical ripening are associated with a greater likelihood of delivery within 24 hours, an increased risk of uterine tachysystole, and no reduction in cesarean delivery when compared to oxytocin or placebo alone [82].

Prepidil® (Pfizer, New York) may be redosed every 6–12 hours, not to exceed three doses, and initiation of oxytocin should be delayed by 6–12 hours after last dosing [83].

The medication in Cervidil is released at a rate of 0.3 mg/h and the insert is sheathed in a thin polyester fabric with a tail, similar to a kite, which allows easy removal of the active insert. The manufacturer of Cervidil recommends removal of the insert when there is onset of active labor or 12 hours after insertion. Additionally, removal may be considered prior to amniotomy, or in the event of a Category II or III fetal heart rate tracing. Oxytocin may be initiated as early as 30 minutes after removal of the insert [33].

4.7 Oxytocin

Oxytocin has been used for decades and is effective alone or in conjunction with other agents, for cervical ripening, labor induction, and augmentation of labor. The cervical and uterine response increases with increasing gestational age, likely due to changes in myometrial oxytocin receptor distribution and activity, and the increase in established gap junctions. Most frequently it is administered intravenously, to allow titration. The plasma half-life is 3–6 minutes and the steady state is reached in 30–40 minutes. The ACOG recommend that all labor and delivery units develop guidelines for the preparation and administration of oxytocin for cervical ripening and induction or augmentation of labor from a quality and patient-safety perspective [33]. Usually 10 units of oxytocin are diluted in 1000 mL of normal saline for a concentration of 10 milliunits per milliliter, using an infusion pump. Variable low- and high-dose oxytocin regimens have been used and studied (Table 4.2). The goal of titration is to use the lowest dose of oxytocin that effects adequate frequency of contractions (every 2–3 minutes) and strength of uterine contractions (200–250 Montevideo units) to allow labor progression. Continuous monitoring of the uterine contractions

Table 4.2 Examples of oxytocin regimens.

		Initial dose (milliunits/min)	Increase by (milliunits/min)	Interval (min) to increase	Endpoints (reduce or discontinue when)
Term gestation	Low dose	0.5–2	0.5–2	15–40	• Vaginal delivery • Tachysystole (> 5 contractions/10 min) • Category II fetal heart rate tracing • Decision for cesarean delivery
	High dose	4–6	3–6	20–40	
Special conditions	Prior cesarean	1–2	0.5–2	15–40	
	Grandmultiparity	1–2	0.5–2	15–40	
	Twin gestation	1–2	0.5–2	15–40	

and fetal heart rate during oxytocin infusion is recommended. Higher dose regimens have been associated with an increased risk of uterine tachysystole, Category II and III fetal heart rate tracings, and cesarean delivery [84]. Pulsatile dosing of oxytocin every 6–10 minutes has also been studied, and shown to be effective, with a lower total dose of oxytocin used, and a lower incidence of uterine tachysystole. However, this method of oxytocin administration requires special equipment and is contemporary, but not common practice [85]. The additional side effects of oxytocin include neonatal hyperbilirubinemia and maternal hypotension and hyponatremia; these are usually associated with higher doses and rapid rates of infusion. Oxytocin is a pituitary hormone similar in structure to, and with some cross-activity with, antidiuretic hormone. For these reasons, an infusion pump with a buretrol is generally used for administration, and high-dose oxytocin should not be mixed in hypotonic solutions such as 5% dextrose with water. Induction of labor in the second trimester typically requires higher dose oxytocin regimens; a more concentrated mixture of oxytocin is used and rest periods are often given between oxytocin administrations to allow for adequate diuresis (Table 4.3).

Oxytocin may be used simultaneously with or after use of balloon catheters, in conjunction with amniotomy, and subsequent to use of prostaglandins (Table 4.4). Oxytocin with amniotomy was shown to shorten the time from amniotomy to delivery than standard care in one study [86]. In another study, no significant differences were found when women were randomized to either immediate oxytocin administration after amniotomy or to amniotomy followed by a 4-hour delay prior to initiation of oxytocin [87], and amniotomy alone may be effective [88].

In one popularized retrospective review of 625,042 live births linked to school records between 1990–1998, the authors found an association between induction and augmentation of labor with the later diagnosis of autism spectrum disorders in childhood [89]. Some experts have expressed concern that the most commonly

Table 4.3 Example of midtrimester oxytocin regimen.

Step	Concentration	Route	Duration	Endpoints
1	50 units oxytocin in 500 mL D5NS **DISCONTINUE INFUSION AND REST for 1 hour**	IV	3 hours	Delivery Oxytocin toxicity (hyponatremia/marked hypotension)
2	60 units oxytocin in 500 mL D5NS **DISCONTINUE INFUSION AND REST for 1 hour**	IV	3 hours	
3	70 units oxytocin in 500 mL D5NS **DISCONTINUE INFUSION AND REST for 1 hour**	IV	3 hours	
4	Continue to increase oxytocin by 10 units in each additional step, mixed in 500 mL D5NS. **REST 1 hour between each bag of oxytocin.**	IV	3 hours/step	MAXIMUM CONCENTRATION: 300 units/500 mL D5NS (1667 milliunits/min)

Table 4.4 Examples of prostaglandin regimens for cervical ripening at term.

Prostaglandin	Medication name	Formulation	Route of administration	Dose	Dosing interval	Interval prior to oxytocin
PGE1	Misoprostol (Cytotec)	100-mcg scored tablet	Vaginal	25–50 mcg (1/4 to 1/2 of tablet)	4–6 hours	4–6 hours
		100-mcg scored tablet	Oral	50–100 mcg (1/2 to 1 tablet)	4–6 hours	4–6 hours
PGE2	Cervidil	Dinoprostone-impregnated insert	Vaginal (posterior fornix)	10 mg	12 hours	30 min after removal
	Prepidil	Dinoprostone gel	Intracervical	0.5 mg/ 2.5 mL gel	6–12 hours MAX: 3 doses	6–12 hours

used agent for induction and augmentation, oxytocin, will be unduly assumed by patients and the media to be causative of autism spectrum disorders [90]. The original study authors have replied that they emphasize in their discussion that the direct cause of autism spectrum disorders remains to be elucidated, and may include obstetrical or medical conditions necessitating induction or augmentation of labor and conditions in labor associated with induction or augmentation, not just the medications used for induction or augmentation [89]. Importantly, the Society for Maternal-Fetal Medicine produced a statement paper to clarify that due to the inherent study design flaws of a retrospective study that links large databases, the findings from this study are not definitive, nor should standard practice be changed with regard to induction or augmentation of labor [91].

4.7.1 Amniotomy

Amniotomy is commonly performed to induce labor or to accelerate labor. It involves mechanically rupturing the amniotic sac by means of an amniotomy hook, spinal needle, scalp electrode, or digital pressure on the bag. Prior to amniotomy, the cervix should be dilated and effaced and the fetal head well applied to the cervix to prevent cord prolapse [88]. If the fetal head is not well applied to the cervix, a 26-gauge needle can be used to puncture the membranes under direct visualization to allow a slow release of amniotic fluid. The fetal heart rate should be evaluated prior to and immediately after the amniotomy procedure.

In a randomized study of 209 women undergoing oxytocin induction of labor to either early amniotomy at 1- to 2-cm cervical dilatation or to late amniotomy at 5 cm, labor was 4 hours shorter in the early amniotomy group [92].

4.8 Active management of labor

In 1969, Kieran O'Driscoll and colleagues at the National Maternity Hospital in Dublin, Ireland, published their prospective study of 1000 women using a standardized protocol of labor management, using oxytocin administration [93,94]. Even in their landmark paper, they stated that, "active management in labour can be conducted only on the basis of individual attention which requires a delivery unit, in effect a special care unit, in which no patient is left unattended and skilled nursing attention and medical supervision are always at hand" [93]. Their goal was delivery within 24 hours, and this was eventually modified to 12 hours [95,96]. At the time, the cesarean delivery rate was near 5%, and the goals were to decrease protracted labor and forceps-assisted vaginal deliveries. Their protocol defined labor as painful contractions with complete effacement, bloody show, and/or ruptured membranes. After the diagnosis of labor was made, women were assessed every hour for the first 3 hours, followed by every 2 hours. If the patient had spontaneous rupture of membranes, oxytocin was initiated 1 hour after admission, if inadequate cervical change was noted. If less than 1 cm of cervical dilatation per hour ensued in those women not ruptured, amniotomy was performed, followed the next hour by oxytocin administration, at a standard concentration of 10 units in one liter of crystalloid, with the rate of infusion determined by the midwife or labor nurse, to attain no more than seven contractions in 15 minutes, and with avoidance of fetal intolerance of labor. The ACOG and the most recent Cochrane review affirm that the use of active management protocols may shorten the duration of labor, but perhaps only modestly the rate of cesarean delivery [97–99].

4.9 Failed induction

Induction of labor usually leads to successful vaginal delivery. Obviously, spontaneous labor has the most success, as, by definition, the condition of the cervix is more likely to have a higher plasticity or Bishop score (Table 4.1). A high Bishop score in a woman undergoing induction of labor indicates a favorable likelihood of successful induction. Conversely, a woman with a low Bishop score requiring induction of labor has the highest risk for failed induction. Although there is no standard definition of failed induction, a workshop comprised of the *Eunice Kennedy Shriver* National Institutes of Child Health and Human Development, the Society for Maternal-Fetal Medicine, and the ACOG proposed that failed induction be considered the inability to generate regular uterine contractions every 3 minutes and cervical change after a minimum of 24 hours of oxytocin administration or 12 hours after membrane rupture [100]. The duration of time for cervical ripening is not included in diagnosing failed induction [100].

Rouse and colleagues in 1999 had proposed that women be allowed at least 4 hours of oxytocin augmentation with adequate contractions, defined as 200 or more Montevideo units, which by definition requires amniotomy and placement of an intrauterine pressure catheter, or 6 hours without adequate contractions prior to consideration of cesarean delivery for arrest of dilatation [101]. In 2001, Rouse and colleagues realized that use of this definition may predispose some women to cesarean delivery, if no cervical change was noted within 2 hours. The authors found, however, that 61% of women who experienced 2 hours of arrest of dilatation would go on to have a successful vaginal delivery if allowed to continue oxytocin augmentation [102].

In contemporary practice, the normal duration of spontaneous labor and time necessary to reach the active phase of cervical dilatation are much longer when compared to the definitions proposed 50 years earlier by Friedman [103,104]. The Consortium on Safe Labor retrospectively reviewed records from 62,415 women with singleton vertex pregnancies at term in spontaneous labor who had a vaginal delivery and a normal perinatal outcome from 19 hospitals across the United States [102]. Based on their analysis, the authors proposed that 6 cm of cervical dilatation is a more appropriate landmark for active phase of labor than the traditionally used definition of 4 cm [105]. In contrast, Hoffman and colleagues found that induction of labor in low-risk multiparous women with and without preinduction cervical ripening had a shorter active phase of labor than women in spontaneous labor [106].

4.10 Safety and quality protocols

All labor and delivery units should have standardized protocols to ensure safe and effective labor induction and augmentation of labor, regardless of whether the induction is performed for medical indications or not. This has been encouraged since the earliest discussions of active management of labor [93] and is even more pertinent in contemporary obstetrics. Such protocols prioritize the indications for induction, gestational age, and need for preinduction cervical ripening. Additionally, systems should be in place to ensure appropriate scheduling, and use of agents during inductions or augmentations of labor. This can be facilitated by the use of patient safety checklists for scheduling induction of labor (Figure 4.3). To ensure patient safety, protocols for medication use, patient and fetal monitoring, and intrauterine resuscitations should be developed and utilized. The ACOG has an example of such checklists [107]. Each hospital may need to individualize protocols based on available local resources and expertise.

There are now institutions implementing hospitalist programs to provide 24-hour dedicated physician coverage of laboring patients to improve patient

A. Call ***-***-**** to schedule inductions with the clinical nurse coordinator

B. Physicians will be notified of the number of inductions already scheduled or if the number exceeds 5 at a later date.

C. Elective inductions will not be scheduled until the woman has reached 38 weeks (for induction at 39 weeks or later).

D. Medical inductions require supporting documentation (e.g. ultrasound report showing oligohydramnios, blood pressure log for hypertension). This is to support accurate triage of inductions as needed.

E. Inductions will be triaged by the OB Hospitalist according to medical necessity on an as needed basis.

Date:__________ **Healthcare provider:** __________

Patient name: __________ **MR number:** __________

Gravida:_____ **Para:**_____ **LMP:**_____ **EDD:**_____

Previous Cesarean delivery: Yes _____ No _____

Proposed date of induction:__________

Indication for induction:

Medical condition: __________

Nonmedical reason: __________

For non-medical induction check if gestational age of 39 0/7 weeks confirmed by Sonogram <20 weeks' gestation:__________

+ FHT documented for 30 weeks' gestation by Doppler sonography:__________

Bishop score:_____ **Group B Strep:**_____ **Hematocrit:** _____

Figure 4.3 Example of guidelines for scheduling induction of labor.

safety and outcomes. A study by Iriye and colleagues compared models of care and found that a dedicated, full-time laborist program was associated with a reduced cesarean delivery rate [108].

4.11 Conclusion

Labor induction and augmentation will likely continue to be one of the most common interventions in obstetrics. Numerous methods of cervical ripening and medication regimens for labor induction have been proven safe and effective when used in accordance with local hospital protocols. Use of checklists and standardization of care has been shown to improve patient safety. In contemporary practice, women must be given adequate time for cervical ripening and labor induction before considering an induction as "failed," particularly as we are becoming aware of the long-term reproductive benefits of preventing the first cesarean delivery and avoiding non-medically indicated inductions prior to 39 weeks of gestation.

References

1 Hamilton BE, Martin JA, and Ventura SJ. Births: preliminary data for 2012. *National Vital Statistics Reports* 2013;**62**(3):1–20.

2 American College of Obstetricians and Gynecologists Committee Opinion No. 560: Medically indicated late-preterm and early-term deliveries. *Obstetrics & Gynecology* 2013;**121**(4): 908–910.

3 American College of Obstetricians and Gynecologists Committee Opinion No. 561: Nonmedically indicated early-term deliveries. *Obstetrics & Gynecology* 2013;**121**(4):911–915.

4 Egarter CH and Husslein P. Biochemistry of myometrial contractility. *Baillière's Clinical Obstetrics and Gynaecology* 1992;**6**(4):755–769.

5 Karteris E, Markovic D, Chen J, Hillhouse EW, and Grammatopoulos DK. Identification of a novel corticotropin-releasing hormone type 1beta-like receptor variant lacking Exon 13 in human pregnant myometrium regulated by estradiol-17beta and progesterone. *Endocrinology* 2010;**151**(10):4959–4968.

6 Zakar T and Mesiano S. How does progesterone relax the uterus in pregnancy? *New England Journal of Medicine* 2011;**364**(10):972–973.

7 Garfield RE and Hayashi RH. Appearance of gap junctions in the myometrium of women during labor. *American Journal of Obstetrics & Gynecology* 1981;**140**(3):254–260.

8 Danforth DN, Veis A, Breen M, Weinstein HG, Buckingham JC, and Manalo P. The effect of pregnancy and labor on the human cervix: changes in collagen, glycoproteins, and glycosaminoglycans. *American Journal of Obstetrics & Gynecology* 1974;**120**(5):641–651.

9 von Maillot K, Stuhlsatz HW, Mohanaradhakrishnan V, and Greiling H. Changes in the glycosaminoglycans distribution pattern in the human uterine cervix during pregnancy and labor. *American Journal of Obstetrics & Gynecology* 1979;**135**(4):503–506.

10 Word RA, Li XH, Hnat M, and Carrick K. Dynamics of cervical remodeling during pregnancy and parturition: mechanisms and current concepts. *Seminars in Reproductive Medicine.* 2007;**25**(1):69–79.

11 Sanchez-Ramos L, Kaunitz AM, and Connor PM. Hygroscopic cervical dilators and prostaglandin E2 gel for preinduction cervical ripening. A randomized, prospective comparison. *Journal of Reproductive Medicine* 1992;**37**(4):355–359.

12 Dale HH. On some physiological actions of ergot. *Journal of Physiology* 1906;**34**(3):163–206.

13 Theobald GW, Graham A *et al.* The use of post-pituitary extract in physiological amounts in obstetrics: a preliminary report. *BMJ* 1948;**2**(4567):123–127.

14 Pierce JG, Gordon S, and Du Vigneaud V. Further distribution studies on the oxytocic hormone of the posterior lobe of the pituitary gland and the preparation of an active crystalline flavianate. *Journal of Biological Chemistry* 1952;**199**(2):929–940.

15 du Vigneaud V RC, Swam JM, Roberts CW, Katsoyannis PG, and Gordon S. The synthesis of an octapeptide amide with the hormonal activity of oxytocin. *Journal of the American Chemical Society* 1953(**75**):4879–4880.

16 Stock SJ, Ferguson E, Duffy A, Ford I, Chalmers J, and Norman JE. Outcomes of elective induction of labour compared with expectant management: population based study. *BMJ* 2012;**344**:e2838.

17 Heimstad R, Romundstad PR, Eik-Nes SH, and Salvesen KA. Outcomes of pregnancy beyond 37 weeks of gestation. *Obstetrics & Gynecology* 2006;**108**(3 Pt 1):500–508.

18 Bukola F, Idi N, M'Mimunya M, Jean-Jose WM, Kidza M, Isilda N *et al.* Unmet need for induction of labor in Africa: secondary analysis from the 2004–2005 WHO global maternal and perinatal health survey (a cross-sectional survey). *BMC Public Health* 2012;**12**:722.

19 Martin JA, Hamilton BE, Ventura SJ, Menacker F, and Park MM. Births: final data for 2000. *National Vital Statistics Reports* 2002;**50**(5):1–101.

20 Martin JA, Osterman MJ, and Sutton PD. Are preterm births on the decline in the United States? Recent data from the National Vital Statistics System. *NCHS Data Brief* 2010 (39):1–8.

21 Rayburn WF and Zhang J. Rising rates of labor induction: present concerns and future strategies. *Obstetrics & Gynecology* 2002;**100**(1):164–167.

22 Davidoff MJ, Dias T, Damus K, Russell R, Bettegowda VR, Dolan S *et al.* Changes in the gestational age distribution among U.S. singleton births: impact on rates of late preterm birth, 1992 to 2002. *Seminars in Perinatology* 2006;**30**(1):8–15.

23 Kuehn BM. Scientists probe the role of clinicians in rising rates of late preterm birth. *Journal of the American Medical Association* 2010;**303**(12):1129–1136.

24 Gyamfi-Bannerman C, Fuchs KM, Young OM, and Hoffman MK. Nonspontaneous late preterm birth: etiology and outcomes. *American Journal of Obstetrics & Gynecology* 2011;**205**(5):456 e1–6.

25 Ananth CV, Gyamfi C, and Jain L. Characterizing risk profiles of infants who are delivered at late preterm gestations: does it matter? *American Journal of Obstetrics & Gynecology* 2008;**199**(4):329–331.

26 March of Dimes Prematurity Prevention Resource Center 2012 [cited 2013 May 12]. Available from: http://www.prematurityprevention.org (accessed May 15, 2015).

27 Spong CY, Mercer BM, D'Alton M, Kilpatrick S, Blackwell S, and Saade G. Timing of indicated late-preterm and early-term birth. *Obstetrics & Gynecology* 2011;**118**(2 Pt 1):323–333.

28 Berghella V, Blackwell SC, Ramin SM, Sibai BM, and Saade GR. Use and misuse of the term "elective" in obstetrics. *Obstetrics & Gynecology* 2011;**117**(2 Pt 1):372–376.

29 Clark SL, Frye DR, Meyers JA, Belfort MA, Dildy GA, Kofford S *et al.* Reduction in elective delivery at <39 weeks of gestation: comparative effectiveness of 3 approaches to change and the impact on neonatal intensive care admission and stillbirth. *American Journal of Obstetrics & Gynecology* 2010;**203**(5):449 e1–6.

30 Donovan EF, Lannon C, Bailit J, Rose B, Iams JD, and Byczkowski T. A statewide initiative to reduce inappropriate scheduled births at 36(0/7)–38(6/7) weeks' gestation. *American Journal of Obstetrics & Gynecology* 2010;**202**(3):243 e1–8.

31 Ehrenthal DB, Hoffman MK, Jiang X, and Ostrum G. Neonatal outcomes after implementation of guidelines limiting elective delivery before 39 weeks of gestation. *Obstetrics & Gynecology* 2011;**118**(5):1047–1055.
32 Oshiro BT, Kowalewski L, Sappenfield W, Alter CC, Bettegowda VR, Russell R *et al.* A multistate quality improvement program to decrease elective deliveries before 39 weeks of gestation. *Obstetrics & Gynecology* 2013;**121**(5):1025–1031.
33 Obstetrics ACoPB. American College of Obstetricians and Gynecologists Practice Bulletin No. 107: Induction of labor. *Obstetrics & Gynecology* 2009;**114**(2 Pt 1):386–397.
34 Baud D, Rouiller S, Hohlfeld P, Tolsa JF, and Vial Y. Adverse obstetrical and neonatal outcomes in elective and medically indicated inductions of labor at term. *Journal of Maternal-Fetal and Neonatal Medicine* 2013.
35 Khireddine I, Le Ray C, Dupont C, Rudigoz RC, Bouvier-Colle MH, and Deneux-Tharaux C. Induction of labor and risk of postpartum hemorrhage in low risk parturients. *PLoS One* 2013;**8**(1):e54858.
36 Shetty A, Burt R, Rice P, and Templeton A. Women's perceptions, expectations and satisfaction with induced labour – a questionnaire-based study. *European Journal of Obstetrics & Gynecology and Reproductive Biology* 2005;**123**(1):56–61.
37 Luthy DA, Malmgren JA, and Zingheim RW. Cesarean delivery after elective induction in nulliparous women: the physician effect. *American Journal of Obstetrics & Gynecology* 2004;**191**(5):1511–1515.
38 Caughey AB, Sundaram V, Kaimal AJ, Gienger A, Cheng YW, McDonald KM *et al.* Systematic review: elective induction of labor versus expectant management of pregnancy. *Annals of Internal Medicine* 2009;**151**(4):252–263, W53–63.
39 Gulmezoglu AM, Crowther CA, Middleton P, and Heatley E. Induction of labour for improving birth outcomes for women at or beyond term. *Cochrane Database of Systematic Reviews* 2012;(**6**):CD004945.
40 Bishop EH. Pelvic scoring for elective induction. *Obstetrics & Gynecology* 1964;**24**:266–268.
41 Baacke KA and Edwards RK. Preinduction cervical assessment. *Clinical Obstetrics and Gynecology* 2006;**49**(3):564–572.
42 Laughon SK, Zhang J, Troendle J, Sun L, and Reddy UM. Using a simplified Bishop score to predict vaginal delivery. *Obstetrics & Gynecology* 2011;**117**(4):805–811.
43 Kolkman DG, Verhoeven CJ, Brinkhorst SJ, van der Post JA, Pajkrt E, Opmeer BC *et al.* The Bishop score as a predictor of labor induction success: a systematic review. *American Journal of Perinatology* 2013;**30**(8):625–630.
44 Tan PC, Vallikkannu N, Suguna S, Quek KF, and Hassan J. Transvaginal sonographic measurement of cervical length vs Bishop score in labor induction at term: tolerability and prediction of Cesarean delivery. *Ultrasound in Obstetrics & Gynecology* 2007; **29**(5):568–573.
45 Garite TJ, Casal D, Garcia-Alonso A, Kreaden U, Jimenez G, Ayala JA *et al.* Fetal fibronectin: a new tool for the prediction of successful induction of labor. *American Journal of Obstetrics & Gynecology* 1996;**175**(6):1516–1521.
46 Jozwiak M, Bloemenkamp KW, Kelly AJ, Mol BW, Irion O, and Boulvain M. Mechanical methods for induction of labour. *Cochrane Database of Systematic Reviews* 2012;(**3**):CD001233.
47 Maslovitz S, Lessing JB, and Many A. Complications of trans-cervical Foley catheter for labor induction among 1,083 women. *Archives of Gynecology and Obstetrics* 2010; **281**(3):473–477.
48 Evaldson GR, Fianu S, Jonasson A, Larsson B, Nord CE, and Olund AR. Does the hygroscopic property of the laminaria tent imply a risk for ascending infection in legal abortions? A microbiological study. *Acta Obstetricia et Gynecologica Scandinavica* 1986;**65**(3):257–261.
49 Lichtenberg ES. Complications of osmotic dilators. *Obstetrical and Gynecological Survey* 2004;**59**(7):528–536.

50 Fox MC and Hayes JL. Cervical preparation for second-trimester surgical abortion prior to 20 weeks of gestation. *Contraception* 2007;**76**(6):486–495.

51 Embrey MP and Mollison BG. The unfavourable cervix and induction of labour using a cervical balloon. *The Journal of Obstetrics and Gynaecology of the British Commonwealth* 1967;**74**(1):44–48.

52 Jonsson M, Hellgren C, Wiberg-Itzel E, and Akerud H. Assessment of pain in women randomly allocated to speculum or digital insertion of the Foley catheter for induction of labor. *Acta Obstetricia et Gynecologica Scandinavica* 2011;**90**(9):997–1004.

53 Heinemann J, Gillen G, Sanchez-Ramos L, and Kaunitz AM. Do mechanical methods of cervical ripening increase infectious morbidity? A systematic review. *American Journal of Obstetrics & Gynecology* 2008;**199**(2):177–187; discussion 87–88.

54 Pennell CE, Henderson JJ, O'Neill MJ, McChlery S, Doherty DA, and Dickinson JE. Induction of labour in nulliparous women with an unfavourable cervix: a randomised controlled trial comparing double and single balloon catheters and PGE2 gel. *BJOG: An International Journal of Obstetrics and Gynaecology* 2009;**116**(11):1443–1452.

55 Delaney S, Shaffer BL, Cheng YW, Vargas J, Sparks TN, Paul K *et al.* Labor induction with a Foley balloon inflated to 30 mL compared with 60 mL: a randomized controlled trial. *Obstetrics & Gynecology* 2010;**115**(6):1239–1245.

56 Fox NS, Saltzman DH, Roman AS, Klauser CK, Moshier E, and Rebarber A. Intravaginal misoprostol versus Foley catheter for labour induction: a meta-analysis. *BJOG: An International Journal of Obstetrics and Gynaecology* 2011;**118**(6):647–654.

57 Sciscione AC, Nguyen L, Manley J, Pollock M, Maas B, and Colmorgen G. A randomized comparison of transcervical Foley catheter to intravaginal misoprostol for preinduction cervical ripening. *Obstetrics & Gynecology* 2001;**97**(4):603–607.

58 Jozwiak M, Oude Rengerink K, Ten Eikelder ML, van Pampus MG, Dijksterhuis MG, de Graaf IM *et al.* Foley catheter or prostaglandin E2 inserts for induction of labour at term: an open-label randomized controlled trial (PROBAAT-P trial) and systematic review of literature. *European Journal of Obstetrics & Gynecology and Reproductive Biology* 2013;**170**(1):137–145.

59 Jozwiak M, Ten Eikelder M, Rengerink KO, de Groot C, Feitsma H, Spaanderman M *et al.* Foley Catheter versus vaginal misoprostol: randomized controlled trial (PROBAAT-M study) and systematic review and meta-analysis of literature. *American Journal of Perinatology* 2013.

60 Levy R, Kanengiser B, Furman B, Ben Arie A, Brown D, and Hagay ZJ. A randomized trial comparing a 30-mL and an 80-mL Foley catheter balloon for preinduction cervical ripening. *American Journal of Obstetrics & Gynecology* 2004;**191**(5):1632–1636.

61 Gibson KS, Mercer BM, and Louis JM. Inner thigh taping vs traction for cervical ripening with a Foley catheter: a randomized controlled trial. *American Journal of Obstetrics & Gynecology* 2013;**209**(3):272 e1–7.

62 Guinn DA, Davies JK, Jones RO, Sullivan L, and Wolf D. Labor induction in women with an unfavorable Bishop score: randomized controlled trial of intrauterine Foley catheter with concurrent oxytocin infusion versus Foley catheter with extra-amniotic saline infusion with concurrent oxytocin infusion. *American Journal of Obstetrics & Gynecology* 2004;**191**(1):225–229.

63 Lin MG, Reid KJ, Treaster MR, Nuthalapaty FS, Ramsey PS, and Lu GC. Transcervical Foley catheter with and without extraamniotic saline infusion for labor induction: a randomized controlled trial. *Obstetrics & Gynecology* 2007;**110**(3):558–565.

64 Levey KA, Arslan AA, and Funai EF. Extra-amniotic saline infusion increases cesarean risk versus other induction methods and spontaneous labor. *American Journal of Perinatology* 2006;**23**(7):435–438.

65 Tan PC, Khine PP, Sabdin NH, Vallikkannu N, and Sulaiman S. Effect of membrane sweeping on cervical length by transvaginal ultrasonography and impact of cervical shortening on cesarean delivery. *Journal of Ultrasound in Medicine* 2011;**30**(2):227–233.

66 Wong SF, Hui SK, Choi H, and Ho LC. Does sweeping of membranes beyond 40 weeks reduce the need for formal induction of labour? *BJOG: An International Journal of Obstetrics and Gynaecology* 2002;**109**(6):632–636.

67 Boulvain M, Stan C, and Irion O. Membrane sweeping for induction of labour. *Cochrane Database of Systematic Reviews* 2005;(**1**):CD000451.

68 Challis JR, Sloboda DM, Alfaidy N, Lye SJ, Gibb W, Patel FA *et al.* Prostaglandins and mechanisms of preterm birth. *Reproduction* 2002;**124**(1):1–17.

69 Ghule VV, Gray C, Galimberti A, and Anumba DO. Prostaglandin-induced cervical remodelling in humans in the first trimester is associated with increased expression of specific tight junction, but not gap junction proteins. *Journal of Translational Medicine* 2012;**10**:40.

70 Platz-Christensen JJ, Pernevi P, Bokstrom H, and Wiqvist N. Prostaglandin E and F2 alpha concentration in the cervical mucus and mechanism of cervical ripening. *Prostaglandins* 1997;**53**(4):253–261.

71 Hofmeyr GJ, Gulmezoglu AM, and Pileggi C. Vaginal misoprostol for cervical ripening and induction of labour. *Cochrane Database of Systematic Reviews* 2010;(**10**):CD000941.

72 Hofmeyr GJ and Gulmezoglu AM. Vaginal misoprostol for cervical ripening and labour induction in late pregnancy. *Birth* 1999;**26**(4):264.

73 Weeks A, Alfirevic Z, Faundes A, Hofmeyr GJ, Safar P, and Wing D. Misoprostol for induction of labor with a live fetus. *International Journal of Gynecology & Obstetrics* 2007;**99** Suppl. 2:S194–197.

74 Wing DA, Lovett K, and Paul RH. Disruption of prior uterine incision following misoprostol for labor induction in women with previous cesarean delivery. *Obstetrics & Gynecology* 1998;**91**(5 Pt 2):828–830.

75 Daskalakis GJ, Mesogitis SA, Papantoniou NE, Moulopoulos GG, Papapanagiotou AA, and Antsaklis AJ. Misoprostol for second trimester pregnancy termination in women with prior caesarean section. *BJOG: An International Journal of Obstetrics and Gynaecology* 2005;**112**(1):97–99.

76 Berghella V, Airoldi J, O'Neill AM, Einhorn K, and Hoffman M. Misoprostol for second trimester pregnancy termination in women with prior caesarean: a systematic review. *BJOG: An International Journal of Obstetrics and Gynaecology* 2009;**116**(9):1151–1157.

77 Bartusevicius A, Barcaite E, and Nadisauskiene R. Oral, vaginal and sublingual misoprostol for induction of labor. *International Journal of Gynecology & Obstetrics* 2005;**91**(1):2–9.

78 Souza AS, Feitosa FE, Costa AA, Pereira AP, Carvalho AS, Paixao RM *et al.* Titrated oral misoprostol solution versus vaginal misoprostol for labor induction. *International Journal of Gynecology & Obstetrics* 2013;**123**(3):207–212.

79 Wing DA, Jones MM, Rahall A, Goodwin TM, and Paul RH. A comparison of misoprostol and prostaglandin E2 gel for preinduction cervical ripening and labor induction. *American Journal of Obstetrics & Gynecology* 1995;**172**(6):1804–1810.

80 Wing DA, Rahall A, Jones MM, Goodwin TM, and Paul RH. Misoprostol: an effective agent for cervical ripening and labor induction. *American Journal of Obstetrics & Gynecology* 1995;**172**(6):1811–1816.

81 Wing DA, Brown R, Plante LA, Miller H, Rugarn O, and Powers BL. Misoprostol vaginal insert and time to vaginal delivery: a randomized controlled trial. *Obstetrics & Gynecology* 2013;**122**(2 Pt 1):201–209.

82 Mozurkewich EL, Chilimigras JL, Berman DR, Perni UC, Romero VC, King VJ *et al.* Methods of induction of labour: a systematic review. *BMC Pregnancy and Childbirth* 2011;**11**:84.

83 Company PaU. Prepidil® Gel 0.5mg Package Insert http://dailymed.nlm.nih.gov/dailymed/lookup.cfm?setid=ab03de5b-782c-4f81-a8dc-7ef9969dd0cf [updated 10/2013; cited 2013 1/30/2013]. Available from: http://dailymed.nlm.nih.gov/dailymed/lookup.cfm?setid=ab03de5b-782c-4f81-a8dc-7ef9969dd0cf.

84 Heuser CC, Knight S, Esplin MS, Eller AG, Holmgren CM, Richards D *et al.* Tachysystole in term labor: incidence, risk factors, outcomes, and effect on fetal heart tracings. *American Journal of Obstetrics & Gynecology* 2013;**209**(1):32 e1–6.

85 Tribe RM, Crawshaw SE, Seed P, Shennan AH, and Baker PN. Pulsatile versus continuous administration of oxytocin for induction and augmentation of labor: two randomized controlled trials. *American Journal of Obstetrics & Gynecology* 2012;**206**(3):230 e1–8.

86 Moldin PG and Sundell G. Induction of labour: a randomised clinical trial of amniotomy versus amniotomy with oxytocin infusion. *BJOG* 1996;**103**(4):306–312.

87 Tan PC, Soe MZ, Sulaiman S, and Omar SZ. Immediate compared with delayed oxytocin after amniotomy labor induction in parous women: a randomized controlled trial. *Obstetrics & Gynecology* 2013;**121**(2 Pt 1):253–359.

88 Macones GA, Cahill A, Stamilio DM, and Odibo AO. The efficacy of early amniotomy in nulliparous labor induction: a randomized controlled trial. *American Journal of Obstetrics & Gynecology* 2012;**207**(5):403 e1–5.

89 Gregory SG, Anthopolos R, Osgood CE, Grotegut CA, and Miranda ML. Association of autism with induced or augmented childbirth in North Carolina Birth Record (1990–1998) and Education Research (1997–2007) databases. *JAMA Pediatrics* 2013;**167**(10):959–966.

90 Vintzileos AM and Ananth CV. Does augmentation or induction of labor with oxytocin increase the risk for autism? *American Journal of Obstetrics & Gynecology* 2013;**209**(6):502–504.

91 SMFM Statement: Labor Induction or Augmentation and Autism Spectrum Disorders [press release]. http://www.smfm.org/attachedfiles/LaborinductionandAutismFinal.pdf2014.

92 Mercer BM, McNanley T, O'Brien JM, Randal L, and Sibai BM. Early versus late amniotomy for labor induction: a randomized trial. *American Journal of Obstetrics & Gynecology* 1995;**173**(4):1321–1325.

93 O'Driscoll K, Jackson RJ, and Gallagher JT. Prevention of prolonged labour. *BMJ* 1969;**2**(5655):477–480.

94 O'Driscoll K, Stronge JM, and Minogue M. Active management of labour. *BMJ* 1973;**3**(5872):135–137.

95 Thornton JG and Lilford RJ. Active management of labour: current knowledge and research issues. *BMJ* 1994;**309**(6951):366–369.

96 O'Driscoll K, Foley M, and MacDonald D. Active management of labor as an alternative to cesarean section for dystocia. *Obstetrics & Gynecology* 1984;**63**(4):485–490.

97 American College of Obstetricians and Gynecologists, Gynecology Committee on Practice B-O Practice Bulletin No. 49, December 2003: Dystocia and augmentation of labor. *Obstetrics & Gynecology* 2003;**102**(6):1445–1454.

98 Brown HC, Paranjothy S, Dowswell T, and Thomas J. Package of care for active management in labour for reducing caesarean section rates in low-risk women. *Cochrane Database of Systematic Reviews* 2008;(4):CD004907.

99 Wei S, Wo BL, Qi HP, Xu H, Luo ZC, Roy C *et al.* Early amniotomy and early oxytocin for prevention of, or therapy for, delay in first stage spontaneous labour compared with routine care. *Cochrane Database of Systematic Reviews* 2013;(8):CD006794.

100 Spong CY, Berghella V, Wenstrom KD, Mercer BM, and Saade GR. Preventing the first cesarean delivery: summary of a joint Eunice Kennedy Shriver National Institute of Child Health and Human Development, Society for Maternal-Fetal Medicine, and American College of Obstetricians and Gynecologists workshop. *Obstetrics & Gynecology* 2012;**120**(5):1181–1193.

101 Rouse DJ, Owen J, and Hauth JC. Active-phase labor arrest: oxytocin augmentation for at least 4 hours. *Obstetrics & Gynecology* 1999;**93**(3):323–328.

102 Rouse DJ, Owen J, Savage KG, and Hauth JC. Active phase labor arrest: revisiting the 2-hour minimum. *Obstetrics & Gynecology* 2001;**98**(4):550–554.

103 Friedman E. The graphic analysis of labor. *American Journal of Obstetrics & Gynecology* 1954;**68**(6):1568–1575.

104 Friedman EA. Primigravid labor: a graphicostatistical analysis. *Obstetrics & Gynecology* 1955;**6**(6):567–589.

105 Zhang J, Landy HJ, Branch DW, Burkman R, Haberman S, Gregory KD *et al.* Contemporary patterns of spontaneous labor with normal neonatal outcomes. *Obstetrics & Gynecology* 2010;**116**(6):1281–1287.

106 Hoffman MK, Vahratian A, Sciscione AC, Troendle JF, and Zhang J. Comparison of labor progression between induced and noninduced multiparous women. *Obstetrics & Gynecology* 2006;**107**(5):1029–1034.

107 American College of Obstetricians and Gynecologists. Patient Safety Checklist No. 5: scheduling induction of labor. *Obstetrics & Gynecology* 2011;**118**(6):1473–1474.

108 Iriye BK, Huang WH, Condon J, Hancock L, Hancock JK, Ghamsary M *et al.* Implementation of a laborist program and evaluation of the effect upon cesarean delivery. *American Journal of Obstetrics & Gynecology* 2013;**209**(3):251 e1–6.

CHAPTER 5
Fetal monitoring and assessment

Alison Cahill
Department of Obstetrics and Gynecology, Washington University School of Medicine, St Louis, MO, USA

5.1 Introduction

The physiologic changes and challenges associated with the intrapartum period can impact both mother and fetus. The importance of assessing fetal well-being during labor and delivery has been recognized for many years, and science regarding the best way to accomplish monitoring for clinical decision making continues to evolve.

5.2 Historical perspectives

5.2.1 Intermittent auscultation to electronic fetal monitoring: evidence-based or not?

The standard of care for intrapartum fetal assessment prior to the introduction of electronic fetal monitoring (EFM) in the mid-20th century was intermittent auscultation of fetal heart tones and fetal scalp pH sampling. Intermittent auscultation was accomplished by the use of a specialized fetal stethoscope by a caregiver, such as an obstetric nurse or midwife, listening to the fetal heart rate and variation through the maternal abdomen. In 1969 Kubli *et al.* [1] published data on the correlation between fetal heart rate patterns and fetal pH, describing 85 patients who underwent continuous EFM and simultaneous fetal scalp pH sampling. He described for the first time correlations between pH and selected fetal heart rate patterns in the 20 minutes prior to sampling. In response to this exciting new technology, which promised to be a non-invasive and much less labor intensive way to monitor the fetal status during labor, large-scale trials to test the impact of EFM on outcomes were undertaken. Further, the expectation of intrapartum EFM quickly stretched beyond correlation with pH to an expectation that EFM would

Management of Labor and Delivery, Second Edition. Edited by George A. Macones.

allow physicians to detect infants at risk for neurologic injury such as cerebral palsy, and even fetal death, and allow intervention to prevent them. Unfortunately, the enthusiasm for EFM could not be quelled and it simultaneously began gaining widespread use. In fact, EFM was never proven to reduce the rate of cerebral palsy and intrapartum death. Just 12 trials have been performed to evaluate the efficacy of EFM since its inception [2–11], and only two of those were deemed to be of high enough quality for the Cochrane meta-analysis [12]. The authors of the Cochrane analysis concluded that while intrapartum EFM (as compared to intermittent auscultation) was associated with a reduction in neonatal seizures, there was no evidence to support a reduction in perinatal death (RR 0.85, 95% CI 0.59–1.23) or cerebral palsy (RR 1.74, 95% CI 0.97–3.11) by EFM. Closer examination of the single piece of evidence associating EFM with a decrease in neonatal seizures [8] has shown it to be statistically unstable [13]. Despite the limitations of the evidence to support the use of EFM, it is ubiquitous and the primary mode of monitoring the fetus during labor in the Unites States today.

5.3 Intrapartum electronic fetal monitoring

5.3.1 Types of fetal heart rate monitors

There are approximately 4 million live births in the United States per year [14]. Over the past 30 years, intrapartum EFM has become the most common obstetric procedure, having been used in the care of 45% of laboring women in 1980, compared to 62% in 1988, and 85% by 2002. In 2005, 97.7% of the 4,198,349 births occurred in a hospital, and it is conservatively estimated that 85.4% underwent intrapartum EFM [15]. Since there are no restrictions to employing EFM, it is typically initiated upon admission to the labor and delivery unit or shortly thereafter. The fetus is most commonly monitored continuously throughout labor until the birth of the infant. EFM, also known as cardiotocography, records changes in and patterns of the fetal heart rate contemporaneously with uterine activity. When EFM technology was introduced in the 1970s [1], it was accomplished non-invasively by placing a Doppler device on the maternal abdomen. Today, EFM can be accomplished as it was originally described, or minimally invasively, by the placement of a small metal electrode on the presenting part of the fetus.

5.3.1.1 External

EFM accomplished non-invasively requires the application of a Doppler ultrasound transducer to the maternal abdominal wall at the level of the enlarged uterus containing the pregnancy. Since ultrasound signals can penetrate human tissue without causing any fetal harm, this technology is ideal for fetal monitoring purposes. The transducer contains both a signal source and a receiver. The ultrasonic beam leaves the transducer and when it encounters a different density that is moving (such as the fetal heart), the signal undergoes a frequency change (referred to as the Doppler

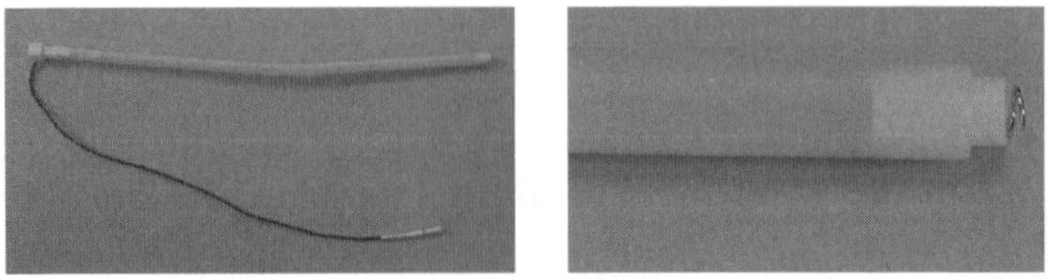

(a) (b)

Figure 5.1 Fetal scalp electrode (FSE). (a) FSE in the plastic introducer; (b) FSE electrode to be applied to the fetal scalp.

shift) which is detected by the transducer and converted to an electronic signal. The electronic signal is then relayed to a receiver (also known as a cardiotachometer) several times per second, and the receiver generates an ongoing paper printout and visual display of the beat-to-beat real-time fetal cardiac heart rate and variation. Disadvantages to this approach to fetal monitoring include artifact, created by movement detected by the transducer on the maternal abdomen that is not the movement of the fetal heart. Under a variety of clinical circumstances, invasive fetal heart rate monitoring may be deemed necessary by the provider.

5.3.1.2 Internal

EFM can be accomplished invasively, with a single lead monitor placed on the infant scalp. For this type of monitoring to be accomplished, the cervix must be dilated and the amniotic sac ruptured. Measurement of the fetal heart rate is acquired by a bipolar electrode which penetrates the skin of the fetal scalp (Figure 5.1a and b). The electrode records the electrical activity of the fetal heart by recording the interval between fetal heart beats (by measuring the R-R interval). The electrical signal is amplified and processed, and the fetal heart rate and variation information is used to generate the same real-time printout and visual display of the fetal heart rate as the Doppler method. In practical application, modern cardiotachometers have the ability to accept fetal heart rate data from either Doppler or fetal electrocardiogram to generate the paper recording of the fetal heart rate and variation used clinically by the caregiver. Obvious disadvantages of this approach include the invasive nature, which introduces the possibility of maternal-fetal fluid exchange and is clinically avoided in cases of maternal infection which can be vertically transmitted. Though rare, fetal scalp electrodes also pose a risk for hematomas and scalp abscesses [16].

5.3.2 Contraction monitoring

Intrapartum fetal monitoring is done in conjunction with the monitoring of uterine activity (Figure 5.2). Uterine contractions are quantified over a 10-minute period, and then averaged over 30 minutes [17]. Besides manual palpation, which can be done at the bedside by trained obstetric nurses and providers, contractions can be monitored automatically using either an external or an internal monitor (below). Regardless of the method used to monitor uterine activity, contraction frequency can be interpreted. The 2008 *Eunice Kennedy Shriver* Nation

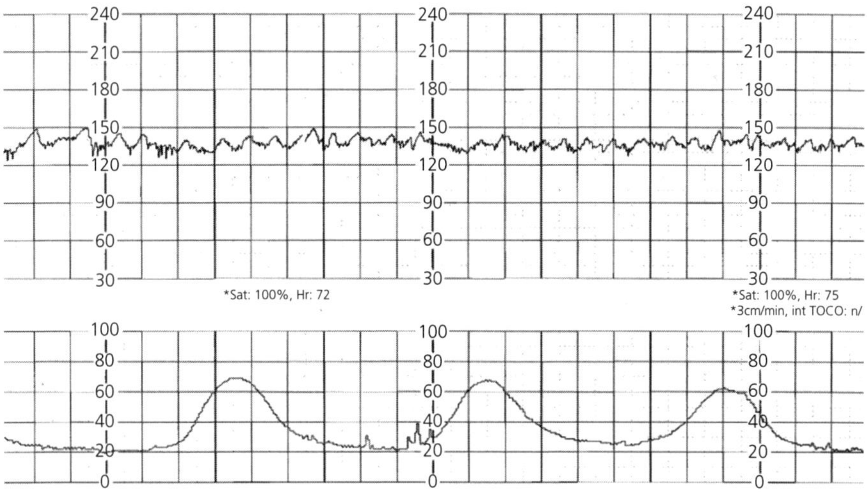

Figure 5.2 Sample of bedside monitoring of EFM and contractions; uterine contractions are found in the lower band.

Institute of Child Health and Human Development (NICHD) specified nomenclature included specific definitions for the visual interpretation of contraction frequency [18]. A *normal* contraction pattern is a contraction frequency of ≤ 5 contractions in 10 minutes. *Tachysystole* is defined as > 5 contractions in 10 minutes, averaged over 30 minutes. Tachysystole should always be further qualified as accompanied by or not accompanied by fetal heart rate decelerations. Quantification of contraction strength requires internal uterine monitoring.

5.3.2.1 External

External uterine monitoring is non-invasive and is accomplished much in the way that external fetal heart rate monitoring is accomplished. A tocodynamometer is applied to the maternal abdomen, typically near the uterine fundus. The device detects movement, and specifically a change in uterine shape, to signify the occurrence of a contraction. The monitor's signal is translated to a receiver at the bedside which prints out real-time contraction data for bedside interpretation. The main advantage of external monitoring is that it is non-invasive and relatively easy to use. Disadvantages include the inability to measure pressure, resulting in a lack of information on contraction strength, and the possibility of signal distortion due to motion and other artifacts, such as adipose of the maternal abdominal wall and maternal movement.

5.3.2.2 Internal

As an alternative to the non-invasive tocodynamometer, an intrauterine pressure catheter (IUPC) can be used to monitor contractions (Figure 5.3). Because the IUPC is an internal, invasive monitor, it requires rupture of the amniotic sac for placement. The IUPC is a flexible catheter with an electronic pressure transducer at the tip which is placed at the time of cervical examination through the dilated cervix

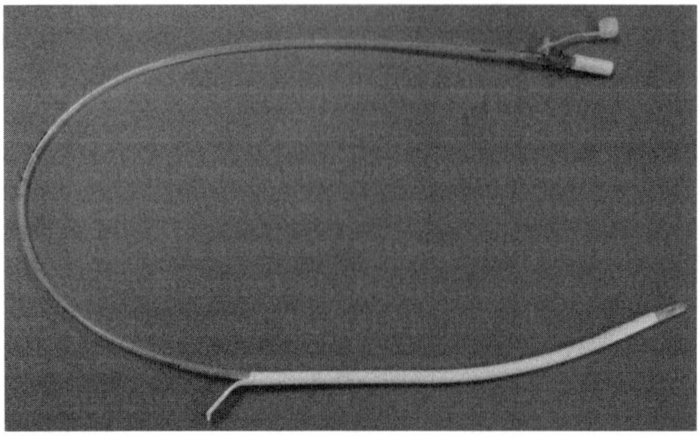

Figure 5.3 An intrauterine pressure catheter (IUPC) inside its plastic guide, ready for insertion.

and advanced to the fundus. The end of the catheter extending out through the cervix is connected to the same bedside transducer as the external monitor, zeroed between contractions, and a similar real-time display of contractions is generated at the bedside. Advantages of IUPCs are that they avoid much of the artifact created by maternal body habitus and movement, they allow interpretation of contraction strength, and they allow initiation of an amnioinfusion (below) when indicated. Disadvantages are that they require rupture of the amniotic sac, and they are invasive. For clinical scenarios in which there is potential for maternal-fetal infectious vertical transmission, such as maternal human immunodeficiency virus (HIV), attempts are made to avoid invasive devices such as IUPCs. There has also been some suggestion that IUPCs may increase the risk for maternal fever and infection [19]. Despite the increase in the relative risk of fever, the absolute risk remains low and thus IUPCs are often used clinically because the potential information gained outweighs the potential infection risk. Besides the use of IUPCs to overcome technical challenges of monitoring contractions with a tocodynamometer in certain clinical situations, IUPCs allow the assessment of contraction strength and thus the calculation of the Montevideo unit (MVU). Early work by Caldeyro-Barcia and Poseiro [20], and later by Krapohl *et al.* [21], using an open-end fluid-filled catheter placed in the uterus, described distributions of MVUs during spontaneous labor. MVUs are calculated during any 10-minute period by multiplying the number of contractions by the average contraction intensity above the baseline pressure. Hauth *et al.* [22], using intrauterine catheters with a pressure transducer at the tip similar to what is used today, described MVUs in women receiving oxytocin for labor induction and augmentation, where infusion was titrated to labor progress and spontaneous vaginal delivery without evidence of fetal heart rate abnormalities. They found that 91% of induced women achieved at least 200–224 MVUs, which led them to recommend that women demonstrate MVUs of at least 200 in the absence of labor progress before arrest is diagnosed. To follow, Hauth *et al.* [23] described a series of 85 women who underwent cesarean for arrest after the vast majority achieved 200 MVUs, and recommended that a minimum of 200 MVUs for 2 hours be achieved without cervical change before a diagnosis of arrest is made; recommendations which were subsequently endorsed by the American College of Obstetricians and Gynecologists (ACOG) [24]. However, while this threshold for sufficient contractions to change the cervix, termed *adequacy*, is still used at the bedside today, scientists are actively working toward a more robust understanding of normal and abnormal contraction patterns given the recent changes in our understanding of normal and abnormal labor progress [25–27].

5.3.3 Nomenclature

It has become widely recognized that the use of common nomenclature when referring to EFM patterns among all obstetric providers is of great importance. Standard definitions of EFM patterns, including the following components, are used for visual EFM interpretation. These definitions have been refined at an EFM consensus workshop [18], and endorsed by ACOG [17] and other clinical entities for universal bedside use.

5.3.3.1 Baseline

The fetal heart rate has a normal baseline rate of 110–160 beats per minute (bpm). It is reported as the mean rate rounded to the nearest increment of 5, over any given 10-minute period. In any given 10-minute period, the baseline must be achieved for at least 2 of the 10 minutes, or the baseline for that 10-minute epoch is said to be indeterminate. A fetal heart rate over 160 bpm is *tachycardia* and a fetal heart rate less than 110 bpm is *bradycardia*.

5.3.3.2 Variability

Fetal heart rate variability is the irregular fluctuations in the amplitude of the fetal heart rate. Variability is visually quantified by the amplitude of the peak-to-trough in bpm, such that 0 bpm is *absent*, 1–5 bpm is *minimal*, 6–25 bpm is *moderate*, and > 25 bpm is *marked*.

5.3.3.3 Accelerations

Accelerations of the fetal heart rate are abrupt rises above the baseline. After 32 weeks, an *acceleration* is a rise of at least 15 bpm above the baseline that lasts at least 15 seconds in duration. Before 32 weeks of gestation, an *acceleration* is a rise in the fetal heart rate of at least 10 bpm, for at least 10 seconds in duration, above the baseline.

5.3.3.4 Decelerations

Heart rate decelerations are decreases in the fetal heart rate below the baseline, and are further classified as *variable*, *early*, *late*, or *prolonged*. *Variable* decelerations are characterized by an abrupt decrease and then return to the fetal heart rate baseline in which the onset to the nadir is less than 30 seconds, and the decrease is at least 15 bpm below the baseline and lasts for at least 15 seconds but no longer than 120 seconds. An *early* deceleration is characterized by a gradual decrease in fetal heart rate below the baseline, taking at least 30 seconds to reach its nadir, and most typically symmetric in shape. A *late* deceleration has a similar shape to an *early* deceleration, taking 30 seconds or more to reach its nadir, but is characterized by its timing relative to the coincident contraction; the onset, nadir, and recovery of the deceleration occur after the beginning, peak, and resolution of the contraction, respectively. *Prolonged* decelerations are decelerations that fall at least 15 beats below the baseline and last more than 120 seconds but less than 10 minutes.

5.3.3.5 Category system

Based on the presence, characteristics, and/or absence of the four components of EFM patterns above (baseline, variability, accelerations, decelerations), a category of EFM is specified for any given 10-minute period of time. Currently, the system for EFM pattern nomenclature endorsed by ACOG, the Society for Maternal-Fetal Medicine (SMFM), and the NICHD specifies three categories [18]. This system replaces the previously used two-category system, describing all patterns as either "reassuring"or "non-reassuring." Since 2008, all EFM patterns are summarized as one of three categories: Category I (normal), Category II (indeterminant), Category III (abnormal) (Table 5.1) [17,18].

Table 5.1 Standard nomenclature – the EFM category system.

Baseline	Variability	Accelerations	Decelerations	Other
Category I (Normal) (must have all of below)				
110–160 bpm	Moderate (ModV)	Present or absent	Absent	None
Category II (Indeterminant) (not Category I or III; may have one of the following features)				
Tachycardia *or* 110–160 bpm *or* Bradycardia *with* variability	Minimal (MinV) *or* Marked(MkV) *or* Absent *without* recurrent decelerations	Absent; even after induced by fetal stimulation	Variable(s) *or* Prolonged(s) *or* Recurrent late with ModV at baseline *or* Recurrent variable with MinV or ModV at baseline	Variable decelerations with "other" characteristics (slow-return, shoulders, etc.)
Category III (Abnormal) (must have all of below)				
110–160 bpm *or* Bradycardia	Absent	Absent	Recurrent late *or* Recurrent variable	Sinusoidal pattern

5.3.4 Electronic fetal monitoring interpretation and management

The three-category system is based on visual EFM pattern interpretation. EFM patterns are to be assessed as Category I, II, or III (Table 5.1) and interpreted within the clinical setting [28]. The presence of specific features may further direct interpretation and management.

5.3.4.1 Prolonged decelerations

Prolonged decelerations, or decelerations lasting more than 2 minutes but less than 10 minutes (Figure 5.4), can occur during labor under a number of circumstances. Clinical assessment after the onset of a prolonged deceleration is noted typically involves several components with a variety of causes in mind, in an effort to resolve the deceleration and allow the heart rate to return to baseline [28]. Prolonged decelerations can be noted during times of rapid cervical change. They can also be a sign of cord prolapse. With both of these possibilities in mind, a cervical exam is prudent. Significant hypotension can result in a prolonged deceleration, and this can frequently occur after placement of a regional anesthetic. Thus it is important to check maternal blood pressure, and a fluid bolus may ameliorate the hypotension. Similarly, given that at or near term, a supine maternal position can compress the inferior vena cava, resulting in decreased venous return and cardiac output as a possible cause for prolonged deceleration, change in maternal position can alleviate this compression. It is also important to interpret the tocometer and examine the maternal abdomen for evidence of tachysystole, in which case a decrease or cessation in any contractile agent such as oxytocin would be warranted [29]. Other less common causes, but some that can be life-threatening, are also important to consider. Significant vaginal bleeding, abdominal pain, and tachysystole along with a prolonged deceleration may be signs of a placental abruption [30–32]. In a woman attempting vaginal birth

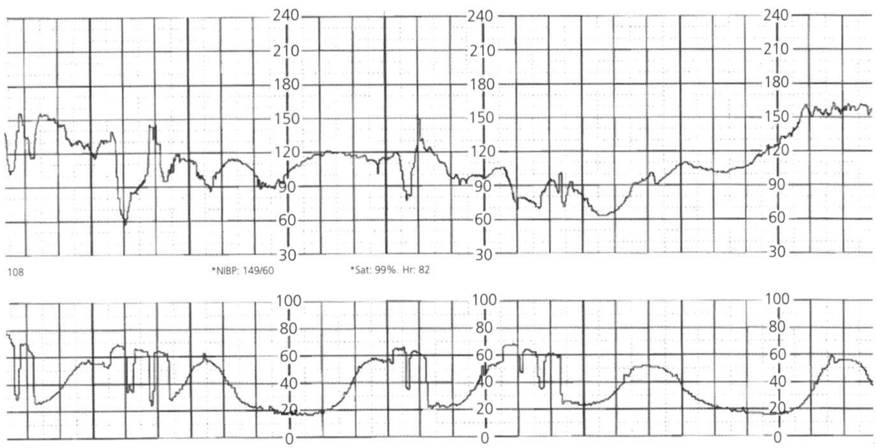

Figure 5.4 A prolonged deceleration; note the fetal heart rate baseline in the 150s.

after a prior cesarean, a prolonged deceleration accompanied by loss of fetal station and abdominal pain may be signs of a uterine rupture [33]. Finally, prolonged deceleration in the setting of vaginal bleeding but in the absence of pain may also be evidence of a vasa previa [34]. The most important components of clinical management of a prolonged deceleration include prompt assessment and consideration of a wide differential in order to facilitate a rapid resolution.

5.3.4.2 Minimal or absent variability

When there is minimal or absent fetal heart rate variability at the baseline, the fetal heart rate category is either II or III and thus warrants additional evaluation. While there are several clinical factors that can result in decreased fetal heart rate variability, such as fetal physiologic sleep cycles [35] or some medication exposures [36], there are often clinical instances when additional measures are taken to assure fetal well-being.

5.3.4.2.1 Scalp stimulation

During periods of minimal or absent EFM variability, or with other patterns when the possibility of acidemia is present, it is possible to perform procedures which induce an EFM response that is correlated with fetal pH. Historically, if the fetal scalp could be accessed, a blood sample could be obtained to enable a direct measure of fetal pH (see below). However, this procedure has fallen out of favor in the United States, in large part due to the discovery of alternative procedures that are non-invasive but yield similar information. The introduction of scalp stimulation was enabled by the observation that when the fetal scalp was sampled, thus "stimulating" the fetal scalp, there was a change in EFM pattern which frequently yielded an acceleration [37–39]. Clark and colleagues [40] then demonstrated that fetal scalp stimulation with an Allis clamp, followed by a fetal heart rate acceleration, was 100% sensitive for a scalp pH ≥ 7.19. Elimian *et al.* [41] published similar findings after digital fetal scalp stimulation of 103 term infants. A fetal heart rate acceleration following scalp stimulation was 100% sensitive for a scalp pH ≥ 7.20. Thus, by achieving a heart rate acceleration following digital scalp stimulation, invasive and more aggressive measures such as scalp sampling for pH and stimulation with Allis clamps quickly fell out of favor. In the setting of EFM patterns raising concern for acidosis, such as minimal or absent variability, digital fetal scalp stimulation that yields a heart rate acceleration is highly sensitive for the absence of acidosis (pH ≥ 7.20).

5.3.4.2.2 Vibro-acoustic stimulation

Vibro-acoustic stimulation, which is performed by applying an artificial larynx to the maternal abdomen between the umbilicus and the pubic symphysis, is a reasonable alternative to digital scalp stimulation in the setting of EFM patterns that necessitate additional fetal reassurance. Preliminary work by Smith and colleagues [42] described transabdominal acoustic stimulation prior to fetal scalp sampling in the setting of concerning EFM patterns and found that all 30 fetuses that responded with a heart rate acceleration had a pH ≥ 7.25. Polzin and colleagues [43] reported that a fetal heart rate acceleration following vibro-acoustic stimulation was 90% sensitive for fetal pH ≥ 7.20, and Ingemarsson and Arulkumaran [44] reported similar findings. Given these findings, vibro-acoustic stimulation is a reasonable alternative to digital scalp stimulation under clinical circumstances that prohibit scalp stimulation, such as a closed cervix. However, as was highlighted in a meta-analysis by Skupski and colleagues [45], while digital scalp and vibro-acoustic stimulation are useful clinical tools to rule out fetal acidosis (pH < 7.20), they are not perfect. Further, if EFM patterns concerning for acidosis persist, repeat testing is indicated.

5.3.4.3 Repetitive variable decelerations

Repetitive decelerations, defined as occurring with greater than 50% of contractions [17], are an EFM periodic pattern clinically encountered (Figure 5.5). Given that variable decelerations are thought to be a physiologic response to compression of the umbilical cord, repetitive variable decelerations are not pathologic per se. However, over time, constant compression of the cord might limit gas exchange, consume the physiologic buffer system, and result in acidemia.

5.3.4.3.1 Amnioinfusion

After it was demonstrated in animal models with oligohydramnios that replenishment with saline fluid could reduce variable decelerations [46], small observational studies in humans described the same [47]. The procedure of replacing normal saline into the uterus via intravenous tubing connected

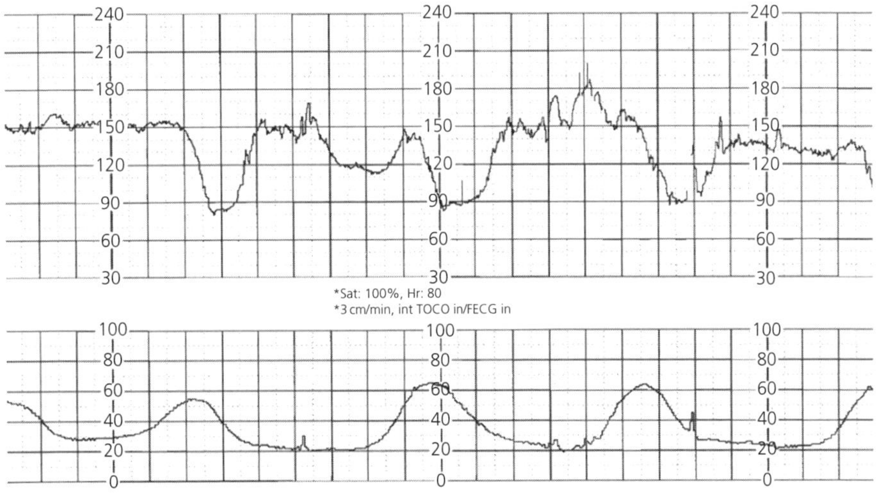

Figure 5.5 Repetitive variable decelerations.

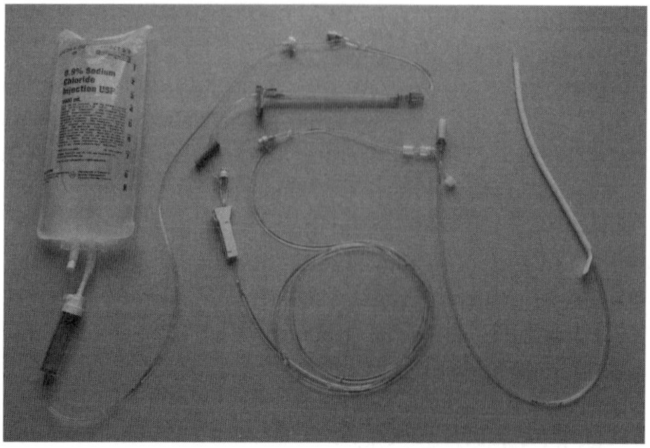

Figure 5.6 Amnioinfusion: intrauterine pressure catheter connected with intravenous tubing to a saline infusion required to start an amnioinfusion.

to an intrauterine pressure catheter came to be known as an amnioinfusion (Figure 5.6). Miyazaki and Nevarez [48] performed a randomized trial of 96 patients (first stage of labor with repetitive variable decelerations who did not respond to oxygen and position change) to amnioinfusion or no amnioinfusion. They reported complete resolution in 51% of the infusion group, but only 4.2% resolution in the non-infusion group ($p < 0.001$), as well as a significant decrease in cesarean for non-reassuring fetal parameters in nulliparous women. Other randomized trials have also demonstrated a reduction in repetitive decelerations [49,50] and cesareans for fetal heart rate parameters [49,51,52]. Most trials demonstrating evidence for efficacy used a bolus of 250–500 cc of normal saline, followed by a continuous infusion if the repetitive variables persisted, through an intrauterine pressure catheter [53]. One small trial by Rinehart and colleagues [54] describes equivalence when using an intermittent infusion technique, but additional evidence has not been published to support this alternative. Puder *et al.* [55] randomized 53 women receiving an amnioinfusion to normal saline or lactated Ringer's solution to test the comparative effect on neonatal electrolytes. They found no difference in neonatal electrolyte profiles between the study groups, which were exposed to equal amounts and durations of the respective infusions. They also reported no cases of hypernatremia or hyperchloremia, further supporting the relative safety of the procedure. Theoretic concerns regarding increases in risks of adverse events such as infectious complications have not been supported by the published evidence. Thus, a reasonable strategy to increase the chance of resolution and decrease the chance of cesarean for non-reassuring fetal heart rate patterns when repetitive variable decelerations are encountered, is initiation of an amnioinfusion.

5.3.4.4 Tachysystole with fetal heart rate changes

Tachysystole is defined as more than five contractions in 10 minutes, averaged over a 30-minute window. Importantly, the term *tachysystole* is to replace any historically used terms to refer to high-frequency contraction patterns, such as *hyperstimulation* or *hypercontractility*. The termination of the use of the latter terms was specified by the 2008 NICHD consensus conference document [18] and subsequent ACOG documents [17,28]. Tachysystole may be accompanied by fetal heart rate decelerations, or may not be, and it is presence of the former that typically requires clinical intervention. In the setting of tachysystole with fetal heart rate decelerations, and with the patient receiving a uterine stimulant for labor induction or augmentation, such as oxytocin, a reduction or cessation of the agent is a reasonable first step in resolution of the decelerations. If the tachysystolic pattern is spontaneous, it may be necessary to use an agent such as terbutaline to reduce the strength and frequency of the contractions. Relatively little published data exist to address the use of acute tocolytics during term labor, despite the frequent use of them in practice. Specifically, beta-adrenergic receptor agonists, magnesium, nitric oxide donors, and oxytocin receptor blockers (no longer commercially available in the United States) have all been considered. Egarter and colleagues [56] described the use of terbutaline as an effective tocolytic in the setting of prostaglandin E2 therapy in 181 women. A small retrospective cohort study by Valenzuela and Foster [57] described the use of magnesium during term labor augmentation with oxytocin for the purposes of normalizing abnormal contraction patterns, which they defined as ≥ 5 contractions in 10 minutes, among other patterns. They described a significantly decreased risk of abnormal contraction frequency in the group exposed to magnesium with oxytocin compared to oxytocin alone, but this was at the potential expense of an increase in rate of cesarean (31.8% magnesium plus oxytocin vs 13.7% oxytocin alone, $p < 0.05$). With no additional supportive evidence in the literature for this practice, the use of magnesium in term labor patients is currently reserved for other obstetric indications. Pacheco and colleagues [58] conducted a small, randomized controlled trial to test the hypothesis that terbutaline could be added to oxytocin without cessation to treat tachysystole at term. They found that cessation of the abnormal uterine contraction patterns was achieved more quickly in the dual therapy group ($p = 0.002$). However, the study was not powered to detect differences in maternal or neonatal birth outcomes. Buhimschi and colleagues [59] conducted a randomized trial of sublingual nitroglycerine compared to placebo to reduce intrauterine pressure and contraction frequency during term labor, but found no evidence for efficacy. They did, however, identify a significant reduction in maternal mean arterial blood pressure in the nitroglycerine group. None of these trials were able to specifically examine efficacy of acute tocolysis in the setting of term labor as it related to fetal heart rate patterns. Heus and colleagues [60] performed a critical review of the literature in 2008, and reported findings which were similar to a Cochrane review by Kulier [61] in

2000 on tocolytics for treatment of tachysystole with fetal heart rate abnormalities. Both found that there were few quality studies to summarize (six by Heus and three by Kulier), and both concluded that the limited available evidence supported the use of beta-adrenergic receptor agonists to improve EFM abnormalities in the setting of tachysystole, though which agent, dose, and whether it should be used alone remained unresolved. In current practice, use of terbutaline (beta-adrenergic receptor antagonist) for the treatment of tachysystole with EFM changes to resolve abnormal EFM patterns that are unresolved with other measures remains reasonable.

5.3.4.5 Fetal tachycardia

Fetal tachycardia, defined as a baseline fetal heart rate greater than 160 bpm, is an element of Category II EFM patterns. Fetal tachycardia can be seen under a variety of clinical circumstances including maternal medication or illicit drug exposure, maternal and/or fetal infection or inflammation, and fetal anemia. Fetal tachycardia has also been associated with acidemia in term infants. Gilstrap *et al.* [62] examined a cohort of low-risk term-born infants and their EFM patterns preceding birth, and found a significantly increased frequency of tachycardia among infants born with an arterial umbilical cord pH < 7.20 compared to those born with a normal pH (22% vs 22%, $p < 0.05$). Others have reported similar results [63–69]. Cahill *et al.* [70] in 2012 published the results of a population-based cohort of consecutive term births, prospectively examining the relationship of the EFM patterns prior to delivery read blind to outcomes, and neonatal acidemia. Among 5388 women, tachycardia occurred infrequently (n = 247; 4.6%). Tachycardia was associated with a more than twofold increase in risk of acidemia (aOR 2.15, 95% CI 1.21–3.82) even after adjusting for nulliparity, fever, prolonged first stage of labor, and obesity. Because the differential diagnosis is wide when fetal tachycardia is observed during term labor, and includes fetal acidemia, additional clinical investigation regarding the underlying cause given the potential for resolution should be undertaken.

5.3.4.6 Medication effects on electronic fetal monitoring patterns

Effects of a variety of frequently used intrapartum medications on term EFM patterns have been described, including opioids, terbutaline, zidovudine, and magnesium sulfate, though the overall body of literature remains relatively limited [71–77]. To date, the impact of magnesium exposure on EFM patterns at term is the medication effect most well-characterized. In 1981, Stallworth *et al.* [78] described the effect of magnesium sulfate on EFM variability in 19 women in term labor with preeclampsia, reporting no significant effect on variability. In the years that followed, a series of reports described conflicting results regarding the impact of magnesium on intrapartum EFM at term, largely limited by sample size and computer interpretation lacking generalizability. Duffy *et al.* [36] reported the results of a large population-based retrospective cohort study of term labor patients. Trained research nurses primarily extracted EFM patterns in the 30 minutes prior to delivery blind to outcomes. The effects of magnesium sulfate on EFM patterns were compared both to women unexposed to magnesium (who by definition did not have preeclampsia) and to those with mild preeclampsia (unexposed to magnesium). They found small but significantly different EFM patterns in women exposed to magnesium compared to the other groups, even after adjusting for confounding factors that could be attributed to magnesium sulfate exposure. Magnesium sulfate was associated with a small decrease in baseline, though still within the normal range (110–160 bpm), fewer prolonged decelerations, and an increase in the frequency of absent or minimal variability (20%). These differences were detected even among infants born without evidence of acidemia, depressed Apgar, or need for advanced nursery admission, suggesting that some of these differences are medication effect as opposed to markers of fetal compromise. Thus, magnesium appears to have an independent effect on term intrapartum EFM patterns, and clinicians should be aware of these effects, though given that the clinical indication for magnesium in term infants is seizure prophylaxis for severe preeclampsia, consideration of the entire clinical picture when interpreting these EFM patterns remains paramount.

5.4 Fetal scalp sampling

Fetal scalp sampling, the procedure by which a fetal blood sample is obtained from the scalp through the dilated cervix in labor and tested for evidence of acidemia, has fallen out of favor in the United States. Advocates for the procedure cite the poor sensitivity of EFM, and argue the value of interpreting EFM patterns to predict pH (which it does poorly) when fetal pH and other measures can be made directly. Opponents highlight the invasive nature of the procedure, the need for frequent quality assessments of the bedside tool to process the samples, and the narrow clinical scenarios in which it might be helpful. In the past 10 years, fetal scalp sampling has become so infrequent that many centers do not perform them and a generation of obstetric providers in training does not have the skill to perform it. Still, the test has continued to have a place in clinical management schema outside the United States and some investigators have described value in scalp samples that are correlated with outcomes. Further, given the weakness of the use of intrapartum EFM patterns alone in predicting adverse outcomes, scalp sampling continues to be considered in algorithms to improve the clinical utility of EFM. In 1999, Kruger and colleagues [79] compared the sensitivity and specificity of pH compared to lactate in fetal scalp samples for low Apgar scores and hypoxic-ischemic encephalopathy (HIE). They found lactate to have a superior sensitivity (100.0% vs 50.0%) but poorer specificity (72.8% vs 80.2%) compared to pH. Westgren and colleagues [80], in a randomized study of women with concerning

EFM patterns that compared lactate to pH analysis from fetal scalp sampling, found that the measures were equivalent in their correlation with fetal arterial cord gas measures at birth and low Apgar scores. Allen *et al.* [81] in a prospective study of women with concerning EFM tracings similarly found that lactate was equivalent to pH, but that both remained poorly sensitive for low Apgar scores and neonatal intensive-care unit admission. Ongoing study, predominantly outside the United States, continues to evaluate this tool as a potential adjunct to aid clinicians in the interpretation of EFM patterns in labor.

5.5 Fetal pulse oximetry

Given that the use of intrapartum fetal heart rate monitoring has persisted in an almost universal fashion despite the relative absence of evidence supporting an improvement in outcomes, either at the trial or the epidemiologic level, with its use, some have suggested that additional devices to assess fetal well-being be employed. In theory, as a group, these could either augment the use of EFM at the bedside in order to improve outcomes, or even replace EFM altogether. One such technology was fetal pulse oximetry. As compared to EFM, an indirect measure of fetal oxygenation and acid-base status, fetal pulse oximetry involves the placement of a non-invasive probe transcervically on the fetal cheek. Garite *et al.* [82] conducted a multicenter, randomized trial to test the hypothesis that for women with a non-reassuring fetal heart rate tracing, the additional information from fetal pulse oximetry would reduce the rate of cesarean without increased adverse outcomes for mother or baby. Among the 1010 women randomized, the technology was deemed safe, with no evidence of increased adverse outcomes in those with pulse oximetry. There was a 50% reduction in the rate of cesarean for non-reassuring fetal parameters in the pulse oximetry group; however, there was no difference in overall cesarean rates between the groups due to a significantly increased rate of cesarean for dystocia in the pulse oximetry group. East *et al.* [83] published similar findings from a multicenter trial in Australia. Klauser and colleagues [84] performed a smaller randomized trial of 360 women, comparing EFM with pulse oximetry to EFM alone, and found that pulse oximetry added to EFM did not decrease the cesarean delivery rate. In 2006, Bloom and colleagues [85] published the results of a multicenter, randomized trial of 5341 nulliparous women comparing rates os cesarean using pulse oximetry plus EFM versus EFM alone, conducted by the National Institute of Child Health and Human Development Maternal-Fetal Medicine Units (MFMU) Network. They found no difference in the rate of cesarean between those with pulse ox plus EFM and those with EFM alone (26.3% vs 27.5%, $p = 0.31$). There was also no difference in the rates of cesarean by indication between the groups. Despite the early data suggesting that fetal intrapartum pulse oximetry might be a non-invasive means for clinicians to improve upon their understanding of fetal oxygenation status and reduce unnecessary cesareans, the trial by the MFMU demonstrated the lack of efficacy, leaving no evidence-based role for fetal pulse oximetry in clinical practice.

5.6 Fetal ST segment analysis

Another tool proposed to improve upon clinical use of EFM, much in the way that fetal pulse oximetry was proposed to, is fetal ST segment analysis. Animal data and data from adult humans demonstrated that the ST segment wave form provided evidence for metabolic acidosis under hypoxic conditions. These data from other biologic models prompted the development of ST waveform analyzer (STAN). STAN adds a continuous ST segment analysis to the ongoing EFM output. Early studies suggested that the use of STAN, compared to EFM alone, might reduce operative interventions for concerning fetal heart rate patterns [86]. Amer-Wahlin and colleagues [87] randomized 4966 women in three centers to EFM plus STAN or EFM alone. They found that the use of STAN in addition to EFM reduced the rate of metabolic acidosis and operative vaginal delivery for fetal distress, but did not reduce the rate of cesarean delivery for fetal distress or adverse neonatal outcomes. Conversely, Dervaitis *et al.* [88] performed an observational study, applying the STAN system to all women in labor but only making the EFM patterns clinically available. After birth, the ST segment analysis was performed, blind to EFM patterns or clinical data. They found that STAN had a poor positive predictive value and a sensitivity of 43% for metabolic acidemia. Ojala and colleagues [89], in a randomized trial of STAN plus EFM versus EFM alone, found no reduction in the rate of cesarean and no improvement in neonatal outcomes with the use of STAN. Similarly, Vayssiere and colleagues [90] performed a randomized trial of STAN plus EFM versus EFM alone, finding no difference in the rate of operative delivery (cesarean or instrumented vaginal) for concerning fetal heart rate patterns. A meta-analysis by Potti and Berghella [91] combined five randomized controlled trials of 15,303 women, comparing STAN plus EFM to EFM alone. They found no improvement in rates of metabolic acidosis, perinatal death, cesarean delivery, and neonatal outcomes with the addition of STAN. They did find that the pooled estimate for rates of operative vaginal delivery were lower with the use of STAN plus EFM compared to EFM alone. The meta-analysis by Becker and colleagues [92] reported similar findings. A Cochrane meta-analysis on the use of STAN was published in 2012 [93]. Pooled estimates showed no evidence for benefit from STAN use for the primary outcomes of the trials: cesarean, metabolic acidosis, neonatal encephalopathy. There was evidence for a reduction in the average number of scalp pH samples performed. In sum, the data published to date do not provide convincing evidence for benefit with the added use of STAN with EFM. While there was evidence in a few of the trials, reflected in the Cochrane meta-analysis, for a reduction in the average number of scalp samples for pH performed, this practice has fallen out of clinical practice in the United States and in parts of Europe, and thus lacks generalizability.

5.7 Research and the future

New understanding of labor, but mechanistically and at the bedside, as well as robust study design and novel analytic techniques are just some of the tools that scientists are currently harnessing to enable providers to improve obstetric care at the bedside with regard to intrapartum fetal assessment and interpretation. A better understanding of EFM patterns, novel tools to augment and improve the interpretation of EFM patterns, or even a replacement of EFM may be in the near future. While evidence-based clinicians continue to care for patients at the beside and implement the existing evidence for best bedside intrapartum fetal assessment, more science and better tools to further improve care and outcomes are anxiously awaited.

References

1 Kubli FW, Hon EH, Khazin AF, and Takemura H. Observations on heart rate and pH in the human fetus during labor. *American Journal of Obstetrics & Gynecology* 1969;**104**:1190–1206.

2 Haverkamp AD, Orleans M, Langendoerfer S, McFee J, Murphy J, and Thompson HE. A controlled trial of the differential effects of intrapartum fetal monitoring. *American Journal of Obstetrics & Gynecology* 1979;**134**:399–412.

3 Haverkamp AD, Thompson HE, McFee JG, and Cetrulo C. The evaluation of continuous fetal heart rate monitoring in high-risk pregnancy. *American Journal of Obstetrics & Gynecology* 1976;**125**:310–320.

4 Herbst A and Ingemarsson I. Intermittent versus continuous electronic monitoring in labour: a randomised study. *BJOG* 1994;**101**:663–668.

5 Kelso IM, Parsons RJ, Lawrence GF, Arora SS, Edmonds DK, and Cooke ID. An assessment of continuous fetal heart rate monitoring in labor. A randomized trial. *American Journal of Obstetrics & Gynecology* 1978;**131**:526–532.

6 Leveno KJ, Cunningham FG, Nelson S *et al.* A prospective comparison of selective and universal electronic fetal monitoring in 34,995 pregnancies. *New England Journal of Medicine* 1986;**315**:615–619.

7 Luthy DA, Shy KK, van Belle G *et al.* A randomized trial of electronic fetal monitoring in preterm labor. *Obstetrics & Gynecology* 1987;**69**:687–695.

8 MacDonald D, Grant A, Sheridan-Pereira M, Boylan P, and Chalmers I. The Dublin randomized controlled trial of intrapartum fetal heart rate monitoring. *American Journal of Obstetrics & Gynecology* 1985;**152**:524–539.

9 Neldam S, Osler M, Hansen PK, Nim J, Smith SF, and Hertel J. Intrapartum fetal heart rate monitoring in a combined low- and high-risk population: a controlled clinical trial. *European Journal of Obstetrics & Gynecology and Reproductive Biology* 1986;**23**:1–11.

10 Renou P, Chang A, Anderson I, and Wood C. Controlled trial of fetal intensive care. *American Journal of Obstetrics & Gynecology* 1976;**126**:470–476.

11 Vintzileos AM, Antsaklis A, Varvarigos I, Papas C, Sofatzis I, and Montgomery JT. A randomized trial of intrapartum electronic fetal heart rate monitoring versus intermittent auscultation. *Obstetrics & Gynecology* 1993;**81**:899–907.

12 Alfirevic Z, Devane D, and Gyte GM. Continuous cardiotocography (CTG) as a form of electronic fetal monitoring (EFM) for fetal assessment during labour. *Cochrane Database of Systematic Reviews* 2006;(3):CD006066.

13 American College of Obstetricians and Gynecologists Practice Bulletin No. 62: Clinical Management Guidelines for Obstetrician-Gynecologists., May 2005. Intrapartum fetal heart rate monitoring. *Obstetrics & Gynecology* 2005;**105**:1161–1169.

14 Martin JA, Hamilton BE, Sutton PD, Ventura SJ, Mathews TJ, and Osterman MJ. Births: final data for 2008. *National Vital Statistics Reports* 2010;**59**:1, 3–71.

15 Martin JA, Hamilton BE, Sutton PD *et al.* Births: final data for 2005. *National Vital Statistics Reports* 2007;**56**:1–103.

16 Cordero L, Anderson CW, and Zuspan FP. Scalp abscess: a benign and infrequent complication of fetal monitoring. *American Journal of Obstetrics & Gynecology* 1983;**146**:126–130.

17 American College of Obstetricians and Gynecologists Practice Bulletin No. 106: Intrapartum fetal heart rate monitoring: nomenclature, interpretation, and general management principles. *Obstetrics & Gynecology* 2009;**114**:192–202.

18 Macones GA, Hankins GD, Spong CY, Hauth J, and Moore T. The 2008 National Institute of Child Health and Human Development workshop report on electronic fetal monitoring: update on definitions, interpretation, and research guidelines. *Obstetrics & Gynecology* 2008;**112**:661–666.

19 Soper DE, Mayhall CG, and Dalton HP. Risk factors for intraamniotic infection: a prospective epidemiologic study. *American Journal of Obstetrics & Gynecology* 1989;**161**:562–566; discussion 6–8.

20 Caldeyro-Barcia R and Poseiro JJ. Oxytocin and contractility of the pregnant human uterus. *Annals of the New York Academy of Sciences* 1959;**75**:813–830.

21 Krapohl AJ, Myers GG, and Caldeyro-Barcia R. Uterine contractions in spontaneous labor. A quantitative study. *American Journal of Obstetrics & Gynecology* 1970;**106**:378–387.

22 Hauth JC, Hankins GD, Gilstrap LC, III, Strickland DM, and Vance P. Uterine contraction pressures with oxytocin induction/augmentation. *Obstetrics & Gynecology* 1986;**68**: 305–309.

23 Hauth JC, Hankins GD, and Gilstrap LC, III. Uterine contraction pressures achieved in parturients with active phase arrest. *Obstetrics & Gynecology* 1991;**78**:344–347.

24 American College of Obstetricians and Gynecologists, Gynecology Committee on Practice B-O Practice Bulletin No. 49, December 2003: Dystocia and augmentation of labor. *Obstetrics & Gynecology* 2003;**102**:1445–1454.

25 Zhang J, Troendle JF, and Yancey MK. Reassessing the labor curve in nulliparous women. *American Journal of Obstetrics & Gynecology* 2002;**187**:824–828.

26 Zhang J, Landy HJ, Branch DW *et al.* Contemporary patterns of spontaneous labor with normal neonatal outcomes. *Obstetrics & Gynecology* 2010;**116**:1281–1287.

27 Zhang J, Troendle J, Mikolajczyk R, Sundaram R, Beaver J, and Fraser W. The natural history of the normal first stage of labor. *Obstetrics & Gynecology* 2010;**115**:705–710.

28 American College of Obstetricians and Gynecologists Practice Bulletin No. 116: Management of intrapartum fetal heart rate tracings. *Obstetrics & Gynecology* 2010;**116**:1232–1240.

29 Stewart RD, Bleich AT, Lo JY, Alexander JM, McIntire DD, and Leveno KJ. Defining uterine tachysystole: how much is too much? *American Journal of Obstetrics & Gynecology* 2012;**207**: 290 e1–6.

30 Higgins SD and Garite TJ. Late abruptio placenta in trauma patients: implications for monitoring. *Obstetrics & Gynecology* 1984;**63**:10S–2S.

31 Ito M, Kawasaki N, Matsui K, and Fujisaki S. Fetal heart monitoring and ultrasound in the management of placental abruption. *International Journal of Gynecology & Obstetrics* 1986;**24**:269–273.

32 Pearlman MD, Klinich KD, Schneider LW, Rupp J, Moss S, and Ashton-Miller J. A comprehensive program to improve safety for pregnant women and fetuses in motor vehicle crashes: a preliminary report. *American Journal of Obstetrics & Gynecology* 2000;**182**:1554–1564.

33 American College of Obstetricians and Gynecologists Practice Bulletin No. 115: Vaginal birth after previous cesarean delivery. *Obstetrics & Gynecology* 2010;**116**:450–463.

34 Kanda E, Matsuda Y, Kamitomo M, Maeda T, Mihara K, and Hatae M. Prenatal diagnosis and management of vasa previa: a 6-year review. *Journal of Obstetrics and Gynaecology Research* 2011;**37**:1391–1396.

35 Petrikovsky BM and Vintzileos AM. Magnesium sulfate and intrapartum fetal behavior. *American Journal of Perinatology* 1990;**7**:154–156.

36 Duffy CR, Odibo AO, Roehl KA, Macones GA, and Cahill AG. Effect of magnesium sulfate on fetal heart rate patterns in the second stage of labor. *Obstetrics & Gynecology* 2012;**119**: 1129–1136.

37 Clark SL, Gimovsky ML, and Miller FC. Fetal heart rate response to scalp blood sampling. *American Journal of Obstetrics & Gynecology* 1982;**144**:706–708.

38 Spencer JA. Predictive value of a fetal heart rate acceleration at the time of fetal blood sampling in labour. *Journal of Perinatal Medicine* 1991;**19**:207–215.

39 Lazebnik N, Neuman MR, Lysikiewicz A, Dierker LR, and Mann LI. Response of fetal heart rate to scalp stimulation related to fetal acid-base status. *American Journal of Perinatology* 1992;**9**:228–232.

40 Clark SL, Gimovsky ML, and Miller FC. The scalp stimulation test: a clinical alternative to fetal scalp blood sampling. *American Journal of Obstetrics & Gynecology* 1984;**148**:274–277.

41 Elimian A, Figueroa R, and Tejani N. Intrapartum assessment of fetal well-being: a comparison of scalp stimulation with scalp blood pH sampling. *Obstetrics & Gynecology* 1997;**89**:373–376.

42 Smith CV, Nguyen HN, Phelan JP, and Paul RH. Intrapartum assessment of fetal well-being: a comparison of fetal acoustic stimulation with acid-base determinations. *American Journal of Obstetrics & Gynecology* 1986;**155**:726–728.

43 Polzin GB, Blakemore KJ, Petrie RH, and Amon E. Fetal vibro-acoustic stimulation: magnitude and duration of fetal heart rate accelerations as a marker of fetal health. *Obstetrics & Gynecology* 1988;**72**:621–626.

44 Ingemarsson I and Arulkumaran S. Reactive fetal heart rate response to vibroacoustic stimulation in fetuses with low scalp blood pH. *BJOG* 1989;**96**:562–565.

45 Skupski DW, Rosenberg CR, and Eglinton GS. Intrapartum fetal stimulation tests: a meta-analysis. *Obstetrics & Gynecology* 2002;**99**:129–134.

46 Gabbe SG, Ettinger BB, Freeman RK, and Martin CB. Umbilical cord compression associated with amniotomy: laboratory observations. *American Journal of Obstetrics & Gynecology* 1976; **126**:353–355.

47 Miyazaki FS and Taylor NA. Saline amnioinfusion for relief of variable or prolonged decelerations. A preliminary report. *American Journal of Obstetrics & Gynecology* 1983;**146**: 670–678.

48 Miyazaki FS and Nevarez F. Saline amnioinfusion for relief of repetitive variable decelerations: a prospective randomized study. *American Journal of Obstetrics & Gynecology* 1985;**153**: 301–306.

49 Strong TH Jr, Hetzler G, Sarno AP, and Paul RH. Prophylactic intrapartum amnioinfusion: a randomized clinical trial. *American Journal of Obstetrics & Gynecology* 1990;**162**:1370–1374; discussion 4–5.

50 MacGregor SN, Banzhaf WC, Silver RK, and Depp R. A prospective, randomized evaluation of intrapartum amnioinfusion. Fetal acid-base status and cesarean delivery. *Journal of Reproductive Medicine* 1991;**36**:69–73.

51 Owen J, Henson BV, and Hauth JC. A prospective randomized study of saline solution amnioinfusion. *American Journal of Obstetrics & Gynecology* 1990;**162**:1146–1149.

52 Macri CJ, Schrimmer DB, Leung A, Greenspoon JS, and Paul RH. Prophylactic amnioinfusion improves outcome of pregnancy complicated by thick meconium and oligohydramnios. *American Journal of Obstetrics & Gynecology* 1992;**167**:117–121.

53 Hofmeyr GJ and Lawrie TA. Amnioinfusion for potential or suspected umbilical cord compression in labour. *Cochrane Database of Systematic Reviews* 2012;(1):CD000013.
54 Rinehart BK, Terrone DA, Barrow JH, Isler CM, Barrilleaux PS, and Roberts WE. Randomized trial of intermittent or continuous amnioinfusion for variable decelerations. *Obstetrics & Gynecology* 2000;**96**:571–574.
55 Puder KS, Sorokin Y, Bottoms SF, Hallak M, and Cotton DB. Amnioinfusion: does the choice of solution adversely affect neonatal electrolyte balance? *Obstetrics & Gynecology* 1994;**84**:956–959.
56 Egarter CH, Husslein PW, and Rayburn WF. Uterine hyperstimulation after low-dose prostaglandin E2 therapy: tocolytic treatment in 181 cases. *American Journal of Obstetrics & Gynecology* 1990;**163**:794–796.
57 Valenzuela GJ and Foster TC. Use of magnesium sulfate to treat hyperstimulation in term labor. *Obstetrics & Gynecology* 1990;**75**:762–764.
58 Pacheco LD, Rosen MP, Gei AF, Saade GR, and Hankins GD. Management of uterine hyperstimulation with concomitant use of oxytocin and terbutaline. *American Journal of Perinatology* 2006;**23**:377–380.
59 Buhimschi CS, Buhimschi IA, Malinow AM, and Weiner CP. Effects of sublingual nitroglycerin on human uterine contractility during the active phase of labor. *American Journal of Obstetrics & Gynecology* 2002;**187**:235–238.
60 de Heus R, Mulder EJ, Derks JB, and Visser GH. Acute tocolysis for uterine activity reduction in term labor: a review. *Obstetrical and Gynecological Survey* 2008;**63**:383–388; quiz 405.
61 Kulier R and Hofmeyr GJ. Tocolytics for suspected intrapartum fetal distress. *Cochrane Database of Systematic Reviews* 2000;CD000035.
62 Gilstrap LC, III, Hauth JC, Hankins GD, and Beck AW. Second-stage fetal heart rate abnormalities and type of neonatal acidemia. *Obstetrics & Gynecology* 1987;**70**:191–195.
63 Agrawal SK, Doucette F, Gratton R, Richardson B, and Gagnon R. Intrapartum computerized fetal heart rate parameters and metabolic acidosis at birth. *Obstetrics & Gynecology* 2003;**102**:731–738.
64 Larma JD, Silva AM, Holcroft CJ, Thompson RE, Donohue PK, and Graham EM. Intrapartum electronic fetal heart rate monitoring and the identification of metabolic acidosis and hypoxic-ischemic encephalopathy. *American Journal of Obstetrics & Gynecology* 2007;**197**: 301 e1–8.
65 Low JA, Victory R, and Derrick EJ. Predictive value of electronic fetal monitoring for intrapartum fetal asphyxia with metabolic acidosis. *Obstetrics & Gynecology* 1999;**93**:285–291.
66 Sameshima H, Ikenoue T, Ikeda T, Kamitomo M, and Ibara S. Unselected low-risk pregnancies and the effect of continuous intrapartum fetal heart rate monitoring on umbilical blood gases and cerebral palsy. *American Journal of Obstetrics & Gynecology* 2004;**190**:118–123.
67 Sameshima H, Ikenoue T, Ikeda T, Kamitomo M, and Ibara S. Association of nonreassuring fetal heart rate patterns and subsequent cerebral palsy in pregnancies with intrauterine bacterial infection. *American Journal of Perinatology* 2005;**22**:181–187.
68 Williams KP and Galerneau F. Fetal heart rate parameters predictive of neonatal outcome in the presence of a prolonged deceleration. *Obstetrics & Gynecology* 2002;**100**:951–954.
69 Williams KP and Galerneau F. Intrapartum fetal heart rate patterns in the prediction of neonatal acidemia. *American Journal of Obstetrics & Gynecology* 2003;**188**:820–823.
70 Cahill AG, Roehl KA, Odibo AO, and Macones GA. Association and prediction of neonatal acidemia. *American Journal of Obstetrics & Gynecology* 2012;**207**:206 e1–8.
71 Hill JB, Alexander JM, Sharma SK, McIntire DD, and Leveno KJ. A comparison of the effects of epidural and meperidine analgesia during labor on fetal heart rate. *Obstetrics & Gynecology* 2003;**102**:333–337.
72 Zimmer EZ, Divon MY, and Vadasz A. Influence of meperidine on fetal movements and heart rate beat-to-beat variability in the active phase of labor. *American Journal of Perinatology* 1988;**5**:197–200.

73 Kopecky EA, Ryan ML, Barrett JF *et al.* Fetal response to maternally administered morphine. *American Journal of Obstetrics & Gynecology* 2000;**183**:424–430.
74 Poehlmann S, Pinette M, and Stubblefield P. Effect of labor analgesia with nalbuphine hydrochloride on fetal response to vibroacoustic stimulation. *Journal of Reproductive Medicine* 1995;**40**:707–710.
75 Mawaldi L, Duminy P, and Tamim H. Terbutaline versus nifedipine for prolongation of pregnancy in patients with preterm labor. *International Journal of Gynecology & Obstetrics* 2008;**100**:65–68.
76 Roth AC, Milsom I, Forssman L, Ekman LG, and Hedner T. Effects of intravenous terbutaline on maternal circulation and fetal heart activity. *Acta Obstetricia et Gynecologica Scandinavica* 1990;**69**:223–228.
77 Blackwell SC, Sahai A, Hassan SS *et al.* Effects of intrapartum zidovudine therapy on fetal heart rate parameters in women with human immunodeficiency virus infection. *Fetal Diagnosis and Therapy* 2001;**16**:413–416.
78 Stallworth JC, Yeh SY, and Petrie RH. The effect of magnesium sulfate on fetal heart rate variability and uterine activity. *American Journal of Obstetrics & Gynecology* 1981;**140**: 702–706.
79 Kruger K, Hallberg B, Blennow M, Kublickas M, and Westgren M. Predictive value of fetal scalp blood lactate concentration and pH as markers of neurologic disability. *American Journal of Obstetrics & Gynecology* 1999;**181**:1072–1078.
80 Westgren M, Kruger K, Ek S *et al.* Lactate compared with pH analysis at fetal scalp blood sampling: a prospective randomised study. *BJOG* 1998;**105**:29–33.
81 Allen RM, Bowling FG, and Oats JJ. Determining the fetal scalp lactate level that indicates the need for intervention in labour. *Australian and New Zealand Journal of Obstetrics and Gynaecology* 2004;**44**:549–552.
82 Garite TJ, Dildy GA, McNamara H *et al.* A multicenter controlled trial of fetal pulse oximetry in the intrapartum management of nonreassuring fetal heart rate patterns. *American Journal of Obstetrics & Gynecology* 2000;**183**:1049–1058.
83 East CE, Brennecke SP, King JF, Chan FY, and Colditz PB, Group FS. The effect of intrapartum fetal pulse oximetry, in the presence of a nonreassuring fetal heart rate pattern, on operative delivery rates: a multicenter, randomized, controlled trial (the FOREMOST trial). *American Journal of Obstetrics & Gynecology* 2006;**194**:606 e1–16.
84 Klauser CK, Christensen EE, Chauhan SP *et al.* Use of fetal pulse oximetry among high-risk women in labor: a randomized clinical trial. *American Journal of Obstetrics & Gynecology* 2005;**192**:1810–1817; discussion 7–9.
85 Bloom SL, Spong CY, Thom E *et al.* Fetal pulse oximetry and cesarean delivery. *New England Journal of Medicine* 2006;**355**:2195–2202.
86 Westgate J, Harris M, Curnow JS, and Greene KR. Plymouth randomized trial of cardiotocogram only versus ST waveform plus cardiotocogram for intrapartum monitoring in 2400 cases. *American Journal of Obstetrics & Gynecology* 1993;**169**:1151–1160.
87 Amer-Wahlin I, Hellsten C, Noren H *et al.* Cardiotocography only versus cardiotocography plus ST analysis of fetal electrocardiogram for intrapartum fetal monitoring: a Swedish randomised controlled trial. *Lancet* 2001;**358**:534–538.
88 Dervaitis KL, Poole M, Schmidt G, Penava D, Natale R, and Gagnon R. ST segment analysis of the fetal electrocardiogram plus electronic fetal heart rate monitoring in labor and its relationship to umbilical cord arterial blood gases. *American Journal of Obstetrics & Gynecology* 2004;**191**:879–884.
89 Ojala K, Vaarasmaki M, Makikallio K, Valkama M, and Tekay A. A comparison of intrapartum automated fetal electrocardiography and conventional cardiotocography – a randomised controlled study. *BJOG: An International Journal of Obstetrics and Gynaecology* 2006;**113**: 419–423.

90 Vayssiere C, David E, Meyer N *et al.* A French randomized controlled trial of ST-segment analysis in a population with abnormal cardiotocograms during labor. *American Journal of Obstetrics & Gynecology* 2007;**197**:299 e1–6.
91 Potti S and Berghella V. ST waveform analysis versus cardiotocography alone for intrapartum fetal monitoring: a meta-analysis of randomized trials. *American Journal of Perinatology* 2012;**29**:657–664.
92 Becker JH, Bax L, Amer-Wahlin I *et al.* ST analysis of the fetal electrocardiogram in intrapartum fetal monitoring: a meta-analysis. *Obstetrics & Gynecology* 2012;**119**:145–154.
93 Neilson JP. Fetal electrocardiogram (ECG) for fetal monitoring during labour. *Cochrane Database of Systematic Reviews* 2012;(4):CD000116.

CHAPTER 6
Operative vaginal delivery

Katherine R. Goetzinger and George A. Macones
Department of Obstetrics and Gynecology, Washington University School of Medicine, St Louis, MO, USA

6.1 Introduction

Operative vaginal delivery is defined as a vaginal delivery achieved by the placement of direct traction on the presenting fetal part with either forceps or a vacuum extractor. The first use of forceps to achieve vaginal delivery of a live infant has been credited to Peter Chamberlin in the 1600s; however, obstetric forceps were not popularized until the 18th century. Since that time, they have undergone many modifications and reinventions, and to date, over 700 types of obstetrical forceps have been described [1]. The concept of a vacuum extractor was originally described by James Yonge in 1705 when he used a cupping glass to assist with vaginal delivery. Malmstrom, however, has been credited with the introduction of the vacuum extractor into modern obstetrics in the early 1950s. Since that time, the vacuum extractor has largely replaced forceps in Europe [2,3].

In contrast to the upward-climbing trend of cesarean section rates in the United States, the rate of operative vaginal delivery has been steadily declining since the mid-1990s. In 2009, the overall rate of operative vaginal delivery was 3.7% (3.0% vacuum deliveries; 0.7% forceps deliveries). This represents a 61% decrease in operative vaginal deliveries since 1995 when the overall incidence of operative vaginal delivery was 9.4% [4]. Controversy regarding maternal and neonatal safety has likely driven this decline; however, the American College of Obstetrics and Gynecology (ACOG) continues to endorse the safety of these instruments in appropriate circumstances [5]. This chapter aims to review the current indications and contraindications for operative delivery, the technical aspects of operative delivery, and the controversy and current evidence surrounding maternal and neonatal safety.

Management of Labor and Delivery, Second Edition. Edited by George A. Macones.

6.2 Indications, contraindications, and prerequisites for operative vaginal delivery

While no indication is absolute, ACOG has recognized a finite number of both maternal and fetal indications that warrant consideration for operative vaginal delivery [5]. These indications are identical for both forceps and vacuum deliveries:

- suspicion of immediate fetal compromise such as in the setting of a non-reassuring fetal heart tracing
- prolonged second stage of labor
- shortening of the second stage for maternal benefit (i.e. such as in the setting of maternal cardiovascular or cerebrovascular disease).

There are few absolute contraindications to operative vaginal delivery. Operative vaginal delivery should be avoided in cases of fetal bleeding disorders such as neonatal alloimmune thrombocytopenia, hemophilia, and von Willebrand's disease, as well as in cases of fetal bone demineralization disorders such as osteogenesis imperfecta and other skeletal dysplasias. Given the potential for a break in the fetal skin barrier with the use of either forceps or vacuum, operative vaginal deliveries are relatively contraindicated in cases of maternal infection such as human immunodeficiency virus (HIV) and hepatitis B and C [6]. Vacuum delivery also is typically avoided in gestations under 34 weeks given the risk for fetal intraventricular hemorrhage; however, forceps deliveries can be safely pursued in gestations under 34 weeks [5]. While vaginal delivery for breech presentation is typically contraindicated in modern obstetric practice, forceps designed for the delivery of the aftercoming head (i.e. Piper forceps) may still be used in experienced hands, especially in the case of breech extraction of the second twin and difficult breech extractions during cesarean sections [1]. In contrast, vacuum extractors are absolutely contraindicated for all nonvertex fetal presentations. Finally, a perceived low likelihood of success of operative vaginal delivery is another relative contraindication. In a 1999 study using data from a California birth registry, Towner and colleagues demonstrated that the risk of intracranial hemorrhage, neonatal convulsions, and requirement for mechanical ventilation was significantly higher in patients undergoing cesarean delivery following a failed operative vaginal delivery attempt compared to the risk of these events observed in patients undergoing spontaneous labor, successful operative vaginal delivery, and cesarean section during labor [7]. Although likelihood of success is a qualitative measure, in the setting of provider concern for cephalopelvic disproportionate and/or limited fetal descent with maternal expulsive efforts, operative vaginal delivery should only be attempted with caution.

Prior to attempting operative vaginal delivery, the fetal head must be engaged in the pelvis, membranes ruptured, and the cervix completely dilated. Additionally, the maternal pelvis should be evaluated for adequacy. Knowledge of fetal presentation, position, lie, and any degree of asynclitism is essential for proper instrument placement and for determination of the proper vector of traction. Operative delivery should be performed with the patient in the dorsal lithotomy position with adequate anesthesia. The bladder should also be drained immediately prior to instrument placement. Given that the only recourse of a failed operative vaginal delivery is cesarean section, operative vaginal delivery only should be attempted in settings where immediate surgical access is feasible.

6.3 Classification system for operative vaginal delivery

Prior to 1988, classification of operative vaginal delivery was based on fetal station described using a scale of 0 to +3. In 1988, ACOG issued a new classification system which divided operative vaginal deliveries into categories of outlet, low, and mid based on fetal station defined as 0–5 cm at or below the level of the maternal ischial spines as well as the degree of rotation. High forceps were no longer included as part of this revised classification system. Table 6.1 displays current criteria for the classification of operative vaginal delivery. This reclassification system was driven by the premise that there is less maternal and fetal risk associated with operative vaginal delivery the lower the fetal head and the less rotation required. This premise and the current ACOG classification scheme have since been validated [8].

Table 6.1 ACOG classification of types of forceps delivery.

Outlet forceps
Scalp is visible at the introitus without separating the labia.
The fetal head has reached the pelvic floor.
The sagittal suture is in anteroposterior diameter or right or left occiput anterior or posterior.
The fetal head is at or on perineum.
Rotation does not exceed 45 degrees.
Low forceps
The leading point of the fetal skull is at ≥ +2 cm station and not on the pelvic floor.
Rotation is 45 degrees or less (left or right occiput anterior to occiput anterior, or left or right occiput posterior to occiput posterior).
Rotation is greater than 45 degrees.
Midforceps
Station is above +2 but head is engaged.
High forceps
Not included in this classification system.

Source: American College of Obstetricians and Gynecologists Practice Bulletin No. 17: Operative vaginal delivery [10]. Reproduced with permission of American College of Obstetricians and Gynecologists.

6.4 Technical aspects of operative vaginal delivery

6.4.1 Forceps

At their most basic level, classical forceps consist of two blades which are each connected to a handle by a shank. The angle at which the blade connects with the shank on the outer side is known as the pelvic curve, corresponding to the curve of the maternal pelvis; whereas, the inner curve of the blade is known as the cephalic curve, corresponding to the curve of the fetal head. Blades can be solid, fenestrated, or pseudo-fenestrated; whereas, the shanks may be overlapping or parallel [1]. These different designs make each type of forceps advantageous for different clinical circumstances (Figures 6.1a and b). For example, overlapping shanks tend to distend the perineum less compared to parallel shanks. In addition, pseudo-fenestrated blades more readily accommodate a fetal head with caput succedaneum and molding. As previously mentioned, over 700 types of forceps have been described; however, there currently exist no randomized controlled trials (RCTs) comparing different types of forceps. While the choice of forceps type is often subjective and based on provider experience and preference, the technical principles of application and traction remain similar.

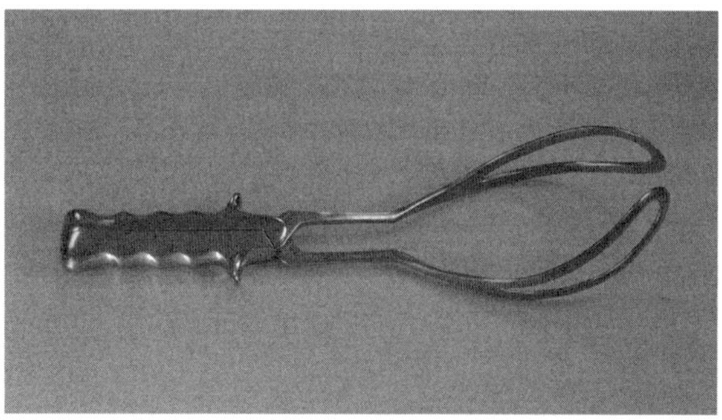

Figure 6.1a Simpson forceps demonstrating fenestrated blades and parallel shanks.

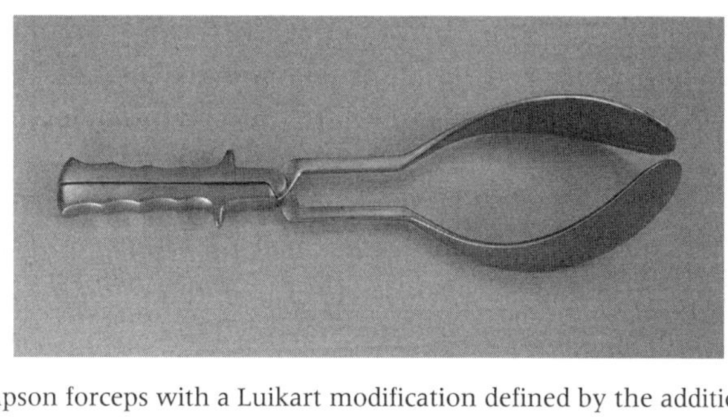

Figure 6.1b Simpson forceps with a Luikart modification defined by the addition of pseudo-fenestrated blades.

Prior to blade placement, the forceps should be positioned, articulated, and de-articulated in order to ensure appropriate function and pairing of the blades. This is often known as a "ghost application." Typically, the left blade is applied first when the sagittal suture lies in the anteroposterior diameter. The left handle is gently grasped by the operator's left thumb and first finger. The operator's right hand is then placed into the left posterior portion of the patient's vagina beside the fetal head. The left blade is then gently slid around the curvature of the fetal head along the palmar surface of the operator's right hand. A similar process is then repeated for the right blade while an assistant holds the left blade in place. Alternatively, when the sagittal suture lies in the oblique diameter (i.e. right occiput anterior [ROA]), the posterior blade is always placed first, providing a cradle for the fetal head to prevent rotation during subsequent blade placement. Application should be such that the blades are evenly placed around the fetal head, therefore allowing the pressure to be evenly distributed with traction. With proper placement, the blades should extend beyond the fetal malar eminences and symmetrically cover the area between the fetal orbit and ear, known as the bimalar biparietal application. Once the blades are successfully placed, the handles are then articulated. Correct placement is checked by ensuring that the sagittal suture runs perpendicular and is equidistant to the plane of the shanks for occiput anterior (OA) position. For occiput posterior (OP) positions, the blades should be equidistant from the midline of the fetal face. No more than a fingertip should be able to be placed between the forceps blade and the fetal head. When correctly placed, the blades should articulate easily. Abnormal blade application such as the common "brow-mastoid" placement typically do not allow for easy articulation and result in slipping of the blades from the fetal head during traction attempts [1,9].

In cases of ROA or LOA position, the fetal head should first be rotated to a direct OA position prior to applying traction. Once this is achieved, traction is applied with one hand grasping the shanks and the other hand grasping the handles. Traction force is applied in a plane which is perpendicular to the plane of the pelvis. As the head descends, the line of traction must then follow the curve of the sacrum and then continue upward through the pelvic outlet. In cases of OP positions, a horizontal force of traction must be maintained until the base of the fetal nose emerges from under the pubic symphysis. The amount of traction force applied should be the least possible to achieve fetal descent. Traction should be steady, coinciding with contraction activity. Progressive descent of the fetal head should be observed with each traction attempt. Once the fetal head is crowning, the blades are disarticulated and removed in the reverse order from that in which they were placed [1,9]. Removal of the blades prior to delivery decreases the risk of deep perineal lacerations [10]. Delivery of the fetal head is then completed, allowing for natural restitution, followed by delivery of the anterior shoulder.

A description of application and traction techniques for specialized forceps, such as Piper forceps for the aftercoming fetal head and Kielland rotational mid-forceps, are beyond the scope of this chapter. As mentioned previously, the use of Piper forceps has virtually become obsolete given that vaginal breech delivery is rarely practiced in modern obstetrics. There is conflicting data regarding maternal and neonatal outcomes following midforceps rotational deliveries with Kielland forceps; however, long-term data seem to suggest no late adverse effects [11–15]. It is important to note that these studies varied widely in their selection of control groups and most were published prior to the reclassification of forceps in 1988. ACOG currently recommends that mid-rotational forceps deliveries be limited to operators with a high level of training in this procedure [5].

6.4.2 Vacuum extraction

The vacuum extractor is comprised of three basic elements: (1) a cup which is applied to the fetal head, (2) a traction device, and (3) tubing which connects the cup and traction device. The vacuum extractor originally described by Malmstrom was comprised of a metal cup; however, this metal cup has largely been replaced by more pliable, soft cups. Hofmeyr and colleagues previously demonstrated that higher traction forces are generated with the rigid, metal cup compared to the soft cup [16]. Consistent with these results, a recent Cochrane review and meta-analysis demonstrated that the metal cup was more likely to result in a successful vaginal delivery compared to the soft cup (RR 1.63, 95% CI 1.17–2.28). However, this same review also demonstrated a higher risk for neonatal cephalohematoma and scalp trauma when using a metal cup [17]. Currently, the two most common vacuum extractors used in the United States include the Kiwi® OmniCup (Clinical Innovations, Murray, Utah) and the Mityvac® (Cooper Surgical, Trumball, Connecticut) (Figure 6.2). Both have a soft cup; however, the Mityvac pump is

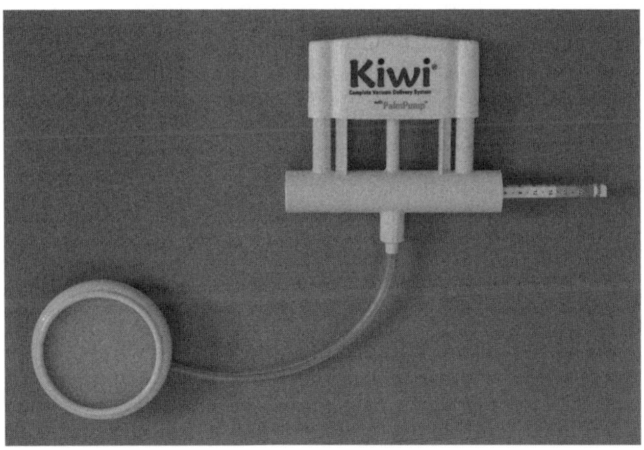

Figure 6.2 Kiwi® OmniCup vacuum extractor: Soft cup with handheld pump designed for single operator use.

operated by an assistant while the operator provides traction; whereas, the Kiwi OmniCup is a handheld device controlled by a single operator.

The vacuum cup is applied along the line of the sagittal suture approximately 3 cm anterior to the posterior fontanelle. Prior to initiating the vacuum, the entire circumference of the cup should be palpated to evaluate for entrapment of maternal soft tissue. Traction vectors are similar to those of forceps, with traction forces ranging between 0.6 and 0.8 kg/cm^2 often quoted as the optimal level of pressure [2]. Traction attempts should be coordinated with maternal expulsive efforts, and manual torque should be avoided in order to minimize the risk of fetal scalp lacerations. There currently is no consensus on the appropriate number of pulls, number of vacuum detachments, or total length of the procedure; however, one study has reported a 28% incidence of neonatal cephalohematoma when the application-to-delivery time exceeded 5 minutes [18]. The vacuum pressure may be either released between traction efforts or maintained throughout the procedure. In a randomized trial, Bofill and colleagues demonstrated that there was no statistically significant difference in maternal or fetal outcomes whether the level of vacuum pressure was decreased between pulls or maintained throughout the procedure [19]. Some argue that continuing the vacuum between contractions may aid in maintaining the gained progress in descent of the fetal head. As with forceps deliveries, progressive fetal descent should be observed with each pull, or abandonment of the procedure should be considered.

6.5 Effectiveness of operative vaginal delivery

There have been multiple studies in the literature comparing forceps delivery to vacuum extraction in terms of rates of maternal morbidity, neonatal morbidity, and effectiveness. It has been hypothesized that forceps are likely to be more effective than vacuum extractors due to the ability of the operator to apply greater force during traction attempts. An early study by Dell and colleagues supported this hypothesis by randomizing 118 patients either to forceps, the silastic vacuum, or the Mityvac vacuum. This study showed a statistically significant increased success rate of forceps (93.3%) compared to the Silastic cup vacuum extractor (72.2%) and the Mityvac (89.2%); however, this study included only primiparous patients and was conducted prior to the 1988 ACOG reclassification system [20]. Two large RCTs have since demonstrated equivalent success rates of vacuum extractors and forceps but have included rotational forceps as well as a variety of different vacuum cups and, therefore, may not be reflective of modern practice [21,22]. Pooling results from the literature, a recent Cochrane review revealed that use of forceps was associated with a 35% decrease in failure of successful vaginal delivery compared to vacuum extraction (RR 0.65, 95% CI 0.45–0.94) [17].

Several authors have attempted to identify maternal and fetal risk factors associated with failed operative vaginal delivery. In a population-based case–control study, Gopalani and colleagues observed that failed operative vaginal delivery was associated with increased maternal age, African American race, higher body mass index (BMI), diabetes, polyhydramnios, induction of labor, dysfunctional labor, and prolonged labor. Patients who failed operative vaginal delivery were also more likely to deliver a low-birthweight infant or a macrosomic infant [23]. In 2007, Ben-Haroush and colleagues published a retrospective cohort study of 83,351 deliveries, of which 5120 (6.1%) were operative vaginal deliveries. The overall failure rate in this study was 8.6% and was significantly more common in vacuum deliveries compared with forceps deliveries (10.0% vs 1.3%, $p < 0.001$). Furthermore, these authors observed that persistent OP fetal head position, absence of anesthesia, and birthweight > 4000 g were independent predictors of a failed operative vaginal delivery [24]. This study highlights the necessity of accurate estimation of fetal weight and evaluation of fetal head position in the selection of appropriate candidates for a trial of operative vaginal delivery.

6.6 Maternal morbidity

It has been well established that forceps deliveries are associated with a higher incidence of maternal perineal trauma compared to vacuum deliveries [21,22,25,26]. In the RCT by Bofill and colleagues, a higher incidence of episiotomy and third- and fourth-degree perineal lacerations was observed with forceps deliveries compared to vacuum. No significant difference in total blood loss or postpartum hemoglobin level was observed [18]. Alternatively, Weerasekera and Premaratne observed no difference in the incidence of third-degree lacerations when comparing forceps to vacuum; however, forceps were associated with a significant increase in cervical lacerations in this study [27]. More recently, Caughey and colleagues performed a large retrospective cohort study comparing 2075 forceps deliveries to 2045 vacuum deliveries. Using multivariate logistic regression analysis, this study demonstrated that delivery by forceps was independently associated with an increased risk for vaginal lacerations (aOR 1.77, 95% CI 1.49–2.11) and third- and fourth-degree perineal lacerations (aOR 1.79, 95% CI 1.52–2.10). Of note, these findings were significant only in primiparous patients. The authors postulated that the downward vector produced with forceps may selectively lead to a greater degree of perineal trauma in primiparous patients compared to multiparous patients [25]. Finally, Baumann and colleagues evaluated the outcomes 40,923 primiparous patients who delivered at term and found that forceps delivery was the factor most strongly associated with anal sphincter laceration (OR 2.68, 95% CI 2.17–3.33) [28]. A summary of studies comparing forceps and vacuum in relation to risk of maternal perineal trauma is shown in Table 6.2.

Table 6.2 Forceps delivery versus vacuum delivery: risk of maternal perineal trauma.

Authors	Year	Design	Injury	Forceps (%)	Vacuum (%)	*p*-value
Johanson *et al.* [21]	1993	RCT	Anal sphincter damage	8.0	5.0	0.15
			Significant vaginal injury	17.0	11.0	0.03
Bofill *et al.* [22]	1996	RCT	Third-degree laceration	21.3	9.6	<0.001
			Fourth-degree laceration	7.3	2.2	0.002
Weerasekera & Premaratne [27]	2002	RCT	Third-degree laceration	1.7	0.9	>0.05
			Cervical laceration	5.0	0.9	0.01
Johnson *et al.* [26]	2004	Retrospective cohort	Third-degree laceration	33.0	23.7	0.03
			Fourth-degree laceration	11.5	4.2	0.003
			Periurethral laceration	0.5	4.2	0.026
Caughey *et al.* [25]	2005	Retrospective cohort	Third- or fourth-degree laceration	36.9	26.8	<0.001
			Vaginal laceration	28.6	22.2	<0.001
			Cervical laceration	3.0	1.5	0.001

Factors that may impact the risk for perineal trauma with operative vaginal delivery have also been evaluated. A retrospective cohort study of 588 forceps-assisted vaginal deliveries demonstrated a threefold increase in risk for third- and fourth-degree perineal lacerations with an OP fetal head position compared to an OA fetal head position [29]. Additionally, the use of midline episiotomy with forceps deliveries has also been found to increase the risk of anal sphincter disruption [30]. Results regarding the use of mediolateral episiotomy with operative vaginal delivery remain conflicting. Hudelist and colleagues demonstrated that routine use of mediolateral episiotomy combined with forceps delivery was significantly associated with severe perineal trauma (OR 5.62, 95% CI 2.16–14.62) [31]. In contrast, de Leeuw and colleagues found that mediolateral episiotomy was significantly protective for anal sphincter injury in both forceps (OR 0.08, 95% CI 0.07–0.11) and vacuum (OR 0.11, 95% CI 00.7–0.11) deliveries. This same study also demonstrated that both primiparity and OP fetal head position were significantly associated with anal sphincter injury, consistent with the results of other authors [32].

It can be argued that the most appropriate comparison of maternal morbidity should be between operative vaginal delivery and cesarean section during the second stage of labor. In a 2001 cohort study, Murphy and colleagues observed an increased incidence of blood loss > 1 liter (aOR 2.82, 95% CI 1.10–7.62) and hospital stay ≥ 6 days (aOR 3.47, 95% CI 1.58–7.62) in those patients who underwent cesarean section during the second stage of labor compared to operative vaginal delivery. Furthermore, they observed no difference in adverse maternal outcome when comparing immediate cesarean delivery during the second stage to cesarean delivery following failed operative delivery attempt [33].

6.7 Pelvic floor dysfunction after operative vaginal delivery

Given the increased risk for anal sphincter injury with operative vaginal delivery, many studies have attempted to evaluate the risk of subsequent pelvic floor dysfunction following operative vaginal delivery. Pelvic floor dysfunction leading to anal incontinence is hypothesized to occur both through direct injury to the anal sphincter and through injury to the pudendal nerve. Multiple observational studies have demonstrated no increase in anal incontinence following operative vaginal delivery compared to spontaneous vaginal delivery [34–37]. However, in a prospective randomized trial comparing forceps delivery to vacuum delivery, the rate of fecal incontinence was significantly higher in those delivered by forceps compared to vacuum (59% vs 33%; RR 2.88, 95% CI 1.41–5.88) [38]. Long-term follow-up studies are few and present conflicting results. A six-year follow-up study demonstrated a significantly increased risk of fecal incontinence after a first delivery by forceps. Additionally, this study also found no protective effect of cesarean section on fecal incontinence [39]. Alternatively, Bollard and colleagues found no significant increase, after 34 years of follow-up, in anal incontinence in patients who underwent forceps delivery [40].

Although these studies are conflicting regarding symptoms of anal incontinence, a deleterious trend toward occult integrity of the anal sphincter has been consistently shown following operative vaginal delivery. Using anal endosonography, Sultan and colleagues demonstrated that 80% of women who underwent forceps delivery had a defect involving at least one of the anal sphincter muscles. Forceps delivery was found to be a significant risk factor for both external and internal anal sphincter defects in multivariate analysis. This study also demonstrated that there was a significant association between any anal sphincter defect and subsequent anal incontinence [41]. Johanson and colleagues observed similar results, citing an 82% incidence of occult sphincter defects following forceps deliveries and a 48% incidence following vacuum deliveries [21]. In 2008, Mahony and colleagues published a case–control study to evaluate the effect of a second vaginal delivery on anal function of patients who underwent a forceps delivery during their first pregnancy. Patients who delivered by forceps in their first pregnancy were more likely to have abnormal endoanal ultrasound and manometry results compared to controls. While there was no difference in anal incontinence between the first and second deliveries comparing the forceps group to controls, 26% of women with abnormal endoanal ultrasound results after their first forceps delivery developed new or worsening incontinence symptoms after their second delivery [42]. It possible that in some circumstances, anal incontinence following operative vaginal delivery may be caused by a "two-hit hypothesis," in which the first operative delivery causes occult anal sphincter injury and the second vaginal delivery further exacerbates this injury leading to overt symptoms.

Urinary incontinence also remains a concern following operative vaginal delivery, occurring in up to 50% of women [43]. Delivery by forceps as well as episiotomy have been shown to increase this risk [34,37]. In a prospective cohort study of women who underwent spontaneous delivery, forceps delivery, and vacuum delivery, the incidence of new-onset urinary incontinence ranged from 12 to 13% and was not significantly different between the three groups. However, at one-year follow-up, both the incidence and the severity of stress urinary incontinence were highest in the forceps group compared to spontaneous and vacuum deliveries [44]. Although the risk of urinary incontinence is increased following vaginal delivery, cesarean delivery has not been shown to completely ameliorate this risk [45]. Liebling and colleagues performed a prospective cohort study comparing women who required operative vaginal delivery to those who had a cesarean section during the second stage of labor. The incidence of any urinary incontinence was significantly higher in the operative vaginal delivery group compared to the cesarean section group at both 6 weeks and 1 year [46]. This increased risk persisted at 3 years as well in a follow-up study [47]. The mechanism of injury remains unclear; however, both bladder neck hypermobility and descent of the bladder neck position at rest have been demonstrated using perineal ultrasound following forceps delivery [48]. While some neuronal injury likely occurs with perineal stretch at the time of complete cervical dilation, compression of the pudendal nerve by the forceps blade with subsequent denervation of the urinary sphincter muscle may contribute to the increased incidence of incontinence observed following forceps delivery.

6.8 Neonatal morbidity

In contrast to maternal morbidity, vacuum deliveries have classically been associated with higher rates of neonatal morbidity compared to forceps deliveries. Multiple RCTs have demonstrated an increased incidence of neonatal cephalohematoma following vacuum delivery compared with forceps delivery [21,22,27]. Bofill and colleagues observed a 37% incidence of cephalohematoma in neonates delivered by vacuum compared to a 19% incidence in those delivered by forceps ($p = 0.015$); however, no statistically significant difference in the incidence of hyperbilirubinemia was observed between the two groups [22]. A large observational study confirmed these findings noting a decreased risk of cephalohematoma with forceps compared to vacuum (aOR 0.25, 95% CI 0.19–0.33); although, this study also demonstrated an increased incidence of neonatal jaundice in the vacuum delivery group. Additionally, this study showed no significant difference in umbilical artery cord gas values between the two groups; however, there was an increased incidence of 5-minute Apgar scores < 7 and neonatal intensive care unit (NICU) admission in the vacuum group [25]. Caput succedaneum and molding as well as neonatal scalp trauma have also been observed more frequently in vacuum deliveries compared to forceps [22,49,50]. Vacuum application lasting longer than 10 minutes has been associated with an increased rate of scalp injury [50]. Finally, Bofill and colleagues observed a trend toward an increased incidence of shoulder dystocia with vacuum compared to forceps delivery ($p = 0.052$), although this study was underpowered to evaluate this outcome [22]. It may initially seem intuitive that forceps would actually be associated with a higher risk of shoulder dystocia given the ability to pull harder with forceps compared to a vacuum. However, Caughey and colleagues proposed that the vector of force during an operative delivery likely contributes more to shoulder dystocia than the magnitude of force. The direct attachment site of the vacuum to the posterior fontanelle produces a vector which is 45 degrees to the floor. This vector may actually produce more traction on the fetal head and pull the anterior shoulder into the pubic symphysis, resulting in a shoulder dystocia. This association was confirmed in his large observational study in which a decreased risk of shoulder dystocia was observed in patients who delivered by forceps compared to vacuum (aOR 0.34, 95% CI 0.20–0.57) [25]. A summary of the current literature evaluating risks of neonatal morbidities when comparing forceps and vacuum is shown in Table 6.3.

Neonatal hemorrhage has been a major concern associated with vacuum deliveries. It has been estimated that the incidence of subgaleal hematomas following vacuum extraction ranges from 26 to 45 per 1000 vacuum deliveries [5]. In a population-based historic cohort study of 305,391 mother-infant dyads, vacuum delivery was associated with an increased risk of subarachnoid hemorrhage (aOR 5.44, 95% CI 1.26–23.43) compared to forceps delivery. No difference in the incidence of intracranial, subdural, or intraventricular hemorrhage was observed between the two groups [51]. In addition, Williams and colleagues observed moderate to severe retinal hemorrhage in 28% of vacuum deliveries compared to 13% of forceps deliveries. Vacuum delivery among small-for-gestational-age infants was closely correlated to increasing degree of severity of the hemorrhage. It is important to note that moderate to severe retinal hemorrhage was also observed in 18% of normal spontaneous vaginal deliveries in this study [52]. In 2007, Simonson and colleagues systematically screened a cohort

Table 6.3 Forceps delivery versus vacuum delivery: neonatal trauma.

Author	Cephalohematoma	Scalp injury	Facial injury/ bruising	Shoulder dystocia	5-minute Apgar < 7	NICU Admission
Broekhuizen 1987[49]	No difference	↑Vacuum	---	↑Vacuum	---	---
Johanson 1993 [21]	↑Vacuum	No difference	No difference	---	No difference	---
Bofill 1996 [22]	↑Vacuum	No difference	---	No difference	---	---
Weerasekera 2002 [26]	↑Vacuum	---	---	---	---	No difference
Johnson 2004 [27]	↑Vacuum	---	↑Forceps		No difference	No difference
Caughey 2005 [25]	↑Vacuum	---	↑Forceps	↑Vacuum	↑Vacuum	↑Vacuum

---, outcome not evaluated.

of 1123 attempted vacuum deliveries using transfontanellar ultrasonography and skull X ray. Cephalohematoma was present in 10.8% of patients, and skull fracture was present in 5.0% of cases, all of which were asymptomatic and did not require therapy. Intracranial hemorrhage occurred in eight patients, of whom seven were asymptomatic. No subgaleal hemorrhages were diagnosed in this cohort. Factors associated with these adverse complications included nulliparity, mid-station vacuum attempt, an extraction requiring more than three traction attempts, and dislodgement of the vacuum cup [53]. Overall, these adverse events were rare, with the majority being incidental findings detected by systematic radiologic screening.

In response to a growing concern over the perceived, serious neonatal morbidity and mortality associated with vacuum delivery, the United States Food and Drug Administration (FDA) issued a Public Health Advisory in 1998 regarding the need for caution when using this instrument [54]. This advisory was based on 12 neonatal deaths and nine serious neonatal injuries which occurred following vacuum delivery over the preceding 4-year period. The FDA cited the following four main recommendations for the use of the vacuum device.

1 Use only when a specific obstetric indication is present.
2 Apply steady traction in the line of the birth canal. Avoid rocking movements or applying torque to the device.
3 Alert those who will be responsible for the neonate's care after delivery.
4 Report reactions associated with the use of the vacuum device to the FDA.

In response to this advisory, ACOG issued a committee opinion during that same year strongly recommending the continued use of vacuum devices by trained practitioners in appropriate clinical circumstances. In this document,

ACOG supported its recommendation by citing the extreme rarity of adverse events (~1 per 45,455 vacuum extractions per year). ACOG also cited concerns that cesarean rates, as well as forceps use by unskilled practitioners, may rise if vacuum delivery were to be abandoned [55].

Although less common, forceps have also been associated with adverse neonatal outcomes. Instrument bruising, corneal abrasions, external ocular trauma, and facial nerve palsy are more common following forceps delivery compared to vacuum delivery [21,25,26,56]. Facial nerve palsy caused by forceps is usually mild and does not require treatment [57]. Long-term ophthalmologic sequelae are rare [56].

6.9 Long-term neonatal outcomes

Although limited, the current evidence suggests no long-term adverse effects for children delivered by vacuum or forceps. Carmody and colleagues assessed babies at the age of 9 months who were randomly assigned to either vacuum or forceps delivery. That study noted no difference in head circumference, weight, hearing, or vision between the two groups [58]. Similarly, Ngan and colleagues found no difference in scholastic performance, speech, self-care ability, or neurologic abnormalities at 10-year follow-up in children delivered by vacuum extraction compared to spontaneous vaginal delivery [59]. To date, the longest follow-up study evaluated 52,282 infants born between 1964 and 1972 in Jerusalem. These children underwent a physical examination and intelligence test at the age of 17. After adjusting for multiple confounders, no difference in mean intelligence score was found in those delivered by vacuum or forceps compared to those delivered spontaneously [60]. In 2007, Bahl and colleagues published a prospective cohort study evaluating the neurodevelopmental outcome of children at 5 years of age delivered by operative vaginal delivery compared to cesarean section in the second stage of labor, an arguably more appropriate comparison group. There was no statistically significant difference in the rates of neurodevelopmental morbidity between the groups. In fact, there were only two cases of significant neurodevelopmental morbidity, both of which were attributed to events unrelated to mode of delivery [61].

6.10 Mode of delivery: sequential instruments versus cesarean section

Given that cesarean section is the only alternative option to operative vaginal delivery, some investigators have attempted to compare neonatal outcomes between operative vaginal delivery and cesarean delivery during the second stage of labor. In a secondary analysis of a *Eunice Kennedy Shriver* National

Institute of Child Health and Human Development–sponsored RCT evaluating fetal pulse oximetry in labor, investigators found no significant differences in umbilical artery cord gas values or Apgar scores among forceps, vacuum, and cesarean deliveries [62]. Other studies have evaluated the effect of various modes of delivery on neonatal outcomes. A large California birth registry study of 583,340 nulliparous patients demonstrated overall low rates of intracranial hemorrhage for all modes of delivery; however, these rates were higher with vacuum, forceps, and cesarean delivery performed during labor compared to spontaneous vaginal deliveries. There was no difference in the risk of intracranial hemorrhage when comparing spontaneous vaginal deliveries to cesarean sections performed *without* labor. This led to the hypothesis that the position of the fetal head in the maternal pelvis during these protracted labors may be an individual risk factor for intracranial hemorrhage since this adverse neonatal outcome was also observed at a higher frequency with cesarean delivery during the second stage. This increased risk of neonatal morbidity may be attributed to the abnormal labor process itself rather than to the instrument used. Most notably in this study, Towner and colleagues also observed an incremental increased risk of intracranial hemorrhage when more than one method of delivery was used (i.e. failed vacuum followed by forceps; failed forceps followed by cesarean delivery). For example, intracranial hemorrhage after failed vacuum delivery followed by successful forceps occurred at a rate that was 7.4 times higher than the spontaneous vaginal delivery rate and 3.4 times higher than the vacuum delivery rate alone [7] (Table 6.4). More recent observational studies have also evaluated neonatal morbidity associated with sequential use of instruments for operative vaginal delivery. Murphy and colleagues observed an increased incidence of third- and fourth-degree perineal lacerations (aOR 2.1, 95% CI 1.2–3.3) and umbilical artery pH values < 7.1 (aOR 3.3, 95% CI 1.7–6.2) when sequential instruments were used compared to a single instrument [63]. Bhide and colleagues compared neonatal morbidity in infants delivered by cesarean section following failed vacuum extraction (n = 85) to infants delivered

Table 6.4 Rate of intracranial hemorrhage by mode of delivery.

Mode of delivery	Rate of intracranial hemorrhage
Spontaneous vaginal delivery	1 in 1900
Cesarean section without labor	1 in 2750
Vacuum extraction	1 in 860
Forceps delivery	1 in 664
Cesarean section with labor and no attempt at operative vaginal delivery	1 in 954
Cesarean section following failed operative delivery	1 in 334
Sequential instruments	1 in 256

Data from Towner *et al.* [7].

by forceps following failed vacuum extraction (n = 257). Results from this study revealed an increased risk of third-degree perineal lacerations when forceps were sequentially used following failed vacuum; however, an increased risk of postpartum hemorrhage was observed with cesarean delivery following failed vacuum. No difference in neonatal morbidity was observed [64]. ACOG currently recommends against the sequential use of instruments to achieve a successful operative vaginal delivery "unless there is a compelling and justifiable reason" [5].

6.11 Subsequent pregnancy outcomes following operative vaginal delivery

There exists a paucity of data regarding patient preference and success rate of mode of delivery in subsequent pregnancies following operative vaginal delivery. In a study comparing primigravidas who underwent mid-cavity operative vaginal delivery versus those who delivered spontaneously, Kadar and Romero observed no significant difference in the incidence of subsequent childbearing between the two groups; however, they did observe an increased incidence of operative vaginal delivery for the indication of cephalopelvic disproportion in those who had an operative vaginal delivery in a previous pregnancy compared to a spontaneous vaginal delivery (11.2% vs 5.0%; $p < 0.005$). Despite this, over 75% of those patients who underwent operative vaginal delivery in their first pregnancy and who delivered a heavier baby in their second pregnancy did so spontaneously [65]. Murphy and colleagues polled a cohort of 393 patients who had an operative vaginal delivery or cesarean section during the second stage of labor. At the time of hospital discharge, over 53% of patients desired to have a future pregnancy, with no significant difference noted between patients who had an operative vaginal compared to a cesarean delivery. However, patients who had an operative vaginal delivery were more likely to prefer a future vaginal delivery than those who delivered by cesarean section (aOR 4.5, 95% CI 2.2–9.2). Although the proportion of patients desiring vaginal delivery did decrease over time, the finding remained statistically significant at 1 year following the index delivery (aOR 3.6, 95% CI 1.6–8.1). Notably, there was no significant difference in patient preference for future mode of delivery in those who delivered by cesarean section following failed operative delivery and those who delivered by immediate cesarean section [66]. In a 3-year follow-up of this same cohort, women who experienced an operative vaginal delivery were more likely to have achieved a subsequent pregnancy than those who delivered by cesarean section (aOR 2.1, 95% CI 1.1–4.3). These women were also more likely to aim for and achieve a successful vaginal delivery if they had experienced a prior operative vaginal delivery (Table 6.5). Of those women who did not desire a future pregnancy, 46% stated that they "could not go through childbirth again."

Table 6.5 Maternal outcomes and preferences regarding subsequent pregnancy following delivery during the second stage of labor by operative vaginal delivery compared to cesarean delivery.

Outcome	Operative vaginal delivery (%)	Cesarean delivery (%)	aOR (95% CI)
	Prior to hospital discharge		
Intention to have a subsequent pregnancy	51	54	1.28 (0.23–6.70)
Desire for future vaginal delivery	79	39	5.50* (2.33–9.01)
	Six weeks after delivery		
Intention to have a subsequent pregnancy	52	53	1.13 (0.20–6.50)
Desire for future vaginal delivery	65	42	3.42* (1.59–7.49)
	One year after delivery		
Intention to have a subsequent pregnancy	55	62	0.61 (0.12–3.23)
Desire for future vaginal delivery	68	42	3.43* (1.42–8.27)
	Three years after delivery		
Achieved a planned subsequent pregnancy	79	67	2.09* (1.10–4.28)
Achieved vaginal delivery for subsequent pregnancy	78	31	9.50* (3.48–25.97)

* Indicates statistically significant finding.
Data from Murphy & Liebling, 2003 [66]; Bahl, Strachan, & Murphy, 2004 [67].

There was no significant difference in this response when comparing patients who underwent operative vaginal delivery to those who underwent cesarean delivery [67].

6.12 The future of operative vaginal delivery

With the declining trend in both forceps and vacuum deliveries, the number of clinicians who are skilled in the use of these instruments has also decreased. This lack of skilled providers has a strong impact on residency training in operative vaginal delivery. In a 1996 survey of North American residency programs, the rate of operative vaginal delivery was 10% or less. Forceps were the primary instrument used in 68% of programs while the vacuum was the preferred instrument in approximately one-third of programs [68]. In a 2007 survey of chief residents, > 90% of residents felt competent to perform vacuum deliveries; whereas, almost half did not feel competent to perform forceps deliveries.

When asked which instrument they would use in practice, only 18.2% of respondents reported that they would predominantly use forceps compared to 48.7% who would predominantly use the vacuum [69].

Over 20% of cesarean deliveries for labor dystocia occur in the second stage of labor [70]. It is possible that many of these could be prevented by more liberal use of operative vaginal delivery. In 2007, Shaffer and Caughey made a call for continued training of obstetricians in the art of operative vaginal delivery, specifically forceps deliveries, in an effort to decrease the primary cesarean section rate [71]. One prior study has shown a positive impact on the amount of resident forceps experience by designating a single, proactive faculty member who is skilled in the use of this instrument to resident teaching on the labor and delivery unit [72]. Additionally, the use of birth simulators to teach proper forceps blade placement has shown promise [73,74]. Finally, it has been shown that formal education and training programs have the potential to improve both maternal and neonatal morbidity associated with operative vaginal delivery [75]. Continued efforts to increase resident exposure and training in both forceps and vacuum deliveries are necessary to ensure that operative vaginal delivery does not become a dying art.

6.13 Conclusion

Operative vaginal delivery continues to have a role in modern obstetric practice. Both forceps and vacuum extractors are acceptable and safe instruments to achieve a successful vaginal delivery. Operator skill and preference should continue to guide decision making regarding which instrument to use. Additionally, maternal and neonatal risks and benefits must be weighed, as well as the risk of failed vaginal delivery, prior to choosing an instrument. With the rising cesarean delivery rate, continued efforts to train clinicians to be skilled in operative vaginal delivery are warranted so that all available modes of delivery can be considered when appropriate during the second stage of labor.

References

1 Dennen PC. *Forceps Deliveries*. 4th edn. Philadelphia, PA: FA Davis Company, 2001.
2 Lucas MJ. The role of vacuum extraction in modern obstetrics. *Clinical Obstetrics and Gynecology* 1994;**37**(4):794–805.
3 Chalmers JA. *The Ventouse: The Obstetric Vacuum Extractor*. Chicago, IL: Year Book Publishers, 1971.
4 Martin JA, Hamilton BE, Ventura SJ *et al.* Births: final data for 2009. *National Vital Statistics Reports* 2011;**60**(1):1–72.
5 American College of Obstetricians and Gynecologists Practice Bulletin No.17: Operative vaginal delivery. Washington, DC: ACOG, 2000.

6 Duff P, Sweet RL, and Edwards RK. Maternal and fetal infections. In: Creasy RK, Resnik R, Iams JD, Lockwood CJ, and Moore TR (eds) *Maternal-Fetal Medicine Principles and Practice*, 6th edn. Saunders Elsevier: Philadelphia, PA, 2009: 739–796.
7 Towner D, Castro MA, Eby-Wilkens E, and Gilbert WM. Effect of mode of delivery in nulliparous women on neonatal intracranial injury. *New England Journal of Medicine* 1999;**341**:1709–1714.
8 Hagadorn-Freathy AS, Yeomans ER, and Hankins GD. Validation of the 1988 ACOG forceps classification system. *Obstetrics & Gynecology* 1991;**77**:356–360.
9 Forceps Delivery and Vacuum Extraction. In: Cunningham FG, Leveno KJ, Bloom SL, Hauth JC, Rouse DJ, and Spong CY (eds) *Williams Obstetrics*, 23rd edn. The McGraw Hill Companies, Inc., 2010: 511–526.
10 Yeomans ER. Operative vaginal delivery. *Obstetrics & Gynecology* 2010;**115**(3):645–653.
11 Bashore RA, Phillips WH Jr, and Brinkman CR, III. A comparison of the morbidity of midforceps and cesarean delivery. *American Journal of Obstetrics & Gynecology* 1990;**162**:1428–1434.
12 Healy DL, Quinn MA, and Pepperell RJ. Rotational delivery of the fetus: Kielland's forceps and two other methods compared. *BJOG* 1982;**89**:501–506.
13 Chiswick ML and James DK. Kielland's forceps: an association with neonatal morbidity and mortality. *BMJ* 1979;**1**:7–9.
14 Robertson PA, Laros RK, and Zhao RL. Neonatal and maternal outcome in low-pelvic and mid-pelvic operative deliveries. *American Journal of Obstetrics & Gynecology* 1990;**162**:1436.
15 Nilsen ST. Boys born by forceps and vacuum extraction examined at 18 years of age. *Acta Obstetricia et Gynecologica Scandinavica* 1984;**63**:549–554.
16 Hofmeyr GJ, Gobitz L, Sonnendecker EW, and Turner MJ. New design rigid and soft vacuum extractor cups: a preliminary comparison of traction forces. *BJOG* 1990;**97**(8):681–685.
17 O'Mahony F, Hofmeyr GJ, and Menon V. Choice of instruments for assisted vaginal delivery. *Cochrane Database of Systematic Reviews* 2010;(**11**):CD005455.
18 Bofill JA, Rust OA, Devidas M, Roberts WE, Morrison JC, and Martin JN Jr. Neonatal cephalohematoma from vacuum extraction. *Journal of Reproductive Medicine* 1997;**42**:565–569.
19 Bofill JA, Rust OA, Schorr SJ, Brown RC, Roberts WE, and Morrison JC. A randomized trial of two vacuum extraction techniques. *Obstetrics & Gynecology* 1997;**89**:758–762.
20 Dell DL, Sightler SE, and Plauche WC. Soft cup vacuum extraction: a comparison of outlet delivery. *Obstetrics & Gynecology* 1985;**66**(5):624–628.
21 Johanson RB, Rice C, Doyle M *et al.* A randomized prospective study comparing the new vacuum extractor policy with forceps delivery. *BJOG* 1993;**100**:524–530.
22 Bofill JA, Rust OA, Schorr SJ et al. A randomized prospective trial of the obstetric forceps versus the M-cup vacuum extractor. *American Journal of Obstetrics & Gynecology* 1996;**175**(5):1325–1330.
23 Gopalani S, Bennett K, and Critchlow C. Factors predictive of failed operative delivery. *American Journal of Obstetrics & Gynecology* 2004;**191**:896–902.
24 Ben-Haroush A, Melamed N, Kaplan B, and Yogev Y. Predictors of failed operative vaginal delivery: a single-center experience. *American Journal of Obstetrics & Gynecology* 2007;**197**:308e1–e5.
25 Caughey AB, Sandberg PL, Zlatnik MG, Thiet MP, Parer JT, and Laros RK Jr. Forceps compared with vacuum: Rates of neonatal and maternal morbidity. *Obstetrics & Gynecology* 2005;**106**(5):908–912.
26 Johnson JH, Figueroa R, Garry D, Elimian A, and Maulik D. Immediate maternal and neonatal effects of forceps and vacuum-assisted deliveries. *Obstetrics & Gynecology* 2004;**103**(3):513–518.
27 Weerasekera DS and Premaratne S. A randomized prospective trial of obstetric forceps versus vacuum extraction using defined criteria. *Journal of Obstetrics and Gynaecology* 2002;**22**(4):344–345.

28 Baumann P, Hammoud AO, McNeely SG, DeRose E, Kudish B, and Hendrix S. Factors associated with anal sphincter laceration in 40,923 primiparous women. *International Urogynecology Journal – Pelvic Floor Dysfunction* 2007;**18**(9):985–990.

29 Benavides L, Wu JM, Hundley AF, Ivester TS, and Visco AG. The impact of occiput posterior fetal head position on the risk of anal sphincter injury in forceps-assisted vaginal deliveries. *American Journal of Obstetrics & Gynecology* 2005;**192**:1702–1706.

30 Kudish B, Blackwell S, Mcneeley G *et al.* Operative vaginal delivery and midline episiotomy: a bad combination for the perineum. *American Journal of Obstetrics & Gynecology* 2006;**195**:749–754.

31 Hudelist G, Gellen, J, Singer C *et al.* Factors predicting severe perineal trauma during childbirth: role of forceps delivery combined with mediolateral episiotomy. *American Journal of Obstetrics & Gynecology* 2005;**192**:875–881.

32 de Leeuw JW, de Wit C, Kuijken JPJA, and Bruinse HW. Mediolateral episiotomy reduces the risk for anal sphincter injury during operative vaginal delivery. *BJOG* 2008;**115**:104–108.

33 Murphy DJ, Liebling RE, Verity L, Swingler R, and Patel R. Early maternal and neonatal morbidity associated with operative delivery in second stage of labour: a cohort study. *Lancet* 2001;**358**;1203–1207.

34 Baydock SA, Flood C, and Shulz JA. Prevalence and risk factors for urinary and fecal incontinence four months after vaginal delivery. *Journal of Obstetrics and Gynaecology Canada* 2009;**31**(1):36–41.

35 Meyer S, Hohlfeld P, Achtari C, Russolo A, and De Grandi P. Birth trauma: short and long term effects of forceps delivery compared with spontaneous delivery on various pelvic floor parameters. *BJOG* 2000;**107**:1360–1365.

36 Schraffordt Koops SE, Vervest HA, and Oostvogel HJ. Anorectal symptoms after various modes of vaginal delivery. *International Urogynecology Journal – Pelvic Floor Dysfunction* 2003;**14**(4):244–249.

37 Casey BM, Schaffer JI, Bloom SL, Heartwell SF, McIntire DD, and Leveno KJ. Obstetric antecedents for postpartum pelvic floor dysfunction. *American Journal of Obstetrics & Gynecology* 2005;**192**:1655–1662.

38 Fitzpatrick M, Beyan M, O'Connell R, and O'Herlihy C. Randomised clinical trial to assess anal sphincter dysfunction following forceps or vacuum assisted vaginal delivery. *BJOG* 2003;**110**:424–429.

39 Macarthur C, Glazener C, Lancashire R, Herbison P, Wilson D, and Grant A. Faecal incontinence and mode of first and subsequent delivery: a six-year longitudinal study. *BJOG* 2005;**112**(8):1075–1082.

40 Bollard RC, Gardiner A, Duthie GS, and Lindow SW. Anal sphincter injury, fecal and urinary incontinence: a 34-year follow-up after forceps delivery. *Diseases of the Colon & Rectum* 2003;**46**(8):1083–1088.

41 Sultan AH, Kamm MA, Nudson CN, Thomas JM, and Bartram CI. Anal-sphincter disruption during vaginal delivery. *New England Journal of Medicine* 1993;**329**(26):1905–1911.

42 Mahony R, Behan M, O'Connell PR, and O'Herlihy C. Effect of second vaginal delivery on anal function in patients at risk of occult anal sphincter injury after first forceps delivery. *Diseases of the Colon & Rectum* 2008;**51**(9):1361–1366.

43 Johanson RB, Heylock E, Carter J, Sultan AH, Walklate K, and Jones PW. Maternal and child health after assisted vaginal delivery: five-year follow-up of a randomized controlled study comparing forceps and ventouse. *BJOG* 1999;**106**(6):544–549.

44 Arya LA, Jackson ND, Myers DL, and Verma A. Risk of new-onset urinary incontinence after forceps and vacuum delivery in primiparous women. *American Journal of Obstetrics & Gynecology* 2001;**185**(6):1318–1323.

45 Rortveit G, Dalveit AK, Hannestad YS, and Hunskaar S. Norwegian EPINCONT study. Urinary incontinence after vaginal delivery or cesarean section. *New England Journal of Medicine* 2003;**348**(10):900–907.

46 Liebling RE, Swingler R, Patel RR, Verity L, Soothill PW, and Murphy DL. Pelvic floor morbidity up to one year after difficult instrumental delivery and cesarean section in the second stage of labor: a cohort study. *American Journal of Obstetrics & Gynecology* 2004;**191**:4–10.

47 Bahl R, Strachan B, and Murphy DL. Pelvic floor morbidity at 3 years after instrumental delivery and cesarean delivery in the second stage of labor and the impact of a subsequent delivery. *American Journal of Obstetrics & Gynecology* 2005;**192**:789–794.

48 Meyer S, Schreyer A, De Grandi P, and Hohlfeld P. The effect of birth on urinary continence mechanisms and other pelvic-floor characteristics. *Obstetrics & Gynecology* 1998;**92**:613–618.

49 Broekhuizen FF, Washington JM, Johnson F, and Hamilton PR. Vacuum extraction versus forceps delivery: Indications and complications, 1979 to 1984. *Obstetrics & Gynecology* 1987;**69**(3):338–342.

50 Teng FY and Sayre JW. Vacuum extraction: does duration predict scalp injury? *Obstetrics & Gynecology* 1997;**89**(2):281–285.

51 Wen SW, Liu S, Kramer MS *et al.* Comparison of maternal and infant outcomes between vacuum extraction and forceps deliveries. *American Journal of Epidemiology* 2001;**153**:103–107.

52 Williams MC, Knuppel RA, O'Brien WF, Weiss A, Spellacy WN, and Pietrantoni M. Obstetric correlates of neonatal retinal hemorrhage. *Obstetrics & Gynecology* 1993;**81**(5):688–694.

53 Simonson C, Barlow P, Dehennin N *et al.* Neonatal complications of vacuum-assisted delivery. *Obstetrics & Gynecology* 2007;**109**(3):626–633.

54 Centers for Devices and Radiological Health: FDA Public Health Advisory: need for caution when using vacuum assisted delivery devices. May 21, 1998.

55 American College of Obstetricians and Gynecologists Committee Opinion No. 208: Delivery by vacuum extraction. Washington, DC: ACOG, 1998.

56 Holden R, Morsman DG, Davidek GM, O'Connor GM, Coles EC, and Dawson AJ. External ocular trauma in instrumental and normal deliveries. *BJOG* 1992;**99**:132–134.

57 Duval M and Daniel SJ. Facial nerve palsy in neonates secondary to forceps use. *Archives of Otolaryngology – Head and Neck Surgery* 2009;**135**(7):634–636.

58 Carmody F, Grant A, Mutch L, Vacca A, and Chalmers I. Follow-up of babies delivered in a randomized controlled comparison of vacuum extraction and forceps delivery. *Acta Obstetricia et Gynecologica Scandinavica* 1986;**65**:763–766.

59 Ngan HY, Miu P, Ko L, and Mah HD. Long-term neurological sequelae following vacuum extractor delivery. *Australian and New Zealand Journal of Obstetrics and Gynaecology* 1990;**30**:111–114.

60 Seidman DS, Laor A, Gale R, Stevenson DK, Mashliach S, and Danon YL. Long-term effects of vacuum and forceps deliveries. *Lancet* 1991;**337**:1583–1585.

61 Bahl R, Patel RR, Swingler R, Ellis M, and Murphy DJ. Neurodevelopmental outcome at 5 years after operative delivery in the second stage of labor: a cohort study. *American Journal of Obstetrics & Gynecology* 2007;**197**:147 e1–6.

62 Contag SA, Clifton RG, Bloom SL *et al.* Neonatal outcomes and operative vaginal delivery versus cesarean delivery. *American Journal of Perinatology* 2010;**27**:493–499.

63 Murphy DJ, Macleod M, Bahl R, and Strachan B. A cohort study of maternal and neonatal morbidity in relation to use of sequential instruments at operative vaginal delivery. *European Journal of Obstetrics & Gynecology and Reproductive Biology* 2011;**156**:41–45.

64 Bhide A, Guven M, Prefumo F, Vankalayapati P, and Thilaganathan B. Maternal and neonatal outcome after failed ventouse delivery: comparison of forceps and cesarean section. *Journal of Maternal-Fetal and Neonatal Medicine* 2007;**20**(7):541–545.

65 Kadar N and Romero R. Prognosis for future childbearing after mid-cavity instrumental deliveries in primigravidas. *Obstetrics & Gynecology* 1983;**62**:166–170.

66 Murphy DL and Liebling RE. Cohort study of maternal views on future mode of delivery after operative delivery in the second stage of labor. *American Journal of Obstetrics & Gynecology* 2003;**188**(2):542–548.

67 Bahl R, Strachan B, and Murphy DL. Outcome of subsequent pregnancy three years after previous operative vaginal delivery in the second stage of labour: a cohort study. *BMJ* 2004;**328**(7435):311.

68 Bofill JA, Rust OA, Perry KG Jr, Roberts WE, Martin RW, and Morrison JC. Forceps and vacuum delivery: a survey of North American residency programs. *Obstetrics & Gynecology* 1996;**88**(4 Pt 1):622–625.

69 Powell J, Gilo N, Foote M, Gil K, and Lavin JP. Vacuum and forceps training in residency: experience and self-reported competency. *Journal of Perinatology* 2007;**27**:343–346.

70 Gifford DS, Morton SC, Fiske M, Keesey J, Keeler E, and Kahn KL. Lack of progress in labor as a reason for cesarean. *Obstetrics & Gynecology* 2000;**95**:589–595.

71 Shaffer BL and Caughey AB. Forceps delivery: potential benefits and a call for continued training. *Journal of Perinatology* 2007;**27**:327–328.

72 Solt I, Jackson S, Moore T, Rotmensch S, and Kim MJ. Teaching forceps: the impact of proactive faculty. *American Journal of Obstetrics & Gynecology* 2011;**204**:448 e1–4.

73 Dupuis O, Moreau R, Pham MT, and Redarce T. Assessment of forceps blade orientations during their placement using an instrumented childbirth simulator. *BJOG* 2009;**119**:327–333.

74 Dupuis O, Decullier E, Clerc J *et al.* Does forceps training on a birth simulator allow obstetricians to improve forceps blade placement? *European Journal of Obstetrics & Gynecology and Reproductive Biology* 2011;**159**:305–309.

75 Cheong YC, Abdullahi H, Lashen H, and Fairlie FM. Can formal education and training improve the outcome of instrumental delivery? *European Journal of Obstetrics & Gynecology and Reproductive Biology* 2004;**113**:139–144.

CHAPTER 7
Cesarean delivery

Methodius G. Tuuli and Molly J. Stout
Department of Obstetrics and Gynecology, Washington University in St Louis, St Louis, MO, USA

7.1 Introduction

Cesarean delivery is the most common major surgical procedure performed on women worldwide. In the United States, nearly 1 in 3 (1.3 million) of the 4 million deliveries annually are by cesarean [1]. Despite the frequency of this procedure, the techniques used have been largely dictated by tradition rather than firm evidence. However, data continues to accumulate on various aspects of cesarean delivery. In this chapter we review the steps of cesarean delivery, with emphasis on evidence-based techniques aimed at reducing morbidity and improving efficiency. We then review postoperative care and considerations for cesarean under special circumstances.

7.2 Cesarean technique

7.2.1 Skin antisepsis

Infectious morbidity is one of the most common complications, affecting 2–20% of cesareans, depending on the population [2]. Because the skin is a major source of organisms responsible for postcesarean wound infection, it is plausible that preoperative skin preparation will reduce wound infection. However, the best type of antiseptic and technique for skin antisepsis at cesarean is unclear. The two most common antiseptics are iodine and chlorhexidine-based solution, usually combined with alcohol and applied in a scrub-and-paint or paint-only fashion. To date, there have been two underpowered trials comparing different antiseptics at cesarean, yielding no significant differences in efficacy. A large multicenter trial and a subsequent meta-analysis in nonobstetric patients

Management of Labor and Delivery, Second Edition. Edited by George A. Macones.

suggested superiority of chlorhexidine alcohol over povidone iodine for surgical antisepsis [3,4]. In contrast, data from before-and-after studies in obstetric patients have yielded mixed results [5–7]. One recent study suggested that scrub-and-paint might be superior to painting alone with iodine [8]. Until results of ongoing large randomized trials provide data to guide clinical practice, both iodine and chlorhexidine-based preparations are acceptable for skin antisepsis at cesarean.

7.2.2 Antibiotic prophylaxis

Antibiotic prophylaxis is the most studied aspect of cesarean delivery. The most recent Cochrane review of 86 studies involving over 13,000 women found that prophylactic antibiotics in women undergoing cesarean substantially reduced the incidence of wound infection (RR 0.39, 95% CI 0.32–0.48), endometritis (RR 0.38, 95% CI 0.34–0.42), and serious maternal infectious complications (RR 0.31, 95% CI 0.19–0.48) [9]. The findings were similar whether the cesarean was elective or non-elective. A meta-analysis of six trials showed that preoperative administration, rather than intraoperative administration (after cord clamp), was associated with a further significant decrease in endometritis and a non-significant reduction in wound infections [10]. There were no differences in neonatal outcomes including neonatal sepsis, sepsis work-up, and neonatal intensive care unit admission, although the studies were not powered to detect differences in neonatal outcomes. Broadening prophylactic antiobiotic coverage may also be beneficial in reducing postcesarean infection [11]. Tita *et al.* found that addition of Azithromycin to the standard first- or second-generation cephalosporins reduced the risk of postoperative endometritis campared with the cephalosporins alone [12]. Results of an ongoing multicenter trial will clarify the role of broading the prophylactic antibiotic spectrum at cesarean. Taken together, the evidence indicates that prophylactic antibiotics should be administered prior to skin incision at cesarean delivery.

7.2.3 Skin Incision and subcutaneous tissue

Transverse skin incision is the most commonly used approach (Figure 7.1). The Pfannenstiel incision is made approximately two fingerbreadths above the symphysis pubis and curved gently upward at the lateral margins. The Joel-Cohen incision consists of a straight skin incision made 3 cm below the anterior superior iliac spines, slightly higher than the location of the Pfannenstiel incision. When compared to a vertical midline incision, a transverse skin incision is associated with less postoperative pain and improved cosmesis [13,14]. The size of the skin incision should be judicious, but adequate to facilitate atraumatic delivery of the fetus. A midline vertical skin incision may be the preferred method for some surgeons in emergent cases. While the vertical approach has been traditionally considered a faster abdominal entry, the predominant use of the transverse incision in modern cesarean suggests most obstetricians may

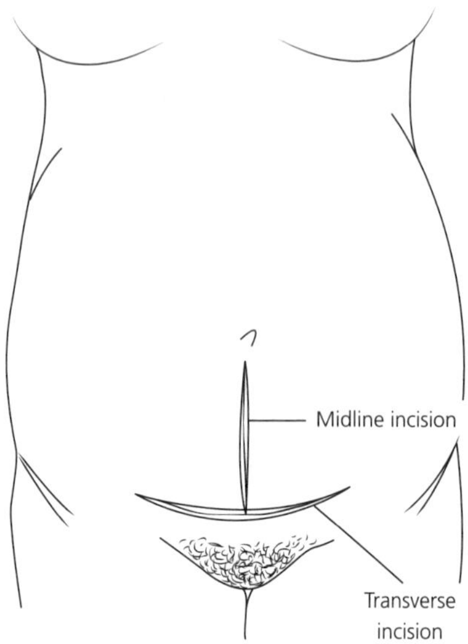

Figure 7.1 Vertical midline and transverse skin incision at cesarean delivery.

prefer this approach even in emergent situations [15]. Importantly, a vertical incision should be considered when additional abdominal exploration is anticipated, as a vertical incision can be extended superiorly to facilitate examination of the mid and upper abdomen.

The subcutaneous tissue can be dissected bluntly or sharply using either the scalpel or electrocautery. Blunt dissection to clear subcutaneous adipose tissue from the underlying rectus fascia may be preferable when possible, to reduce bleeding. There is no evidence to suggest superiority of scalpel compared to electrosurgical techniques for the subcutaneous tissue, and either may be used as necessary.

7.2.4 Fascial and peritoneal entry

The fascia is commonly entered through a transverse incision in the midline followed by sharp or blunt dissection laterally. The fascia is commonly dissected off the rectus muscles and may provide increased lateral space for surgical access and delivery by allowing independent movement of the fascial and muscle layers. However, evidence for its benefit is lacking. Furthermore, when a Maylard incision (transection of the rectus muscles after ligation of the inferior epigastric vessels) is used, the rectus muscles should not be dissected off the fascia because the muscles will no longer be invested with adequate blood supply.

The rectus muscles are usually separated in the midline to expose the underlying peritoneum. However, partial transection of the rectus muscles may be necessary, especially at repeat cesareans. Care should be taken to assure hemostasis using electrocautery or suture ligation of blood vessels. Entry of the peritoneum may be performed bluntly or sharply. Either way, it should be done with sufficient cephalad movement to prevent incidental bladder injury. Sharp entry is performed by elevating the peritoneum and incising it with the Metzenbaum scissors. This may be particularly necessary when there is concern for intra-abdominal adhesions. While sharp entry does not completely eliminate the risk of visceral injury, a sharp injury (as opposed to digital or electrocautery) is more easily repaired. Extension of the peritoneal incision can be performed using simultaneous bilateral blunt traction by the surgeon and assistant.

7.2.5 Bladder flap

Creation of the bladder flap is part of the standard cesarean technique. It is created by grasping the vesico-uterine peritoneum with the dissecting forceps, incising it about 2 cm above the bladder reflection and extending the incision laterally in both directions. The loose tissue plane between the uterus and the bladder is then digitally dissected and a bladder blade is inserted to retract the bladder away from the lower uterine segment. The rationale in the pre-antibiotic era was that its creation and subsequent closure prevented spread of infection from the uterus to the intraperitoneal cavity. It was also intended to allow access to the lower uterine segment without injury to the bladder.

Three randomized trials and a subsequent meta-analysis suggest the bladder flap is unnecessary at cesarean [16–18]. Omission was associated with decreased incision-to-delivery interval, total operating time, and postoperative pain and increased postoperative hemoglobin [16,17]. One trial showed decreased adhesions at repeat cesarean when the bladder flap was omitted at the initial cesarean delivery [19]. There were no differences in bladder injury, although bladder injury was rare. Further, some retrospective studies implicate difficulty creating the bladder flap in the causation rather than prevention of bladder injury. Thus, the data suggest that creation of the bladder flap may be unnecessary, and increases operative time and adhesions.

7.2.6 Uterine incision and expansion

The uterus may be incised in various ways at cesarean (Figure 7.2). While the low-transverse and classical incisions are most common, others such as high-transverse, low-vertical, T-incision, and J-incision are sometimes used. No matter the type of incision made, the size of the hysterotomy should be sufficient for atraumatic delivery. The low-transverse hysterotomy is the preferred uterine incision type if the lower uterine segment is adequately developed. A low-transverse hysterotomy allows for consideration of trial of labor for appropriate candidates in future pregnancies. Because the lower uterine segment is relatively less muscular than the uterine body and fundus, the risk for uterine rupture during subsequent labor is significantly reduced. If the lower uterine segment is too narrow to allow safe transverse incision, a classical vertical or low-vertical incision should be performed.

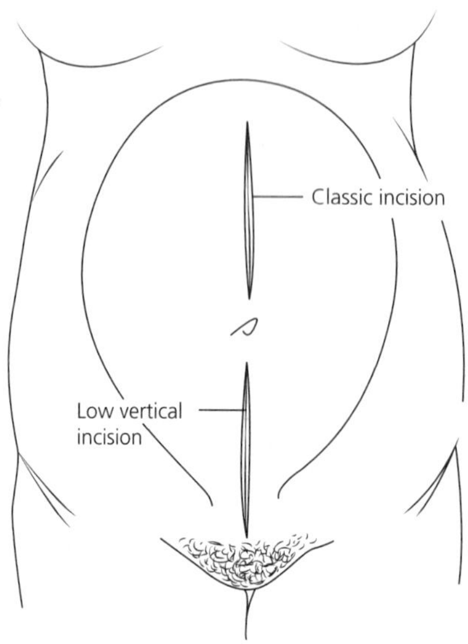

Figure 7.2 Low-transverse, low-vertical, and classical uterine incisions.

The low-transverse uterine incision may be extended laterally with blunt digital pressure or sharply with the scissors. One study comparing sharp versus blunt expansion of a low-transverse hysterotomy found no differences in the risk of inadvertent extension into vessels and blood loss [20]. Two subsequent randomized trials found that blunt digital traction was associated with less blood loss, improved postoperative hematocrit, and less need for blood transfusion [21,22]. Cromi *et al.* showed that the direction of blunt traction may influence outcomes. Digital traction in the cephalad–caudad direction was associated with decreased risk of vascular extension and decreased blood loss compared to lateral–cephalad traction [23].

7.2.7 Delivery of fetus and placenta

To deliver the fetus the surgeon's hand closest to the maternal pelvis is inserted into the hysterotomy and advanced around the fetal head. The fetal head is then lifted out of the pelvis toward the hysterotomy. Excessive flexion of the wrist during this maneuver risks injury to the lower uterine segment and uterine arteries. When the patient has been in labor prior to the cesarean, especially in the case of arrest of descent in the second stage of labor, elevation of the fetal head out of the pelvis may require the assistance of a vaginal hand. When the fetus is in breech presentation, the fetal buttocks or hips are elevated out of the maternal pelvis, and the hips are grasped and brought to the incision to deliver the buttocks. After delivery of the legs, a sterile moist towel is wrapped around the fetal trunk to deliver the body to the level of the scapulae. Fetal arms are delivered with the assistance of rotation of the fetal body if necessary.

The head is delivered by placing two fingers on the forehead or maxilla, flexing the chin toward the chest and applying gentle traction.

For the fetus in the transverse position it is important to know the location of the fetal spine. If the spine is toward the uterine fundus ("back up"), a low-transverse hysterotomy may be performed. The presence of fetal arms and legs toward the hysterotomy facilitates traction of the fetus into the breech or vertex presentation for delivery. On the other hand, if the fetus is transverse with spine toward the maternal cervix ("back down") a classical hysterotomy should be considered as no fetal parts are present to facilitate version of the fetus into a breech or vertex presentation for delivery.

After delivery of the infant, placental delivery can be accomplished by either cord traction with uterine fundal massage or manual extraction. Cord traction for delivery of the placenta is preferred because it is associated with significant reduction in postoperative endometritis, blood loss, and hospital stay [24].

Uterine contraction is the primary mechanism to decrease uterine bleeding after delivery of the placenta. Oxytocin is the first line uterotonic agent to prevent postpartum hemorrhage. While it is commonly administered during or immediately after delivery of the placenta, the optimal timing, dose, rate, and duration of administration have not been definitively established. One study found an oxytocin dose of 0.35 international units per minute to be effective in 90% of healthy women undergoing elective cesarean delivery at term without a priori risk factors for uterine atony [25]. In a cohort of patients undergoing cesarean delivery for labor arrest, the minimum effective oxytocin dose was 3 IU per minute by rapid intravenous infusion [26]. Tita *et al.* showed in a three-arm trial that 10, 40, and 80 units of prophylactic oxytocin administered in 500 mL over 1 hour were not significantly different for the prevention of postpartum hemorrhage at vaginal delivery [27]. While the term uterus is highly sensitive to oxytocin, significant receptor desensitization occurs with oxytocin exposure. Thus, women who have been in labor or have been augmented with oxytocin will likely require higher doses for the same uterotonic effect than women who have cesarean delivery before the onset of labor. The American College of Obstetricians and Gynecologists and the Royal College of Obstetricians and Gynecologists suggest 10–40 units of oxytocin in 500–1000 mL of Lactated Ringers administered at a rate of 125 mL/h for post-delivery hemorrhage prevention.

7.2.8 Hysterotomy closure

While the optimal technique for closure of the hysterotomy is controversial, the primary aim is to achieve excellent hemostasis (Figure 7.3). Single-layer, double-layer, locked, and unlocked suture techniques have been investigated. A recent meta-analysis of 20 randomized trials comparing single versus double layers and locking versus unlocked sutures for uterine closure of low-transverse cesarean found all types of closure comparable for short-term maternal outcomes, except for shorter operative time with single-layer closure, compared to double-layer

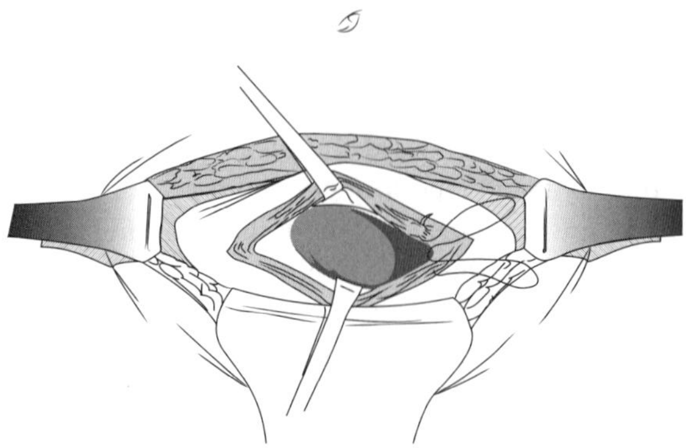

Figure 7.3 Closure of low-transverse uterine after delivery of the fetus and placenta with continuous suture.

closure [28]. Single-layer and locked first-layer closure were associated with lower residual myometrial thickness. Two studies assessing long-term outcomes found no significant differences between single- and double-layer closure for uterine dehiscence. There were no cases of uterine rupture in either group. Thus, current evidence based on randomized trials does not support a specific type of uterine closure for optimal maternal outcomes and is insufficient to conclude about the risk of uterine rupture. Until more data on long-term outcomes are available, both single- and double-layer closures are acceptable techniques.

Exteriorization of the uterus during hysterotomy closure is often employed to optimize visualization and surgical accessibility. Studies evaluating hysterotomy repair *in situ* as compared to exteriorization show no significant difference in clinical outcomes [29–31]. Thus, the decision to exteriorize or leave the uterus *in situ* should be based on maternal anatomy, visualization, presence of adhesive disease, and personal preference.

7.2.9 Intraperitoneal irrigation

The peritoneal cavity is often irrigated to remove amniotic fluid, blood clots, and other debris with the goal of decreasing the risk of infectious morbidity and postoperative pain. However, recent studies suggest peritoneal irrigation does not reduce postoperative pain or infectious morbidity [32,33]. A trial of more than 200 patients found that peritoneal irrigation was associated with increased intraoperative nausea, in addition to no decrease in postoperative febrile morbidity [34]. Taken together, the data suggest that intraperitoneal irrigation for cesarean delivery is an unnecessary step that may increase risk of nausea.

7.2.10 Closure of visceral and parietal peritoneum

Visceral and parietal peritoneal closure is advocated by some to restore normal anatomy and decrease risk of adhesive disease [32]. However, recent data suggest that nonclosure is associated with decreased operative time and no significant increase in postoperative maternal morbidity [33]. One randomized trial of closure versus nonclosure of the visceral and parietal peritoneum reported similar severity of adhesive disease at repeat cesarean and time from skin incision to delivery [34]. This suggests that closure of the peritoneal layers at cesarean is unnecessary.

7.2.11 Rectus fascia closure

Closure of the rectus fascia is an unarguably critical step because the fascia is the major structure responsible for integrity of the anterior abdominal wall. General surgical principles suggest closure of midline abdominal incisions with delayed absorbable monofilament suture in a running-unlocked fashion at stitch intervals of ≤ 1 cm [35]. While there is little data specific to closure of transverse incisions, this principle should be followed at cesarean.

7.2.12 Subcutaneous and skin closure

A meta-analysis of five randomized trials showed a significant 34% decrease in wound disruption when subcutaneous dead space greater than 2 cm was closed with delayed absorbable suture (RR 0.66, 95% CI 0.48–0.91). This reduction seems to be largely a result of decreased wound seromas (RR 0.42, 95% CI 0.24–0.75). The number needed to treat was 16. There was no benefit of closure for subcutaneous depth of 2 cm or less (RR 1.01, 95% CI 0.46–2.20) [36]. Two meta-analyses suggest there is no additional benefit to the placement of subcutaneous drains in the prevention of wound seromas [37,38].

The skin can be closed with subcuticular suture or staples. A meta-analysis of six studies found that closure with staples was associated with a twofold higher risk of wound infection or separation compared with subcuticular suture closure (13.4% vs 6.6%, pooled OR 2.06, 95% CI 1.43–2.98) [39]. The number needed to treat was 16. No significant differences were found with respect to postoperative pain, cosmesis, or patient satisfaction. Two subsequent large randomized trials have confirmed these findings [40,41]. However, because most studies excluded women at high risk of wound infection, the optimal skin closure technique in high-risk women, such as those with diabetes, chorioamnionitis, and morbid obesity, requires further study.

7.2.13 Bundle techniques and factorial trials

While the steps of cesarean delivery are often evaluated separately, there are complete sets of techniques for cesarean delivery including the Joel-Cohen, Pfannenstiel, Misgav-Ladach, and Pelosi methods. A meta-analysis of randomized trials of intention to perform cesarean using the different techniques suggests the Joel-Cohen-based methods are superior to Pfannenstiel-based techniques [42]. The Pelosi method was shown in one study to result in significantly decreased operative time, blood loss, and overall cost and improved patient outcome over traditional local cesarean technique [43]. While these bundle techniques appear attractive, it is not possible to identify the most effective aspects of the techniques. Further, the techniques are inevitably modified in different ways by different surgeons and it is unclear how that affects outcomes.

Two large factorial randomized trials evaluated several aspects of cesarean delivery simultaneously [33,44]. The CAESAR trial was a 2×2×2 factorial trial conducted in the United Kingdom and involved 3033 women randomized to three alternative surgical techniques: single- versus double-layer closure of the uterine incision, closure versus nonclosure of the pelvic peritoneum, and liberal versus restricted use of a subrectus sheath drain [33]. There were no differences between any of the arms of the trial for the primary outcome (maternal infectious morbidity) or any of the secondary outcomes. The CORONIS trial was a 2×2×2×2×2 international trial that randomized 15,935 women to five alternative surgical strategies: blunt versus sharp abdominal entry, exteriorization of the uterus versus intra-abdominal repair, single-layer versus double-layer closure of the uterus, closure versus nonclosure of the peritoneum, and chromic catgut versus polyglactin-910 for uterine repair [44]. There were also no statistically significant differences within any of the intervention pairs for the primary outcome (a composite of death, maternal infectious morbidity, further operative procedures, or > 1 unit blood transfusion). These surprising results have attracted criticism with regards to the choice of techniques tested, biologic plausibility of the primary outcome measures, and suitability of the factorial design. Follow-up studies are underway to assess the effects of these techniques on long-term outcomes.

7.3 Postcesarean delivery care

7.3.1 Pain control

Pain after cesarean delivery occurs via somatic pain sensation of the superficial and deep abdominal wall as well as visceral pain from the uterus transmitted through the hypogastric plexus. Adequate pain control is important to hasten recovery time, decrease risk for pulmonary complications, improve ambulation, facilitate adequate maternal rest, and allow bonding between the mother and newborn. Cesarean delivery may be performed under spinal, epidural, or general anesthesia, and the type of anesthesia used intraoperatively may affect the optimal postoperative pain control therapies.

When neuraxial anesthesia is used, intrathecal opiates may be administered for postoperative pain control. For patients who received neuraxial anesthesia, the obstetrician and anesthesiologist must communicate and coordinate pain control in the immediate postoperative period. Intravenous opiates may be used after cesarean either by nurse-administered injections or patient-controlled analgesic pumps. Oral analgesics are also safe within several hours of completion of cesarean delivery. Thus, as the patient is able to tolerate oral fluids and food, oral pain control options are appropriate. Oral opiates can be administered at regular time intervals with additional doses available as needed to obtain adequate pain control. Tramadol is a weak opioid agonist with additional activity in the serotonin, GABA, and norepinephrine pathways. It can be used as an adjunct in oral pain medication regimens. Both opiates and tramadol are safe in breastfeeding mothers [45,46].

Nonsteroidal anti-inflammatory drugs (NSAIDS) including ibuprofen, diclofenac, and ketorolac are useful in postcesarean pain control and are particularly effective for the visceral uterine pain associated with involution [47]. The use of NSAIDs may also minimize the doses of opiates required to achieve adequate pain control [48]. NSAIDs have well-known effects on the renal, hematologic, and gastrointestinal systems and should be used with caution, or avoided, in patients with specific medical conditions. Acetaminophen may be used and is often combined with an oral opiate. Organ dysfunction and death may occur with acetaminophen overdose. Thus, the maximal daily dose of 4 g should not be exceeded. If combination acetaminophen-opiate formulation is used, breakthrough pain control should be achieved with oral opiates alone or other non-acetaminophen medications to avoid the risk of acetaminophen overdose.

Transverse abdominis plane (TAP) nerve blockade has been used to decrease afferent nociception from anterior abdominal wall incisions. Local anesthetic is injected into the tissue plane between the internal oblique and transversus abdominis muscles. Studies assessing TAP nerve block for postcesarean pain control have been mixed, but it may be a useful adjunct in patients who have contraindications to opiates or NSAIDs [49–52].

7.3.2 Ambulation, diet and Foley catheter

The immediate postpartum period is a high-risk period for development of thromboembolism. Pelvic surgery is also associated with a high risk of thromboembolic complication. The combination of prothrombotic changes associated with pregnancy and cesarean delivery put postcesarean women at risk of deep vein thrombosis and pulmonary embolism in the immediate postoperative period. As soon as patients have recovered from regional anesthesia, they should be encouraged to get out of bed to a chair and ambulate several times per day. Early ambulation has been shown to decrease time to tolerate regular diet and return of flatus and bowel function [53,54]. However, the risk–benefit ratio of routine heparin administration for deep vein thrombosis prophylaxis postcesarean is unclear.

Clinical studies of gastrointestinal motility have shown that small bowel motility resumes within hours of surgery, while gastric motility and colonic function return within 24 and 48–72 hours, respectively [55,56]. Diet advancement after routine cesarean section should not be delayed until the passage of flatus. A regular diet can be provided per the patient's wishes on the day of surgery or on postoperative day 1. Postoperative and postanesthetic nausea is common and patients will most often be able to self-regulate their oral intake.

Withholding oral intake or only offering clear liquids is unnecessary and may in fact delay return of normal bowel activity [57,58]. Notably, the etiology of postoperative ileus is complex and likely multifactorial related to surgical manipulation, opiate, and anesthesia effects.

A urinary catheter is routinely placed at the time of cesarean to facilitate complete bladder drainage and move the bladder inferiorly away from the lower uterine segment. The catheter should be removed as soon as the patient can ambulate to either a bedside commode or the bathroom. Urinary retention should be considered if the patient is unable to void 6–8 hours after a urinary catheter has been removed. The urinary catheter may need to be reinserted and a void trial re-attempted 24 hours later. Longer duration of bladder drainage may be necessary for bladder injury.

7.3.3 Incision care

The dressing placed at the completion of surgery can be left in place for one or two days. However, if the dressing is soaked with blood it should be removed, and a new bandage reapplied as needed. The incision site should be examined daily by medical staff to verify that the wound appears to be healing well without erythema or other signs of infection. If staples are used they are often removed on postoperative day 3–4 for Pfannenstiel incisions. Removal may be delayed until day 7–10 for vertical incisions and in patients at high risk of wound separation such as the obese. A recent non-inferiority trial comparing early to delayed staple removal in obese women undergoing cesarean failed to demonstrate non-inferiority, suggesting that delayed removal of staples should remain the accepted standard in obese women [59].

7.4 Considerations for cesarean under special scenarios

7.4.1 Emergency cesarean delivery

Performing an emergency cesarean delivery for either maternal or fetal compromise is an essential skill for practicing obstetricians. The "30-minute rule" is commonly invoked suggesting that for cesarean deliveries performed emergently for fetal compromise, the decision-to-incision (or decision-to-delivery) time should be 30 minutes or less. The 30-minute guideline is based on expert opinion, and differences in fetal benefit are likely more influenced by clinical factors such as severity of fetal heart rate abnormalities, gestational age, fetal growth, and maternal condition than the exact duration from decision to delivery [60–63]. Nonetheless, when emergency delivery is indicated for either maternal or fetal benefit, it should be performed both as expeditiously and as safely as possible. If regional anesthesia is not in place, clinical decision making as to regional or general endotracheal anesthesia should be based on clinical acuity.

Several surgical steps can be omitted for emergency cesarean deliveries. Prophylactic antibiotics should be administered as soon as the decision is made to perform cesarean delivery [64]. Blunt extension of the fascia and entry into the peritoneal cavity are used for efficiency. Once the peritoneal cavity is entered, care should be taken while making the uterine incision to avoid injury to the bladder, uterine vessels, and the fetus.

7.4.2 Classical cesarean delivery

Low-transverse hysterotomy has replaced classical as the preferred uterine incision technique at cesarean. Nonetheless, classical cesarean uterine incisions may be indicated when the lower uterine segment is not adequately developed, for transverse fetal lie with back-down, for perimortem cesarean delivery, and when the lower uterine segment is inaccessible due to extensive adhesions, uterine leiomyomas, and prominent vasculature and other lesions. Because classical cesarean involves a vertical incision through the contractile part of the myometrium, patients should be counseled postoperatively about the need for repeat cesarean delivery without labor in subsequent pregnancies due to the risk of uterine rupture.

7.4.3 Cesarean during labor

Cesarean delivery may be indicated during labor for arrest disorders, nonreassuring fetal status, or other intrapartum complications. As opposed to scheduled cesarean delivery performed prior to labor, intrapartum cesarean has additional challenges. Typically the lower uterine segment is thinner during labor and thus the hysterotomy should be made carefully to avoid laceration to the fetus. In addition, lateral extension to the uterine vessels can occur more easily through an attenuated lower uterine segment. If the fetal station has descended into the maternal pelvis, elevation of the fetal head to the level of the hysterotomy can also cause trauma to the lower uterine segment and uterine vasculature. Cesarean deliveries performed in labor, particularly in the second stage of labor, are at a higher risk of endometritis, although it is unclear what specific interventions are indicated [65].

7.4.4 Repeat cesarean delivery

As the number of cesarean deliveries continues to rise, so will the number of repeat cesareans. Adhesive disease and surgical complications increase with increasing number of prior cesarean deliveries. In a study of 83,000 cesarean deliveries at multiple centers in the United States, Rouse *et al.* reported an increased risk for placenta accreta, hysterectomy, packed red blood cell transfusion, bladder injury, bowel injury, and longer operating room time with increasing number of prior cesarean deliveries. With four prior cesarean deliveries the risk for hysterectomy was 2.4%, blood transfusion 3.7%, bladder injury 1.7%, and bowel injury 0.3% [66]. The possibility for adhesive disease and complications including need for transfusion as well as injury to surrounding organs should be discussed. Importantly, the surgical technique often needs to be modified including using careful sharp dissection as necessary.

7.4.5 Cesarean in obese patients

Obesity continues to rise in the United States with more than one-third of the population meeting criteria for obesity (BMI ≥ 30 kg/m^2) and an increasing population of patients in the superobese category (BMI ≥ 50 kg/m^2). Obesity increases the risk for operative complications during and after cesarean delivery in addition to the known pregnancy complications. Further, obesity is associated with an increased risk of needing cesarean delivery [67]. While optimization of maternal and fetal outcomes should involve preconception maternal weight loss, obstetricians should be familiar with surgical considerations and complications unique to patients with obesity.

An operating table and instruments of appropriate size are necessary for successful surgery in obese women. The optimal incision type in the obese patient is still unclear. Incision underneath the fold of a large panniculus may increase the risk for wound infection. However, incision through the panniculus often involves dissection through a thick layer of adipose tissue that heals poorly. In a retrospective cohort study comparing low-transverse skin incision to vertical skin incision in more than 400 pregnant patients with BMI ≥ 35 kg/m^2, there was no difference in the risk of wound infection or breakdown. However, there was an increased risk for classical uterine incision in patients with vertical skin incision, suggesting that access to the lower uterine segment may be limited with vertical skin incisions [68]. In a cohort of patients with BMI ≥ 50 kg/m^2, one-third of the patients had a wound complication and 25% required readmission to the hospital. The main risk factors for wound complications were maternal smoking and placement of subcutaneous drain, suggesting that subcutaneous tissue drains may increase, not decrease, the risk for wound infection. Furthermore, despite traditional teaching, vertical skin incisions may not be superior to Pfannenstiel incisions in obese patients [69].

While antibiotic prophylaxis is the best strategy for preventing postcesarean infection, there are special challenges in obese women. A prospective study of patients undergoing non-emergent cesarean delivery examined concentration of cefazolin in incisional adipose tissue after a 2-g cefazolin dose 30–60 minutes prior to surgery. Tissue specimens had adequate antibiotic inhibitory concentrations for gram positive cocci, but obese and extremely obese patients had inadequate tissue concentrations of cefazolin for gram negative bacteria. This suggests that inadequate tissue antibiotic concentration may contribute to increase wound morbidity in obese patients [70]. However, the extent to which reduced tissue penetration in obese women can be overcome by higher doses of antibiotics is unknown.

References

1 Hamilton BE, Martin JA, and Ventura SJ. Births: preliminary data for 2012. *National Vital Statistics Reports* 2013;**62**(3). Available from: http://www.cdc.gov/nchs/data/nvsr/nvsr62/nvsr62_03.pdf (accessed May 15, 2015).

2 Smaill F and Hofmeyr GJ. Antibiotic prophylaxis for cesarean section. *Cochrane Database of Systematic Reviews* 2002:CD000933.

3 Darouiche RO, Wall MJ Jr., Itani KM *et al.* Chlorhexidine-alcohol versus povidone-iodine for surgical-site antisepsis. *New England Journal of Medicine* 2010;**362**:18–26.

4 Noorani A, Rabey N, Walsh SR, and Davies RJ. Systematic review and meta-analysis of preoperative antisepsis with chlorhexidine versus povidone-iodine in clean-contaminated surgery. *British Journal of Surgery* 2010;**97**:1614–1620.

5 Menderes G, Athar Ali N, Aagaard K, and Sangi-Haghpeykar H. Chlorhexidine-alcohol compared with povidone-iodine for surgical-site antisepsis in cesarean deliveries. *Obstetrics & Gynecology* 2012;**120**:1037–1044.

6 Amer-Alshiek J, Alshiek T, Almog B *et al.* Can we reduce the surgical site infection rate in cesarean sections using a chlorhexidine-based antisepsis protocol? *Journal of Maternal-Fetal and Neonatal Medicine* 2013;**26**:1749–1752.

7 Rauk PN. Educational intervention, revised instrument sterilization methods, and comprehensive preoperative skin preparation protocol reduce cesarean section surgical site infections. *American Journal of Infection Control* 2010;**38**:319–323.

8 Weed S, Bastek JA, Sammel MD, Beshara M, Hoffman S, and Srinivas SK. Comparing postcesarean infectious complication rates using two different skin preparations. *Obstetrics & Gynecology* 2011;**117**:1123–1129.

9 Smaill FM and Gyte GM. Antibiotic prophylaxis versus no prophylaxis for preventing infection after cesarean section. *Cochrane Database of Systematic Reviews* 2010:CD007482.

10 Baaqeel H and Baaqeel R. Timing of administration of prophylactic antibiotics for caesarean section: a systematic review and meta-analysis. *BJOG* 2013;**120**:661–669.

11 Tita AT, Rouse DJ, Blackwell S, Saade GR, Spong CY, and Andrews WW. Emerging concepts in antibiotic prophylaxis for cesarean delivery: a systematic review. *Obstetrics & Gynecology* 2009;**113**:675–682.

12 Tita AT, Hauth JC, Grimes A, Owen J, Stamm AM, and Andrews WW. Decreasing incidence of postcesarean endometritis with extended-spectrum antibiotic prophylaxis. *Obstetrics & Gynecology* 2008;**111**:51–56.

13 Franchi M, Ghezzi F, Raio L *et al.* Joel-Cohen or Pfannenstiel incision at cesarean delivery: does it make a difference? *Acta Obstetricia et Gynecologica Scandinavica* 2002;**81**:1040–1046.

14 Mathai M, Ambersheth S, and George A. Comparison of two transverse abdominal incisions for cesarean delivery. *International Journal of Gynecology & Obstetrics* 2002;**78**:47–49.

15 Wylie BJ, Gilbert S, Landon MB *et al.* Comparison of transverse and vertical skin incision for emergency cesarean delivery. *Obstetrics & Gynecology* 2010;**115**:1134–1140.

16 Hohlagschwandtner M, Ruecklinger E, Husslein P, and Joura EA. Is the formation of a bladder flap at cesarean necessary? A randomized trial. *Obstetrics & Gynecology* 2001;**98**:1089–1092.

17 Tuuli MG, Odibo AO, Fogertey P, Roehl K, Stamilio D, and Macones GA. Utility of the bladder flap at cesarean delivery: a randomized controlled trial. *Obstetrics & Gynecology* 2012;**119**:815–821.

18 O'Neill HA, Egan G, Walsh CA, Cotter AM, and Walsh SR. Omission of the bladder flap at caesarean section reduces delivery time without increased morbidity: a meta-analysis of randomised controlled trials. *European Journal of Obstetrics & Gynecology and Reproductive Biology* 2014;**174**:20–26.

19 Malvasi A, Tinelli A, Guido M *et al.* Effect of avoiding bladder flap formation in caesarean section on repeat caesarean delivery. *European Journal of Obstetrics & Gynecology and Reproductive Biology* 2011;**159**:300–304.

20 Rodriguez AI, Porter KB, and O'Brien WF. Blunt versus sharp expansion of the uterine incision in low-segment transverse cesarean section. *American Journal of Obstetrics & Gynecology* 1994;**171**:1022–1025.

21 Sekhavat L, Dehghani Firouzabadi R, and Mojiri P. Effect of expansion technique of uterine incision on maternal blood loss in cesarean section. *Archives of Gynecology and Obstetrics* 2010;**282**:475–479.

22 Magann EF, Chauhan SP, Bufkin L, Field K, Roberts WE, and Martin JN Jr. Intra-operative haemorrhage by blunt versus sharp expansion of the uterine incision at caesarean delivery: a randomised clinical trial. *BJOG: An International Journal of Obstetrics and Gynaecology* 2002;**109**:448–452.

23 Cromi A, Ghezzi F, Di Naro E, Siesto G, Loverro G, and Bolis P. Blunt expansion of the low transverse uterine incision at cesarean delivery: a randomized comparison of 2 techniques. *American Journal of Obstetrics & Gynecology* 2008;**199**:292 e1–6.

24 Anorlu RI, Maholwana B, and Hofmeyr GJ. Methods of delivering the placenta at caesarean section. *Cochrane Database of Systematic Reviews* 2008:CD004737.

25 Carvalho JC, Balki M, Kingdom J, and Windrim R. Oxytocin requirements at elective cesarean delivery: a dose-finding study. *Obstetrics & Gynecology* 2004;**104**:1005–1010.

26 Balki M, Ronayne M, Davies S *et al.* Minimum oxytocin dose requirement after cesarean delivery for labor arrest. *Obstetrics & Gynecology* 2006;**107**:45–50.

27 Tita AT, Szychowski JM, Rouse DJ *et al.* Higher-dose oxytocin and hemorrhage after vaginal delivery: a randomized controlled trial. *Obstetrics & Gynecology* 2012;**119**:293–300.

28 Roberge S, Demers S, Berghella V, Chaillet N, Moore L, and Bujold E. Impact of single- vs double-layer closure on adverse outcomes and uterine scar defect: a systematic review and metaanalysis. *American Journal of Obstetrics & Gynecology* 2014;**211**(5):453–460.

29 Jacobs-Jokhan D and Hofmeyr G. Extra-abdominal versus intra-abdominal repair of the uterine incision at caesarean section. *Cochrane Database of Systematic Reviews* 2004:CD000085.

30 Siddiqui M, Goldszmidt E, Fallah S, Kingdom J, Windrim R, and Carvalho JC. Complications of exteriorized compared with in situ uterine repair at cesarean delivery under spinal anesthesia: a randomized controlled trial. *Obstetrics & Gynecology* 2007;**110**:570–575.

31 Coutinho IC, Ramos de Amorim MM, Katz L, and Bandeira de Ferraz AA. Uterine exteriorization compared with in situ repair at cesarean delivery: a randomized controlled trial. *Obstetrics & Gynecology* 2008;**111**:639–647.

32 Lyell DJ, Caughey AB, Hu E, and Daniels K. Peritoneal closure at primary cesarean delivery and adhesions. *Obstetrics & Gynecology* 2005;**106**:275–280.

33 Caesarean section surgical techniques: a randomised factorial trial (CAESAR). *BJOG: An International Journal of Obstetrics and Gynaecology* 2010;**117**:1366–1376.

34 Kapustian V, Anteby EY, Gdalevich M, Shenhav S, Lavie O, and Gemer O. Effect of closure versus nonclosure of peritoneum at cesarean section on adhesions: a prospective randomized study. *American Journal of Obstetrics & Gynecology* 2012;**206**:56 e1–4.

35 Ceydeli A, Rucinski J, and Wise L. Finding the best abdominal closure: an evidence-based review of the literature. *Current Surgery* 2005;**62**:220–225.

36 Chelmow D, Rodriguez EJ, and Sabatini MM. Suture closure of subcutaneous fat and wound disruption after cesarean delivery: a meta-analysis. *Obstetrics & Gynecology* 2004;**103**:974–980.

37 Hellums EK, Lin MG, and Ramsey PS. Prophylactic subcutaneous drainage for prevention of wound complications after cesarean delivery – a metaanalysis. *American Journal of Obstetrics & Gynecology* 2007;**197**:229–235.

38 Ramsey PS, White AM, Guinn DA *et al.* Subcutaneous tissue reapproximation, alone or in combination with drain, in obese women undergoing cesarean delivery. *Obstetrics & Gynecology* 2005;**105**:967–973.

39 Tuuli MG, Rampersad RM, Carbone JF, Stamilio D, Macones GA, and Odibo AO. Staples compared with subcuticular suture for skin closure after cesarean delivery: a systematic review and meta-analysis. *Obstetrics & Gynecology* 2011;**117**:682–690.

40 Figueroa D, Jauk VC, Szychowski JM *et al.* Surgical staples compared with subcuticular suture for skin closure after cesarean delivery: a randomized controlled trial. *Obstetrics & Gynecology* 2013;**121**:33–38.

41 Mackeen AD, Khalifeh A, Fleisher J *et al.* Suture compared with staple skin closure after cesarean delivery: a randomized controlled trial. *Obstetrics & Gynecology* 2014;**123**:1169–1175.

42 Hofmeyr JG, Novikova N, Mathai M, and Shah A. Techniques for cesarean section. *American Journal of Obstetrics & Gynecology* 2009;**201**:431–444.

43 Wood RM, Simon H, and Oz AU. Pelosi-type vs. traditional cesarean delivery. A prospective comparison. *Journal of Reproductive Medicine* 1999;**44**:788–795.

44 Abalos E, Addo V, Brocklehurst P *et al.* Caesarean section surgical techniques (CORONIS): a fractional, factorial, unmasked, randomised controlled trial. *Lancet* 2013;**382**:234–248.

45 Ilett KF, Paech MJ, Page-Sharp M *et al.* Use of a sparse sampling study design to assess transfer of tramadol and its O-desmethyl metabolite into transitional breast milk. *British Journal of Clinical Pharmacology* 2008;**65**:661–666.

46 Hendrickson RG and McKeown NJ. Is maternal opioid use hazardous to breast-fed infants? *Clinical Toxicology (Phila)* 2012;**50**:1–14.

47 Nauta M, Landsmeer ML, and Koren G. Codeine-acetaminophen versus nonsteroidal anti-inflammatory drugs in the treatment of post-abdominal surgery pain: a systematic review of randomized trials. *American Journal of Surgery* 2009;**198**:256–261.

48 Kenny GN, McArdle CS, and Aitken HH. Parenteral ketorolac: opiate-sparing effect and lack of cardiorespiratory depression in the perioperative patient. *Pharmacotherapy* 1990;**10**:127S–131S.

49 Eslamian L, Jalili Z, Jamal A, Marsoosi V, and Movafegh A. Transversus abdominis plane block reduces postoperative pain intensity and analgesic consumption in elective cesarean delivery under general anesthesia. *Journal of Anesthesia* 2012;**26**:334–338.

50 McMorrow RC, Ni Mhuircheartaigh RJ, Ahmed KA *et al.* Comparison of transversus abdominis plane block vs spinal morphine for pain relief after Caesarean section. *British Journal of Anaesthesia* 2011;**106**:706–712.

51 Costello JF, Moore AR, Wieczorek PM, Macarthur AJ, Balki M, and Carvalho JC. The transversus abdominis plane block, when used as part of a multimodal regimen inclusive of intrathecal morphine, does not improve analgesia after cesarean delivery. *Regional Anesthesia and Pain Medicine* 2009;**34**:586–589.

52 Loane H, Preston R, Douglas MJ, Massey S, Papsdorf M, and Tyler J. A randomized controlled trial comparing intrathecal morphine with transversus abdominis plane block for post-cesarean delivery analgesia. *International Journal of Obstetric Anesthesia* 2012;**21**:112–118.

53 Oldmeadow LB, Edwards ER, Kimmel LA, Kipen E, Robertson VJ, and Bailey MJ. No rest for the wounded: early ambulation after hip surgery accelerates recovery. *ANZ Journal of Surgery* 2006;**76**:607–611.

54 Sindell S, Causey MW, Bradley T, Poss M, Moonka R, and Thirlby R. Expediting return of bowel function after colorectal surgery. *American Journal of Surgery* 2012;**203**:644–648.

55 Nachlas MM, Younis MT, Roda CP, and Wityk JJ. Gastrointestinal motility studies as a guide to postoperative management. *Annals of Surgery* 1972;**175**:510–522.

56 Jeffery KM, Harkins B, Cresci GA, and Martindale RG. The clear liquid diet is no longer a necessity in the routine postoperative management of surgical patients. *The American Surgeon* 1996;**62**:167–170.

57 Kovavisarach E and Atthakorn M. Early versus delayed oral feeding after cesarean delivery. *International Journal of Gynecology & Obstetrics* 2005;**90**:31–34.
58 Warren J, Bhalla V, and Cresci G. Postoperative diet advancement: surgical dogma vs evidence-based medicine. *Nutrition in Clinical Practice* 2011;**26**:115–125.
59 Nuthalapaty FS, Lee CM, Lee JH, Kuper SG, and Higdon HL, III. A randomized controlled trial of early versus delayed skin staple removal following caesarean section in the obese patient. *Journal of Obstetrics and Gynaecology Canada* 2013;**35**:426–433.
60 Schauberger CW and Chauhan SP. Emergency cesarean section and the 30-minute rule: definitions. *American Journal of Perinatology* 2009;**26**:221–226.
61 Holcroft CJ, Graham EM, and Penning DH. Cord gas analysis, decision-to-delivery interval and the 30-minute rule for emergency cesareans. *Journal of Perinatology* 2005;**25**:616.
62 Hillemanns P, Strauss A, Hasbargen U *et al.* Crash emergency cesarean section: decision-to-delivery interval under 30 min and its effect on Apgar and umbilical artery pH. *Archives of Gynecology and Obstetrics* 2005;**273**:161–165.
63 American College of Obstetricians and Gynecologists Practice Bulletin No. 116: Management of intrapartum fetal heart rate tracings. *Obstetrics & Gynecology* 2010;**116**:1232–1240.
64 American College of Obstetricians and Gynecologists Practice Bulletin No. 120: Use of prophylactic antibiotics in labor and delivery. *Obstetrics & Gynecology* 2011;**117**:1472–1483.
65 Tuuli MG, Liu L, Longman RE, Odibo AO, Macones GA, and Cahill AG. Infectious morbidity is higher after second-stage compared with first-stage cesareans. *American Journal of Obstetrics & Gynecology* 2014; **211**(4):410 e1–6.
66 Rouse DJ, MacPherson C, Landon M *et al.* Blood transfusion and cesarean delivery. *Obstetrics & Gynecology* 2006;**108**:891–897.
67 Marshall NE, Guild C, Cheng YW, Caughey AB, and Halloran DR. Maternal superobesity and perinatal outcomes. *American Journal of Obstetrics & Gynecology* 2012;**206**:417 e1–6.
68 Bell J, Bell S, Vahratian A, and Awonuga AO. Abdominal surgical incisions and perioperative morbidity among morbidly obese women undergoing cesarean delivery. *European Journal of Obstetrics & Gynecology and Reproductive Biology* 2011;**154**:16–19.
69 Alanis MC, Villers MS, Law TL, Steadman EM, and Robinson CJ. Complications of cesarean delivery in the massively obese parturient. *American Journal of Obstetrics & Gynecology* 2010;**203**:271 e1–7.
70 Pevzner L, Swank M, Krepel C, Wing DA, Chan K, and Edmiston CE Jr. Effects of maternal obesity on tissue concentrations of prophylactic cefazolin during cesarean delivery. *Obstetrics & Gynecology* 2011;**117**:877–882.

CHAPTER 8
Trial of labor after cesarean

William Grobman and Emily Miller
Department of Obstetrics and Gynecology, Feinberg School of Medicine, Northwestern University Medical School, Chicago, IL, USA

8.1 Background

8.1.1 Rates of cesarean section

Over the past 40 years, cesarean section rates have dramatically increased in the United States. Attention to this trend led to a transient decline in cesareans in the mid-1990s. However, rates have begun to rise again and have now increased by over 50% over the past decade. In 2007, 32% of all deliveries occurred by cesarean, a frequency far above the Healthy People 2010 goal of 15% [1]. This increased frequency has occurred for both primary and repeat cesareans. However, repeat cesarean birth is the largest single indication for cesarean, contributing to nearly 40% of cesareans annually [1].

8.1.2 Trends in trial of labor after cesarean utilization

8.1.2.1 Rates and patterns

One pivotal cause for the increase in repeat cesareans over time is the declining number of women undergoing a trial of labor after cesarean (TOLAC). Initial studies of TOLAC noted that the majority of women experienced a vaginal birth, and that the frequency of adverse outcomes was low. Thus, TOLAC was recommended as a reasonable option by the American College of Obstetrics and Gynecology (ACOG) for all women with one prior low-transverse cesarean section [2]. Correspondingly, by the mid-1990s, nearly 30% of all live births were a result of a vaginal birth after cesarean (VBAC) [3]. Concomitantly, cesarean rates decreased from 22.7 to 20.7% between 1990 and 1996.

Over the subsequent decade, however, TOLAC rates began to decline precipitously, from 70% in 1997 to just under10% in 2006 [4]. A number of

Management of Labor and Delivery, Second Edition. Edited by George A. Macones.

reasons for this decline, including both medical and non-medical factors, have been posited. Regardless of the etiology, however, the decline is one of the contributors to the rising cesarean rate. One goal of Healthy People 2020 is to increase the frequency of VBAC by 10% [5].

8.1.2.2 Non-medical influences of trial of labor after cesarean utilization

Multiple non-medical factors have been shown to influence TOLAC utilization. These consist of provider factors, systems factors, and patient factors. In terms of provider influences, the risk of litigation has been cited as a reason for performing a repeat cesarean [6,7]. In one survey of obstetricians, over 60% of providers reported changes in practice as a direct response to litigation [8]. Of those who reported change, 26% responded that one change was to stop offering TOLAC. This reported relationship is supported by evidence that the institution of malpractice caps is associated with increased utilization of TOLAC and decreased cesarean rates [7].

Even if a provider wishes to offer a TOLAC, they sometimes are unable to because of the system in which they practice. For example, in 1999, ACOG issued a statement that a physician capable of an emergency cesarean must be "immediately available" for women in active labor undergoing TOLAC [9]. Hospitals that felt they could not reliably meet this criterion began to forego the offer of TOLAC to their patients, and the number of hospitals that supported TOLAC declined by 30% [10,11].

Patient preferences for elective repeat cesarean versus TOLAC are complex and involve both an assessment of medical risk and the personal values that are attributed to different outcomes (e.g. the "value" of having a vaginal delivery). Qualitative data have shown that familial obligations, level of involvement of a woman's partner, and the strength of the wish to experience vaginal delivery all influence a woman's decision to attempt a TOLAC [12–14].

8.2 Risks of trial of labor after cesarean

Medical factors that influence the frequency of TOLAC include those of maternal and neonatal risks, although these risks at times are in conflict with each other. This concept of competing risks is exemplified in the systematic review by Guise and colleagues [15]. Using data derived from their analysis of the existing literature, they concluded that for every 100,000 women undergoing an elective repeat cesarean, nine additional maternal deaths would be incurred (i.e. 11,111 TOLACs would need to be done to prevent one maternal death). Conversely, for every 100,000 women undergoing a TOLAC, 83 additional perinatal deaths would occur (i.e. 1205 elective repeat cesareans would need to be performed to prevent one perinatal death).

8.2.1 Maternal morbidity

Most of the incremental increase in maternal morbidity occurs when a TOLAC fails and a woman requires a repeat cesarean in labor [16–19]. Women with a successful TOLAC have less frequent morbidity than women who undergo an elective repeat cesarean [16–18,20]. Thus, predictors of a VBAC are intrinsically related to risks of morbidity. Maternal risks to be considered include hemorrhage, infection, operative injury, uterine rupture, hysterectomy, and maternal death. Observational studies comparing women undergoing a TOLAC versus women undergoing a planned repeat cesarean can be used to guide the assessment of these risks.

The largest of these studies, sponsored by the Maternal-Fetal Medicine Units (MFMU) Network of the *Eunice Kennedy Shriver* National Institute of Child Health and Human Development (NICHD), included women with a prior cesarean at 19 academic medical centers [17]. Of these women, 17,898 underwent a TOLAC and 15,801 underwent a planned cesarean. The absolute frequency of maternal and neonatal risks associated with either approach to delivery was low. These findings have been corroborated by others and have afforded the obstetric community useful guidelines for patient counseling [21,22]. An overview of the published risks can be found in Table 8.1.

8.2.1.1 Hemorrhage

The existing data regarding whether hemorrhage is more common after TOL or after planned cesarean are conflicting. Landon and colleagues demonstrated an increased risk of blood transfusion in their TOLAC cohort (1.7% vs 1.0%, aOR 1.7, 95% CI = 1.4–2.1) [17]. However, a meta-analysis pooling results from five studies that assessed blood transfusion demonstrated no difference between the two approaches to delivery (1.7% vs 1.2%) [22]. Notably, any increased risk of transfusion is predominantly associated with women who fail TOLAC and thus assessment of success remains an integral aspect of counseling [17,22,23].

8.2.1.2 Infection

Similar to hemorrhage, the women in the MFMU Network Cesarean Registry who underwent TOLAC more commonly experienced endometritis than those undergoing an elective repeat cesarean (2.9% vs 1.8%, aOR 1.6, 95% CI = 1.4–1.9) [17]. Again, this risk appears to be predominantly driven by the risk of endometritis in women with a repeat cesarean in labor. However, this finding has not been replicated in all studies, and some investigators have identified increased risks of endometritis in women undergoing elective cesarean [18,24].

8.2.1.3 Operative injury

Operative injury has been defined variably, although definitions often include injury to the urinary system and bowel, and in some studies, laceration of the uterine artery [17,20,25,26]. These studies have been inconsistent with regard to whether operative injury is more frequent among women undergoing

Table 8.1 Maternal risks by route of delivery in women with a prior cesarean.

Maternal morbidity										
	Bais (27)		Blanchette (26)		Gregory (19)		Hibbard (16)		Kwee (21)	
	TOLAC (n = 184)	Elective cesarean (n = 68)	TOLAC (n = 754)	Elective cesarean (n = 727)	TOLAC (n = 11,480)	Elective cesarean (n = 29,970)	TOLAC (n = 1324)	Elective cesarean (n = 431)	TOLAC (n = 3274)	Elective cesarean (n = 1295)
Transfusion	8 (4%)	4 (6%)	3 (0.4%)	2 (0.3%)	63 (0.55%)	153 (0.51%)	11 (0.8%)	6 (1.4%)	–	–
Endometritis	–	–	11 (1.5%)	9 (1.2%)	–	–	108 (8.2%)	38 (8.8%)	–	–
Operative injury	–	–	2 (0.3%)	3 (0.4%)	–	–	–	–	2 (0.1%)	0 (0.0%)
Uterine rupture	1 (0.5%)	1 (2%)	12 (1.6%)*	0 (0.0%)	78 (0.68%)	38 (0.013%)	10 (0.8%)	0 (0.0%)	49 (1.1%)	0 (0.0%)
Hysterectomy	0 (0%)	0 (0%)	2 (0.3%)	0 (0.0%)			6 (0.5%)	0 (0.0%)	3 (0.1%)	0 (0.0%)
Maternal death	0 (0%)	0 (0%)	0 (0.0%)	0 (0.0%)	0 (0.0%)	2 (0.007%)	0 (0.0%)	0 (0.0%)	–	–

*denotes a statistically significant difference.

TOLAC or those with a planned cesarean. Nevertheless, as with other adverse outcomes, it is clear that operative injury occurs significantly more frequently when a TOLAC fails. This increased risk is predominantly due to women requiring a repeat cesarean in labor as women with a successful TOLAC have low rates of operative injury (3.0% vs 0.1%, aOR 5.1, 95% CI = 2.5–10.7) [20].

8.2.1.4 Uterine rupture or dehiscence

One risk of a TOLAC that has been a focus of attention is that of uterine rupture, defined as a disruption of the myometrium as well as of the overlying serosa with an associated maternal or neonatal morbidity requiring a change in clinical care. This is differentiated from uterine dehiscence, in which there are no adverse maternal or perinatal sequelae. The type of uterine scar is the factor most associated with uterine rupture, with frequencies of less than 1% reported in the setting of TOLAC for women with a prior low-transverse scar. In contrast, substantially higher rates have been reported for women undergoing TOLAC with prior classical cesarean scars [16–19,21,24–28]. Even women who plan for an elective repeat cesarean may have a uterine rupture, as a rupture can occur prior to or in early labor, but the frequency of rupture among these women is significantly less than that among women undergoing a TOLAC.

Landon (17)		Loebel (28)		Macones (18)		Tan (25)		Wen (24)	
TOLAC (n = 17,898)	Elective cesarean (n = 15,801)	TOLAC (n = 927)	Elective cesarean (n = 481)	TOLAC (n = 13,706)	Elective cesarean (n = 11,299)	TOLAC (n = 768)	Elective cesarean (n = 232)	TOLAC (n = 128,960)	Elective cesarean (n = 179,795)
304 (1.7%)*	158 (1.0%)	12 (1.3%)	3 (0.6%)	96 (0.7%)*	136 (1.2%)	36 (4.7%)	17 (7.3%)	245 (0.19%)*	268 (0.15%)
517 (2.9%)*	285 (1.8%)	–	–	1288 (9.4%)*	1469 (13.0%)	–	–	487 (0.38%)*	837 (0.47%)
64 (0.4%)	52 (0.3%)	4 (0.4%)	2 (0.4%)	178 (1.3%)	113 (1.0%)	6 (0.9%)	0 (0.0%)	–	–
124 (0.7%)*	0 (0.0%)	4 (0.4%)	2 (0.4%)	134 (0.9%)*	1 (0.004%)	2 (0.3%)	0 (0.0%)	843 (0.65%)*	453 (0.25%)
41 (0.2%)	47 (0.3%)	–	–	–	–	2 (0.3%)	2 (0.9%)	245 (0.19%)*	268 (0.15%)
3 (0.02%)	7 (0.04%)	0 (0.0%)	0 (0.0%)	–	–	0 (0.0%)	0 (0.0%)	2 (0.002%)	10 (0.006%)

8.2.1.5 Hysterectomy

Hysterectomy is another rare complication associated with childbirth. Although uterine rupture is one risk factor for a hysterectomy, elective repeat cesarean delivery is associated with an increased risk compared to successful TOLAC. Thus overall, TOLAC does not appear to increase the risk of hysterectomy compared to elective repeat cesarean [16,17,21,24–27].

8.2.1.6 Maternal death

Maternal mortality occurs at an overall rate of 10.1/100,000 for women with a prior cesarean delivery [29]. The largest cohort of women undergoing TOLAC versus repeat cesarean did not demonstrate a difference in maternal mortality between the two groups [17]. However, when multiple studies were summarized by a comprehensive review, a small but statistically significant increase in mortality rates was seen in women undergoing elective repeat cesarean delivery compared to TOLAC (0.013% vs 0.004%, RR 0.33, 95% CI = 0.13–0.88) [29].

8.2.2 Neonatal morbidity

Neonatal consequences related to delivery after a prior cesarean also need to be considered in patient counseling. Uterine rupture is the adverse outcome that places the fetus at greatest risk of adverse short- and long-term outcomes. Outcomes that have been examined commonly in the literature include Apgar

Table 8.2 Neonatal risks by route of delivery in women with a prior cesarean.

Neonatal morbidity										
	Bais (27)		Blanchette (26)		Bujold (35)		Hook (31)		Kamath (33)	
	TOLAC (n = 184)	Elective cesarean (n = 68)	TOLAC (n = 755)	Elective cesarean (n = 737)	TOLAC (n = 6718)	Elective cesarean (n = 1862)	TOLAC (n = 492)	Elective cesarean (n = 497)	TOLAC (n = 343)	Elective cesarean (n = 329)
5-Minute Apgar < 7	3 (2%)	0 (0%)	12 (1.6%)	11 (1.5%)	–	–	48 (10%)*	20 (4%)	–	–
NICU admission	13 (7%)	4 (6%)	36 (4.8%)	31 (4.2%)	–	–	6 (2%)	17 (3%)	16 (4.9%)*	32 (9.3%)
HIE/Asphyxia	–	–	–	–	–	–	–	–	–	–
Perinatal death	3 (2%)	0 (0%)	2 (0.2%)	0 (0%)	4 (0.06%)	2 (0.11%)	1 (0.2%)	0 (0%)	–	–

*denotes a statistically significant difference.

scores, as well as frequency of neonatal intensive care unit (NICU) admission, hypoxic-ischemic encephalopathy, and perinatal death. Because of the absence of any randomized controlled trials, observational studies guide our assessment of these risks. An overview of the published risks can be found in Table 8.2.

8.2.2.1 Apgar scores

Five-minute Apgar scores are often reported as a proxy for evidence of perinatal depression, although they are poor predictors of the risk of future neurologic compromise [30]. The existing literature has not consistently demonstrated a difference in mean Apgar scores or the risk of a low Apgar score (e.g. less than 7 at 5 minutes) in newborns of women who have undergone a TOLAC compared to those who have undergone planned repeat cesarean [29].

8.2.2.2 Neonatal intensive care unit admission

In many of the studies that have compared women undergoing TOLAC to those who have undergone elective repeat cesarean there is no evidence of a difference in the frequency of NICU admission [25–28,31,32]. In the studies in which a statistically significant difference was identified, the women who underwent elective repeat cesarean were found to have increased rates of NICU admissions (9.3% vs 4.9%, $p = 0.025$) [33]. This was predominantly related to either increased frequency of hypoglycemia or of supplemental oxygen in neonates born by planned cesarean.

8.2.2.3 Hypoxic-ischemic encephalopathy/asphyxia

Hypoxic-ischemic encephalopathy (HIE) refers to a perinatal asphyxial event that leads to both immediate and long-term neurologic morbidity. Richardson *et al.* did not study HIE directly, but used umbilical cord arterial pH as a surrogate

Landon (17)		Loebel (28)		Richardson (32)		Smith (36)		Tan (25)	
TOLAC (n = 15,338)	Elective cesarean (n = 15,014)	TOLAC (n = 927)	Elective cesarean (n = 481)	TOLAC (n = 2646)	Elective cesarean (n = 843)	TOLAC (n = 15,515)	Elective cesarean (n = 9014)	TOLAC (n = 768)	Elective cesarean (n = 232)
–	–	–	–	26 (1%)	13 (1.5%)	–	–	6 (0.8%)	0 (0%)
–	–	39 (4.2%)	27 (5.6%)	220 (8.3%)	74 (8.8%)	–	–	51 (6.6%)	14 (6.0%)
12 (0.08%)*	0 (0.0%)	–	–	–	–	–	–	–	–
47 (0.3%)*	20 (0.1%)	1 (0.1%)	1 (0.2%)	3 (0.11%)	0 (0%)	20 (0.13%)	1 (0.01%)	3 (0.4%)	0 (0%)

marker for asphyxia; they found a higher point estimate of pH < 7.0, (0.5% vs 0.1%, OR = 0.3, 95% CI = 0.1–1.8) among women undergoing TOLAC, but this difference did not reach statistical significance [32]. Data from the study of Landon and colleagues demonstrate a slightly higher frequency of HIE in neonates of women undergoing TOLAC compared to those having an elective cesarean (0.1% vs 0.0%, $p < 0.001$) [17]. When women experienced a uterine rupture, the frequency of HIE was 6.2%. When including women in the elective cesarean group who desired repeat cesarean but presented in labor, rates of HIE in the cesarean group were 0.013% [34]. Similarly, Richardson used umbilical cord arterial pH to assess for academia; they found a higher point estimate of pH < 7.0 (0.5% vs 0.1%, OR = 0.3, 95% CI = 0.1–1.8), but this difference did not reach statistical significance [32].

8.2.2.4 Perinatal death

Perinatal death is defined as fetal death beyond 20 weeks of gestation or neonatal death at less than 28 days of life, capturing both antenatal and intrapartum events. In the NICHD-sponsored MFMU study, perinatal mortality rates were 0.29% in the TOLAC cohort and 0.13% in the repeat cesarean group. In the context of a uterine rupture, the frequency of perinatal death was 1.8%. It should be noted that the study by Landon *et al.* excluded women who desired an elective cesarean if they presented in spontaneous labor. When these women were included in a secondary analysis, the presence of labor increased the frequency of perinatal death in the elective cesarean cohort [34]. These data suggest that, even though women may plan to have a repeat cesarean, obstetric events can occur prior to their scheduled cesarean that can increase their risks of adverse outcomes. Also, it is not clear that all perinatal deaths associated with a TOLAC were a result of the choice to undergo TOLAC. The possibility exists that cases of women with intrauterine fetal demise were encouraged to undergo TOLAC after the stillbirth was recognized antenatally. This possibility would result in the frequency of stillbirth associated with TOLAC appearing higher than it actually is.

8.2.3 Risks in subsequent pregnancies

Importantly, the risks documented above for both maternal and neonatal health only estimate the risks in the current pregnancy. Yet, additional cesarean deliveries magnify both maternal and perinatal risks in subsequent pregnancies. Future abnormal placentation is one aspect that contributes to these risks, given that each subsequent cesarean increases the risk of placenta previa and accreta, which both increase maternal risks (transfusion, operative injury, hysterectomy, and even maternal death) [37]. Furthermore, for women with placenta previa the median gestational age at delivery decreases, with a corresponding increase in risks of prematurity [37].

Repeat pregnancy after uterine rupture remains another clinical concern. Historic practice was to perform permanent sterilization after uterine rupture if the uterus could be preserved given the suspected increased risk of uterine rupture in subsequent pregnancies [38]. While limited numbers guide the estimates, if a woman undergoes labor, recurrent uterine rupture rates range from 4 to 33%, depending on the location of the prior rupture [38–41]. Thus, if a woman is pregnant after a uterine rupture, repeat cesarean should be performed before labor ensues with consideration toward delivery at 37–39 weeks to reduce the risk of recurrent rupture [42].

8.3 Predictors of vaginal birth after cesarean

The frequency of a successful vaginal birth after cesarean (VBAC) has ranged in most studies from 60 to 80% [17–20,43,44]. Demographic, historical, and pregnancy characteristics influence the chance of success and may be used to help with individualized counseling. As previously noted, TOLACs that result in repeat cesarean are responsible for the majority of the morbidity associated with TOLAC. Thus, the likelihood of success is correlated with the likelihood of morbidity, and counseling about the individual likelihood of VBAC gives insight into whether a woman is at greater risk of morbidity from undergoing a TOLAC [45,46].

8.3.1 Demographic characteristics

Various demographic characteristics have been studied for their association with TOLAC success, including maternal race, age, and BMI. Race, for example, has repeatedly been shown to be associated with VBAC. While women of Hispanic and African American race are more likely to undergo TOLAC, they are over

30% less likely to have a VBAC compared with white women [47,48]. The exact reasons for this racial disparity remain uncertain. Maternal age is linked to VBAC frequency as well, with younger women being more likely to experience a vaginal delivery [20,49–51]. Maternal body mass index is also predictive of VBAC, with a higher BMI being associated with increasing risks of failure [51–53]. In addition to lower maternal BMI, lower weight gain in pregnancy seems to be associated with a greater chance of VBAC success; women who gain less than 40 pounds are more likely to achieve vaginal delivery [54].

8.3.2 Historical factors

Multiple maternal factors related to a woman's medical and obstetric history also give insight into the chance of VBAC. A prior vaginal delivery has been strongly associated with an increased chance of TOLAC in multiple studies [36,47,50,51,55–58]. The order of the prior vaginal deliveries also seems to be important, with increased success in women when a vaginal delivery has occurred after the cesarean. The chance of success also seems to rise with each successive VBAC achieved [59].

The indication for prior cesarean also is related to the chance of VBAC. Women with non-recurrent indications, such as malpresentation or non-reassuring fetal status, for their prior cesarean are more likely to have a VBAC compared to women diagnosed with arrest disorders of labor [47,51,55,60–62].

Multiple investigators have noted that women with maternal diseases (defined variably as including diabetes, asthma, thyroid disease, seizure disorder, hypertension, renal disease, and/or connective tissue disease) have decreased success of VBAC [47,49,55].

Analyses of two large cohorts have been conducted assessing the chance of VBAC with one versus more than one prior uterine incision [63,64]. Macones and colleagues did not demonstrate any difference in vaginal delivery rates between the two groups. In contrast, Landon *et al.* demonstrated a slightly decreased chance of VBAC for women with multiple prior cesareans compared to those with just one prior cesarean (74% vs 66%, $p < 0.001$).

8.3.3 Factors related to the current pregnancy

8.3.3.1 Fetal size

Birthweight is associated with the chance of VBAC in women undergoing TOLAC, with larger infants associated with a lower likelihood of success [47]. In women with a prior cesarean for labor dystocia, greater fetal size than in a prior pregnancy reduces the chance of a vaginal delivery as well [65]. It should be noted, however, that the studies that have evaluated the association between fetal size and VBAC have relied upon birthweights, not estimated weights, for their analyses. In addition, the adverse impact of macrosomia (a birthweight of > 4000 g) may be mitigated by a prior vaginal delivery. In one study, success rates in women with a prior vaginal delivery were not affected by fetal size [66].

8.3.3.2 Multiple gestation

Management of a pregnancy in which the prior cesarean was for twin gestation and management of a multiple gestation after prior cesarean have both been studied. Women with a singleton and a prior cesarean for a multifetal gestation have a higher chance of VBAC compared to those with a prior cesarean of a singleton gestation (86% vs 73%, OR = 2.2, 95% CI = 1.7–2.8) [67]. Women with a prior cesarean who currently have a multifetal gestation are less likely to choose a TOLAC; however, those who do proceed with TOLAC have the same chance of VBAC as those with singletons [68,69].

8.3.3.3 Induction of labor

The chance of VBAC consistently has been shown to be lower for women who are induced than for women who are undergoing spontaneous labor. This is particularly true when women are induced with an unfavorable cervix [29,70]. However, it should be noted that most studies that have analyzed women with a prior cesarean undergoing labor induction have compared them to women undergoing spontaneous labor, and it remains uncertain whether and to what degree labor induction decreases the chance of VBAC when compared to the actual clinical alternative, namely expectant management.

8.3.3.4 Gestational age

Several investigators have studied whether VBAC success is lower when TOLAC is attempted after the estimated date of delivery (EDD) [71–73]. Some of these studies demonstrated an increased risk of failure when delivery occurred after the EDD, while others demonstrated slightly lower chance of VBAC when delivery occurred after 41 weeks of gestation. It should be noted, however, that in these studies success rates among those who delivered after their EDD remained relatively high (approximately 65%) [71–73].

8.3.4 Predictors of success models

The existence of the many associations that have been described does not necessarily translate into the ability of any one factor to accurately predict VBAC [74]. Moreover, women do not have just one factor but many combinations of different factors, and thus a predictive model must account for these different combinations. Several investigators have developed models to predict VBAC [51,56,60,61,75–79]. Grobman *et al.*, using a contemporary cohort from the MFMU Cesarean Registry, designed a model for women with term pregnancies with one prior low-transverse cesarean that incorporates variables known only at the first prenatal visit, in order that women can begin to be counseled at the beginning of their prenatal care [51]. Additionally, a second model is available that can incorporate new information that becomes available only as pregnancy progresses (e.g. the need for labor induction) [79]. This model has been externally validated in populations other than that in which it was developed, and is available online at http://www.bsc.gwu.edu/mfmu/vagbirth.html [80].

8.4 Uterine rupture

8.4.1 Factors association with uterine rupture

One feared risk of a TOLAC is uterine rupture, with its attendant maternal and neonatal morbidity. Various characteristics of a woman and her pregnancy are associated with this risk. However, even understanding these relationships offers limited ability to accurately predict uterine rupture based on either individual or a combination of characteristics [81,82].

8.4.1.1 Demographic characteristics

Demographic factors such as maternal race, age, and BMI have all been evaluated as risk factors for uterine rupture. White race, increasing maternal age, and obesity have all been associated with an increased risk of uterine rupture [18,53,54,81,83].

8.4.1.2 Historical factors

Historical factors that have been studied in the context of uterine rupture include prior vaginal delivery, inter-delivery interval, prior postpartum febrile morbidity, and the presence of uterine anomalies. The studies that have examined the association of prior vaginal delivery have consistently shown that this obstetric history lowers the chance of uterine rupture (ORs ranging from 0.2 to 0.6) [64,82,84–86]. Similarly, a prior VBAC seems be protective of uterine rupture [64]. Conversely, shorter inter-delivery intervals, such as less than 2 years, have been associated with a higher chance of uterine rupture [64,84,87]. The relationship between endomyometritis at the time of a prior cesarean and subsequent uterine rupture has been studied as well. One nested case–control study that examined the relationship between postpartum febrile morbidity and uterine rupture demonstrated fourfold increased odds of uterine rupture in women who experienced postpartum fever after their prior cesarean [88]. Results of one study suggested that women with Müllerian anomalies were at higher risk of uterine rupture [89]. However, these results were confounded due to a higher frequency of induction among women with Müllerian anomalies. More recent evidence suggests that, once induction is adequately controlled for, women with a prior cesarean and Müllerian anomalies are not any more likely to experience uterine rupture [90].

8.4.1.2.1 Prior cesarean uterine scar

The type of the prior hysterotomy scar is strongly associated with the chance of uterine rupture. Three types of uterine incisions are utilized primarily. The majority of cesareans occur via a low-transverse uterine incision. A low-vertical incision is a vertical incision that exists only within the non-contractile lower aspect of the uterus, whereas a classical incision is a vertical incision that extends beyond the limits of the lower segment.

While limited, the existing data do not support a difference in the rate of uterine rupture when comparing a low-transverse incision to a low-vertical incision [91,92]. Labor in the setting of a classical incision has been reported to result in a significantly higher frequency of uterine rupture. Spong and colleagues, reporting on women who were in the MFMU Cesarean Registry, reported frequencies of uterine rupture ranging from 0.75% with a low-transverse incision to 1.59% with classical or T-incisions [34]. Other investigators have reported a frequency of rupture in women with a prior classical scar that is greater than 5% [93]. Given the high risk of uterine rupture associated with a classical scar, this type of incision is considered a contraindication to planned TOLAC.

There does not appear to be a risk of uterine rupture significantly greater than that associated with a low-transverse incision when TOLAC is undertaken in the setting of an unknown type of uterine incision [94–96]. This lack of difference reflects the fact that the majority of unknown incisions are most likely of the low-transverse type. Thus, unless there is a high suspicion of a prior classical incision based on clinical information, an unknown scar is not a contraindication to TOLAC.

8.4.1.2.2 Layers of prior closure

Uterine closure at the time of initial cesarean can be performed in either one or two layers. Closure in one layer decreases operative time and blood loss at the initial cesarean, but some have questioned whether this technique could affect the chance of uterine rupture in future pregnancies [97]. While some studies have demonstrated an increased risk of rupture when a single-layer closure is used, others have not confirmed this association [98,99]. Of note, in the study by Bujold *et al.*, the surgical technique for hysterotomy closure utilized predominantly a chromic locking suture, while in the latter study a vicryl unlocking stitch was placed. It is possible, then, that the suture type and technique, and not the number of layers closed, may be most relevant to whether the chance of rupture is increased. Ultimately, sufficient data are not available to elucidate the relationship between surgical technique in a prior cesarean and chance of rupture in a subsequent TOLAC.

8.4.1.2.3 Multiple cesareans

The risk of uterine rupture as it relates to the number of prior cesareans has been assessed in several studies, with some reporting that the chance of rupture was significantly higher (3.7%) with two prior cesareans [63,64,100,101]. The two recent large multicenter studies, however, did not discern a difference of such magnitude. Macones *et al.* noted that the risk of rupture was statistically higher for women with two prior cesareans as compared to one prior cesarean (1.8% vs 0.9%, aOR 2.3, 95% CI = 1.37–3.85), although the absolute difference was relatively small. Landon *et al.* did not find any difference in the frequency of rupture when women with two or more cesareans were compared to those with only one prior cesarean (0.9% vs 0.7%, $p = 0.37$). Given the results of the most recent analyses, ACOG considers TOLAC in women with two prior cesareans a reasonable option [42].

8.4.1.3 Current pregnancy

8.4.1.3.1 Birthweight

Data on the relationship between birthweight and the risk of rupture are inconsistent. One study demonstrated an increased risk of uterine rupture in women without a prior vaginal delivery who delivered a neonate with a birthweight over 4000 g (2.8% vs 1.2%, $p = <0.001$) [66]. This finding, however, has not been reproduced in other studies [64,87,88]. Given the lack of consistency within the existing literature, as well as the use of actual birthweight versus antenatally known fetal weight assessments in the analyses, there is not a strong evidence base to suggest that clinicians can use estimated fetal weight to clarify the risk of uterine rupture during a TOLAC.

8.4.1.3.2 Multiple gestation

Multiple studies have assessed whether a uterine rupture is more likely during a TOLAC with a twin gestation [67–69,102–104]. Most of these studies, including the two largest, do not demonstrate an increased risk of rupture when a twin gestation is present.

8.4.1.3.3 Induction of labor

Several studies have noted that the frequency of uterine rupture is approximately twofold higher when a TOLAC is the result of induction as compared to spontaneous labor [17,18,47,51,105–107]. It should be noted, however, that the absolute risk of this increase is less than 1%. Moreover, this increased risk has not been demonstrated to exist among women who have had a prior vaginal delivery [70].

The type of induction agent used also may play a role in the risk of rupture. Initial studies of prostaglandins (prostaglandin E_1 or prostaglandin E_2) demonstrated a three- to fivefold increased risk of uterine rupture compared to spontaneous labor [47,105,106]. Because of limited data, it remains unknown whether this risk is shared equally among all prostaglandin types. Also, some have suggested that it is not the prostaglandin itself, but the type of induction in which the prostaglandin is used – namely, an induction in a woman with an unfavorable cervix in whom sequential methods are employed – that determines the risk of uterine rupture. Macones *et al.*, for example showed that when prostaglandins were not used with other induction agents, the risk of rupture was not as high as had been previously reported [18]. Landon *et al.*, however, did not find a particularly higher risk when prostaglandins were used in concert with other agents, and Grobman *et al.* did not find that induction with an unfavorable cervix significantly increased risk of rupture compared to induction with a favorable cervix [17,70]. Based on the existing data, ACOG has issued the statement that misoprostol should not be used in patients with a prior cesarean [42]. Transcervical Foley catheter placement, another frequently used cervical ripening technique, does not appear to be associated with an increased risk of uterine rupture [106,108–110].

Oxytocin may be used as either an induction or an augmentation agent in women undergoing TOLAC. Similar to other induction agents, data on its association with uterine rupture are conflicting. Landon reported that when oxytocin alone is used to induce labor the risk of rupture is 1.1% and is increased in comparison to spontaneous labor (0.4%, aOR 3.01, 95% CI = 1.66–5.46) [47]. A similar increased risk occurred with the use of oxytocin for augmentation (0.9% vs 0.4%, aOR 2.42, 95% CI = 1.49–3.93). However, Macones did not find an increased risk of uterine rupture when oxytocin was used without prostaglandins.[18] Two studies have attempted to quantify a dose–response effect of oxytocin on rates of uterine rupture and have identified an association between higher doses of oxytocin and increased rates of uterine rupture, although one specific threshold has not been identified [111,112].

8.4.1.3.4 Post-dates

One prospective cohort demonstrated a sixfold increased risk of uterine rupture in women who delivered after 40 weeks of gestation, compared to women who delivered before 40 weeks (2.1% vs 0.3%, aOR 6.3, 95% CI = 1.9–20.2) and this association held true whether labor was spontaneous or induced [71]. However, a larger secondary analysis of a retrospective cohort failed to demonstrate this association [72]. Interestingly, a systematic review of induction of labor suggests that the increased risk of rupture associated with induction is predominantly the effect of induction after 40 weeks of gestational age, as this effect is not observed when induction occurs before the EDD [29].

8.4.1.3.5 Predictors of rupture models

As with prediction of a successful TOLAC, researchers have attempted to combine different risk factors for uterine rupture in order to determine whether an accurate prediction model could be derived that would help to guide clinical decision making [36,81,82,84]. Unfortunately, none of these models accurately predict rupture. Thus, while women can be counseled with respect to their risk factors for rupture, an important aspect of this counseling is the unpredictability of this rare event.

8.4.2 Signs and symptoms of uterine rupture

The most common sign associated with uterine rupture is an abnormal fetal heart rate tracing. Specific patterns reported include significant variable decelerations, late decelerations, or bradycardia [113–115]. Other signs and symptoms of uterine rupture include vaginal bleeding, loss of fetal station, and/or severe abdominal pain. Some had theorized that the use of epidural analgesia could mask the abdominal pain associated with uterine rupture, thereby delaying the diagnosis. However, this concern has not been validated in clinical practice, as investigators have shown that women who have uterine rupture diagnosed do feel pain, as manifested by complaint or by their request for and/or use of additional pain medication. For example, Cahill *et al.* demonstrated frequent epidural redosing occurred in temporal proximity to a uterine rupture being diagnosed [116]. Thus, the concern of "masking" a uterine rupture with epidural analgesia has not been substantiated, and epidural analgesia should not be withheld from women undergoing TOLAC who desire this form of pain control [42].

8.5 Pregnancy management

8.5.1 Antenatal management

8.5.1.1 Counseling

A woman with a prior cesarean is at increased risk of complications in a subsequent pregnancy, regardless of approach to delivery. Antenatal counseling on route of delivery requires a thorough discussion of complications related to TOLAC as well as complications related to a repeat cesarean. Important risks include not only risks in this current pregnancy, but also risks throughout the reproductive lifespan associated with the chosen route of delivery.

Counseling on short-term risks includes an assessment of the chance of success and risk of adverse outcomes based on individual characteristics. A VBAC success calculator using information available antenatally is available at http://www.bsc.gwu.edu/mfmu/vagbirth.html. This calculator can help to inform early discussions about approach to delivery. As pregnancy evolves, other factors, such as possible need for induction, can be woven into the decision making. An individualized and accurate uterine rupture prediction model has, conversely, not been established. However, information about certain factors that have been associated with the chance of uterine rupture, such as type of prior uterine scar, can be used in counseling a woman about her risk.

The ultimate decision to undergo a TOLAC must be one made by a woman and her healthcare provider based on her individual preferences. The counseling and decision should be documented in the medical records. Because of the lack of clear superiority of TOLAC versus repeat cesarean, ACOG considers global mandates for or against TOLAC to be inappropriate [42].

8.5.1.2 External cephalic version

Data on outcomes of external cephalic version (ECV) in women with a prior cesarean are limited to case series, all of which report successful version rates akin to those of women without a prior cesarean [117–121]. Safety data are also reassuring, with no cases of uterine rupture in the 192 reported ECV attempts in these case series.

8.5.2 Intrapartum management

8.5.2.1 Fetal monitoring

As noted earlier, a concerning change in the fetal heart rate tracing is the most common sign of a uterine rupture. Thus, based on expert opinion, continuous fetal monitoring once labor is diagnosed has been recommended [42]. If an adequate tracing can be obtained with external monitoring, there is no need for a fetal scalp electrode. External tocometry is also sufficient, as there are no consistent data suggesting improved outcomes with intrauterine pressure catheters [122,123].

8.5.2.2 Induction or augmentation of labor

Induction of labor is an option for women undergoing a TOLAC. However, the potential decreased chance of VBAC success and the increased risk of rupture, particularly for women with a prior vaginal delivery, compared to spontaneous labor, should be noted. Other individualized factors, such as the favorability of the cervix, should be taken into account when counseling about the benefits and risks of induction of labor. Similarly, labor augmentation with oxytocin has been reported in several studies to be associated with a slightly increased risk of uterine rupture. However, the absolute risk increase is small [17,18]. Also, it is not just oxytocin use but the amount of oxytocin used that is related to the risk of uterine rupture [112]. Based on their analysis of data from a multicenter study, one group of investigators has recommended particular caution at higher oxytocin doses [112].

8.5.2.3 Epidural analgesia

There has not been consistent evidence that the use of epidural analgesia by women undergoing TOLAC affects their chance of VBAC or the risk of uterine rupture [35,47,61,64,87,124,125]. Also, as noted previously, there is not good evidence to substantiate the concern that use of epidural analgesia will lead to a delay in diagnosis of uterine rupture and worse obstetric outcomes. Thus, ACOG recommends maternal request as a sufficient indication for epidural analgesia in labor and notes that this recommendation should not be altered by the presence of a prior cesarean delivery [42].

8.5.2.4 Suspected uterine rupture

When a uterine rupture is suspected, delivery of the fetus should be accomplished as expeditiously and as safely as is possible. How quickly delivery must occur in order avoid an adverse perinatal outcome remains poorly understood. In one recent study, Holmgren *et al.* found that those neonates who were delivered within 18 minutes of suspected rupture did not experience asphyxial injury [126]. However, the total number of neonates in the entire study group was 36, with only 17 being delivered within 18 minutes. Consequently, it cannot be known with certainty whether this threshold is fully protective.

When uterine rupture occurs, repair of the defect is possible the majority of the time. However, in approximately 10–20% of cases, hysterectomy is required to achieve hemostasis [20,127].

8.5.2.5 Delivery

Vaginal delivery in a woman undergoing a TOLAC should be approached no differently than in a woman without a prior cesarean. There are no good data to suggest that routine scar inspection by palpation, in asymptomatic women, is beneficial [128]. Furthermore, repair of asymptomatic uterine dehiscence has not been shown to improve clinical outcomes [42]. However, after delivery, if there is clinical suspicion of rupture, such as signs of maternal hypovolemia or excessive vaginal bleeding, exploration is warranted.

8.5.3 Second trimester delivery

Prostaglandin E1 (PGE1) is a commonly used agent for labor induction in the second trimester. Its use in the second trimester in women with a prior cesarean has not been associated with increased risks of rupture in comparison to other induction agents [129]. While the data are limited to case series, the frequency of uterine rupture among women undergoing induction with PGE1 in the second trimester has been reported to be 0.3–0.4% in women with one prior cesarean, which is a range comparable to that of women in spontaneous labor at term [130,131].

Rates of failed induction and time to delivery intervals among women undergoing second trimester labor inductions seem to be equivalent for women with and without a prior cesarean [132–134]. Among a general population, the addition of mifepristone before misoprostol induction seems to shorten the interval to delivery and improve vaginal delivery rates in second trimester inductions [129]. While data are limited, the use of mifepristone in women with a prior cesarean seems to be safe [135].

8.5.4 Intrauterine fetal demise

The mode of delivery for patients with a prior cesarean diagnosed with an intrauterine fetal demise (IUFD) in the third trimester requires an explicit focus on maternal outcomes. Thus TOLAC should be encouraged in women with an IUFD and a prior low-transverse cesarean section. It is appropriate to avoid prostaglandin E1 in the third trimester, given its association with increased risk of uterine rupture. A transcervical Foley may represent a safer cervical ripening choice if induction is required.

References

1 Menacker F and Hamilton BE. Recent trends in cesarean delivery in the United States. *NCHS Data Brief* 2010;**35**:1–8.

2 American College of Obstetricians and Gynecologists Committee Opinion No. 64: Guidelines for vaginal delivery after a previous cesarean birth. Washington, DC: ACOG, 1988.

3 National Institutes of Health State-of-the-Science Conference Statement: Cesarean delivery on maternal request. *NIH Consensus and State-of-the-Science Statements* **23**:5, 2006.

4 Martin JA, Hamilton BE, Sutton PD, Ventura SJ, Menacker F, Kirmeyer S *et al.* Births: final data for 2006. *National Vital Statistics Reports* 2009;**57**(7):1–104.

5 Healthy People 2020. http://www.healthypeople.gov/ (accessed May 15, 2015).

6 Coleman VH, Erickson K, Schulkin J, Zinberg S, and Sachs BP. Vaginal birth after cesarean delivery: practice patterns of obstetrician-gynecologists. *Journal of Reproductive Medicine* 2005;**50**(4):261–266.

7 Yang YT, Mello MM, Subramanian SV, and Studdert DM. Relationship between malpractice litigation pressure and rates of cesarean section and vaginal birth after cesarean section. *Medical Care* 2009;**47**(2):234–242.

8 Klagholz J and Strunk AL. Overview of the 2009 ACOG Survey on Professional Liability. http://www.acog.org/-/media/Departments/Professional-Liability/2012PLSurveyNational.pdf (accessed June 10, 2015).

9 American College of Obstetricians and Gynecologists Practice Bulletin No.5: Vaginal birth after previous cesarean delivery. Washington, DC: ACOG, 1999.

10 Shihady IR, Broussard P, Bolton LB *et al.* Vaginal birth after cesarean: do California hospital policies follow national guidelines? *Journal of Reproductive Medicine* 2007;**52**:349–358.

11 Roberts RG, Deutchman M, King VJ, Fryer GE, and Miyoshi TJ. Changing policies on vaginal birth after cesarean: impact on access. *Birth* 2007;**34**(4):316–322.

12 Eden KB, Hashima JN, Osterweil P, Nygren P, and Guise JM. Childbirth preferences after cesarean birth: A review of the evidence. *Birth* 2004:**31**;49–60.

13 Moffat MA, Bell JS, Porter MA, Lawton S, Hundley V, Danielian P *et al.* Decision making about mode of delivery among pregnant women who have previously had a caesarean section: a qualitative study. *BJOG* 2007;**114**:86–93.

14 Cleary-Goldman J, Cornelisse L, Simpson LL, and Robinson JN. Previous cesarean delivery: understanding and satisfaction with mode of delivery in a subsequent pregnancy in patients participating in a formal vaginal birth after cesarean counseling program. *American Journal of Perinatology* 2005;**22**:217–221.

15 Guise JM, Denman MA, Emeis C, Marshall N, Walker M, Fu R *et al.* Vaginal birth after cesarean: new insights on maternal and neonatal outcomes. Obstetrics & Gynecology 2010; **115**:1627–1678.

16 Hibbard JU, Ismail MA, Wang Y, Te C, and Karrison T. Failed vaginal birth after a cesarean section: how risky is it? I. Maternal morbidity. *American Journal of Obstetrics & Gynecology* 2001;**184**:1365–1371.

17 Landon MB, Hauth JC, Leveno KJ *et al.* Maternal and perinatal outcomes associated with a trial of labor after prior cesarean delivery. *New England Journal of Medicine.* 2004;**351**(25): 2581–2589.

18 Macones GA, Peipert J, Nelson DB *et al.* Maternal complications with vaginal birth after cesarean delivery: a multicenter study. *American Journal of Obstetrics & Gynecology* 2005; **193**(5):1656–1662.

19 Gregory KD, Korst LM, Cane P, Platt LD, and Kahn K. Vaginal birth after cesarean and uterine rupture rates in California. *Obstetrics & Gynecology* 2002;**100**:749–753.

20 McMahon MJ, Luther ER, Bowes WA Jr, and Olshan AF. Comparisons of a trial of labor with an elective second cesarean section. *New England Journal of Medicine* 1996;**335**:689–695.

21 Kwee A, Bots ML, Visser GHA, and Bruinse HW. Obstetric management and outcome of pregnancy in women with a history of cesarean section in the Netherlands. *European Journal of Obstetrics & Gynecology and Reproductive Biology* 2007;**132**:171–176.

22 Rossi AC and D'Addario V. Maternal morbidity following a trial of labor after cesarean section vs elective repeat cesarean delivery: a systematic review with meta-analysis. *American Journal of Obstetrics & Gynecology* 2008;**199**:224–231.

23 El-Sayed YY, Watkins MM, Fix M, Druzin ML, Pullen KM, and Caughey AB. Perinatal outcomes after successful and failed trials of labor after cesarean delivery. *American Journal of Obstetrics & Gynecology* 2007;**196**:583 e581–585.

24 Wen SW, Rusen ID, Walker M, Liston R, Kramer MS, Baskett T *et al.* Comparison of maternal mortality and morbidity between trial of labor and elective cesarean section among women with previous cesarean delivery. *American Journal of Obstetrics & Gynecology* 2004;**191**:1263–1269.

25 Tan PC, Subramaniam RN, and Omar SZ. Labour and perinatal outcome in women at term with one previous lower-segment caesarean: a review of 1000 consecutive cases. *Australian and New Zealand Journal of Obstetrics and Gynaecology* 2007;**47**:31–36.

26 Blanchette H, Blanchette M, McCabe J, and Vincent S. Is vaginal birth after cesarean safe? Experience at a community hospital. *American Journal of Obstetrics & Gynecology* 2001;**184**:1478–1484.

27 Bais JM, van der Borden DM, Pel M, Bonsel GJ, Eskes M, van der Slikke HJ *et al.* Vaginal birth after caesarean section in a population with a low overall caesarean section rate. *European Journal of Obstetrics & Gynecology and Reproductive Biology* 2001;**96**:158–162.

28 Loebel G, Zelop CM, Egan JFX, and Wax J. Maternal and neonatal morbidity after elective repeat Cesarean delivery versus a trial of labor after previous cesarean delivery in a community teaching hospital. *Journal of Maternal-Fetal and Neonatal Medicine* 2004;**15**: 243–246.

29 Guise JM, Eden K, Emeis C, Denman MA, Marshall N, Fu RR *et al.* Vaginal birth after cesarean: new insights. *Evidence Report/Technology Assessment* 2010;**191**:1–397.

30 American College of Obstetricians and Gynecologists Committee Opinion No. 333: The Apgar score. Washington, DC: ACOG, 2006.

31 Hook B, Kiwi R, Amini SB, Fanaroff A, and Hack M. Neonatal morbidity after elective repeat cesarean and trial of labor. *Pediatrics* 1997;**100**:348–353.

32 Richardson BS, Czikk MJ, daSilva O, and Natale R. The impact of labor at term on measures of neonatal outcome. *American Journal of Obstetrics & Gynecology* 2005;**192**:219–226.

33 Kamath BD, Todd TK, Glazner JE, Lezontte D, and Lynch AM. Neonatal outcomes after elective cesarean delivery. *Obstetrics & Gynecology* 2009;**113**:1231–1238.

34 Spong CY, Landon MB, Gibert S, Rouse DJ, Leveno KJ, Varner MW *et al.* Risk of uterine rupture and adverse perinatal outcome at term after cesarean delivery. *Obstetrics & Gynecology* 2007;**110**:801–807.

35 Bujold E and Gauthier RJ. Neonatal morbidity associated with uterine rupture: what are the risk factors? *American Journal of Obstetrics & Gynecology* 2002;**186**(2):311–314.

36 Smith GC, White IR, Pell JP, and Dobbie R. Predicting cesarean section and uterine rupture among women attempting vaginal birth after prior cesarean section. *PLoS Medicine* 2005; **2**:871–878.

37 Grobman WA, Gersnoviez R, Landon MB, Spong CY, Leveno KJ, Rouse DJ *et al.* Pregnancy outcomes for women with placenta previa in relation to the number of prior cesarean deliveries. *Obstetrics & Gynecology* 2007;**110**:1249–1255.

38 Al Qahtani NH and Hajeri FA. Pregnancy outcome and fertility after complete uterine rupture: a report of 20 pregnancies and a review of literature. *Archives of Gynecology and Obstetrics* 2011;**284**:1123–1126.

39 Lim AC, Kwee A, and Bruinse HW. Pregnancy after uterine rupture: a report of 5 cases and a review of the literature. *Obstetrical and Gynecological Survey* 2005;**60**:613–617.

40 Ritchie EH. Pregnancy following simple repair of the ruptured gravid uterus. *BJOG* 1989;**96**:1361.

41 Usta IM, Hamdi MA, Musa AA, and Nassar AH. Pregnancy outcome in patients with previous uterine rupture. *Acta Obstetricia et Gynecologica Scandinavica* 2007;**86**:172–176.

42 American College of Obstetricians and Gynecologists Practice Bulletin No.115: Vaginal birth after previous cesarean delivery. Washington, DC: ACOG, 2010.

43 Flamm BL, Newman LA, Thomas SJ, Fallon D, and Yoshida MM. Vaginal birth after cesarean delivery: results of a 5-year multicenter collaborative study. *Obstetrics & Gynecology* 1990;**76**:750–754.

44 Miller DA, Diaz FG, and Paul RH. Vaginal birth after cesarean: a 10-year experience. *Obstetrics & Gynecology* 1994;**84**:255–258.

45 Cahill AG, Stamilio DM, Odibo AO, Peipert JF, Ratcliffe SJ, Stevens EJ *et al.* Is vaginal birth after cesarean (VBAC) or elective repeat cesarean safer in women with a prior vaginal delivery? *American Journal of Obstetrics & Gynecology* 2006;**195**:1143–1147.

46 Grobman WA, Lai Y, Landon MB, Spong CY, Leveno KJ, Rouse DJ *et al.* Can a prediction model for vaginal birth after cesarean also predict the probability of morbidity related to a trial of labor? *American Journal of Obstetrics & Gynecology* 2009;**200**:56 e1–6.

47 Landon MB, Leindecker S, Spong CY, Hauth JC, Bloom S, Varner MW *et al.* The MFMU cesarean registry: factors affecting the success of trial of labor after previous cesarean delivery. *American Journal of Obstetrics & Gynecology* 2005;**193**:1016–1023.

48 Cahill AG, Stamilio DM, Odibo AO, Peipert J, Stevens E, and Macones GA. Racial disparity in the success and complications of vaginal birth after cesarean delivery. *Obstetrics & Gynecology* 2008;**111**:654–658.

49 Srinivas SK, Stamilio DM, Sammel MD, Stevens EJ, Peipert JF, Odibo AO *et al.* Vaginal birth after cesarean delivery: does maternal age affect safety and success? *Paediatric and Perinatal Epidemiology* 2007;**21**:114–120.

50 Cameron CA, Roberts CL, and Peat B. Predictors of labor and vaginal birth after cesarean section. *International Journal of Gynecology & Obstetrics* 2004;**85**:267–269.

51 Grobman WA, Lai Y, Landon MB, Spong CY, Leveno KJ, Rouse DJ *et al.* Development of a nomogram for prediction of vaginal birth after cesarean delivery. *Obstetrics & Gynecology* 2007;**109**:806–812.

52 Goodall PT, Ahn JT, Chapa JB, and Hibbard JU. Obesity as a risk factor for failed trial of labor in patients with previous cesarean delivery. *American Journal of Obstetrics & Gynecology* 2005;**192**:1423–1426.

53 Hibbard JU, Gilbert S, Landon MB, Hauth JC, Leveno KJ, and Spong CY. Trial of labor or repeat cesarean delivery in women with morbid obesity and previous cesarean delivery. *Obstetrics & Gynecology* 2006;**108**:125–3013.

54 Juhasz G, Gyamfi C, Gyamfi P, Tocce K, and Stone JL. Effect of body mass index and excessive weight gain on success of vaginal birth after cesarean delivery. *Obstetrics & Gynecology* 2005;**106**:741–746.

55 Gyamfi C, Juhasz G, Gyamfi P, and Stone JL. Increased success of trial of labor after previous vaginal birth after cesarean. *Obstetrics & Gynecology* 2004;**104**:715–719.

56 Flamm BL and Geiger AM. Vaginal birth after cesarean delivery: an admission scoring system. *Obstetrics & Gynecology* 1997;**90**:907–910.

57 Macones GA, Hausman N, Edelstein R, Stamilio DM, and Marder SJ. Predicting outcomes of trials of labor in women attempting vaginal birth after cesarean delivery: a comparison of

multivariate methods with neural networks. *American Journal of Obstetrics & Gynecology* 2001;**184**:409–413.

58 Caughey AB, Shipp TD, Repke JT, Zelop C, Cohen A, and Lieherman E. Trial of labor after cesarean: the effect of previous vaginal delivery. *American Journal of Obstetrics & Gynecology* 1998;**179**:938–941.

59 Mercer BM, Gilbert S, Landon MB, Spong CY, Leveno KJ, Rouse DJ *et al.* Labor outcomes with increasing number of prior vaginal births after cesarean delivery. *Obstetrics & Gynecology* 2008;**111**:285–291.

60 Weinstein D, Benshushan A, Tanos V, Zilberstein R, and Rojansky N. Predictive score for vaginal birth after cesarean. *American Journal of Obstetrics & Gynecology* 1996;**174**:192–198.

61 Gonen R, Tamir A, Degani S, and Ohel G. Variables associated with successful vaginal birth after one cesarean section: a proposed vaginal birth after cesarean score. *American Journal of Perinatology* 2004;**21**:447–453.

62 Spaans WA, Sluijs MB, van Roosmalen J, and Bleker OP. Risk factors at caesarean section and failure of subsequent trial of labor. *European Journal of Obstetrics & Gynecology and Reproductive Biology* 2002;**100**:163–166.

63 Macones GA, Cahill A, Pare E, Stamilio DM, Ratcliffe S, Stevens E *et al.* Obstetric outcomes in women with two prior cesarean deliveries: is vaginal birth after cesarean delivery a viable option? *American Journal of Obstetrics & Gynecology* 2005;**192**:1223–1229.

64 Landon MB, Spong CY, Thom E, Hauth JC, Bloom SL, Varner MW *et al.* Risk of uterine rupture with a trial of labor in women with multiple and single prior cesarean delivery. *Obstetrics & Gynecology* 2006;**108**:12–20.

65 Peaceman AM, Gersnoviez R, Landon MB, Spong CY, Leveno KJ, Varner MW *et al.* The MFMU Cesarean Registry: impact of fetal size on trial of labor success for patients with previous cesarean for dystocia. *American Journal of Obstetrics & Gynecology* 2006; **195**:1127–1131.

66 Elkousy MA, Sammel M, Stevens E, Peipert JF, and Macones G. The effect of birth weight on vaginal birth after cesarean delivery success rates. *American Journal of Obstetrics & Gynecology* 2003;**188**:824–830.

67 Varner MW, Thom E, Spong CY, Landon MB, Leveno KJ, and Rouse DJ. Trial of labor after one previous cesarean delivery for multifetal gestation. *Obstetrics & Gynecology* 2007;**110**: 814–819.

68 Cahill A, Stamilio DM, Pare E, Peipert JP, Stevens EJ, Nelson DB *et al.* Vaginal birth after cesarean (VBAC) attempt in twin pregnancies: is it safe? *American Journal of Obstetrics & Gynecology* 2005;**193**:1050–1055.

69 Sansregret A, Bujold E, and Gauthier RJ. Twin delivery after a previous caesarean: twelve-year experience. *Journal of Obstetrics and Gynaecology Canada* 2003;**25**:294–298.

70 Grobman WA, Gilbert S, Landon MB, Spong CY, Leveno KJ, Rouse DJ *et al.* Outcomes of induction of labor after one prior cesarean. *Obstetrics & Gynecology* 2007;**109**:262–269.

71 Kiran TS, Chui YK, Bethel J, and Bhal PS. Is gestational age an independent variable affecting uterine scar rupture rates? *European Journal of Obstetrics & Gynecology and Reproductive Biology* 2006;**126**:68–71.

72 Coassolo KM, Stamilio DM, Pare E, Peipert JF, Stevens E, Nelson DB *et al.* Safety and efficacy of vaginal birth after cesarean attempts at or beyond 40 weeks of gestation. *Obstetrics & Gynecology* 2005;**106**:700–706.

73 Zelop CM, Shipp TD, Cohen A, Repke JT, and Lieberman E. Trial of labor after 40 weeks' gestation in women with a prior cesarean. *Obstetrics & Gynecology* 2001;**97**:391–393.

74 Grobman WA and Stamilio DM. Methods of clinical prediction. *American Journal of Obstetrics & Gynecology* 2006;**194**:888–894.

75 Troyer LR and Parisi VM. Obstetric parameters affecting success in a trial of labor: designation of a scoring system. *American Journal of Obstetrics & Gynecology* 1992;**167**:1099–1104.

76 Pickhardt MG, Martin JN, Meydrech EF, Blake PG, Martin RW, Perry KG *et al.* Vaginal birth after cesarean delivery: are there useful and valid predictors of success or failure? *American Journal of Obstetrics & Gynecology* 1992;**166**:1811–1815.

77 Hashima JN and Guise JM. Vaginal birth after cesarean: a prenatal scoring tool. *American Journal of Obstetrics & Gynecology* 2007;**196**:e22–23.

78 Srinivas SK, Stamilio DM, Stevens EJ, Odibo AO, Peipert JF, and Macones GA. Predicting failure of a vaginal birth attempt after cesarean delivery. *Obstetrics & Gynecology* 2007;**109**:800–805.

79 Grobman WA, Lai Y, Landon MB, Spong CY, Leveno KJ, and Rouse DJ. Does information available at admission for delivery improve prediction of vaginal birth after cesarean? *American Journal of Perinatology* 2009;**26**:693–701.

80 Costantine MM, Fox KA, Pacheco LD, Mateus J, Hankins GD, Grobman WA *et al.* Does information available at delivery improve the accuracy of predicting vaginal birth after cesarean? Validation of the published models in an independent patient cohort. *American Journal of Perinatology* 2011;**28**:293–298.

81 Macones GA, Cahill AG, Stamilio DM, Odibo A, Peipert J, and Stevens EJ. Can uterine rupture in patients attempting vaginal birth after cesarean delivery be predicted? *American Journal of Obstetrics & Gynecology* 2006;**195**:1148–1152.

82 Grobman WA, Lai Y, Landon MB, Spong CY, Leveno KJ, and Rouse DJ. Prediction of uterine rupture associated with attempted vaginal birth after cesarean delivery. *American Journal of Obstetrics & Gynecology* 2008;**199**:30e1–30e5.

83 Shipp TD, Zelop C, Repke JT, Cohen A, Caughey AB, and Lieberman E. The association of maternal age and symptomatic uterine rupture during a trial of labor after prior cesarean delivery. *Obstetrics & Gynecology* 2002;**99**:585–588.

84 Shipp TD, Zelop C, and Lieberman E. Assessment of the rate of uterine rupture at the first prenatal visit: a preliminary evaluation. *Journal of Maternal-Fetal and Neonatal Medicine* 2008;**21**:129–133.

85 Caughey AB, Shipp TD, Repke JT, Zelop CM, Cohen A, and Lieberman E. Rate of uterine rupture during a trial of labor in women with one or two prior cesarean deliveries. *American Journal of Obstetrics & Gynecology* 1999;**181**:872–876.

86 Zelop CM, Shipp TD, Repke JT, Cohen A, and Lieberman E. Effect of previous vaginal delivery on the risk of uterine rupture during a subsequent trial of labor. *American Journal of Obstetrics & Gynecology* 2000;**183**:1184–1186.

87 Bujold E, Mehta SH, Bujold C, and Gauthier RJ. Interdelivery interval and uterine rupture. *American Journal of Obstetrics & Gynecology* 2002;**187**:1199–1202.

88 Shipp TD, Zelop C, Cohen A, Repke JT, and Lieberman E. Post-cesarean delivery fever and uterine rupture in a subsequent trial of labor. *Obstetrics & Gynecology* 2003;**101**:136–139.

89 Ravasia DJ, Brain PH, and Pollard JK. Incidence of uterine rupture among women with mullerian duct anomalies who attempt vaginal birth after cesarean delivery. *American Journal of Obstetrics & Gynecology* 1999;**181**:877–881.

90 Erez O, Dukler D, Novack L, Rozen A, Zolotnik L, Bashiri A *et al.* Trial of labor and vaginal birth after cesarean section in patients with uterine mullerian anomalies: a population-based study. *American Journal of Obstetrics & Gynecology* 2007;**196**:537 e1–11.

91 Shipp TD, Zelop CM, Repke JT, Cohen A, Caughey AB, and Lieberman E. Intrapartum uterine rupture and dehiscence in patients with prior lower uterine segment vertical and transverse incisions. *Obstetrics & Gynecology* 1999;**94**:735–740.

92 Martin JN, Perry KG, Roberts WE, and Meydrech EF. The case for trial of labor in the patient with a prior low-segment vertical cesarean incision. *American Journal of Obstetrics & Gynecology* 1997;**117**:144–148.

93 de Costa C. Vaginal birth after classical caesarean section. *Australian and New Zealand Journal of Obstetrics and Gynaecology* 2005;**45**:182–186.

94 Pruett KM, Kirshon B, Cotton DB, and Piondexter AN. Is vaginal birth after two or more cesarean sections safe? *Obstetrics & Gynecology* 1988;**72**:163–165.

95 Beall M, Eglinton GS, Clark SL, and Phelan JP. Vaginal delivery after cesarean section in women with unknown types of uterine scar. *Journal of Reproductive Medicine* 1984; **29**:31–35.

96 Leung AS, Farmer RM, Leung EK, Medearis AL, and Paul RH. Risk factors associated with uterine rupture during trial of labor after cesarean delivery: a case-control study. *American Journal of Obstetrics & Gynecology* 1993;**168**:1358–1363.

97 Dodd, JM, Anderson ER, and Gates S. Surgical techniques for uterine incision and uterine closure at the time of caesarean section. *Cochrane Database of Systematic Reviews* 2008.

98 Bujold E, Bujold C, Hamilton EF, Harel F, and Gauthier RJ. The impact of a single-layer or double-layer closure on uterine rupture. *American Journal of Obstetrics & Gynecology* 2002;**186**(6):1326–1330.

99 Durnwald C and Mercer B. Uterine rupture, perioperative and perinatal morbidity after single-layer and double-layer closure at cesarean delivery. *American Journal of Obstetrics & Gynecology* 2003;**189**:925–929.

100 Asakura H and Myers SA. More than one previous cesarean delivery: a 5-year experience with 435 patients. *Obstetrics & Gynecology* 1995;**85**:924–929.

101 Caughey AB, Shipp TD, Repke JT, Zelop CM, Cohen A, and Lieberman E. Rate of uterine rupture during a trial of labor in women with one or two prior cesarean deliveries. *American Journal of Obstetrics & Gynecology* 1999;**181**(4):872–876.

102 Miller DA, Mullin P, Hou D, and Paul RH. Vaginal birth after cesarean section in twin gestation. *American Journal of Obstetrics & Gynecology* 1996;**175**:194–198.

103 Strong TH, Phelan JP, Ahn MO, and Sarno AP. Vaginal birth after cesarean delivery in the twin gestation. *American Journal of Obstetrics & Gynecology* 1989;**161**:29–32.

104 Myles T. Vaginal birth of twins after a previous cesarean section. *Journal of Maternal-Fetal and Neonatal Medicine* 2001;**10**:171–174.

105 Lydon-Richelle M, Holt VL, Easterling TR, and Martin DP. Risk of uterine rupture during labor among women with a prior cesarean delivery. *New England Journal of Medicine* 2001;**345**:3–8.

106 Ravasia DJ, Wood SL, and Pollard JK. Uterine rupture during induced trial of labor among women with previous cesarean delivery. *American Journal of Obstetrics & Gynecology* 2000;**183**:1176–1179.

107 Zelop CM, Shipp TD, Repke JT, Cohen A, Caughey AB, and Liberman E. Uterine rupture during induced or augmented labor in gravid women with one prior cesarean delivery. *American Journal of Obstetrics & Gynecology* 1999;**181**:882–886.

108 Ben-Aroya Z, Hallak M, Segal D, Friger M, Katz M, and Mazor M. Ripening of the uterine cervix in a post-cesarean parturient: prostaglandin E2 versus Foley catheter. *Journal of Maternal-Fetal and Neonatal Medicine* 2002;**12**:42–45.

109 Bujold E, Blackwell SC, Hendler I, Berman S, Sorokin Y, and Gauthier RJ. Modified Bishop's score and induction of labor in patients with a previous cesarean delivery. *American Journal of Obstetrics & Gynecology* 2004;**19**:1644–1648.

110 Khotaba S, Volfson M, Tarazova L, Odeh M, Barenboym R, Fait V *et al.* Induction of labor in women with previous cesarean section using the double balloon device. *Acta Obstetricia et Gynecologica Scandinavica* 2001;**80**:1041–1042.

111 Goetzl L, Shipp TD, Cohen A, Zelop CM, Repke JT, and Lieberman E. Oxytocin dose and the risk of uterine rupture in a trial of labor after cesarean. *Obstetrics & Gynecology* 2001; **97**:381–384.

112 Cahill AG, Waterman BM, Stamilio DM, Odibo AO, Allsworth JE, Evanoff B *et al.* Higher maximum doses of oxytocin are associated with an unacceptably high risk for uterine

rupture in patients attempting vaginal birth after cesarean delivery. *American Journal of Obstetrics & Gynecology* 2008;**199**:32 e1–5.

113 Craver-Pryor E, Mertz HL, Beaver BW, Koontz G, Martinez-Borges A, Smith JG *et al.* Intrapartum predictors of uterine rupture. *American Journal of Perinatology* 2007;**24**: 317–321.

114 Ridgeway JJ, Weyrich DL, and Benedetti TJ. Fetal heart rate changes associated with uterine rupture. *Obstetrics & Gynecology* 2004;**103**:506–512.

115 Leung AS, Leung E, and Paul RH. Uterine rupture after previous cesarean delivery: maternal and fetal consequences. *American Journal of Obstetrics & Gynecology* 1993; **169**:945–950.

116 Cahill AG, Odibo AO, Allsworth JE, and Macones GA. Frequent epidural dosing as a marker for impending uterine rupture in patients who attempt vaginal birth after cesarean delivery. *American Journal of Obstetrics & Gynecology* 2010;**202**:355 e1–5.

117 Flamm BL, Fried MW, Lonky NM, and Giles WS. External cephalic version after previous cesarean section. *American Journal of Obstetrics & Gynecology* 1991;**165**:370–372.

118 Abenhaim HA, Varin J, and Boucher M. External cephalic version among women with a previous cesarean delivery: report on 36 cases and review of the literature. *American Journal of Perinatology* 2009;**37**:156–160.

119 de Meeus JB, Ellia F, and Magnin G. External cephalic version after previous cesarean section: a series of 38 cases. *European Journal of Obstetrics & Gynecology and Reproductive Biology* 1998;**81**:65–68.

120 Clock C, Kurtzman J, White H, and Chung JH. Cesarean risk after successful external cephalic version: a matched, retrospective analysis. *Journal of Perinatology* 2009;**29**: 96–100.

121 Schachter M, Kogan S, and Blickstein I. External cephalic version after previous cesarean section – a clinical dilemma. *International Journal of Gynecology & Obstetrics* 1994;**45**:17–20.

122 Devoe LD, Croom CS, Youssef AA, and Murray C. The prediction of "controlled" uterine rupture by the use of intrauterine pressure catheters. *Obstetrics & Gynecology* 1992;**80**: 626–629.

123 Rodriguez MH, Masaki DI, Phelan JP *et al.* Uterine rupture: are intrauterine pressure catheters useful in the diagnosis? *American Journal of Obstetrics & Gynecology* 1989;**161**: 666–669.

124 McNally OM and Turner MJ. Induction of labour after 1 previous caesarean section. *Australian and New Zealand Journal of Obstetrics and Gynaecology* 1999;**39**:425–429.

125 Barger MK, Weiss J, Nannini A, Werler M, Heeren T, and Stubblefield G. Risk factors for uterine rupture among women who attempt a vaginal birth after a previous cesarean: a case-control study. *Journal of Reproductive Medicine* 2011;**56**:313–320.

126 Holmgren C, Scott JR, Porter TF, Esplin MS, and Bardsley T. Uterine rupture with attempted vaginal birth after cesarean delivery: decision-to-delivery time and neonatal outcome. *Obstetrics & Gynecology* 2012;**119**:725–731.

127 Miller DA, Goodwin TM, Gherman RB, and Paul RH. Intrapartum rupture of the unscarred uterus. *Obstetrics & Gynecology* 1997;**89**:671–673.

128 Lurie S, Hagay Z, Goldschmit R, and Insler V. Routine previous cesarean scar exploration following successful vaginal delivery. Is it necessary? *European Journal of Obstetrics & Gynecology and Reproductive Biology* 1992;**45**:185–186.

129 Hammond C. Recent advances in second-trimester abortion: an evidence-based review. *American Journal of Obstetrics & Gynecology* 2009;**200**:347–356.

130 Berghella V, Airoldi J, O'Neill AM, Einhorn K, and Hoffman M. Misoprostol for second trimester pregnancy termination in women with prior caesarean: a systematic review. *BJOG* 2009;**116**:1151–1157.

131 Gotal V. Uterine rupture in second-trimester misoprostol-induced abortion after cesarean delivery: a systematic review. *Obstetrics & Gynecology* 2009;**113**:1117–1123.
132 Bhattacharjee N, Ganguly RP, and Saha SP. Misoprostol for termination of mid-trimester post-caesarean pregnancy. *Australian and New Zealand Journal of Obstetrics and Gynaecology* 2007;**47**:23–25.
133 Marinoni E, Santoro M, Vitagliano MP, Patella A, Cosmi EV, and Di Iorio R. Intravaginal gemeprost and second-trimester pregnancy termination in the scarred uterus. *International Journal of Gynecology & Obstetrics* 2007;**97**:35–39.
134 Dickinson JE. Misoprostol for second-trimester pregnancy termination in women with a prior cesarean delivery. *Obstetrics & Gynecology* 2005;**105**:352–356.
135 Lelaidier C, Baton C, Benifla JL, Fernandez H, Bourget P, and Prydman R. Mifepristone for labour induction after previous caesarean section. *BJOG* 1994;**101**:501–503.

CHAPTER 9
Malpresentation and malposition

Yvonne W. Cheng[1] and Aaron B. Caughey[2]
[1] *Department of Obstetrics, Gynecology, and Reproductive Sciences, University of California, San Francisco, CA, USA*
[2] *Department of Obstetrics and Gynecology, Oregon Health and Science University, Portland, OR, USA*

9.1 Introduction

While the large majority of fetuses are head down with a flexed head and in the occiput anterior position and vertex presentation, there are others which either do not present head down or do not present in the optimal position. When there is a noncephalic, nonvertex presentation, it is considered *malpresentation*. When there is a fetus that is rotated so that it is in the transverse or posterior position, it is considered a *malposition*. These malpresentations and malpositions lead to higher rates of perinatal complications, most commonly cesarean delivery. In the following chapter we explore the epidemiology and outcomes related to the malpresentations and malpositions as well as potential modes of management.

9.2 Malpresentation

The presentation of a fetus refers to the anatomical part that is leading into the pelvic inlet or birth canal. The head is usually presenting, thus labeled cephalic presentation. When evaluated on a standard ultrasound or on Leopold's or a vaginal exam with a minimally dilated cervix, often the specific attitude of the head (its flexion) cannot be assessed, so cephalic is as specific as can be determined. However, in labor, with greater cervical dilation, the fontanelles can be palpated to determine the flexion of the fetal head, and most commonly, the presenting part is the top of the fetal head just in front of the posterior fontanelle – also known as the fetal vertex, or vertex presentation. Fetal malpresentation thus describes a condition where the presenting part is any other than the vertex.

Management of Labor and Delivery, Second Edition. Edited by George A. Macones.

9.2.1 Breech presentation

Breech is the most common type of fetal malpresentation [1,2], and can be categorized based on the relationship between the lower extremities and the buttocks of the fetus. Frank breech describes the fetus whose lower extremities are flexed at the hips but extended at the knees such that the feet are close to the head. Complete breech describes the fetus whose lower extremities are flexed at the hip as well as the knees, thus the feet are next to the buttocks. Incomplete breech describes the fetus with one or both hips that are not flexed and one or both legs that are not flexed such that either the foot or the knee lies lower than the buttocks. Footling breech is a type of incomplete breech where one or both feet become the presenting part.

9.2.1.1 Epidemiology

Breech presentation occurs in approximately 3–4% of all deliveries [3,4]. In 2008, 4.8% of singleton live births between 24 and 42 weeks of gestations were delivered in breech presentation in the US [5], with decreasing incidence of breech as the gestational age increases. For example, the proportion of live births between 24 and 26 weeks of gestation born via breech presentation was 22–28%. Between 28 and 30 weeks of gestational age, the proportion of breech deliveries was 17–20%, while the proportion of breech deliveries was 9–12% between 32 and 34 weeks, and 6–10% between 34 and 36 weeks. At term, only 3–5% of singleton live births were delivered in breech presentation (Table 9.1). Compared to neonates born in vertex presentation, studies have suggested that neonates born in breech presentation have higher incidence rates of perinatal and infant morbidity and mortality, even after controlling for preterm birth and congenital malformations [6–10]. With respect to causality, it has been suggested that a subset of fetuses that do not "vert" to cephalic may have baseline neurologic issues. While data on long-term consequences of birth in breech presentation remains sparse, one cohort study that linked birth registry data with data collected during evaluation for military services in Denmark suggests a negative association between breech delivery and long-term cognitive outcome [11]. According to a large population-based study, the rate of recurrent breech in a second consecutive pregnancy was 9.9%; the recurrence rate was 27.5% in a third consecutive pregnancy (after two prior breech deliveries) [12,13]. Whether this is related to maternal or neonatal factors has not been elucidated.

9.2.1.2 Risk factors

One of the strongest risk factors for breech presentation is prematurity. Certainly, the prevalence of breech presentation is greater with earlier gestational age, thus a breech presentation in the setting of preterm birth is not particularly surprising. Studies which examined fetal presentation in the second and third trimesters also suggest that abnormal presentation detected in early third trimester (between 28 and 32 weeks of gestation) carries a 22–43% chance of persistent

Table 9.1 Proportion of singleton live births that were delivered in breech presentation in the US in 2008, with stratification by gestational age.

Among singletons only			
Gestational age	**Vertex (no.;%)**	**Breech (no.;%)**	**Total (no.;%)**
24	2,157	1,023	3,180
	67.83	32.17	100.00
25	2,354	1,115	3,469
	67.86	32.14	100.00
26	2,777	1,063	3,840
	72.32	27.68	100.00
27	3,237	1,037	4,274
	75.74	24.26	100.00
28	4,081	1,122	5,203
	78.44	21.56	100.00
29	4,638	1,162	5,800
	79.97	20.03	100.00
30	6,285	1,312	7,597
	82.73	17.27	100.00
31	7,955	1,446	9,401
	84.62	15.38	100.00
32	12,498	1,719	14,217
	87.91	12.09	100.00
33	18,399	2,331	20,730
	88.76	11.24	100.00
34	34,515	3,655	38,170
	90.42	9.58	100.00
35	61,195	5,058	66,253
	92.37	7.63	100.00
36	135,331	9,541	144,872
	93.41	6.59	100.00
37	320,579	19,318	339,897
	94.32	5.68	100.00
38	791,682	42,391	834,073
	94.92	5.08	100.00
39	1,219,608	59,749	1,279,357
	95.33	4.67	100.00
40	886,412	28,924	915,336
	96.84	3.16	100.00
41	248,221	7,424	255,645
	97.10	2.90	100.00
42	18,549	615	19,164
	96.79	3.21	100.00
Total	3,780,473	190,005	3,970,478
	95.21	4.79	100.00

malpresentation at term [14,15]. While other etiologies of breech presentation may be multifactorial and less clear, some studies suggest diminished muscle tone or abnormal motor function as contributing factors. It was observed that infants with neuromuscular disorders were more likely to be delivered in breech presentation [16]. Other fetal risk factors include small fetal size, congenital malformations, aneuploidy, female fetal sex, and multiple gestations [7,17]. Maternal characteristics associated with breech presentation include increased maternal age [4,18], uterine anomalies (such as uterine septum, unicornuate or bicornuate uterus [19–21], and space-occupying uterine myomas [22,23]), contracted pelvis [24], multiparity [25], and previous history of cesarean delivery [26,27]. Additionally, placenta previa and abnormal amniotic fluid volume (polyhydramnios as well as oligohydramnios) have also been associated with higher incidence of breech presentation [12,28,29].

9.2.1.3 Management and outcome

The diagnosis of breech presentation is usually made by physical examination using Leopold's maneuvers by experienced clinicians or by ultrasonography [30,31]. If breech presentation persists near term or if the fetal presentation is uncertain, sonographic examination is recommended for confirmation and to determine the type of breech as well as the estimated fetal weight. Some of the risks during labor and delivery to the fetus that presents breech include prolapse of the umbilical cord (particularly with footling or incomplete breech) in the setting of ruptured membranes, prolonged umbilical cord compression, head entrapment in the presence of incompletely dilated cervix or cephalopelvic disproportion, and birth trauma related to breech maneuvers such as hyperextension of the neck [32–35]. Thus, options other than vaginal delivery of the breech are often considered in much of the developed world.

9.2.1.4 External cephalic version

External cephalic version (ECV) is a procedure in which the fetus with a noncephalic presentation is rotated or "verted" to the cephalic presentation by manipulation through the mother's gravid abdomen. The goal of ECV is to reduce the incidence of breech presentation at the onset of labor and thus decrease the probability of cesarean delivery. The American College of Obstetricians and Gynecologists (ACOG) recommends that all women near term with a singleton breech fetus be offered an attempt at ECV [36]. Compared to scheduled cesarean delivery for singleton term breech presentation, ECV has been shown to be cost saving if the success rate is greater than 63%; however, ECV is not cost-effective if the success rate is < 32%. Between 32 and 64%, ECV costs more than cesarean but is associated with higher quality-adjusted life-years (QALYs) such that a trial of ECV remains a reasonable cost-effective option [37].

Typically performed at or near term in non-laboring women, studies have shown that the overall success of ECV is around 50–65% [38–43], and is dependent on

Table 9.2 Factors associated with success/failure of external cephalic version.

Favorable factors	Unfavorable factors
Multiparity	Nulliparity
Posterior placenta	Anterior or laternal placenta
Normal amniotic fluid volume	Low amniotic fluid
Unengaged presenting part	Descent of the breech into the pelvis
Earlier gestation	Maternal obesity
Regional anesthesia	Advanced gestation
	Excessive estimated fetal weight
	Posterior located fetal spine

clinician's skills as well as maternal/pregnancy factors. A number of maternal and obstetric characteristics have been identified as factors associated with a successful ECV [40–45] (Table 9.2). As low amniotic fluid volume is associated with decreased likelihood of successful ECV, it has also been shown that amnioinfusion after initial failure does not improve eventual success [46]. Since ECV at term is associated with decreased likelihood of success, studies comparing ECV performed in the late-preterm gestation (34–36 weeks) versus at term (37–38 weeks) report that early ECV is associated with higher rates of cephalic presentation in labor [47,48]. However, another trial demonstrated that early ECV did not decrease the rate of cesarean and may actually increase the risk of preterm birth [49]. While women with singleton breech presentation at or near term should be offered ECV, some relative contraindications to ECV include: uterine anomalies, third-trimester bleeding, multiple gestation, oligohydramnios, rupture of membranes, and onset of labor [36]. Overall the risks of ECV are relatively low, with a composite complication rate of approximately 6%, according to a systematic review that included 84 studies and 12,955 women, and include: emergency cesarean, placental abruption, cord prolapse, vaginal bleeding, and rupture of the membranes [50].

Recent systematic reviews of the impact of interventions such as tocolysis, fetal acoustic stimulation, regional anesthesia, transabdominal amnioinfusion, or systematic opioids on the success of ECV for breech presentation at term revealed that beta-mimetics (such as terbutaline) increased the frequency of cephalic presentation in labor and reduced cesarean delivery [51,52]. A number of randomized controlled trials found that regional analgesia in combination with tocolytic was more effective than tocolytic alone in increasing the success rate of ECV [53–57]. While the success of version was validated in a systematic review [58], there was, however, no difference in cephalic presentation in labor, nor in cesarean delivery, in another meta-analysis [51].

Although ECV decreases the frequency of cesarean compared to no ECV, studies have shown that the risk of cesarean (for labor dystocia and fetal intolerance of labor) is higher in women after successful ECV compared to the general obstetric population [59–61].

9.2.1.5 Planned cesarean delivery versus planned vaginal delivery in term gestations

While cesarean delivery for breech presentation to improve perinatal morbidity and mortality has been suggested as early as 1959 [62], vaginal delivery remained the most common mode of delivery in the US until the mid-1970s and 1980s when cesarean delivery became more frequent with the goal of improving fetal well-being [63,64]. Cesarean delivery for the indication of breech presentation in the US rose from 12% in 1970 to 87% in 2003 [65,66]. Similar increases in cesarean delivery performed for breech presentation have been seen worldwide, particularly in developed countries [67–69].

The changes in practice pattern regarding mode of delivery for singleton breech presentation at term were initially gradual and in response to emerging data from a number of retrospective cohort studies and small prospective randomized controlled trials suggesting a small but statistically significant increase in the risk of perinatal mortality and morbidity in women who had vaginal breech deliveries in the 1980s and 1990s [70–76]. In 2000, Hannah and colleagues published the results of an international, multicenter, randomized controlled study (Term Breech Trial) that compared the perinatal outcomes of term breech deliveries by mode of delivery [77]. In this landmark study, 2088 women with a singleton fetus in frank or complete breech presentation were randomly assigned to either planned cesarean or planned vaginal delivery. The risk of perinatal mortality, neonatal mortality, and serious neonatal morbidity was lower among women who had planned cesarean (17 of 1039 [1.6%]) compared to women who had planned vaginal delivery (52 of 1039 [5.0%]; RR 0.33, 95% CI 0.19–0.59; $p < 0.0001$), while there was no significant difference in maternal mortality [77]. Criticism of this study included the heterogeneous environments in which it was conducted and the lack of CT or MRI pelvimetry. Subsequently, in 2001, the ACOG recommended that planned vaginal delivery of singleton term breech was no longer appropriate [78]. As such, the proportion of women with singleton term breech presentation that undergo cesarean delivery has drastically increased worldwide [65,67,79].

Following the completion of the Term Breech Trial, the authors published additional follow-up studies that examined maternal outcomes at 3 months postpartum, as well as outcomes for mothers and children 2 years after birth. While at 3 months post-delivery the incidence of urinary incontinence was lower in women who had planned cesarean delivery [80], there was no difference in maternal outcome at 2-year follow-up [81]. Further, for 923 of the 1159 children (79.6%) who were followed to 2 years of age, the risk of death or neurodevelopmental delay was not different for those who had planned cesarean and those who had planned vaginal births [82]. In this cohort, 17 of the 18 children diagnosed with serious morbidity at birth in the original trial were deemed normal at the 2-year follow-up. It could be that the follow-up study lacked statistical power to detect a clinically significant benefit from planned cesarean delivery or the potential benefit was only short-term. Another explanation may be that the use of pooled outcome measure at the time of birth (perinatal mortality + neonatal mortality + serious neonatal morbidity) overestimated the true long-term risk of vaginal delivery among singleton term breech births [83]. Other studies have corroborated that the long-term outcomes of infants who were singleton breech at term were not significantly different for those who were delivered vaginally and those who had cesarean delivery [84,85].

Further, some studies suggest that the attempt of vaginal breech delivery under strict protocols may yield good neonatal outcome without evidence of increased perinatal morbidity or mortality [86–89]. Criteria for selecting appropriate candidates for trial of vaginal singleton breech delivery include: spontaneous onset of labor, gestational age greater than 37 weeks, frank or complete breech presentation, no fetal anomalies on ultrasound examination, adequate maternal pelvis (with clinical pelvimetry or objective assessment by radiographic evaluation via X ray, CT, or MRI), estimated fetal weight between 2500 and 4000 g, and flexed fetal head. Thresholds for maternal pelvis to be considered "adequate" include: (1) Transverse diameter of the inlet measurement of 12 cm or greater; (2) Anteroposterior (AP) diameter of the inlet measurement of 11 cm or greater and AP diameter of the outlet measurement of 10 cm or greater; and (3) interspinous diameter measurement of 9 cm or greater [90–92]. Additionally, some regimens have described not utilizing oxytocin augmentation of labor and the importance of ensuring the presence of normal labor progression [86–89,93]. Beside the above criteria, the attendance of an experienced obstetrician skilled at vaginal breech maneuvers, sound judgment, and willingness to abandon the attempt in case of abnormal progression or non-reassuring fetal surveillance are all vital to a safe vaginal delivery of a breech fetus at term.

The ACOG subsequently modified its recommendation regarding management of term singleton breech presentation, stating that "the decision regarding the mode of delivery should depend on the experience of the health care provider" and that "planned vaginal delivery of a term singleton breech fetus may be reasonable under hospital specific protocol guidelines for both eligibility and labor management" [83]. It further notes that "women should be informed that the risk of perinatal or neonatal mortality or short-term neonatal morbidity may be higher than if a cesarean is planned and that in instances in which breech vaginal delivery is pursued, great caution should be exercised, and detailed patient informed consent should be documented" [83]. Thus, counseling should be individualized as there may be situations in which the risk of cesarean or the mother's desire to avoid cesarean could outweigh the potential risk of perinatal morbidity/mortality associated with the attempt of vaginal breech delivery.

9.2.1.6 Planned cesarean delivery versus planned vaginal delivery preterm

Fewer data exist regarding optimal mode of delivery for singleton breech in the preterm gestation. Due to concern for head entrapment as preterm fetuses tend to have a larger head circumference-to-abdominal circumference ratio, cesarean delivery is generally accepted as the preferred method of delivery [94]. There have been few randomized controlled trials to examine this question, due to low recruitment as the clinicians were reluctant to enroll eligible women [95,96]. Some studies suggest that routine cesarean delivery of breech fetuses born in the extremely preterm gestation (24–26 weeks) has not improved neonatal outcome, likely due to the inherent high morbidity and mortality associated with extreme prematurity and very low birthweight (VLBW) [97–100].

9.2.2 Shoulder presentation

Shoulder presentation is a result of an oblique or transverse fetal lie and occurs in approximately 1 in 300 deliveries [101,102]. Prematurity and high parity are the most common risk factors for transverse lie; other risk factors include: uterine anomalies, placenta previa, polyhydramnios, and multiple gestations [103,104]. Compared to cephalic presentation, fetuses in shoulder presentation are at higher risk of morbidity and mortality, partly due to the likelihood of concurrent low-birthweight and preterm birth [105]. Additionally, umbilical cord prolapse occasionally occurs with the fetus in transverse lie and can be associated with high rates of perinatal death and birth asphyxia, particularly if cord prolapse occurs outside of the hospital where immediate cesarean delivery is not readily feasible [106,107].

Management of shoulder presentation depends on the concurrent clinical situation. If the diagnosis of shoulder presentation is confirmed and the mother is either in labor or has rupture of the membranes, then cesarean delivery is indicated. If the membranes are intact and there is no contraindication to ECV, then ECV may be offered [105].

9.2.3 Funic presentation

Funic presentation refers to the clinical scenario where portions of the umbilical cord are the presenting part of the fetus and are thus closest to the cervix. While routine ultrasound surveillance to assess umbilical cord position is not recommended, the diagnosis of funic presentation can be made antepartum with ultrasonography and color Doppler when clinical suspicion arises [108,109]. In one cohort of women with breech presentation, weekly routine ultrasound after 36 weeks detected funic presentation in 4% of the study population [110]. When funic presentation is identified as an incidental finding prior to onset of labor, follow-up evaluation is recommended as many cases of funic presentation detected antepartum will resolve [109–111]. If funic presentation persists, scheduled cesarean delivery has been considered as funic presentation is a harbinger for cord prolapse and can be associated with high perinatal morbidity and mortality [110,111].

Umbilical cord prolapse occurs in 0.14–0.62% of deliveries [112–114]. Fetal malpresentation, particularly shoulder or footling presentation, is one of the strongest risk factors for cord prolapse [109–111]. However, cord prolapse can still occur in pregnancies with cephalic presentation as the overall incidence of nonvertex presentation is low. Other risk factors include prematurity, multiparity, polyhydramnios, rupture of the membranes, and low-lying placenta [110,115,116]. Thus, patients with preterm premature rupture of the membrane whose fetus is noncephalic are particularly at risk of umbilical cord prolapse. Obstetric interventions, such as artificial rupture of the membranes, particularly prior to engagement of the fetal head, fetal scalp electrode placement, intrauterine catheter insertion, and manual rotation of the fetal head also contribute to the occurrence of cord prolapse [117]. One sign of cord prolapse can be fetal bradycardia or severe variable decelerations on fetal heart tracing; at times, it can also be detected on cervical examination.

Once the diagnosis of cord prolapse is confirmed, prompt cesarean delivery is recommended to minimize perinatal morbidity and mortality [114,115,118]. While funic reduction has been reported as a management of umbilical cord prolapse, it can lead to intrapartum asphyxia or fetal death and thus may be considered only if cesarean delivery cannot be performed or if vaginal delivery is imminent [119]. Other resuscitative efforts in the case of cord prolapse include reducing or alleviating cord compression, including elevating the presenting part of the cord, placing patient in steep Trendelenburg position, and back-filling of maternal bladder as the distended bladder can elevate the presenting part [120,121]. While historically umbilical cord prolapse is associated with high risk of perinatal morbidity and mortality, studies suggest that outcomes in recent decades have improved, likely due to improved neonatal care/resuscitation and availability of cesarean, and because a high proportion of cord prolapses are due to iatrogenic obstetric procedures (such as artificial rupture of the membranes) in the hospital, where such interventions are readily available [117,122,123].

9.2.4 Face and brow presentation

9.2.4.1 Face presentation

Despite being head-down, nonvertex fetuses are still considered to have a malpresentation. Face presentation, with the fetal neck extended, is relatively rare, with an estimated incidence rate that ranges between 1 in 600 and 1 in 1250 deliveries [124,125]. Face presentation is more likely to occur in multiparous women than in nulliparous women [125,126]; other associated factors include black race/ethnicity, prematurity, low birthweight (<2500 g), fetal macrosomia, and cephalopelvic disproportion [124,127,128]. Additionally, fetal anomaly, particularly anencephaly and anterior neck mass, are risk factors for face presentation [125,126,129]. Typically diagnosed during labor, face presentation is further characterized as mentum anterior, mentum transverse, or mentum posterior position. Fetuses that present with mentum anterior position may be closely monitored and a vaginal delivery may be attempted, as the majority of these do achieve spontaneous vaginal delivery (~85%) [126,127,130]. While fetuses in mentum transverse position may rotate to anterior and thus deliver vaginally, cesarean delivery should be considered for fetuses with persistent mentum posterior position [127]. Variable decelerations are often noted in labor, as is longer duration of labor, and neonatal Apgar score of < 7 at 5 minutes, though there is no difference in base excess or other short-term neonatal outcome [126,127]. Of note, fetuses that have labored in the face presentation, particularly those that have experienced the pressures of second stage of labor, have faces that exhibit edema, bruising, and abrasions. It is important to warn patients of this fact so they are not shocked at the time of delivery.

9.2.4.2 Brow presentation

Similar to face presentation, the incidence rate of brow presentation is rare, estimated to be between 1 in 500 and 1 in 1700 [129,131]. The fetus presenting with the brow has an extended neck, but not to the degree of that in face presentation. While brow presentation is in itself not compatible with vaginal delivery, fetuses that present with their brow early in labor may either further extend their necks to face presentation or flex their necks and revert to vertex presentation. Thus, women with a clinically adequate pelvis may be managed expectantly with close monitoring, with cesarean delivery if abnormal labor or fetal intolerance of labor occurs [132,133]. Similar to face presentations, brow presenting fetuses may have bruising, edema, and abrasions of their faces, which should be mentioned to patients.

9.3 Malposition

While fetal presentation describes the presenting part of a fetus, fetal position describes the relation of the presenting part relative to the maternal pelvis. In the setting of a vertex presentation, the fetal occiput relative to the maternal pelvis is used to describe the fetal position. More specifically, the fetal occiput can be either in anterior (occiput anterior, or OA), posterior (occiput posterior, or OP), or transverse (occiput transverse, or OT) position. The fetal position in the transverse position can be further specified relative to maternal left or right side, so LOT or ROT. Further, if the presentation is between LOT and OA on the left side of the maternal pelvis it is described as left occiput anterior, or LOA. Similarly, a fetal presentation between ROT and OP on the right side of the maternal pelvis would be described as ROP.

9.3.1 Epidemiology

The diagnosis of fetal malposition is usually made by digital vaginal examination; bedside ultrasound may be used to confirm diagnosis if fetal position remains uncertain by clinical exam [134]. Persistent occiput posterior position (OP) is the most common malposition at delivery [135], with an incidence ranging between 2 and 13% [136,137]. It has been demonstrated that more fetuses actually enter labor in either OP or OT position and undergo rotation of the fetal head during the labor process such that most malpositions are a manifestation of intrapartum "malrotation" or lack of rotation during labor [134,138,139].

9.3.2 Risk factors

Factors associated with fetal malposition include nulliparity, maternal age greater than 35 years, African American race, macrosomia (birthweight > 4000 g), induction of labor, and epidural use [136–138,140–142]. The association between the use of epidural anesthesia in labor and fetal malposition has been examined widely and many studies report a higher rate of persistent OP position with epidural use [134,135,143]. However, other studies argue that the association between epidural and malposition may not be causal as the incidence rate of fetal malposition has remained relatively constant over time despite a dramatic increase in the use of epidural for labor analgesia over the past decades [135,136]. On the other hand, prospective studies that have examined changes in fetal position during labor in nulliparous women using serial ultrasound examinations observed that the proportion of fetal OP position was equivalent at the time of epidural placement and in early active labor (4 hours after admission) in women who did not have epidural analgesia; however, women who had epidural analgesia had a higher proportion of OP malposition at delivery (12.9%) compared to those without epidural (3.3%) [134,143]. It is thus hypothesized that epidural analgesia promotes pelvic muscle relaxation and thus inhibits fetal head rotation in labor, leading to higher likelihood of persistent OP position at delivery [134,143].

9.3.3 Perinatal outcomes with malposition

Fetal malposition has been associated with both increased maternal and increased neonatal complications. There are a number of studies that have found that OP position is associated with prolonged labor, increased rates of third- or fourth-degree perineal lacerations, postpartum hemorrhage, chorioamnionitis and operative deliveries, both operative vaginal delivery and cesarean delivery [139–141,145]. Specifically, it has been reported that only 15–29% of nulliparas and 55% of multiparas in persistent OP position achieved spontaneous vaginal delivery without operative interventions [136,139,141,144].

Neonates delivered in the OP position have been observed to have higher risks of adverse neonatal outcomes including acidemic umbilical cord gases (pH < 7.0 and/or base excess < −12), meconium-stained amniotic fluid (but not meconium aspiration syndrome), birth trauma, and admission to the neonatal intensive care nursery [144]. Neonates delivered in the OP position had lower 1-minute Apgar scores but not lower 5-minute Apgar scores when compared to those born in the OA position [136,141,145,146]. Interestingly, while it has been described that neonates delivering in the OP position have a lower rate of shoulder dystocia, they have a higher rate of brachial plexus injuries, which speaks to an etiology related to malposition in labor as opposed to birth trauma at the time of delivery.

9.3.4 Management

There are widely held beliefs about non-interventional ways to prevent OP position or to resolve OP position in labor. In the antepartum setting, there was a recent large, multicenter, randomized controlled trial in which the investigators assigned 2547 women at 36–37 weeks to exercise programs to examine whether a specific exercise regimen would facilitate anterior rotation of the fetal head to promote OA position in labor. One group was assigned to take a daily walk while the other group was asked to assume a hands-and-knees position with slow pelvic rocking for 10minutes twice daily until onset of labor. For both groups, the occurrence of OP position in labor was no different (~8%) [147]. Thus, to date there is no known effective intervention to minimize OP position prior to labor. A variety of maternal positions during labor to facilitate the resolution of OP position have been described in the nursing and midwifery literature, but to date have not been examined in prospective, randomized controlled trials.

Malposition is associated with labor dystocia, increased cesarean delivery and operative vaginal delivery as well as higher risk of maternal and neonatal morbidity; yet, rotational forceps are reserved for clinicians experienced and skilled in their application and fewer practitioners are adequately trained to offer such operative delivery and maneuvers [148]. Alternatively, manual rotation of the fetal occiput from OP/OT position to OA position was first described as an alternative intervention in 1971 by Walkowiak [149]. Because the fetal head can rotate on its own during labor, manual rotation should be avoided during the first stage of labor to avoid unnecessary intervention and minimize cervical laceration – a risk of manual rotation [150]. Recent studies further suggest manual rotation as a safe and effective intervention in the setting of labor arrest, particularly in the second stage, with a high rate of successful rotation ranging between 74 and 93% among those who underwent a trial of rotation [151,152]. Compared to expectant management of labor, women whose fetus was in OP or OT position undergoing successful manual rotation to OA position were less likely to deliver by cesarean or operative (forceps or vacuum-assisted) vaginal deliveries [150,152,153]. Women who had successful manual rotation from OP/OT position to OA position also had a shorter second stage of labor, and were less likely to have severe perineal lacerations (third- or fourth-degree perineal lacerations) and postpartum hemorrhage [154]. Maternal characteristics associated with higher likelihood of a successful rotation include multiparous women, and women younger than 35 years [150,152]. Additionally, rotational attempts are more likely to be successful when performed at time of diagnosis of malposition early in second stage (i.e. prophylactic rotation) than when arrest of descent has occurred [152]. However, because fetuses in OP/OT position early in second stage may rotate to the OA position spontaneously during the second stage and rotation attempt is associated with higher risk of cervical laceration, routine prophylactic rotation may not be warranted [152]. However, a recent, small, prospective, randomized trial demonstrated a shorter second stage of labor in women who underwent prophylactic rotation, though there was no effect on mode of delivery.

9.4 Conclusions

Fetal malpresentation and malposition are common challenges facing the obstetric clinician. One of the most important aspects of care for these abnormalities is to have a complete understanding of the risks and benefits of various management plans to be able to adequately counsel patients. Another important feature is actually making the diagnosis of these complications so that appropriate intervention can be taken. For example, diagnosis of breech presentation should be made at 35–36 weeks of gestation so that ECV can occur in a timely fashion as success rates are higher with an earlier gestational age. Similarly, malpresentations and malpositions in labor should be diagnosed earlier as well. For those who have challenges diagnosing malposition with a vaginal exam, ultrasound is a useful adjunct. While there is little to do in the setting of malpresentation in labor to effect change, delivery management will vary. Malposition is important to diagnose in labor so that an attempt at manual (or forceps) rotation may be affected to reduce complications and operative deliveries.

References

1 Demol S, Bashiri A, Furman B, Maymon E, Shoham-Vardi I, and Mazor M. Breech presentation is a risk factor for intrapartum and neonatal death in preterm delivery. *European Journal of Obstetrics & Gynecology and Reproductive Biology* 2000; **93**(1):47–51.

2 Benson WL, Boyce DC, and Vaughn DL. Breech delivery in the primigravida. *Obstetrics & Gynecology* 1972;**40**(3):417–428.

3 Hickok DE, Gordon DC, Milberg JA, Williams MA, and Daling JR. The frequency of breech presentation by gestational age at birth: a large population-based study. *American Journal of Obstetrics & Gynecology* 1992;**166**(3):851.

4 Martin JA, Hamilton BE, Sutton PD, Ventura SJ, Menacker F, Kirmeyer S *et al.* Division of Vital Statics. Birth: Final data for 2006. *National Vital Statistics Reports* 2009;**57**(7)1–102.

5 Martin JA, Hamilton BE, Sutton PD, Ventura SJ, Mathews TJ, and Osterman MJK. Division of Vital Statistics. Births: Final data for 2008. *National Vital Statistics Reports* 2010;**59**(1):1–72.

6 Luterkort M, Polberger S, Weldner BM, Persson PH, and Bjerre I. Growth in breech presentation. Ultrasound and post-partal assessment of growth in 225 fetuses presenting by the breech in the 33rd gestational week. *American Journal of Obstetrics & Gynecology* 1986;**65**(2):157–160.

7 Sherer DM, Spong CY, Minior VK, and Salafia CM. Increased incidence of fetal growth restriction in association with breech presentation in preterm deliveries <32 weeks. *American Journal of Perinatology* 1997;**14**(1):35–37.

8 Schutte MF, van Hemel OJ, van de Berg C, and van de Pol A. Perinatal mortality in breech presentations as compared to vertex presentations in singleton pregnancies: an analysis based upon 57,819 computer-registered pregnancies in the Netherlands. *European Journal of Obstetrics & Gynecology and Reproductive Biology* 1985;**19**(6):391–400.

9 De Crespigny LJ and Pepperell RJ. Perinatal mortality and morbidity in breech presentation. *Obstetrics & Gynecology* 1979;**53**(2):141–145.

10 Krebs L and Langhoff-Roos J. The relation of breech presentation at term to epilepsy in childhood. *European Journal of Obstetrics & Gynecology and Reproductive Biology* 2006;**127**(1):26–28.

11 Sørensen HT, Steffensen FH, Olsen J, Sabroe S, Gillman MW, Fischer P, and Rothman KJ.Long-term follow-up of cognitive outcome after breech presentation at birth. *Epidemiology* 1999;**10**(5):554–556.

12 Ford JB, Roberts CL, Nassar N, Giles W, and Morris JM. Recurrence of breech presentation in consecutive pregnancies. *BJOG* 2010;**117**(7):830–836.

13 Albrechtsen S, Rasmussen S, Dalaker K, and Irgens LM. Reproductive career after breech presentation: subsequent pregnancy rates, interpregnancy interval, and recurrence. *Obstetrics & Gynecology* 1998;**92**(3):345.

14 Fox AJ and Chapman MG. Longitudinal ultrasound assessment of fetal presentation: a review of 1010 consecutive cases. *Australian and New Zealand Journal of Obstetrics and Gynaecology* 2006;**46**(4):341–344.

15 Westgren M, Edvall H, Nordström L, Svalenius E, and Ranstam J. Spontaneous cephalic version of breech presentation in the last trimester. *British Journal of Obstetrics and Gynaecology* 1985;**92**(1):19–22.

16 Axelrod FB, Leistner HL, and Porges RF. Breech presentation among infants with familial dysautonomia. *Journal of Pediatrics* 1974;**84**(1):107–109.

17 Roberts CL, Algert CS, Peat B, and Henderson-Smart D. Small fetal size: a risk factor for breech birth at term. *International Journal of Gynecology & Obstetrics* 1999;**67**(1):1–8.

18 Ludford I, Scheil W, Tucker G, and Grivell R. Pregnancy outcomes for nulliparous women of advanced maternal age in South Australia, 1998–2008. *Australian and New Zealand Journal of Obstetrics and Gynaecology* 2012;**52**(3):217–219.

19 Ben-Rafael Z, Seidman DS, Recabi K, Bider D, and Mashiach S. Uterine anomalies. A retrospective, matched-control study. *Journal of Reproductive Medicine* 1991;**36**(10):723.

20 Michalas SP. Outcome of pregnancy in women with uterine malformation: evaluation of 62 cases. *International Journal of Gynecology & Obstetrics.* 1991;**35**(3):215.

21 Hua M, Odibo AO, Longman RE, Macones GA, Roehl KA, and Cahill AG. Congenital uterine anomalies and adverse pregnancy outcomes. *American Journal of Obstetrics & Gynecology* 2011;**205**(6):558 e1–5. Epub 2011 Jul 22.

22 2Stout MJ, Odibo AO, Graseck AS, Macones GA, Crane JP, and Cahill AG. Leiomyomas at routine second-trimester ultrasound examination and adverse obstetric outcomes. *Obstetrics & Gynecology* 2010;**116**(5):1056–1063.

23 Qidwai GI, Caughey AB, and Jacoby AF. Obstetric outcomes in women with sonographically identified uterine leiomyomata. *Obstetrics & Gynecology* 2006;**107**(2 Pt 1):376–382.

24 Lam MH, Chan LY, Wong SF, Tam W, and Lau TK. Relationship between maternal pelvic parameters and idiopathic term breech presentation. *European Journal of Obstetrics & Gynecology and Reproductive Biology* 2005;**118**(2):267–268.

25 Karp LE. Breech presentation and parity: the proof of the pelvis. *Journal of the American Medical Association*. 1983;**249**(5):647.
26 Vendittelli F, Rivière O, Crenn-Hébert C, Rozan MA, Maria B, and Jacquetin B; AUDIPOG Sentinel Network. Is a breech presentation at term more frequent in women with a history of cesarean delivery? *American Journal of Obstetrics & Gynecology* 2008;**198**(5):521 e1–6.
27 Kalogiannidis I, Masouridou N, Dagklis T, Masoura S, Goutzioulis M, Prapas Y, and Prapas N. Previous cesarean section increases the risk for breech presentation at term pregnancy. *Clinical and Experimental Obstetrics & Gynecology* 2010;**37**(1):29–32.
28 Fianu S and Václavínková V. The site of placental attachment as a factor in the aetiology of breech presentation. *American Journal of Obstetrics & Gynecology* 1978;**57**(4):371.
29 Gemer O and Segal S. Incidence and contribution of predisposing factors to transverse lie presentation. *International Journal of Gynecology & Obstetrics* 1994;**44**(3):219–221.
30 Lydon-Rochelle M, Albers L, Gorwoda J, Craig E, and Qualls C. Accuracy of Leopold maneuvers in screening for malpresentation: a prospective study. *Birth* 1993;**20**(3):132–135.
31 Thorp JM Jr, Jenkins T, and Watson W. Utility of Leopold maneuvers in screening for malpresentation. *Obstetrics & Gynecology* 1991;**78**(3 Pt 1):394–396.
32 Daniel Y, Fait G, Lessing JB, Jaffa A, Gull I, Shenav M, Peyser MR, and Kupferminc MJ. Umbilical cord blood acid-base values in uncomplicated term vaginal breech deliveries. *American Journal of Obstetrics & Gynecology* 1998;**77**(2):182–185.
33 Christian SS and Brady K. Cord blood acid-base values in breech-presenting infants born vaginally. *Obstetrics & Gynecology* 1991;**78**(5 Pt 1):778–781.
34 Wigglesworth JS and Husemeyer RP. Intracranial birth trauma in vaginal breech delivery: the continued importance of injury to the occipital bone. *British Journal of Obstetrics and Gynaecology* 1977;**84**(9):684–691.
35 Rietberg CC, Elferink-Stinkens PM, Brand R, van Loon AJ, Van Hemel OJ, and Visser GH. Term breech presentation in the Netherlands from 1995 to 1999: mortality and morbidity in relation to the mode of delivery of 33,824 infants. *BJOG* 2003;**110**(6):604–609.
36 American College of Obstetricians and Gynecologists Practice Patterns No. 4, July 1997: External cephalic version. *International Journal of Gynecology & Obstetrics* 1997;**59**(1):73–80.
37 Tan JM, Macario A, Carvalho B, Druzin ML, and El-Sayed YY. Cost-effectiveness of external cephalic version for term breech presentation. *BMC Pregnancy Childbirth* 2010;**10**:3.
38 Burgos J, Cobos P, Rodriguez L, Pijoán JI, Fernández-Llebrez L, Martínez-Astorquiza T, and Melchor JC. Clinical score for the outcome of external cephalic version: a two-phase prospective study. *Australian and New Zealand Journal of Obstetrics and Gynaecology* 2012;**52**(1):59–61.
39 Aisenbrey GA, Catanzarite VA, and Nelson C. External cephalic version: predictors of success. *Obstetrics & Gynecology* 1999;**94**(5 Pt 1):783–786.
40 Lau TK, Lo KW, Wan D, and Rogers MS. Predictors of successful external cephalic version at term: a prospective study. *British Journal of Obstetrics and Gynaecology* 1997;**104**(7):798.
41 Brocks V, Philipsen T, and Secher NJ. A randomized trial of external cephalic version with tocolysis in late pregnancy. *British Journal of Obstetrics and Gynaecology* 1984;**91**(7):653.
42 Kok M, Cnossen J, Gravendeel L, van der Post J, Opmeer B, and Mol BW. Clinical factors to predict the outcome of external cephalic version: a meta-analysis. *American Journal of Obstetrics & Gynecology* 2008;**199**(6):630 e1.
43 Fortunato SJ, Mercer LJ, and Guzick DS. External cephalic version with tocolysis: factors associated with success. *Obstetrics & Gynecology* 1988;**72**(1):59.
44 Newman RB, Peacock BS, VanDorsten JP, and Hunt HH. Predicting success of external cephalic version. *American Journal of Obstetrics & Gynecology* 1993;**169**(2 Pt 1):245–249.
45 Boucher M, Bujold E, Marquette GP, and Vezina Y. The relationship between amniotic fluid index and successful external cephalic version: a 14-year experience. *American Journal of Obstetrics & Gynecology* 2003;**189**(3):751–754.

46 Adama van Scheltema PN, Feitsma AH, Middeldorp JM, Vandenbussche FP, and Oepkes D. Amnioinfusion to facilitate external cephalic version after initial failure. *Obstetrics & Gynecology* 2006;**108**(3 Pt 1):591–592.

47 Hutton EK, Kaufman K, Hodnett E, Amankwah K, Hewson SA, McKay D, Szalai JP, and Hannah ME. External cephalic version beginning at 34 weeks' gestation versus 37 weeks' gestation: a randomized multicenter trial. *American Journal of Obstetrics & Gynecology* 2003;**189**(1):245–254

48 Hutton EK and Hofmeyr GJ. External cephalic version for breech presentation before term. *Cochrane Database of Systematic Reviews* 2006;(**1**):CD000084. Review.

49 Hutton EK, Hannah ME, Ross SJ, Delisle MF, Carson GD, Windrim R *et al.* Early ECV2 Trial Collaborative Group. The Early External Cephalic Version (ECV) 2 Trial: an international multicentre randomised controlled trial of timing of ECV for breech pregnancies. *BJOG.* 2011;**118**(5):564–577. DOI: 10.1111/j.1471-0528.2010.02837.x. Epub 2011 Feb 4.

50 Grootscholten K, Kok M, Oei SG, Mol BW, and van der Post JA. External cephalic version-related risks: a meta-analysis. *Obstetrics & Gynecology* 2008;**112**(5):1143.

51 Cluver C, Hofmeyr GJ, Gyte GM, and Sinclair M. Interventions for helping to turn term breech babies to head first presentation when using external cephalic version. *Cochrane Database of Systematic Reviews* 2012;(**1**):CD000184.

52 Hofmeyr GJ. Interventions to help external cephalic version for breech presentation at term. *Cochrane Database of Systematic Reviews* 2004;(**1**):CD000184.

53 Dugoff L, Stamm CA, Jones OW, III, Mohling SI, and Hawkins JL. The effect of spinal anesthesia on the success rate of external cephalic version: a randomized trial. *Obstetrics & Gynecology* 1999;**93**(3):345–349.

54 Weiniger CF, Ginosar Y, Elchalal U, Sela HY, Weissman C, and Ezra Y. Randomized controlled trial of external cephalic version in term multiparae with or without spinal analgesia. *British Journal of Anaesthesia* 2010;**104**(5):613–618. Epub 2010 Mar 25.

55 Sullivan JT, Grobman WA, Bauchat JR, Scavone BM, Grouper S, McCarthy RJ *et al.* A randomized controlled trial of the effect of combined spinal-epidural analgesia on the success of external cephalic version for breech presentation. *International Journal of Obstetric Anesthesia* 2009;**18**(4):328–334.

56 Weiniger CF, Ginosar Y, Elchalal U, Sharon E, Nokrian M, and Ezra Y. External cephalic version for breech presentation with or without spinal analgesia in nulliparous women at term: a randomized controlled trial. *Obstetrics & Gynecology* 2007;**110**(6):1343–1350.

57 Mancuso KM, Yancey MK, Murphy JA, and Markenson GR. Epidural analgesia for cephalic version: a randomized trial. *Obstetrics & Gynecology* 2000;**95**(5):648–651.

58 Goetzinger KR, Harper LM, Tuuli MG, Macones GA, and Colditz GA. Effect of regional anesthesia on the success rate of external cephalic version: a systematic review and meta-analysis. *Obstetrics & Gynecology* 2011;**118**(5):1137–1144.

59 Vézina Y, Bujold E, Varin J, Marquette GP, and Boucher M. Cesarean delivery after successful external cephalic version of breech presentation at term: a comparative study. *American Journal of Obstetrics & Gynecology* 2004;**190**(3):763–768.

60 Lau TK, Lo KW, and Rogers M. Pregnancy outcome after successful external cephalic version for breech presentation at term. *American Journal of Obstetrics & Gynecology* 1997;**176** (1 Pt 1):218–223. Review.

61 Chan LY, Leung TY, Fok WY, Chan LW, and Lau TK. High incidence of obstetric interventions after successful external cephalic version. *BJOG* 2002;**109**(6):627–631.

62 Wright RC. Reduction of perinatal mortality and morbidity in breech delivery through routine use of cesarean delivery. *Obstetrics & Gynecology* 1959;**14**:758–763.

63 Ghosh MK. Breech presentation: evolution of management. *Journal of Reproductive Medicine* 2005;**50**(2):108–116.

64 Bowes WA Jr, Taylor ES, O'Brien M, and Bowes C. Breech delivery: evaluation of the method of delivery on perinatal results and maternal morbidity. *American Journal of Obstetrics & Gynecology* 1979;**135**(7):965–973.

65 Martin JA, Hamilton BE, Sutton PD, Ventura SJ, Menacker F, and Munson ML. Division of Vital Statistics. Birth: Final data for 2003. *National Vital Statistics Reports* 2005;**54**(2):1–116.

66 Lee HC, El-Sayed YY, and Gould JB. Population trends in cesarean delivery for breech presentation in the United States, 1997–2003. *American Journal of Obstetrics & Gynecology* 2008;**199**(1):59 e1–8.

67 Rietberg CC, Elferink-Stinkens PM, and Visser GH. The effect of the Term Breech Trial on medical intervention behaviour and neonatal outcome in the Netherlands: an analysis of 35,453 term breech infants. *BJOG* 2005;**112**(2):205–209.

68 Pradhan P, Mohajer M, and Deshpande S. Outcome of term breech births: 10-year experience at a district general hospital. *BJOG* 2005;**112**(2):218–222.

69 Pasupathy D, Wood AM, Pell JP, Fleming M, and Smith GC. Time trend in the risk of delivery-related perinatal and neonatal death associated with breech presentation at term. *International Journal of Epidemiology* 2009;**38**(2):490–498.

70 Irion O, Hirsbrunner Almagbaly P, and Morabia A. Planned vaginal delivery versus elective caesarean section: a study of 705 singleton term breech presentations. *British Journal of Obstetrics and Gynaecology* 1998;**105**(7):710–717.

71 Lindqvist A, Nordén-Lindeberg S, and Hanson U. Perinatal mortality and route of delivery in term breech presentations. *British Journal of Obstetrics and Gynaecology* 1997; **104**(11):1288–1291.

72 Kiely JL. Mode of delivery and neonatal death in 17,587 infants presenting by the breech. *British Journal of Obstetrics and Gynaecology* 1991;**98**(9):898–904.

73 Thorpe-Beeston JG, Banfield PJ, and Saunders NJ. Outcome of breech delivery at term. *BMJ* 1992;**305**(6856):746–747.

74 Roman J, Bakos O, and Cnattingius S. Pregnancy outcomes by mode of delivery among term breech births: Swedish experience 1987–1993. *Obstetrics & Gynecology* 1998; **92**(6):945–950.

75 Obwegeser R, Ulm M, Simon M, Ploeckinger B, and Gruber W. Breech infants: vaginal or cesarean delivery? *American Journal of Obstetrics & Gynecology* 1996;**75**(10):912–916.

76 Collea JV, Chein C, and Quilligan EJ. The randomized management of term frank breech presentation: a study of 208 cases. *American Journal of Obstetrics & Gynecology* 1980; **137**(2):235–244.

77 Hannah ME, Hannah WJ, Hewson SA, Hodnett ED, Saigal S, and Willan AR. Planned caesarean section versus planned vaginal birth for breech presentation at term: a randomised multicentre trial. *Term Breech Trial Collaborative Group. Lancet.* 2000;**356**(9239):1375–1383.

78 American College of Obstetricians and Gynecologists, Committee on Obstetric Practice Committee Opinion No. 265, December 2001: Mode of term singleton breech delivery. *International Journal of Gynecology & Obstetrics* 2002;**77**(1):65–66.

79 Hartnack Tharin JE, Rasmussen S, and Krebs L. Consequences of the Term Breech Trial in Denmark. *Acta Obstetricia et Gynecologica Scandinavica* 2011;**90**(7):767–771.

80 Hannah ME, Hannah WJ, Hodnett ED, Chalmers B, Kung R, Willan A *et al.* Term Breech Trial 3-Month Follow-up Collaborative Group. Outcomes at 3 months after planned cesarean vs planned vaginal delivery for breech presentation at term: the international randomized Term Breech Trial. *Journal of the American Medical Association.* 2002;**287**(14):1822–1831.

81 Hannah ME, Whyte H, Hannah WJ, Hewson S, Amankwah K, Cheng M *et al.* Term Breech Trial Collaborative Group. Maternal outcomes at 2 years after planned cesarean section versus planned vaginal birth for breech presentation at term: the international randomized Term Breech Trial. *American Journal of Obstetrics & Gynecology* 2004;**191**(3):917–927.

82 Whyte H, Hannah ME, Saigal S, Hannah WJ, Hewson S, Amankwah K *et al.* Term Breech Trial Collaborative Group. Outcomes of children at 2 years after planned cesarean birth versus planned vaginal birth for breech presentation at term: the International Randomized Term Breech Trial. *American Journal of Obstetrics & Gynecology* 2004;**191**(3): 864–871.

83 American College of Obstetricians and Gynecologists Committee Opinion No. 340, July 2006: Mode of term singleton breech delivery. *Obstetrics & Gynecology* 2006;**108**:235–237.

84 Munstedt K, von Georgi R, Reucher S, Zygmundt M, and Lang U. Term breech and long-term morbidity – cesarean section versus vaginal breech delivery. *European Journal of Obstetrics & Gynecology and Reproductive Biology* 2001;**96**(2):163–167.

85 Danielian PJ, Wang J, and Hall MH. Long-term outcome by method of delivery of fetuses in breech presentation at term: population-based follow-up. *BMJ* 1996;**312**(7044):1451–1453.

86 Alarab M, Regan C, O'Connell MP, Keane DP, O'Herlihy C, and Foley ME. Singleton vaginal breech delivery at term: still a safe option. *Obstetrics & Gynecology* 2004;**103**:407–412.

87 Guiliani A, Scholl WM, Basver A, and Tamussino KF. Mode of delivery and outcomes of 699 term singleton breech deliveries in a single center. *American Journal of Obstetrics & Gynecology* 2002;**187**:1694–1698.

88 Hopkins LM, Esakoff T, Noah MS, Moore DH, Sawaya GF, and Laros RK Jr. Outcomes associated with cesarean section versus vaginal breech delivery at a university hospital. *Journal of Perinatology* 2007;**27**(3):141–146.

89 Goffinet F, Carayol M, Foidart JM, Alexander S, Uzan S, Subtil D, and Bréart G; PREMODA Study Group. Is planned vaginal delivery for breech presentation at term still an option? Results of an observational prospective survey in France and Belgium. *American Journal of Obstetrics & Gynecology* 2006;**194**(4):1002–1011.

90 Laros RK Jr, Flanagan TA, and Kilpatrick SJ. Management of term breech presentation: a protocol of external cephalic version and selective trial of labor. *American Journal of Obstetrics & Gynecology* 1995;**172**(6):1916–1923.

91 Russell JGB and Richards B. A review of the pelvimetry data. *British Journal of Radiology* 1971;**44**:780–784.

92 Jeyabalan A, Larkin RW, and Landers DV. Vaginal breech deliveries selected using computed tomographic pelvimetry may be associated with fewer adverse outcomes. *Journal of Maternal-Fetal and Neonatal Medicine* 2005;**17**(6):381–385.

93 Hauth JC and Cunningham FG. Vaginal breech delivery is still justified. *Obstetrics & Gynecology* 2002;**99**(6):1115–1116.

94 Robilio PA, Boe NM, Danielsen B, and Gilbert WM. Vaginal vs cesarean delivery for preterm breech presentation of singleton infants in California: a population-based study. *Journal of Reproductive Medicine* 2007;**52**(6):473.

95 Penn ZJ, Steer PJ, and Grant A. A multicentre randomised controlled trial comparing elective and selective caesarean section for the delivery of the preterm breech infant. *British Journal of Obstetrics and Gynaecology* 1996;**103**(7):684.

96 Zlatnik FJ. The Iowa premature breech trial. *American Journal of Perinatology* 1993;**10**(1):60.

97 Stohl HE, Szymanski LM, and Althaus J. Vaginal breech delivery in very low birth weight (VLBW) neonates: experience of a single center. *Journal of Perinatal Medicine* 201;**39**(4):379–383.

98 Cibils LA, Karrison T, and Brown L. Factors influencing neonatal outcomes in the very-low-birth-weight fetus (<1500 grams) with a breech presentation. *American Journal of Obstetrics & Gynecology* 1994;**171**(1):35–42.

99 Malloy MH, Onstad L, and Wright E. The effect of cesarean delivery on birth outcome in very low birth weight infants. National Institute of Child Health and Human Development Neonatal Research Network. *Obstetrics & Gynecology* 1991;**77**(4):498–503.

100 Main DM, Main EK, and Maurer MM. Cesarean section versus vaginal delivery for the breech fetus weighing less than 1500 grams. *American Journal of Obstetrics & Gynecology* 1983;**146**(5):580–584.

101 Seeds JW and Cefalo RC. Malpresentations. *Clinical Obstetrics and Gynecology* 1982;**25**(1):145–156. Review.

102 Gemer O and Segal S. Incidence and contribution of predisposing factors to transverse lie presentation. *International Journal of Gynecology & Obstetrics* 1994;**44**(3):219.

103 Nassar N, Roberts CL, Cameron CA, and Olive EC. Diagnostic accuracy of clinical examination for detection of non-cephalic presentation in late pregnancy: cross sectional analytic study. *BMJ* 2006;**333**(7568):578.

104 Kawathekar P, Kasturilal MS, Srinivas P, and Sudha G. Etiology and trends in the management of transverse lie. *American Journal of Obstetrics & Gynecology* 1973;**117**(1):39–44.

105 Hankins GD, Hammond TL, Snyder RR, and Gilstrap LC, III. Transverse lie. *American Journal of Perinatology* 1990;**7**(1):66.

106 Ylä-Outinen A, Heinonen PK, and Tuimala R. Predisposing and risk factors of umbilical cord prolapse. *American Journal of Obstetrics & Gynecology* 1985;**64**(7):567.

107 Uygur D, Kiş S, Tuncer R, Ozcan FS, Erkaya S. Risk factors and infant outcomes associated with umbilical cord prolapse. *International Journal of Gynecology & Obstetrics* 2002;**78**(2):127.

108 Raga F, Osborne N, Ballester MJ, and Bonilla-Musoles F. Color flow Doppler: a useful instrument in the diagnosis of funic presentation. *Journal of the National Medical Association* 1996;**88**(2):94–96.

109 Lange IR, Manning FA, Morrison I, Chamberlain PF, and Harman CR. Cord prolapse: is antenatal diagnosis possible? *American Journal of Obstetrics & Gynecology* 1985;**151**(8):1083–1085.

110 Kinugasa M, Sato T, Tamura M, Suzuki H, Miyazaki Y, and Imanaka M. Antepartum detection of cord presentation by transvaginal ultrasonography for term breech presentation: potential prediction and prevention of cord prolapse. *Journal of Obstetrics and Gynaecology Research* 2007;**33**(5):612–618.

111 Ezra Y, Strasberg SR, and Farine D. Does cord presentation on ultrasound predict cord prolapse? *Gynecologic and Obstetric Investigation* 2003;**56**(1):6.

112 Dilbaz B, Ozturkoglu E, Dilbaz S, Ozturk N, Sivaslioglu AA, and Haberal A. Risk factors and perinatal outcomes associated with umbilical cord prolapse. *Archives of Gynecology and Obstetrics* 2006;**274**(2):104–107.

113 Koonings PP, Paul RH, and Campbell K. Umbilical cord prolapse. A contemporary look. *Journal of Reproductive Medicine* 1990;**35**(7):690.

114 Murphy DJ and MacKenzie IZ. The mortality and morbidity associated with umbilical cord prolapse. *British Journal of Obstetrics and Gynaecology* 1995;**102**(10):826.

115 Kahana B, Sheiner E, Levy A, Lazer S, and Mazor M. Umbilical cord prolapse and perinatal outcomes. *International Journal of Gynecology & Obstetrics* 2004;**84**(2):127.

116 Oyelese Y, Yeo L, Kinzler W, Smulian J, and Vintzileos AM. Persistent funic presentation resulting from marginal cord insertion into a low-lying placenta. *Ultrasound in Obstetrics & Gynecology* 2004;**24**(6):692–693.

117 Usta IM, Mercer BM, and Sibai BM. Current obstetrical practice and umbilical cord prolapse. *American Journal of Perinatology* 1999;**16**(9):479.

118 Critchlow CW, Leet TL, Benedetti TJ, and Daling JR. Risk factors and infant outcomes associated with umbilical cord prolapse: a population-based case-control study among births in Washington State. *American Journal of Obstetrics & Gynecology* 1994;**170**(2):613–618.

119 Barrett JM. Funic reduction for the management of umbilical cord prolapse. *American Journal of Obstetrics & Gynecology* 1991;**165**(3):654–657.

120 Runnebaum IB and Katz M. Intrauterine resuscitation by rapid urinary bladder instillation in a case of occult prolapse of an excessively long umbilical cord. *European Journal of Obstetrics & Gynecology and Reproductive Biology* 1999;**84**(1):101–102.

121 Katz Z, Shoham Z, Lancet M, Blickstein I, Mogilner BM, and Zalel Y. Management of labor with umbilical cord prolapse: a 5-year study. *Obstetrics & Gynecology* 1988;**72**(2):278.

122 Boyle JJ and Katz VL. Umbilical cord prolapse in current obstetric practice. *Journal of Reproductive Medicine* 2005;**50**(5):303–306.

123 Khan RS, Naru T, and Nizami F. Umbilical cord prolapse – a review of diagnosis to delivery interval on perinatal and maternal outcome. *Journal of Pakistan Medical Association* 2007;**57**(10):487–491.

124 Duff P. Diagnosis and management of face presentation. *Obstetrics & Gynecology* 1981;**57**(1):105.

125 Benedetti TJ, Lowensohn RI, and Truscott AM. Face presentation at term. *Obstetrics & Gynecology* 1980;**55**(2):199–202.

126 Schwartz Z, Dgani R, Lancet M, and Kessler I. Face presentation. *Australian and New Zealand Journal of Obstetrics and Gynaecology* 1986;**26**(3):172–176.

127 Shaffer BL, Cheng YW, Vargas JE, Laros RK Jr, and Caughey AB. Face presentation: predictors and delivery route. *American Journal of Obstetrics & Gynecology* 2006;**194**(5):e10–2. Epub 2006 Apr 21.

128 Bhal PS, Davies NJ, and Chung T. A population study of face and brow presentation. *Journal of Obstetrics and Gynaecology* 1998;**18**(3):231–235.

129 Bashiri A, Burstein E, Bar-David J, Levy A, and Mazor M. Face and brow presentation: independent risk factors. *Journal of Maternal-Fetal and Neonatal Medicine* 2008;**21**(6):357.

130 Barger MK. What do you do when the baby is winking at you? Case report of a face presentation. *Journal of Midwifery & Womens Health* 2002;**47**(6):487–489.

131 Gardberg M, Leonova Y, and Laakkonen E. Malpresentations – impact on mode of delivery. *American Journal of Obstetrics & Gynecology* 2011;**90**(5):540–542.

132 Stitely ML and Gherman RB. Labor with abnormal presentation and position. *Obstetrics and Gynecology Clinics of North America* 2005;**32**(2):165–179.

133 Levy DL. Persistent brow presentation: a new approach to management. *Southern Medical Journal* 1976;**69**(2):191–192.

134 Leiberman E, Davidson K, Lee-Parritz A, and Shearer E. Changes in fetal position during labor and their association with epidural anesthesia. *Obstetrics & Gynecology* 2005;**105**:974–982.

135 Yancy MK, Zhang J, Schweitzer DL, Schwarz J, and Klebanoff MA. Epidural anesthesia and fetal head malposition at vaginal delivery. *Obstetrics & Gynecology* 2001;**97**:608–612.

136 Sizer AR and Nirmal DM. Occipitoposterior position: associated factors and obstetric outcomes in nulliparas. *Obstetrics & Gynecology* 2000;**96**:749–752.

137 Gardberg M and Tuppurainen M. Persistent occiput posterior presentation – a clinical problem. *American Journal of Obstetrics & Gynecology* 1994;**73**:45–47.

138 Akmal S, Tsoi E, Howard R, Osei E, and Nicolaides KH. Investigation of OP delivery by intrapartum sonography. *Ultrasound in Obstetrics & Gynecology* 2004;**24**:425–428.

139 Gardberg M, Laakkonen E, and Sälevaara M. Intrapartum sonography and persistent occiput posterior position: A study of 408 deliveries. *Obstetrics & Gynecology* 1998; **91**:746–749.

140 Cheng YW, Shaffer BL, and Caughey AB. Associated factors and outcomes of persistent occiput posterior position: A retrospective cohort study from 1976–2001. *Journal of Maternal-Fetal and Neonatal Medicine* 2006;**19**(9):563–568.

141 Fitzpatrick M, McQuillan K, and O'Herlihy C. Influence of persistent occiput posterior position on delivery outcome. *Obstetrics & Gynecology* 2001;**98**:1027–1031.

142 Souka AP, Haritos T, Basayiannis K, Niokokyri N, and Antsaklis A. Intrapartum ultrasound for the examination of the fetal head position in normal and obstructed labor. *Journal of Maternal-Fetal and Neonatal Medicine* 2003;**13**:59–63.

143 Robinson CA, Macones GA, Roth NW, and Morgan MA. Does station of the fetal head at epidural placement affect the position of the fetal vertex at delivery? *American Journal of Obstetrics & Gynecology* 1996;**175**:991–994.

144 Cheng YW, Shaffer BL, and Caughey AB. The association between persistent occiput posterior position and neonatal outcomes. *Obstetrics & Gynecology* 2006;**107**(4):837–844.

145 Floberg J, Belfrage P, and Ohlsen H. Influence of the pelvic outlet capacity on fetal head presentation at delivery. *American Journal of Obstetrics & Gynecology* 1987;**66**:127–130.

146 Senécal J, Xiong X, and Fraser WD, for the PEOPLE Study Group. Effect of fetal position on second-stage duration and labor outcome. *Obstetrics & Gynecology* 2005;**105**:763–772.

147 Kariminia A, Chamberlain ME, Keogh J, and Shea A. Randomised controlled trial of effect of hands and knees posturing on incidence of occiput posterior position at birth. *BMJ* 2004;**328**(7438):490.

148 Park JS, Robinson JN, and Norwitz ER. Rotational forceps: should these procedures be abandoned? *Seminars in Perinatology* 2003;**27**(1):112–120.

149 Walkowiak RG. Manual rotation of the transverse posterior occiput. *Obstetrics & Gynecology* 1971;**37**:464–467.

150 Shaffer BL, Cheng YW, Varagas JE, Laros RK, and Caughey AB. Manual rotation of the fetal occiput: predictors of success and delivery. *American Journal of Obstetrics & Gynecology* 2006;**194**:37–39.

151 Cargill YM, MacKinnon CJ, Arsenault MY, Bartellas E, Daniels S, Gleason T *et al.* Clinical Practice Obstetrics Committee. Guidelines for operative vaginal birth. *Journal of Obstetrics and Gynaecology Canada* 2004;**26**:747–761.

152 Le Ray C, Serres P, Schmitz T, Cabrol D, and Goffinet F. Manual rotation in occiput posterior or transverse position: risk factors and consequences on cesarean delivery rate. *Obstetrics & Gynecology* 2007;**110**:873–879.

153 Reichman O, Gdansky E, Latinsky B, Labi S, and Samueloff A. Digital rotation from occiputo-posterior to occipito-anterior decreases the need for cesarean section. *European Journal of Obstetrics & Gynecology and Reproductive Biology* 2008;**136**:25–28.

154 Shaffer BL, Cheng YW, Vargas JE, and Caughey AB. Manual rotation to reduce cesarean delivery in persistent occiput posterior or transverse position. *Journal of Maternal-Fetal and Neonatal Medicine* 2010;**24**(1):65–72.

CHAPTER 10
Multiple gestations

Laura Houston and Roger Newman
Maternal-Fetal Medicine, Medical University of South Carolina, Charleston, SC, USA

10.1 Introduction

The incidence of multifetal gestations continues to rise in the United States. The highest rate of twin births was reported in 2009, at 33.2/1000 live births, a 2% rise from the previous year. There has been a continuous increase in twin births since 1980, with a more gradual rise since 2004. These increasing rates of twin births have varied across ethnicities, ranging from a 62% rise in non-Hispanic white women, to a 42% in non-Hispanic black women, and a 25% in Hispanic women in the past two decades [1].

Similarly, an increase in the rate of triplet and higher order gestations was noted in 2009, at 153.5/100,000 births. Overall, a 400-fold increase has occurred since the 1980s, with the highest incidence reported in 1998. While variable, the rate has been decreasing since that peak. In absolute numbers, 137,217 twins and 5905 triplets were born in the United States in 2009 [1].

The increasing incidence of multiple gestations has largely been attributed to delayed maternal childbearing and assisted reproductive technologies (ART) [2]. In 2006, 17% of all twins and 38% of triplets and higher order multiple gestations in the United States were related to assisted technologies [3].

10.2 Perinatal and maternal complications

While representing a little over 3% of pregnancies, multiple gestations are associated with a disparate proportion of perinatal morbidity and mortality. In 2005, the fetal mortality rate was 2.7-fold higher for twins, compared to singletons. This increased to fivefold higher when considering higher order multiple

Management of Labor and Delivery, Second Edition. Edited by George A. Macones.

gestations [4]. The increased risk of premature birth is related to both spontaneous preterm labor and indicated preterm birth. According to 2005 data from the Centers for Disease Control, the mean gestational age at birth was 35.2 weeks for twins and 31.9 weeks for triplets in the United States [5]. In 2009, the mean birthweight was 2336 g for twins and 1660 g for triplets [1].

The relationship of perinatal morbidity and mortality beyond the association with premature birth and growth restriction, however, is not completely clear. Numerous studies have reported an increase in mortality among multiple gestations, compared to singletons [6,7]. When considering the late preterm period beyond 34 weeks, risks of perinatal complications such as respiratory distress syndrome and sepsis were greater in twins when compared to singletons of a similar gestational age [8]. In a study comparing growth restricted singletons and twins, the twins were noted to have an increased risk of morbidity and mortality [9]. Conversely, other studies have reported similar outcomes for multiple gestations when matched with singletons by gestational age [10,11]. When considering extremely low-birthweight twins and triplets (401–1000 g), increased risks of mortality and neurodevelopmental delay have been reported [12,13]. However, a study of very low-birthweight (VLBW) multiples (<1500 g) found similar rates of morbidity, with the exception of an increased risk for apnea and patent ductus arteriosus [14].

Overall, rates of neurodevelopmental disability such as cerebral palsy are higher for multiples, compared to singleton gestations [7,15]. One study reported that 1.5% of twin pregnancies result in at least one child with cerebral palsy, compared to 8% of triplets and 43% of quadruplets [16]. Monochorionicity has been reported as a risk factor as well [17]. In a study of over 1 million births from Australian and American data, the overall rate of cerebral palsy was fourfold higher in twins than in singletons. This rate was similar regardless of birth order and same or different sex pairs. A higher rate was noted in the surviving twin whose co-twin had died in utero or in the neonatal period [7]. Similar to mortality, the risk for cerebral palsy is related to gestational age and birthweight. A literature review in 2009 stratified risk of cerebral palsy by birthweight and found no differences in singletons and twins with birthweight < 2500 g. A higher rate of cerebral palsy, however, was noted in twins born > 2500 g, compared to singletons of the same birthweight [18].

Additional antepartum considerations in multiple gestations include risks of monochorionicity, monoamnionicity, twin-to-twin transfusion, congenital anomalies, and abnormalities of fetal growth, including growth discordance and growth restriction [19–22]. Early ultrasound is important in order to establish accurate dating and chorionicity, as are follow-up ultrasounds to define anatomic normality and assess fetal growth. Multiple gestations are at higher risk for hospitalization during pregnancy [23]. Complications such as gestational diabetes, urinary tract infections, anemia, and pruritic urticarial papules and plaques of pregnancy (PUPP) are seen more commonly in multiple gestations [24–26].

Intrapartum risks include preterm labor, premature rupture of membranes, placental abruption, hypertensive disorders, malpresentation, and increased rate of cesarean delivery [27–29]. A prospective trial found a twofold increased risk of gestational hypertension and 2.6-fold higher risk of preeclampsia in twin pregnancies compared to singletons. Higher rates of preterm birth were reported in these pregnancies [30]. Similar risks were seen in retrospective data inclusive of over 100,000 twin pregnancies. However, twins with gestational hypertension were not found to have an increased risk of adverse outcomes compared with singleton pregnancies [31]. The incidence of abruption is higher in multiple gestations. This was confirmed in a large retrospective study of singleton and multiple pregnancies [32]. Interestingly, the rate of perinatal mortality related to abruption was noted to decrease with increasing fetal number. Although speculative, this may be related to the shorter duration of pregnancy with greater plurality. When growth discordance is present, however, abruption does magnify the risk of adverse outcomes [33].

Postpartum hemorrhage, likely a consequence of uterine overdistention, is a significant consideration in the immediate postpartum period. With vaginal delivery, the use of pitocin and prolonged labor are additive risk factors for uterine atony [34]. Several trials have found an increased risk for peripartum hysterectomy in multiple gestations [35,36]. One study, however, reported no increased risk after controlling for mode of delivery [37]. The maternal and fetal risks associated with multiple gestations are summarized in Table 10.1.

Table 10.1 Maternal-fetal risks of multiple gestations.

Antepartum
- perinatal mortality
- neurodevelopmental disability
- monochorionicity/twin-to-twin transfusion
- congenital anomalies
- growth discordance
- growth restriction
- hospitalization
- gestational diabetes
- urinary tract infections
- anemia
- pruritic urticarial papules and plaques of pregnancy (PUPP)

Intrapartum
- preterm labor
- premature rupture of membranes
- hypertensive disorders
- malpresentation
- abruption
- cesarean delivery

Postpartum
- uterine atony
- postpartum hemorrhage
- peripartum cardiomyopathy

10.3 Intrapartum preparation

Preparation is fundamental to the successful delivery of a multiple gestation (Table 10.2). Obstetrical providers with experience in delivery of multiples should be present, as well as a pediatric or neonatology team capable of neonatal resuscitation. Obstetrical anesthesia should be immediately available during labor and present for delivery. An experienced nursing staff is also necessary, given the difficulty sometimes encountered in fetal monitoring and potential for maternal complications during delivery.

Ultrasound at presentation should confirm fetal presentation, as well as assessment of fetal weight. A portable ultrasound device is recommended, so that ultrasound can be used in the operating room during delivery. It should be cautioned that determining the fetal lie of twins in a term or near term laboring woman is not always an easy task. This can be a critical decision point, and the fetal lie should be confirmed by an experienced sonologist.

Continuous monitoring of each fetus should be performed throughout labor. External fetal monitoring is acceptable; however, care must be taken to ensure that each fetus is being monitored separately. If monitoring is questionable and rupture of membranes is feasible, an internal scalp electrode can be placed on the presenting twin. Continuous uterine tocometry is also important. Assessment

Table 10.2 Intrapartum preparation in multiple gestations.

Teams
• obstetric
• neonatal
• anesthesia
• nursing
Fetal monitoring
• external fetal monitoring and tocometry
• availability of internal monitors
• portable ultrasound machine
Maternal resuscitation
• large-bore (16–18 gauge) IV
• availability of blood products
• uterotonics
o methylergonovine (Methergine)
o 15-methyl prostaglandin $F_{2\alpha}$ (Hemabate)
o oxytocin
Operating room
Delivery
• vacuum or forceps, including Piper forceps
• uterine tocolytics
o nitroglycerine
o terbutaline

of fetal decelerations is made in relation to contractions, and pitocin administration can be titrated to adequate contraction frequency but avoidance of uterine tachysystole.

Availability of an operating room and blood bank is essential for the safe delivery of multiples. Adequate IV access with a large-bore (16–18 gauge) IV at presentation is recommended, with assessment of initial hemoglobin and platelet count. Blood should be readily available for the patient, given the risk of uterine atony. All uterotonics, such as methylergonovine (Methergine), 15-methyl prostaglandin $F_{2\alpha}$ (Hemabate), and oxytocin, should be accessible. Conversely, uterine tocolytics, such as nitroglycerine and terbutaline, should be present in the event that uterine relaxation is needed. Delivery in an operating room is recommended with all teams present. This "double set-up" allows for emergent cesarean to be performed if necessary during delivery. Epidural anesthesia is recommended for labor, which permits immediate fetal manipulation or cesarean if complications are encountered.

10.4 Timing of delivery

The optimal gestational age for delivery of multiples must balance complications of prematurity with risk of fetal death as pregnancy continues. An increased risk of third-trimester stillbirth is seen at earlier gestational ages in twins compared to singletons (Figure 10.1). Numerous studies have reported that the nadir of

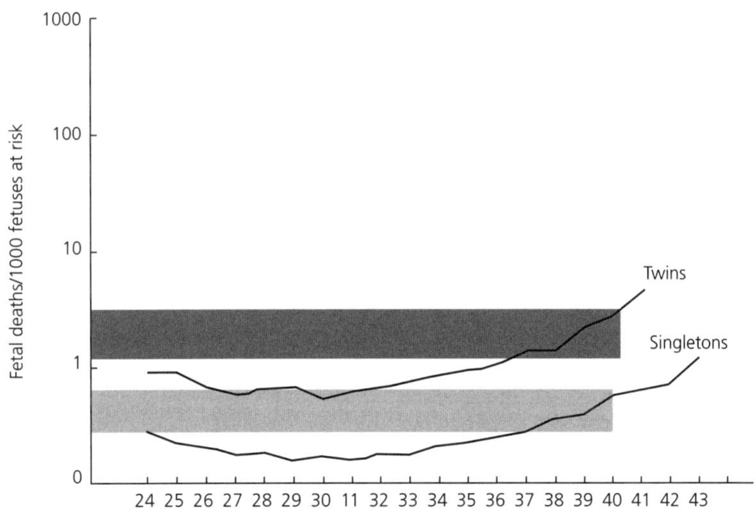

Figure 10.1 Fetal death rate and prospective risk of fetal death (stillbirth) for singleton and twin gestations. *Source*: Kahn *et al.*, 2003 [44]. Adapted with permission from Lippincott Williams & Wilkins.

perinatal mortality in twins occurs between 37 and 38 weeks of gestation, compared to later gestational ages in singletons [38–40].

A consensus conference sponsored by the Eunice Kennedy Shriver National Institute of Child Health and Human Development (NICHD) and Society for Maternal-Fetal Medicine (SMFM) in 2011 offered consensus-based recommendations for multiple gestations [41]. The proposed gestational age of 38 weeks for delivery of uncomplicated dichorionic twins has been fairly consistent with prior recommendations as the optimal time to minimize both fetal and neonatal risk [42,43]. Earlier delivery would be indicated for maternal or fetal complications, such as non-reassuring fetal testing, significant growth restriction, oligohydramnios, or abnormal Doppler studies. Delivery could be extended to, but no later than, 39 weeks with normal, concordant growth and amniotic fluid, reassuring fetal testing, and thorough patient counseling [44]. Optimal timing for monochorionic twins is less clear. Monochorionicity appears to be associated with higher risk of unanticipated stillbirth during the late preterm and early term gestational periods [45,46]. The NICHD/SMFM workshop proposed a delivery interval for monochorionic twins of 34–37 weeks of gestation [41]. This recommendation has been challenged in a recent publication in press by Robinson *et al.*, which employs a decision analysis and concludes that delivery of monochorionic twins between 36 and 38 weeks of gestation is associated with optimal outcomes [47]. Delivery recommendations for additional high-risk multiple gestations, such as monoamniotic twins and higher order multiples, should be individualized in consultation with a Maternal-Fetal Medicine specialist experienced in multiple gestations.

10.5 Delivery

Decisions regarding mode of delivery require consideration of multiple factors. Fetal presentation, fetal weight and concordance, prior obstetrical history, maternal stability, and fetal status are all important aspects of that decision. Operator experience and infrastructure capabilities are also essential elements in the development of a delivery plan. If the delivering obstetrician does not perform breech vaginal deliveries, for example, this will limit options available for the patient. Patient counseling remains central to the development of an effective delivery plan.

Regrettably, there is a paucity of strong clinical data regarding the delivery of multiples. Few large prospective or randomized trials are available to guide clinical decision making. Much of current obstetrical practice results from a combination of large experiential reviews, retrospective cohort studies, and expert consensus. Given the methodologic shortcomings of this data type, it is unclear whether differences, or lack thereof, seen in obstetrical and neonatal outcomes result from true differences in mode of delivery, or can be largely attributed to bias and confounding in the trials.

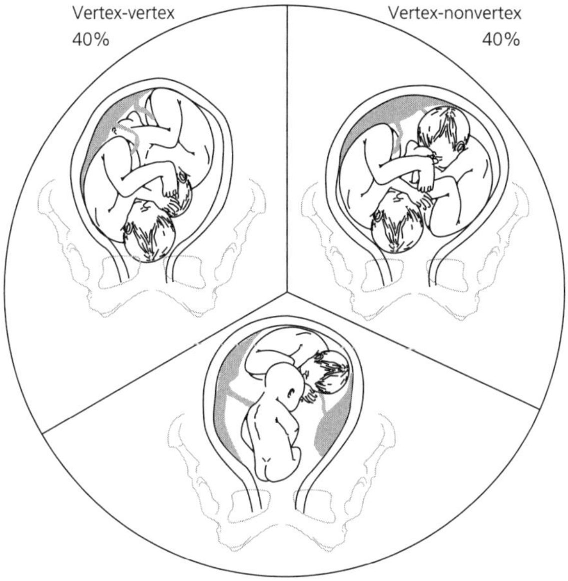

Figure 10.2 Three presentation alternatives encountered in twin gestations and their relative frequencies.

A useful way to conceptualize the various delivery options for multiple gestations is to consider the variable presentation alternatives (Figure 10.2).

10.6 Vertex/vertex

General obstetrical opinion supports a trial of labor with vertex/vertex presentation, occurring in 38–48% of twins [48]. A high rate of success with vaginal delivery, up to 81–91%, is reported in the literature [49,50].

There does not appear to be neonatal benefit from routine cesarean delivery for either normal or VLBW vertex/vertex twins. An earlier retrospective study suggested that vaginally delivered vertex second twins under 1500 g experienced greater morbidity than those delivered by cesarean [51]. While some authors have reported similar findings [48,52], this trend has been contradicted by others [53], including a population-based study conducted between 1995 and 1999 that did not find any neonatal benefit to cesarean delivery if birthweight was less than 1500 g [54]. A retrospective study conducted between 1994 and 1999 not only failed to find a benefit to cesarean delivery for VLBW twins, but reported a higher incidence of respiratory distress syndrome (RDS) in vertex/vertex twins who had undergone cesarean compared to vaginal delivery [55]. Morales and colleagues also reported an increased rate of RDS in vertex/vertex twins under 1500 g delivered by cesarean [56].

Historically, delivery of the second twin within 30 minutes of the first has been advised. Studies have been inconsistent regarding this recommendation. An older study found no difference in 5-minute Apgars in vaginally delivered vertex-vertex twins; this included delivery intervals greater than 20 minutes [57]. More recent studies have focused on a trend toward decreasing umbilical cord pH values and Apgar scores with an increasing delivery interval [58]. In a study from 2002, the median delivery interval was 16.5 minutes. Decreasing arterial and venous pH and base excess values were reported with increasing inter-delivery times. All second twins born within 15 minutes of their co-twin had umbilical arterial pH values greater than 7. Of note, all twins with pH values less than 7 had abnormalities seen on their intrapartum tracing [59]. There is a paucity of long-term data related to the delivery interval; as such, the implications of these short-term findings are unknown. Setting a fixed time limit on delivery of the second twin will increase the risk of iatrogenic intervention. With reassuring continuous fetal monitoring, an absolute time limit is not necessary. However, it is important to be mindful of the interval and the potential for complications during this time period.

Following delivery of the presenting twin, close monitoring of both position and fetal heart rate of the second twin is important. The availability of an assistant skilled in ultrasound is useful so the position of the second twin can be followed closely. Ultrasound findings are confirmed by pelvic examination, and the fetal heart monitor is then repositioned on the second twin for continuous monitoring. Ultrasound and pelvic exam are important to assess fetal descent and cervical dilation, and for exclusion of complications, such as a compound presentation or cord prolapse. Once position and a reassuring heart rate have been confirmed, pitocin can be increased or initiated if contractions are not sufficient. This can occur within 10 minutes of delivery of the first twin if contractions have not resumed. Amniotomy can be performed in the usual fashion if the fetal vertex is well applied to the cervix, or leaked slowly with a spinal needle, with close monitoring of fetal descent. This is ideally performed during a contraction to facilitate application of the fetal vertex to the cervix.

Delivery in an operating room enhances preparedness in the event of a complication during delivery, with availability of obstetrical, neonatal, anesthesia, and nursing staff. If a complication develops following delivery of the presenting twin, options include emergent cesarean delivery of the second twin, operative vaginal delivery, or internal podalic version with subsequent breech extraction. The safety of internal podalic version in an emergent circumstance is unknown, and this option is rarely undertaken due to the limited experience and training in this skill and to the rapid availability of cesarean delivery. Similarly, high operative vaginal delivery should be avoided in favor of an emergent cesarean. If the option of cesarean is unavailable, an emergent mid or high operative vaginal delivery should be performed only by an experienced obstetrician.

A large US population-based study analyzed over 42,000 vertex second twins, following vaginal delivery of the presenting twin. The authors reported an 8.3% operative vaginal delivery rate of the second twin, with an additional 6.3% delivered by cesarean [60]. Non-reassuring fetal status, cord prolapse, maternal complications, abnormal labor, and birthweight discordance with the second twin weighing 25% more than the presenting twin were associated with an increased risk of either an operative vaginal or a cesarean delivery. Cord prolapse and non-reassuring fetal status were more strongly associated with cesarean delivery [60].

10.7 Vertex/nonvertex

Approximately 40% of twin gestations will have a vertex/nonvertex presentation. The majority of these are vertex/breech, with a smaller proportion vertex/transverse and vertex/oblique. The optimal mode of delivery for vertex/nonvertex twins is unknown and remains a controversial issue in obstetrics. Study findings are inconsistent, and conclusive practice recommendations are difficult to make given variations in comparison groups and study populations. Additionally, this literature is largely retrospective and observational, with only one randomized trial for consideration.

Many authors have advocated the safety of vaginal delivery in vertex/nonvertex twin gestations (Table 10.3). In 1982, Acker reported a comparison between 74 nonvertex second twins who underwent cesarean and 76 second twins delivered vaginally by breech extraction. No difference in mortality or 5-minute Apgar scores < 7 was noted [61]. In 1985, Chervenak found no difference in neonatal death, respiratory distress syndrome, intraventricular hemorrhage, or 5-minute Apgar scores < 6 between 112 vertex second twins and 80 nonvertex second twins delivered vaginally. One neonatal death occurred following cesarean delivery in their cohort of 362 twin gestations. Three neonatal injuries were reported: Erb's palsy and cephalohematoma, both in presenting vertex twins, and a clavicular/humerus fracture in a second twin delivered by breech extraction [57]. Similar findings have been reported by other authors [62–64]. One randomized trial from Israel was published in 1987. Thirty-three vertex/nonvertex twins over 35 weeks of gestation were randomized to vaginal delivery, and 27 to cesarean. No differences in neonatal morbidity were reported [65].

In a prospective study of 266 vertex/nonvertex twin gestations, neonatal benefits were associated with vaginal delivery for both infants. A lower incidence of pulmonary and infectious complications was found for nonvertex second twins delivered by breech extraction, compared to external cephalic version and cesarean delivery [69]. In 2002, Caukwell and Murphy reported a retrospective comparison of 237 vertex and 185 nonvertex second twins. Admission to the neonatal intensive care unit was noted to be higher in vertex second twins

Table 10.3 Nonvertex second twin-similar outcomes for cesarean and vaginal delivery.

Study	Comparison groups (second twin)	Outcome
Acker *et al.* 1982 [61]	74 nonvertex-cesarean 76 nonvertex-vaginal breech	No difference in mortality
Chervenak *et al.* 1985 [57]	112 vertex-vaginal 80 nonvertex-vaginal breech	No difference in neonatal death, RDS, IVH
Mazor *et al.* 1986 [62]	89 vertex 89 nonvertex	No difference in perinatal morbidity
Gocke *et al.* 1989 [63]	41 nonvertex-ECV 55 nonvertex-vaginal breech 40 nonvertex-cesarean	No difference in neonatal morbidity and mortality
Rabinovici *et al.* 1987 [65] (only RCT)	33 nonvertex-vaginal 27-cesarean	No difference in neonatal morbidity
Mauldin *et al.* 1998 [69]	41 nonvertex-vaginal 19-ECV, vaginal 24-cesarean	↓ pulmonary, infectious complications for vaginal breech delivery
Caukwell and Murphy 2002 [70]	237 vertex 185 nonvertex	No difference in perinatal death, RDS ↑ NICU admission-vertex, cesarean
Schmitz *et al.* 2008 [71]	657 planned vaginal 101 planned cesarean	No difference in neonatal morbidity
Adam *et al.* 1991 [64]	146 vertex 120 nonvertex	No difference in neonatal morbidity overall 1 perinatal death and 3 IVH-breech vaginal < 1500 g or < 32 weeks
Fishman *et al.* 1993 [66]	207 vertex 193 nonvertex	No difference in neonatal outcomes
Greig *et al.* 1992 [67]	416 total twins 54 nonvertex-vaginal	No differences in neonatal outcomes, except ↓ 1-minute Apgar scores in second nonvertex vaginal delivery
Davison *et al.* 1992 [68]	54 nonvertex-vaginal 43 nonvertex-cesarean	No difference in neonatal morbidity

RDS = respiratory distress syndrome; IVH = intraventricular hemorrhage; ECV = external cephalic version; RCT = randomized controlled trial; NICU = neonatal intensive care unit.

delivered by cesarean, although it is unclear how the indication for cesarean may confound this finding. Five-minute Apgar scores < 7, respiratory distress syndrome, and perinatal death rates were similar [70]. In 2006, a retrospective study of over 600 twin gestations in France revealed no difference in neonatal morbidity between second twins delivered vaginally or by cesarean [49]. In 2008,

Table 10.4 Studies favoring cesarean for delivery of nonvertex second twin.

Study	Comparison groups (second twin)	Outcome
Yang *et al.* 2005 [72]	5723 nonvertex-cesarean 7113-nonvertex-vaginal 2349 nonvertex-cesarean following vaginal delivery of A	↑ neonatal mortality in vaginally delivered
Usta *et al.* 2005 [73]	138 nonvertex-vaginal 79 nonvertex-cesarean	↑ neonatal morbidity and mortality in vaginally delivered If > 1500 g, no difference in neonatal death
Armson *et al.* 2006 [74]	733 vertex 454 nonvertex	↑ perinatal mortality and neonatal morbidity in second twins born vaginally
Herbst *et al.* 2008 [75]	2638 cesarean deliveries 13,353 vaginal deliveries	↑ neonatal morbidity when second twin delivered vaginally (<34 weeks)

a retrospective study of 758 twin pairs over 35 weeks of gestation compared the outcomes of second twins from 657 planned vaginal deliveries and 101 planned cesareans. Overall, neonatal morbidity was higher in the planned cesarean group, but no differences were noted after controlling for pregnancy complications [71].

Conversely, multiple authors have suggested that cesarean is the preferred mode of delivery when the second twin is nonvertex (Table 10.4). In 2005, a retrospective study of over 15,000 vertex/nonvertex twin pairs was published from the US matched multiple birth dataset. A higher neonatal mortality rate was found in twins delivered vaginally compared to those delivered by cesarean [72]. In the same year, a retrospective study of 217 vertex/nonvertex twins revealed that neonatal morbidity and mortality was higher among vaginally delivered twins, compared to those born by cesarean. When limiting the analysis to those twins greater than 1500 g, 5-minute Apgar scores and the neonatal death rate were no longer significantly different, while 1-minute Apgar scores < 4 remained greater in the vaginal group [73]. Composite morbidity and mortality in more than 1500 twin pairs was higher in second twins born vaginally, compared to first twins born vaginally in a retrospective analysis published in 2006. Conversely, outcomes were similar for first and second twins born by planned cesarean over 37 weeks and under 34 weeks. Second twins, however, experienced more adverse outcomes when delivered between 34 and 36 weeks by planned cesarean. Thirty-three cesareans were needed to avoid one composite adverse outcome [74]. In 2008, over 22,000 twin pairs from a Swedish national medical registry were analyzed. When both twins were born vaginally, a higher rate of neonatal mortality and 5-minute Apgar scores < 7 were noted in the second twin, compared to second twins born by cesarean. When stratifying by gestational age, both findings remained significant for second twins born before 34 weeks. Only 5-minute Apgar scores < 7 remained significant over 34 weeks of gestation [75].

Differing conclusions can be found regarding the issue of VLBW second twins in nonvertex presentation. In 1982, a retrospective study found an increased risk of mortality among nonvertex second twins weighing 601–999 g born vaginally, compared to their vaginally delivered presenting co-twin. For birthweight 1000–1499 g, increased morbidity was found for second twins delivered vaginally. No differences were seen in twins born by cesarean [51]. Rydhstrom reported no differences in mortality when assessing presentation in over 800 twins weighing less than 1500 g. The cesarean delivery rate for malpresentation increased significantly during the study period (from 6 to 60%); however, no differences in cerebral palsy or mental retardation were found [53]. Zhang *et al.* reported a benefit of cesarean delivery on morbidity and mortality for twins weighing less than 1000 g [52]. Similarly, Ziadeh and Badria reported decreased mortality among 40 vertex/nonvertex twins with birthweights less than 1500 g when the mode of delivery was cesarean [55]. Alternatively, a retrospective study in 2004 by Shinwell and colleagues did not find a difference in neonatal outcomes for twins less than 1500 g delivered by cesarean or vaginally [54].

When preparing for vaginal delivery of a vertex/nonvertex twin pair, the skill level of the obstetrician is paramount. If the obstetrician does not perform breech extraction, a cesarean delivery would be recommended. Patient consent to breech extraction of the second twin is necessary. Availability of immediate cesarean delivery, uterine tocolytics, and adequate anesthesia are essential as well. Epidural anesthesia is recommended so patient discomfort does not prevent appropriate interventions. Ultrasound at admission should be performed to estimate fetal weight in addition to presentation. Definitions of significant fetal weight discordance are variable in the literature. Some definitions are based on percentage of weight difference, while others use absolute estimated weight differences. A study using the US matched multiple birth dataset reported an impact of mode of delivery on mortality only for discordance over 40% [76]. A study in 2003 reported overall similar neonatal outcomes in vaginally delivered twins who differed by as much as 250 g, where the second twin was larger [77]. Technical difficulty may be encountered, however, if the second twin is larger by 500 g or more.

Following delivery of the presenting twin, the presentation of the second twin should be immediately assessed by vaginal exam and ultrasonography. If the second twin is in the frank breech presentation and is engaged, artificial rupture of membranes can be performed during a uterine contraction, assisted with fundal pressure. The infant should be allowed to spontaneously deliver to the level of the umbilicus with assisted breech extraction subsequently performed, carefully maintaining the body in a neutral position. With rotation, each shoulder is swept out, flexing each antecubital fossa. Delivery of the head is then achieved with flexion of the head using the Mauriceau–Smellie–Veit maneuver. Piper forceps can also assist delivery of the head. Delivery of a footling or complete breech presentation is best achieved by total breech extraction. Using a vaginal hand, the feet are grasped, if possible while membranes are intact. Difficulty may be encountered if a hand is confused for a foot.

Once the feet have been carried well down into the vaginal canal, the membranes are ruptured during a contraction, and the infant is delivered with breech maneuvers. The routine use of 50– 100 μg of nitroglycerine to relax the lower uterine segment is advised to assist with all breech extractions. If a transverse lie is encountered, options for vaginal delivery include internal podalic version with breech extraction or external cephalic version and vertex vaginal delivery.

Care must be taken in assessing appropriate candidates for vaginal delivery of the nonvertex presenting second twin. A relatively recent phenomenon has been the increasing frequency of combined delivery (cesarean delivery of the second twin following vaginal delivery of the first twin). Estimates for this occurrence have varied widely (0–24.8%) [72,78,79]. Analysis of the US matched multiple birth database reported an increased risk of neonatal mortality among vertex/breech infants born by the combined vaginal-cesarean route, compared with both born by cesarean or vertex/vertex born vaginally [80]. Increased neonatal morbidity, such as lower Apgar scores and increased risks of ventilation and seizure, has been reported in other studies of combined delivery as well [81,82].

10.8 Nonvertex first twin

A nonvertex presenting twin is less commonly encountered – generally, in less than 20% of twin pairs. Data regarding optimal mode of delivery is limited. Cesarean is strongly indicated for a transverse presentation of the first twin. Following the results of the Term Breech Trial [83], suggesting a reduced risk of singleton neonatal morbidity and mortality with cesarean compared to breech vaginal delivery, cesarean has also been increasingly favored as the mode of delivery for a breech presenting first twin. Small retrospective studies have been published, which report similar outcomes for breech-vertex vaginal delivery compared to cesarean; however, these studies suffer from a lack of sufficient sample size to draw powerful conclusions. Blickstein *et al.* reported similar morbidity and mortality among 24 vaginally delivered breech/vertex twins, compared to 35 delivered by cesarean [84]. In France, planned vaginal delivery was retrospectively compared with planned cesarean in approximately 200 patients with a breech presenting twin, over 35 weeks of gestation. Of 124 patients in the planned vaginal delivery group, 48% delivered vaginally. No differences in adverse neonatal composite outcome were noted. Venous thromboembolism was higher in the planned cesarean group [85].

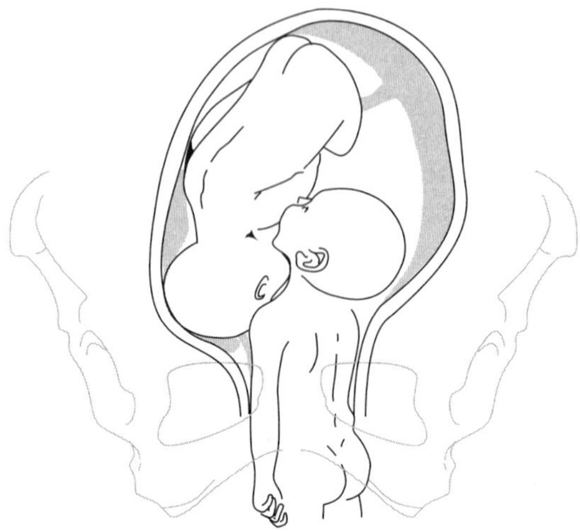

Figure 10.3 Interlocking chins of a breech/vertex twin gestation resulting in an impacted delivery.

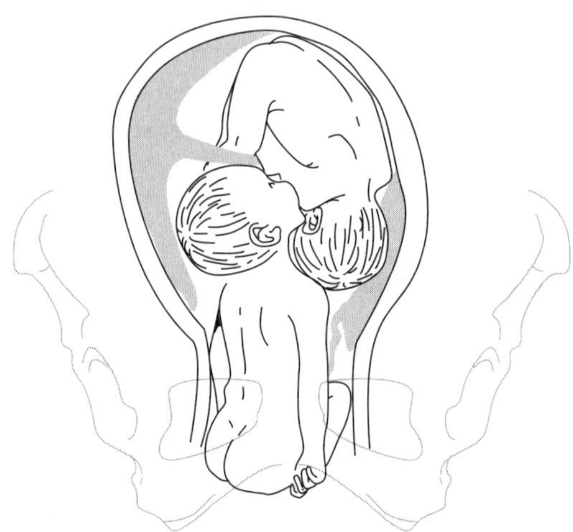

Figure 10.4 Deflexion of the head of breech twin A due to the influence of the vertex of twin B.

A rare but perilous outcome of vaginal delivery in breech/vertex twins is impaction or interlocking of the two infants (Figure 10.3). As the presenting breech twin descends into the pelvis, its chin can become impacted against the neck or chin of the second vertex twin. This appears to be quite rare in the literature (1 in 645 to 817 twin deliveries); however, it is potentially catastrophic for the presenting twin, as delivery will be obstructed [86,87]. Even if interlocking does not occur, there is still the possibility that the second twin could induce extension of the first twin's head, increasing the risk of head entrapment, cervical injury, labor dystocia, or cord prolapse during delivery (Figure 10.4). Kelsick and

Minkoff reported a 4.2% perinatal loss rate with vaginal delivery of a breech first twin compared to 2.4% when delivery was by cesarean [88].

While vaginal delivery is not absolutely contraindicated for breech/vertex twins, strong consideration should be given to cesarean delivery. If vaginal delivery is planned, risks and benefits should be thoroughly discussed with the patient, and a skilled obstetrician present for delivery.

10.9 Cesarean delivery

Although cesarean delivery of both twins eliminates the risks of a combined vaginal/cesarean birth, it does not eliminate maternal and neonatal risks during delivery. While some authors have reported an increase in respiratory morbidity with cesarean delivery of multiples, this has not been observed by others. In a retrospective review of 126 twins delivered by cesarean after 36 weeks of gestation, Chasen *et al.* reported an increased risk of respiratory complications only in twins born prior to 38 weeks of gestation [89]. A study from 2010 assessed the risk of transient tachypnea of the newborn after 37 weeks of gestation in relation to an increasing rate of elective cesareans performed at their institution (from an 18% rate of elective cesarean to 25–48%). No difference was found among the three time periods assessed [90].

Similar to vaginal delivery, intrapartum preparation for cesarean delivery of multiples requires planning and availability of resources. Large-bore IV access (16–18 gauge) is recommended, and availability of blood products should be confirmed with the blood bank. Uterotonics, including methylergonovine (Methergine), 15-methyl prostaglandin $F_{2\alpha}$ (Hemabate), and oxytocin, should be present in the operating room given the risk of uterine atony and postpartum hemorrhage. Availability of uterine tocolytics, such as nitroglycerine or terbutaline, is also necessary in the event difficulty is encountered with intrauterine fetal manipulation during delivery. Relaxation of uterine tone may help reduce fetal injury and unnecessary uterine incisions or lacerations. A skilled anesthesia team should be present, as well as nursing staff and pediatric teams prepared for each infant.

Decision making regarding the type of uterine incision requires consideration of infant presentation, birthweight, thickness or development of the lower uterine segment, and proficiency of the obstetrician. A low-transverse uterine incision is generally favored if the lower uterine segment is developed. By the third trimester, most twins will demonstrate development of the lower uterine segment. However, if the lower uterine segment is thick, estimated birthweight is less than 1500 g, and malpresentation is noted, difficulty may be encountered delivering through a low-transverse incision, and a vertical hysterotomy should be considered. Concerns include the possibility of head entrapment or a contraction band occurring between the upper and lower uterine segments, contributing to a difficult delivery.

If difficulty is encountered once a low-transverse incision has been made, options include extending the incision and/or administering uterine tocolytics. A low-transverse incision can be extended either in a J fashion, from one or both edges with bandage scissors, or by creating a vertical uterine incision from the middle, a T-incision. A J-incision may provide better exposure and ultimately closes as a stronger uterine repair. Our preference would be the immediate administration of 50–100 μg of nitroglycerine given intravenously. Alternatively, 0.25–0.50 mg of terbutaline can be given subcutaneously for uterine relaxation, although in our experience this does not work as completely or as quickly as nitroglycerine.

Avoiding rupture of membranes with creation of the hysterotomy can be beneficial. The incision may be extended either by manual stretch or bandage scissors. In a labored uterus or with a well-developed lower uterine segment, manual stretch often provides an adequate hysterotomy. If unlabored or thick, bandage scissors may be needed. If the first fetus is vertex, a hand is placed under the head, which is lifted upward toward the hysterotomy. Rupture of membranes is performed. Rotating the head for delivery to an occiput anterior presentation reduces the risk of hysterotomy extension. Delivery is facilitated with fundal pressure. If frank breech is noted, the hips are grasped and elevated toward the hysterotomy. Membranes are ruptured, and steady traction on the hips is applied with the infant's back facing upward until the scapulae are visible. Usual breech maneuvers are then used to deliver the arms and head. If the presenting twin is footling or complete breech or transverse, the feet are grasped first, ideally while membranes are intact. Once the feet have reached the hysterotomy, membranes can be ruptured, and the infant is delivered by breech extraction. Piper forceps can be used to assist with delivery of the after-coming head if needed.

Following delivery of the first twin, attention should be turned to the second twin's presentation. Delivery is achieved similarly to that of the first twin. Minimizing time to delivery of the second twin is beneficial, given the risk of uterine contraction and changes in uterine pressure and perfusion following delivery of the presenting twin.

10.10 Special cases

10.10.1 Trial of labor after prior cesarean

In well-selected patients with twins, a trial of labor after prior cesarean (TOLAC) can be a safe option. Similar contraindications should be respected as in singletons, such as a prior vertical hysterotomy, myomectomy, uterine rupture, or usual obstetrical contraindications to labor. Vertex/vertex presentation, prior vaginal delivery, and spontaneous labor are the most favorable predictors of success, although these elements are not absolutely required for a trial of labor.

Small retrospective studies have reported 70–80% success rates with TOLAC in twin pregnancies, which is a similar success rate to that for singleton gestations. These studies include relatively small numbers of patients and are subject to bias and confounding [91,92]. A larger prospective study published in 1996 assessed the outcomes of 210 women with twin pregnancies and prior cesarean section. Of those, 56% underwent elective repeat c-section, and the remaining 92 patients attempted a trial of labor. Sixty-four patients (70%) successfully delivered both twins vaginally. Sixteen per cent failed trial of labor and delivered both twins by cesarean, whereas 14% underwent combined vaginal and cesarean delivery. An increased rate of endomyometritis was found in women who had an elective repeat cesarean, and one maternal death in the study occurred due to pulmonary embolism following repeat cesarean. No uterine ruptures occurred following trial of labor. After controlling for prematurity and obstetrical complications, no differences were seen in neonatal morbidity or mortality [93].

A 4-year, prospective multicenter trial performed within the NICHD Maternal-Fetal Medicine Units Network reported the results of 412 women with twin gestation and at least one prior cesarean section. Fifty-five per cent underwent elective repeat cesarean, with 186 women undergoing TOLAC. The success rate for vaginal delivery of both twins was 65%. Of the 66 women who failed trial of labor, 45% had combined delivery and 55% delivered both twins by cesarean. Just over 50% of women undergoing a trial of labor had a previous vaginal delivery; however, rates of success were not found to be different with or without a prior vaginal delivery. When presentation was assessed, a decreased likelihood of successful trial of labor was found with vertex/nonvertex twins. A 1.1% risk of uterine rupture was noted in the trial of labor group; however, this was not statistically different from either singletons undergoing a trial of labor or twins delivered by repeat cesarean. A higher proportion of extremely preterm twins was noted in the trial of labor group, with higher rates of fetal and neonatal complications reported in this group. When assessing twins delivered after 34 weeks of gestation, neonatal outcomes were similar [94].

Conventional wisdom regarding an increased risk of uterine rupture in multiples due to uterine overdistention has not been confirmed by the clinical evidence (Table 10.5). However, these trials have smaller sample sizes compared to available singleton reviews and lack sufficient power to conclusively answer this question.

10.10.2 Monoamniotic twins

Given its infrequent occurrence, recommendations regarding monoamniotic twins are based upon case series and expert opinion. Differing views are published regarding antepartum and intrapartum management, such as appropriate antenatal testing schedule, inpatient versus outpatient status, and timing of delivery. Monoamnionicity occurs in approximately 1–3% of monozygotic twin gestations, although the estimated frequency is quite variable in the literature,

Table 10.5 Trial of labor after cesarean (TOLAC) in twins.

Study	Number of twins	Success rate (%)	Uterine rupture (%)	Maternal complications
Myles [91]	19	84.2	0	5.3% uterine dehiscence, postpartum hemorrhage rates
Delaney and Young [92]	38	73.7	0	↑ infectious morbidity-elective cesarean ($p = 0.04$); ↑ early postpartum hemorrhage- trial of labor ($p = 0.01$)
Miller *et al.* [93]	92	70	0	↑ endomyometritis- elective cesarean ($p = 0.04$)
Varner *et al.* [94]	186	64.5	1.1	No difference- endomyometritis, transfusion, intensive care admission
Odeh *et al.* [95]	21	80.9	0	↑ length of hospitalization- cesarean
Wax *et al.* [96]	12	83.3	0	↑ length of NICU stay in second twin-trial of labor ($p = 0.04$)

NICU = neonatal intensive care unit.

from 1 in 1650 to as rare as 1 in 93,000 deliveries [97]. The associated perinatal mortality rate also ranges widely in the literature. Older literature reports a 30–70% mortality rate [98,99]. With prenatal diagnosis, antenatal testing, earlier delivery, and improvements in neonatal intensive care, lower mortality estimates ranging from 8 to 35% have been published [97,100,101]. When fetal anomalies are excluded, the perinatal mortality rate may now be as low as 11%, based on a review of recent literature [102].

There has been some suggestion of improved neonatal outcome with inpatient admission. In 2005, Heyborne *et al.* reported the outcomes of 43 women with monoamniotic twin gestations admitted for elective inpatient monitoring at a median gestational age of 26.5 weeks, compared to 44 women managed in the outpatient setting. The inpatient non-stress test schedule was two to three times daily, whereas the outpatient twins underwent antenatal testing between one and three times each week. No neonatal deaths occurred in the inpatient group, but 13 fetal deaths occurred in the outpatient group [103]. Similar findings were reported in a smaller retrospective study in 2006. No fetal deaths occurred among 11 pregnancies managed with continuous inpatient monitoring initiated between 24 and 28 weeks. Three deaths occurred among 12 pregnancies managed as outpatients, with antenatal testing at least three times weekly [104].

Timing of delivery is also disputed in the literature, with some authors reporting no fetal deaths after 30 weeks of gestation [105] and successful pregnancy outcomes until 40 weeks of gestation [97]. More commonly, however, authors recommend earlier delivery, documenting a continuing risk of unanticipated stillbirth with advancing gestational age, typically from lethal cord entanglement. Elective delivery at 32–34 weeks of gestation was proposed by the NICHD/SMFM workshop in 2011 [41], and this recommendation is concordant with the suggestion of multiple authors [101,103,106]. Continuing a monoamniotic pregnancy past 34 weeks is not contraindicated; however, this should be limited to well-counseled, carefully selected patients being managed as inpatients with close antenatal surveillance.

There is minimal information regarding mode of delivery for monoamniotic twins. Most authors recommend cesarean as the planned mode of delivery. Concerns with vaginal delivery include cord entanglement leading to acute, severe non-reassuring fetal status during labor or premature cord clamping of the second twin once the presenting twin has delivered due to cord entanglement. However, with continuous intrapartum monitoring and vertex/vertex presentation, a trial of labor may be reasonable for selected monoamniotic twins.

10.10.3 Conjoined twins

Conjoined twins are a rare consequence of the twinning process, with an estimated incidence of 1 in 50–100,000 births [107]. This occurs when the zygote splits more than 12 or 13 days after fertilization. The type of conjoining is described based upon which area of the body is fused. Thoracopagus twins are the most common and are joined anteriorly at the thorax and/or upper abdomen. If the heads are also joined, the union is referred to as cephalothoracopagus. Omphalopagus twins are united anteriorly at the umbilicus and lower abdomen. Pygopagus conjoined twins are fused posteriorly at the sacrum. Ischiopagus twins are united caudally at the pelvis and/or lower abdominal wall, and the spinal cord may be shared as well. The least common type is craniopagus, where the heads are fused. This may occur in any cranial area (frontal, parietal, temporoparietal, or occipital), with varying degrees of brain tissue shared [108].

With the common use of ultrasound, conjoined twins are frequently diagnosed prenatally. In addition to ultrasound and Doppler flow, MRI may be helpful in delineating anatomical junctions [109]. Prognosis depends upon which organs are shared, and to what extent separation is possible. Mode of delivery depends largely upon gestational age and anticipated prognosis. If delivered prior to 20 weeks of gestation, a vaginal delivery may be feasible. Delivery thereafter usually requires cesarean. If a possibility of postnatal survival exists, monitoring through labor would not be possible. Even if the prognosis is poor, however, cesarean may still be necessary given the physical limitations of the cervix and pelvis once the conjoined twins reach a certain size.

10.10.4 Higher order multiple gestations

The increased maternal and neonatal risks in higher order gestations are well known.

Higher rates of preterm labor, premature rupture of membranes, growth restriction, and preeclampsia are among these risks. In 2009, 5905 triplets and

355 quadruplets were born in the United States, representing a 4% increase from the previous year. More than 94% of higher order multiples were delivered prior to 37 weeks, and 37% of triplets were born prior to 32 weeks [1]. Similar to the question of inpatient versus outpatient management of monoamniotic twins, the optimal antepartum management of triplets in the third trimester remains complex. Several authors have reported a later gestational age at delivery and thus higher birthweights in triplets managed as inpatients [110,111]. However, while acknowledging a potential trend toward higher birthweight with elective admission, a recent Cochrane review did not find differences in maternal and neonatal outcomes between inpatient and outpatient admission [112].

The optimal gestational age for delivery is not known. A significant portion of higher order multiples will spontaneously deliver preterm, and a large remaining proportion will require indicated preterm delivery for maternal or fetal complications. If a triplet gestation with concordant growth and reassuring fetal testing remains undelivered, it is reasonable to consider elective delivery by 35–36 weeks of gestation given an increasing risk of stillbirth with advancing gestation. A population-based study reported a nadir in fetal mortality with a delivery interval of 34–35 weeks for triplet gestations [113].

The majority of higher order multiple gestations are delivered by cesarean section. Depending upon obstetrician skill level, and with appropriately chosen patients, some triplets may be candidates for vaginal delivery. Small retrospective case series have reported favorable outcomes in vaginally delivered triplets with high rates of success [114,115]. Similar principles as with twin vaginal delivery candidates would apply. Availability of a skilled obstetrician comfortable with vertex and breech vaginal delivery is paramount. All teams, including anesthesia and neonatology, should be present. Concordant growth within 500 g, overall birthweight greater than 1500 g, and vertex presenting first and second triplet at a minimum would be optimal.

10.11 Special procedures

10.11.1 Intrapartum external cephalic version

An intrapartum management option for a breech or transverse second twin is external cephalic version (ECV) with subsequent vertex vaginal delivery. Small case series and retrospective studies have reported good success with ECV of the malpresenting second twin. In 1983, Chervenak reported an overall success rate of 72% for 25 attempted versions. Slightly more second twins were transverse than breech, and success rates were 71% and 73%, respectively. Success was unaffected by gestational age or parity. While birthweight did not impact the overall success rate, external version was unsuccessful when the second twin weighed 500 g more than its co-twin [116]. In 1989, a study of 136 vertex-nonvertex twin pairs greater than 1500 g was published by Gocke *et al.* Neonatal morbidity and mortality were noted to be similar regardless of mode of delivery, when external version, breech extraction, and primary cesarean were compared. External version was less likely, however, to result in a successful vaginal delivery than breech extraction (46% vs 96%). This failure rate was partially explained by a greater rate of complications in the ECV group, such as non-reassuring fetal status, cord prolapse, and compound presentation, even when a vertex presentation was achieved [63]. In another study, ECV was successful in 89% and 92% of 18 breech and 12 transverse presentations greater than 35 weeks of gestation, following vaginal delivery of the first twin. All but one twin had 1- and 5-minute Apgar scores greater than 7. Three-quarters of their patients had epidural anesthesia, and the remainder delivered with pudendal or local blocks [117]. Kaplan *et al.* reported a 75% success rate in 96 vertex/nonvertex vaginal deliveries with birthweight greater than 1500 g [118].

Chauhan retrospectively reviewed the outcomes of 112 vertex/nonvertex twin pairs. Approximately half delivered by cesarean, 23 delivered by breech extraction, and 21 underwent external cephalic version. Successful vaginal delivery occurred more frequently in the breech extraction group compared to those undergoing ECV. Higher rates of persistent breech presentation and non-reassuring fetal status occurred in the ECV group. In the authors' review of the literature, they estimated a 58% rate of success and 10% complication rate for ECV in second twins. Reported complications included non-reassuring fetal status, compound presentation, cord prolapse, and placental abruption [119]. An additional consideration is the potential cost-effectiveness of each management option. Mauldin *et al.* reported outcomes of 84 vertex/nonvertex twin pairs in 1998. Sixty twin sets delivered vaginally; 41 had successful breech extraction of the second twin, and 19 second twins underwent ECV. Twenty-four twins delivered by cesarean. Lowest maternal and neonatal charges and the shortest maternal hospital stays were noted in the breech extraction group. Infants delivered vaginally vertex and by breech extraction had lower rates of pulmonary and infectious disease, compared to the other modes of delivery. Clinical and cost outcomes were found to be most favorable for breech extraction of the second twin, following vaginal delivery of the presenting twin [69].

When considering the delivery options for a nonvertex second twin, clinical and cost data suggest there may be benefits associated with breech extraction. While the available trials are small and observational, there may be a higher complication and ultimate failure rate associated with external cephalic version. In appropriately chosen patients with a skilled obstetrician and availability of necessary resources, consideration should be given to breech extraction of the nonvertex second twin.

However, external cephalic version remains a management option for obstetricians who do not perform breech extraction, or if the second twin is not a good candidate for breech extraction, such as a twin with birthweight discordance (>500 g) or a VLBW twin. Anesthesia should be present at the delivery, with available staffing and set-up for emergent cesarean if needed. The patient should

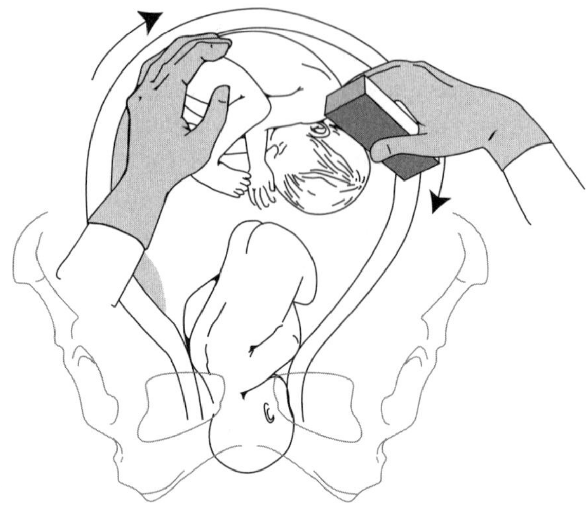

Figure 10.5 During the delivery of twin A, an assistant uses the ultrasound transducer to identify the lie of twin B and initiates efforts to induce the fetal version to a cephalic presentation.

be counseled regarding the possibility of cesarean if complications develop or if ECV is unsuccessful.

The availability of a skilled assistant is important for external version. As the first twin is delivering, ultrasound should confirm presentation of the second twin. Epidural anesthesia is beneficial during this procedure for patient comfort and relaxation of the abdominal wall. If the second twin is transverse or an oblique breech as the first twin is delivering, the assistant can initiate the version of the second twin (Figure 10.5). The assistant can use the ultrasound transducer to help guide the fetal head toward the pelvis. Following delivery of the first twin, external cephalic version should be initiated immediately by the operator. ECV is most successful with intact membranes and before a presenting part has engaged into the pelvis. The operator uses both hands abdominally to perform the version (Figure 10.6). A forward or backward roll can be used, whichever produces the smallest distance for the vertex to reach the pelvis. It is not uncommon for the second twin to remain unengaged following successful version. Maternal pushing, fundal pressure, and oxytocin administration can be used to facilitate engagement of the fetal vertex following successful version. Ultrasound should assess the fetal heart rate and vaginal exam should rule out complications such as a compound presentation or cord prolapse. Following reassurance, rupture of membranes can be performed, and vaginal delivery achieved with maternal pushing and oxytocin if necessary.

10.11.2 Internal podalic version

Internal podalic version, with subsequent breech extraction of a previously non-breech second twin, is uncommonly performed in the United States. Using a combination of ultrasound and internal exam, the position of the fetus is

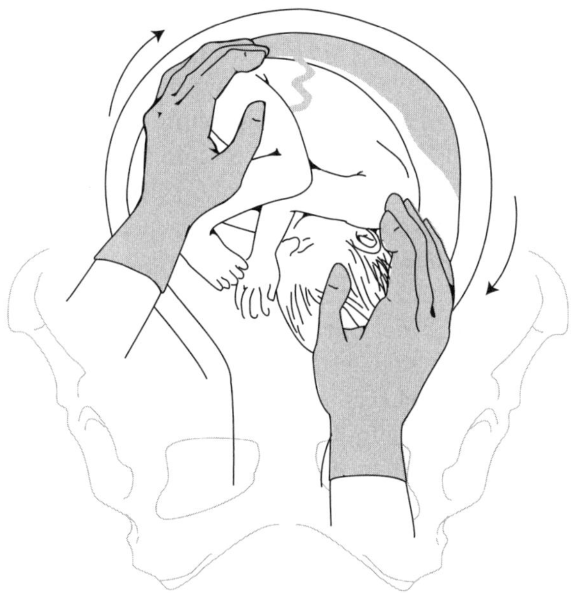

Figure 10.6 Following delivery of twin A, the operator uses both hands to perform a forward roll into a cephalic presentation.

assessed. Fetal presentation may be ventral, vertex, or scapular. In a ventral presentation, the face and chest will be facing the cervix.

Internal version is most straightforward when the fetus is in the ventral position because the feet can generally be grasped without additional maneuvers. The operator's hand is introduced into the uterus, and the fetal feet are identified. The feet are brought through the cervix, followed by the body, and the infant is delivered with breech maneuvers. If the infant is noted to be in vertex presentation, additional maneuvers are required. One hand is placed abdominally, while the other hand of the operator is within the uterus. The intrauterine hand elevates the head from the cervix into the abdominal hand, guiding it toward the fundus. The intrauterine hand then grasps the feet and brings them toward the cervix. Ideally, this is performed with the amniotic sac intact. This allows the uterus to remain distended, and the amniotic fluid enhances mobility of the fetus. If only one foot can be identified, the other will become accessible as the body is descending into the pelvis. It is possible at this stage to confuse a foot with an arm. Once the feet have been clearly identified and brought down into the cervix, the membranes are ruptured, and the infant is delivered as in breech presentation.

If the infant's right or left shoulder (scapular) is presenting, more difficulty may be encountered when attempting internal podalic version. Similar to the vertex presentation, the intrauterine hand elevates the shoulder out of the pelvis into the abdominal hand. It may be difficult to maneuver the resulting transverse lie if the back is facing downward. Ultimately, the back must be rotated upward, and the feet grasped and brought toward the cervix. Again, an arm may be confused for a foot, or an arm may prolapse downward while the body is transverse. Uterine relaxation with terbutaline or nitroglycerine is recommended, given the difficulty with these manipulations. Patient comfort with adequate anesthesia is crucial. In the absence of an obstetrician highly skilled in this intrauterine fetal manipulation, cesarean delivery may be the preferred management option.

If uterine relaxation is needed, 50–100 μg of nitroglycerine intravenously can be administered by anesthesia. Concomitant preparation for emergent cesarean is recommended in the event that uterine relaxation is not successful in facilitating vaginal delivery. An alternative option is 0.25–0.50 mg of terbutaline subcutaneously. Following delivery of both infants, the placenta may be delivered either spontaneously or manually. If anesthesia remains adequate and the uterus is relaxed, manual removal can be performed, with a uterine sweep afterward to verify the removal of all products and to assess for uterine injury. Postpartum pitocin should be initiated following delivery of the placenta. Additional uterotonics may be needed if uterine atony is encountered.

Because internal podalic version and breech delivery are less commonly performed today, fewer obstetricians are skilled in this procedure. Research experience is also limited to small retrospective studies and case series. There is minimal information regarding urgent version of a previously vertex second twin. More commonly, internal podalic version is reported for transverse lie of a second twin. A small prospective study reported favorable outcomes of 11 second twins in transverse lie, who underwent internal podalic version. Gestational age was greater than 35 weeks, and birthweights were over 1880 g. All infants had 5-minute Apgar scores of 7 or higher [120]. Twenty-five twin pairs, in whom the second twin was born following internal podalic version, were followed between 2 and 12 years after birth. No statistically significant differences were reported between the first and second twins; however, the two children in the study diagnosed with cerebral palsy had both been born by breech extraction at gestational ages less than 32 weeks [121]. There is a scarcity of evidence regarding the safety of internal podalic version in VLBW infants. Given a lack of evidence and clinical experience, cesarean should be considered if the second twin is estimated to be < 1500 g.

10.11.3 Delayed interval delivery

When one fetus of a multiple gestation delivers vaginally, especially at an extremely premature gestational age, one management possibility includes delayed interval delivery of the remaining fetus(es). This plan is considered a relatively extreme option in order to potentially improve the remaining fetuses' survival given a pre- or periviable gestational age. This potential benefit is balanced against significant maternal and fetal risks, such as infectious morbidity, abruption, and postpartum hemorrhage. Monochorionicity is typically considered a contraindication to delayed interval delivery, given the potential negative hemodynamic impact on the remaining co-twin [122].

Literature on this subject not surprisingly consists of small series. A literature review published in 1999 identified 48 twin gestations managed with delayed interval delivery. When stratifying by first birth prior to 24 weeks, 35 twins were found. The interval ranged from 3 to 143 days between deliveries with a median of 35 days. Tocolytics, antibiotics, and cerclage were used often in the trials identified, and no differences in outcome were found when stratifying for these interventions [123]. Two studies assessed delayed interval delivery using the US matched multiple birth database. One study matched 200 delayed deliveries with 374 nondelayed deliveries. With a median interval between delivery of 6 days (range 2–107 days), delayed second twins showed a higher gestational age at delivery and improved survival, particularly when the first delivery occurred between 24 and 29 weeks [124]. Another study using the same database identified 258 twins born between 22 and 28 weeks, where delivery occurred with at least a 1-week interval between each neonate. When the first delivery occurred between 22 and 23 weeks, perinatal mortality improved with delayed delivery up to 3 weeks. Of note, an increasing rate of small-for-gestational-age births was noted when at least 4 weeks passed between deliveries [125]. A study of 29 multiples in 2005 reported a median inter-delivery time of 19.6 days. While short-term improvements were found in neonatal morbidity and mortality, no significant differences were seen in neurodevelopment outcome among the small number of children followed up to 2 years [126].

Maternal risks associated with this intervention must also be considered. Six of 19 women (32%) attempting delayed interval delivery experienced significant morbidity. These included postpartum hemorrhage (two required transfusion, one required cesarean hysterectomy) and infectious morbidity (four with sepsis, two with clostridium difficile) [122]. These risks are crucial considerations when counseling a patient regarding this option.

There is no consensus regarding the use of tocolytics, antibiotics, inpatient monitoring, or cerclage placement. Most studies use some combination, if not all, of these interventions. One small study of seven patients reported a longer delivery interval with the use of cerclage (9 vs 26 days). This remained significant after controlling for antibiotics and tocolytics. The incidence of chorioamnionitis was 36%, and maternal sepsis occurred in 5% of patients. Cerclage was not associated with an increased risk of infection [127].

Delayed interval delivery is achieved by clamping and tying the cord of the delivered twin high into the cervix, so that it is drawn back into the uterus. If a rescue cerclage is planned, 5 mm Mersilene is most often used to provide more cervical support and reduce the likelihood of tearing through the cervix. If prolapsing membranes occur, approximately 300–500 mL of sterile water can be used to backfill the bladder. The anterior and posterior lips of the cervix are grasped with ring forceps, while another ring forceps with a moist sponge can be used to gently elevate the membranes. McDonald cerclage is usually the preferred technique. Tocolysis, broad-spectrum antibiotics, and inpatient observation can be considered over the next 7–10 days, with close maternal monitoring for the development of complications necessitating delivery.

10.12 Conclusion

With the incidence of multiple gestations increasing and their perinatal impact significant, principles for optimal intrapartum management are an important obstetrical focus. Labor and delivery of multiples require preparation and availability of numerous teams, including obstetricians skilled in their delivery. Multiple gestations present numerous maternal and fetal risks, which must be appreciated at the time of delivery. Current literature offers a guide in their management, but is limited by observational, largely retrospective data with small study samples. This chapter provides a summary of the literature currently available and a guide to principles central to the delivery of multiple gestations.

References

1. Martin JA, Hamilton BE, Ventura SJ *et al.* Births: Final data for 2009. *National Vital Statistics Reports* 2011;**60**:1–104.
2. Reynolds MA, Schieve LA, Martin JA, Jeng G, and Macaluso M. Trends in multiple births conceived using assisted reproductive technology, United States, 1997–2000. *Pediatrics* 2003;**111**:1159–1162.
3. Sunderam S, Chang J, and Flowers L. Assisted reproductive technology surveillance-United States, 2006. *MMWR Surveillance Summaries* 2009;**58**:1–25.
4. MacDorman MF and Kirmeyer S. Fetal and perinatal mortality, United States, 2005. *National Vital Statistics Reports* 2009;**57**:1–19.
5. Centers for Disease Control. QuickStats: Mean gestational age, by plurality-United States, 2005. *MMWR Morbidity and Mortality Weekly Report* 2008;**57**:238.
6. Luke B and Keith LG. The contribution of singletons, twins and triplets to low birth weight, infant mortality and handicap in the United States. *Journal of Reproductive Medicine* 1992;**37**:661–666.
7. Scher AI, Petterson B, Blair E *et al.* The risk of mortality or cerebral palsy in twins: a collaborative population-based study. *Pediatric Research* 2002;**52**:671–681.
8. Refuerzo JS, Momirova V, Peaceman AM *et al.* Neonatal outcomes in twin pregnancies delivered moderately preterm, late preterm, and term. *American Journal of Perinatology* 2010;**27**:537–542.
9. Odibo AO, McDonald RE, Stamilio DM, Ural SH, and Macones GA. Perinatal outcomes in growth-restricted twins compared with age-matched growth-restricted singletons. *American Journal of Perinatology* 2005;**22**:269–273.
10. Garite TJ, Clark RH, Elliott JP, and Thorp JA. Twins and triplets: the effect of plurality and growth on neonatal outcome compared with singleton infants. *American Journal of Obstetrics & Gynecology* 2004;**191**:700–707.

11 Ballabh P, Kumari J, Alkouatly HB *et al.* Neonatal outcome of triplet versus twin and singleton pregnancies: a matched case control study. *European Journal of Obstetrics & Gynecology and Reproductive Biology* 2003;**107**:28–36.
12 Wadhawan R, Oh W, Perritt RL *et al.* Twin gestation and neurodevelopmental outcome in extremely low birth weight infants. *Pediatrics* 2009;**123**:e220–227.
13 Wadhawan R, Oh W, Vohr BR *et al.* Neurodevelopmental outcomes of triplets or higher-order extremely low birth weight infants. *Pediatrics* 2011;**127**:e654–660.
14 Kirkby S, Genen L, Turenne W, and Dysart K. Outcomes and milestone achievement differences for very low-birth-weight multiples compared with singleton infants. *American Journal of Perinatology* 2010;**27**:439–444.
15 Petterson B, Nelson KB, Watson L, and Stanley F. Twins, triplets and cerebral palsy in births in Western Australia in the 1980s. *BMJ* 1993;**307**:1239–1243.
16 Yokoyama Y, Shimizu T, and Hayakawa K. Prevalence of cerebral palsy in twins, triplets and quadruplets. *International Journal of Epidemiology* 1995;**24**:943–948.
17 Burguet A, Monnet E, Pauchard JY *et al.* Some risk factors for cerebral palsy in very premature infants: importance of premature rupture of membranes and monochorionic twin placentation. *Biology of the Neonate* 1999;**75**:177–186.
18 Pharoah PO and Dundar Y. Monozygotic twinning, cerebral palsy and congenital anomalies. *Human Reproduction Update* 2009;**15**:639–648.
19 Sperling L, Kiil C, Larsen LU *et al.* Detection of chromosomal abnormalities, congenital abnormalities and transfusion syndrome in twins. *Ultrasound in Obstetrics & Gynecology* 2007;**29**:517–526.
20 Gao Y, He Z, Luo Y *et al.* Selective and non-selective intrauterine growth restriction in twin pregnancies: high-risk factors and perinatal outcome. *Archives of Gynecology and Obstetrics* 2012;**285**:973–978.
21 Campbell KH, Copel JA, and Ozan Bahtiyar M. Congenital heart defects in twin gestations. *Minerva Ginecologica* 2009;**61**:239–244.
22 Doyle PE, Beral V, Botting B, and Wale CJ. Congenital malformations in twins in England and Wales. *Journal of Epidemiology and Community Health* 1991;**45**:43–48.
23 Haas JS, Berman S, Goldenberg AB, Lee LW, and Cook EF. Prenatal hospitalization and compliance with guidelines for prenatal care. *American Journal of Public Health* 1996;**86**:815–819.
24 Rauh-Hain JA, Rana S, Tamez H *et al.* Risk for developing gestational diabetes in women with twin pregnancies. *Journal of Maternal-Fetal and Neonatal Medicine* 2009;**22**:293–299.
25 Elling SV, McKenna P, and Powell FC. Pruritic urticarial papules and plaques of pregnancy in twin and triplet pregnancies. *Journal of the European Academy of Dermatology and Venereology* 2000;**14**:378–381.
26 Chowdhury S and Hussain MA. Maternal complications in twin pregnancies. *Mymensingh Medical Journal* 2011;**20**:83–87.
27 Gardner MO, Goldenberg RL, Cliver SP, Tucker JM, Nelson KG, and Copper RL. The origin and outcome of preterm twin pregnancies. *Obstetrics & Gynecology* 1995;**85**:553–557.
28 Ananth CV, Smulian JC, Demissie K, Vintzileos AM, and Knuppel RA. Placental abruption among singleton and twin births in the United States: risk factor profiles. *American Journal of Epidemiology* 2001;**153**:771–778.
29 Santolaya J, Sampson M, Abramowicz JS, and Warsof SL. Twin pregnancy. Ultrasonographically observed changes in fetal presentation. *Journal of Reproductive Medicine* 1992;**37**:328–330.
30 Sibai BM, Hauth J, Caritis S *et al.* Hypertensive disorders in twin versus singleton gestations. National Institute of Child Health and Human Development Network of Maternal-Fetal Medicine Units. *American Journal of Obstetrics & Gynecology* 2000;**182**:938–942.

31 Luo ZC, Simonet F, An N, Bao FY, Audibert F, and Fraser WD. Effect on neonatal outcomes in gestational hypertension in twin compared with singleton pregnancies. *Obstetrics & Gynecology* 2006;**108**:1138–1144.

32 Salihu HM, Bekan B, Aliyu MH, Rouse DJ, Kirby RS, and Alexander GR. Perinatal mortality associated with abruptio placenta in singletons and multiples. *American Journal of Obstetrics & Gynecology* 2005;**193**:198–203.

33 Ananth CV, Demissie K, and Hanley ML. Birth weight discordancy and adverse perinatal outcomes among twin gestations in the United States: the effect of placental abruption. *American Journal of Obstetrics & Gynecology* 2003;**188**:954–960.

34 Suzuki S, Kikuchi F, Ouchi N *et al.* Risk factors for postpartum hemorrhage after vaginal delivery of twins. *Journal of Nippon Medical School* 2007;**74**:414–417.

35 Whiteman MK, Kuklina E, Hillis SD *et al.* Incidence and determinants of peripartum hysterectomy. *Obstetrics & Gynecology* 2006;**108**:1486–1492.

36 Knight M, Kurinczuk JJ, Spark P, and Brocklehurst P, United Kingdom Obstetric Surveillance System Steering Committee. Cesarean delivery and peripartum hysterectomy. *Obstetrics & Gynecology* 2008;**111**:97–105.

37 Bodelon C, Bernabe-Ortiz A, Schiff MA, and Reed SD. Factors associated with peripartum hysterectomy. *Obstetrics & Gynecology* 2009;**114**:115–123.

38 Sairam S, Costeloe K, and Thilaganathan B. Prospective risk of stillbirth in multiple-gestation pregnancies: a population-based analysis. *Obstetrics & Gynecology* 2002;**100**:638–641.

39 Dodd JM, Robinson JS, Crowther CA, and Chan A. Stillbirth and neonatal outcomes in South Australia, 1991–2000. *American Journal of Obstetrics & Gynecology* 2003;**189**:1731–1736.

40 Luke B. Reducing fetal deaths in multiple births: optimal birthweights and gestational ages for infants of twin and triplet births. *Acta Geneticae Medicae et Gemellologiae (Roma)* 1996;(45):333–348.

41 Spong CY, Mercer BM, D'alton M, Kilpatrick S, Blackwell S, and Saade G. Timing of indicated late-preterm and early-term birth. *Obstetrics & Gynecology* 2011;**118**:323–333.

42 Newman RB and Unal ER. Multiple gestations: timing of indicated late preterm and early-term births in uncomplicated dichorionic, monochorionic, and monoamniotic twins. *Seminars in Perinatology* 2011;**35**:277–285.

43 Breathnach FM, McAuliffe FM, Geary M, Perinatal Ireland Research Consortium *et al.* Optimum timing for planned delivery of uncomplicated monochorionic and dichorionic twin pregnancies. *Obstetrics & Gynecology* 2012;**119**:50–59.

44 Kahn B, Lumey LH, Zybert PA *et al.* Prospective risk of fetal death in singleton, twin, and triplet gestations: implications for practice. *Obstetrics & Gynecology* 2003;**102**:685–692.

45 Sebire NJ, Snijders RJ, Hughes K, Sepulveda W, and Nicolaides KH. The hidden mortality of monochorionic twin pregnancies. *BJOG* 1997;**104**:1203–1207.

46 Lee YM, Wylie BJ, Simpson LL, and D'Alton ME. Twin chorionicity and the risk of stillbirth. *Obstetrics & Gynecology* 2008;**111**:301–308.

47 Robinson BK, Miller RS, D'Alton ME, and Grobman WA. Effectiveness of timing strategies for delivery of monochorionic diamniotic twins. *American Journal of Obstetrics & Gynecology* 2012;**207**(1):53 e1–7.

48 Yang Q, Wen SW, Chen Y, Krewski D, Fung Kee Fung K, and Walker M. Neonatal mortality and morbidity in vertex-vertex second twins according to mode of delivery and birth weight. *Journal of Perinatology* 2006;**26**:3–10.

49 Sibony O, Touitou S, Luton D, Oury JF, and Blot P. Modes of delivery of first and second twins as a function of their presentation. Study of 614 consecutive patients from 1992 to 2000. *European Journal of Obstetrics & Gynecology and Reproductive Biology* 2006;**126**:180–185.

50 Salim R, Lavee M, Nachum Z, and Shalev E. Outcome of twins delivery; predictors for successful vaginal delivery: a single center experience. *Twin Research and Human Genetics* 2006;**9**:685–690.

51 Barrett JM, Staggs SM, Van Hooydonk JE, Growdon JH, Killam AP, and Boehm FH. The effect of type of delivery upon neonatal outcome in premature twins. *American Journal of Obstetrics & Gynecology* 1982;**143**:360–367.

52 Zhang J, Bowes WA Jr, Grey TW, and McMahon MJ. Twin delivery and neonatal and infant mortality: a population-based study. *Obstetrics & Gynecology* 1996;**88**:593–598.

53 Rydhstrom H. Prognosis for twins with birth weight less than 1500 gm: the impact of cesarean section in relation to fetal presentation. *American Journal of Obstetrics & Gynecology* 1990;**163**:528–533.

54 Shinwell ES, Blickstein I, Lusky A, and Reichman B. Effect of birth order on neonatal morbidity and mortality among very low-birthweight twins: a population-based study. *Archives of Disease in Childhood – Fetal Neonatal Edition* 2004;**89**:F145–148.

55 Ziadeh SM and Badria LF. Effect of mode of delivery on neonatal outcome of twins with birthweight under 1500 g. *Archives of Gynecology and Obstetrics* 2000;**264**:128–130.

56 Morales WJ, O'Brien WF, Knuppel RA, Gaylord S, and Hayes P. The effect of mode of delivery on the risk of intraventricular hemorrhage in nondiscordant twin gestations under 1500 g. *Obstetrics & Gynecology* 1989;**73**:107–110.

57 Chervenak FA, Johnson RE, Youcha S, Hobbins JC, and Berkowitz RL. Intrapartum management of twin gestation. *Obstetrics & Gynecology* 1985;**65**:119–124.

58 Suh YH, Park KH, Hong JS *et al.* Relationship between twin-to-twin delivery interval and umbilical artery acid-base status in the second twin. *Journal of Korean Medical Science* 2007;**22**:248–253.

59 Leung TY, Tam WH, Leung TN, Lok IH, and Lau TK. Effect of twin-to-twin delivery interval on umbilical cord blood gas in the second twins. *BJOG* 2002;**109**:63–67.

60 Yang Q, Wen SW, Chen Y, Krewski D, Fung Kee Fung K, and Walker M. Occurrence and clinical predictors of operative delivery for the vertex second twin after normal vaginal delivery of the first twin. *American Journal of Obstetrics & Gynecology* 2005;**192**:178–184.

61 Acker D, Lieberman M, Holbrook RH, James O, Phillippe M, and Edelin KC. Delivery of the second twin. *Obstetrics & Gynecology* 1982;**59**:710–711.

62 Mazor M, Leiberman JR, Dreval D, Wiznitzer A, Alyagon A, and Insler V. Management and outcome of vertex-breech and vertex-vertex presentation in twin gestation: a comparative study. *European Journal of Obstetrics & Gynecology and Reproductive Biology* 1986;**22**:69–75.

63 Gocke SE, Nageotte MP, Garite T, Towers CV, and Dorcester W. Management of the nonvertex second twin: primary cesarean section, external version, or primary breech extraction. *American Journal of Obstetrics & Gynecology* 1989;**161**:111–114.

64 Adam C, Allen AC, and Baskett TF. Twin delivery: influence of the presentation and method of delivery on the second twin. *American Journal of Obstetrics & Gynecology* 1991;**165**:23–27.

65 Rabinovici J, Barkai G, Reichman B, Serr DM, and Mashiach S. Randomized management of the second nonvertex twin: vaginal delivery or cesarean section. *American Journal of Obstetrics & Gynecology* 1987;**156**:52–56.

66 Fishman A, Grubb DK, and Kovacs BW. Vaginal delivery of the nonvertex second twin. *American Journal of Obstetrics & Gynecology* 1993;**168**:861–864.

67 Greig PC, Veille JC, Morgan T, and Henderson L. The effect of presentation and mode of delivery on the neonatal outcome in the second twin. *American Journal of Obstetrics & Gynecology* 1992;**167**:901–906.

68 Davison L, Easterling TR, Jackson JC, and Benedetti TJ. Breech extraction of low-birth-weight second twins: can cesarean section be justified? *American Journal of Obstetrics & Gynecology* 1992;**166**:497–502.

69 Mauldin, JG, Newman RB, and Mauldin PD. Cost-effective delivery management of the vertex and nonvertex twin gestation. *American Journal of Obstetrics & Gynecology* 1998; **179**:864–869.

70 Caukwell S and Murphy DJ. The effect of mode of delivery and gestational age on neonatal outcome of the non-cephalic presenting second twin. *American Journal of Obstetrics & Gynecology* 2002;**187**:1356–1361.

71 Schmitz T, Carnavalet Cde C, Azria E, Lopez E, Cabrol D, and Goffinet F. Neonatal outcomes of twin pregnancy according to the planned mode of delivery. *Obstetrics & Gynecology* 2008;**111**:695–703.

72 Yang Q, Wen SW, Chen Y, Krewski D, Fung Kee Fung K, and Walker M. Neonatal death and morbidity in vertex-nonvertex second twins according to mode of delivery and birth weight. *American Journal of Obstetrics & Gynecology* 2005;**192**:840–847.

73 Usta IM, Rechdan JB, Khalil AM, and Nassar AH. Mode of delivery for vertex-nonvertex twin gestations. *International Journal of Gynecology & Obstetrics* 2005;**88**:9–14.

74 Armson BA, O'Connell C, Persad V, Joseph KS, Young DC, and Baskett TF. Determinants of perinatal mortality and serious neonatal morbidity in the second twin. *Obstetrics & Gynecology* 2006;**108**:556–564.

75 Herbst A and Kallen K. Influence of mode of delivery on neonatal mortality in the second twin, at and before term. *BJOG* 2008;**115**:1512–1517.

76 Kontopoulos EV, Ananth CV, Smulian JC, and Vintzileos AM. The influence of mode of delivery on twin neonatal mortality in the US: variance by birth weight discordance. *American Journal of Obstetrics & Gynecology* 2005;**192**:252–256.

77 Usta IM, Nassar AH, Abu Musa AA, Awwad JT, Yunis KA, and Seoud MA. Perinatal outcome of vaginally delivered twin gestations with a larger twin B. *Journal of Perinatology* 2003;**23**:409–413.

78 Fox NS, Silverstein M, Bender S, Klauser CK, Saltzman DH, and Rebarber A. Active second-stage management in twin pregnancies undergoing planned vaginal delivery in a U.S. population. *Obstetrics & Gynecology* 2010;**115**:229–233.

79 Ginsberg NA and Levine EM. Delivery of the second twin. *International Journal of Gynecology & Obstetrics* 2005;**91**:217–220.

80 Kontopoulos EV, Ananth CV, Smulian JC, and Vintzileos AM. The impact of route of delivery and presentation on twin neonatal and infant mortality: a population-based study in the USA, 1995–97. *Journal of Maternal-Fetal and Neonatal Medicine* 2004;**15**:219–224.

81 Bjelic-Radisic V, Pristauz G, Haas J *et al.* Neonatal outcome of second twins depending on presentation and mode of delivery. *Twin Research and Human Genetics* 2007;**10**:521–527.

82 Wen SW, Fung Kee Fung K, Oppenheimer L, Demissie K, Yang Q, and Walker M. Neonatal morbidity in second twin according to gestational age at birth and mode of delivery. *American Journal of Obstetrics & Gynecology* 2004;**191**:773–777.

83 Hannah ME, Hannah WJ, Hewson SA, Hodnett ED, Saigal S, and Willan AR. Planned caesarean section versus planned vaginal birth for breech presentation at term: a randomised multicentre trial. Term Breech Trial Collaborative Group. *Lancet* 2000;**356**:1375–1383.

84 Blickstein I, Weissman A, Ben-Hur H, Borenstein R, and Insler V. Vaginal delivery of breech-vertex twins. *Journal of Reproductive Medicine* 1993;**38**:879–882.

85 Sentilhes S, Goffinet F, Talbot A *et al.* Attempted vaginal versus planned cesarean delivery in 195 breech first twin pregnancies. *Acta Obstetricia et Gynecologica Scandinavica* 2007; **86**:55–60.

86 Cohen M, Kohl SG, and Rosenthal AH. Fetal interlocking complicating twin gestation. *American Journal of Obstetrics & Gynecology* 1965;**91**:407–412.

87 Rydhstrom H and Cullberg G. Pregnancies with growth-retarded twins in breech-vertex presentation at increased risk for entanglement during delivery. *Journal of Perinatal Medicine* 1990;**18**:45–50.

88 Kelsick F and Minkoff H. Management of the breech second twin. *American Journal of Obstetrics & Gynecology* 1982;**144**:783–786.

89 Chasen ST, Madden A, and Chervenak FA. Cesarean delivery of twins and neonatal respiratory disorders. *American Journal of Obstetrics & Gynecology* 1999;**181**:1052–1056.
90 Suzuki S, Yamashita E, Inde Y, Hiraizumi Y, and Satomi M. Increased rate of elective cesarean delivery and neonatal respiratory disorders in twin pregnancies. *Journal of Nippon Medical School* 2010;**77**:93–96.
91 Myles T. Vaginal birth of twins after a previous cesarean section. *Journal of Maternal-Fetal and Neonatal Medicine* 2001;**10**:171–174.
92 Delaney T and Young DC. Trial of labour compared to elective caesarean in twin gestations with a previous caesarean delivery. *Journal of Obstetrics and Gynaecology Canada* 2003;**25**:289–292.
93 Miller DA, Mullin P, Hou D, and Paul RH. Vaginal birth after cesarean section in twin gestation. *American Journal of Obstetrics & Gynecology* 1996;**175**:194–198.
94 Varner MW, Leindecker S, Spong CY *et al.* The Maternal-Fetal Medicine Unit cesarean registry: trial of labor with a twin gestation. *American Journal of Obstetrics & Gynecology* 2005;**193**:135–140.
95 Odeh M, Tarazova L, Wolfson M, and Oettinger M. Evidence that women with a history of cesarean section can deliver twins safely. *Acta Obstetricia et Gynecologica Scandinavica* 1997;**76**:663–666.
96 Wax JR, Philput C, Mather J, Steinfeld JD, and Ingardia CJ. Twin vaginal birth after cesarean. *Connecticut Medicine* 2000;**64**:205–208.
97 Tessen JA and Zlatnik FJ. Monoamniotic twins: a retrospective controlled study. *Obstetrics & Gynecology* 1991;**77**:832–834.
98 Quigley JK. Monoamniotic twin pregnancy. *American Journal of Obstetrics & Gynecology* 1935;**29**:354–362.
99 Timmons JD and Dealvarez RR. Monoamniotic twin pregnancy. *American Journal of Obstetrics & Gynecology* 1963;**86**:875–881.
100 Rodis JF, McIlveen PF, Egan JF, Borgida AF, Turner GW, and Campbell WA. Monoamniotic twins: improved perinatal survival with accurate prenatal diagnosis and antenatal fetal surveillance. *American Journal of Obstetrics & Gynecology* 1997;**177**:1046–1049.
101 Roqué H, Gillen-Goldstein J, Funai E, Young BK, and Lockwood CJ. Perinatal outcomes in monoamniotic gestations. *Journal of Maternal-Fetal and Neonatal Medicine* 2003; **13**:414–421.
102 Allen VM, Windrim R, Barrett J, and Ohlsson A. Management of monoamniotic twin pregnancies: a case series and systematic review of the literature. *BJOG* 2001;**108**:931–936.
103 Heyborne KD, Porreco RP, Garite TJ, Phair K, and Abril D, Obstetrix/Pediatrix Research Study Group. Improved perinatal survival of monoamniotic twins with intensive inpatient monitoring. *American Journal of Obstetrics & Gynecology* 2005;**192**:96–101.
104 DeFalco LM, Sciscione AC, Megerian G *et al.* Inpatient versus outpatient management of monoamniotic twins and outcomes. *American Journal of Perinatology* 2006;**23**:205–211.
105 Carr SR, Aronson MP, and Coustan DR. Survival rates of monoamniotic twins do not decrease after 30 weeks' gestation. *American Journal of Obstetrics & Gynecology* 1990;**163**: 719–722.
106 Beasley E, Megerian G, Gerson A, and Roberts NS. Monoamniotic twins: case series and proposal for antenatal management. *Obstetrics & Gynecology* 1999;**93**:130–134.
107 Edmonds LD and Layde PM. Conjoined twins in the United States, 1970–1977. *Teratology* 1982;**25**:301–308.
108 Kaufman MH. The embryology of conjoined twins. *Child's Nervous System* 2004;**20**: 508–525.
109 Spielmann AL, Freed KS, and Spritzer CE. MRI of conjoined twins illustrating advances in fetal imaging. *Journal of Computer Assisted Tomography* 2001;**25**:88–90.

110 Skrablin S, Kuvacic I, Jukic P, Kalafatic D, and Peter B. Hospitalization vs outpatient care in the management of triplet gestations. *International Journal of Gynecology & Obstetrics* 2002;**77**:223–229.

111 Adams DM, Sholl JS, Haney EI, Russell TL, and Silver RK. Perinatal outcome associated with outpatient management of triplet pregnancy. *American Journal of Obstetrics & Gynecology* 1998;**178**:843–847.

112 Crowther CA and Han S. Hospitalisation and bed rest for multiple pregnancy. *Cochrane Database of Systematic Reviews* 2010;(**7**):CD000110.

113 Luke B. Reducing fetal deaths in multiple births: optimal birthweights and gestational ages for infants of twin and triplet births. *Acta Geneticae Medicae et Gemellologiae (Roma)* 1996;**45**:333–348.

114 Grobman WA, Peaceman AM, Haney EI, Silver RK, and MacGregor SN. Neonatal outcomes in triplet gestations after a trial of labor. *American Journal of Obstetrics & Gynecology* 1998;**179**:942–945.

115 Alamia V Jr, Royek AB, Jaekle RK, and Meyer BA. Preliminary experience with a prospective protocol for planned vaginal delivery of triplet gestations. *American Journal of Obstetrics & Gynecology* 1998;**179**:1133–1135.

116 Chervenak FA, Johnson RE, Berkowitz RL, and Hobbins JC. Intrapartum external version of the second twin. *Obstetrics & Gynecology* 1983;**62**:160–165.

117 Tchabo JG and Tomai T. Selected intrapartum external cephalic version of the second twin. *Obstetrics & Gynecology* 1992;**79**:421–423.

118 Kaplan B, Peled Y, Rabinerson D, Goldman GA, Nitzan Z, and Neri A. Successful external version of B-twin after the birth of A-twin for vertex—non-vertex twins. *European Journal of Obstetrics & Gynecology and Reproductive Biology* 1995;**58**:157–160.

119 Chauhan SP, Roberts WE, McLaren RA, Roach H, Morrison JC, and Martin JN Jr. Delivery of the nonvertex second twin: breech extraction versus external cephalic version. *American Journal of Obstetrics & Gynecology* 1995;**173**:1015–1020.

120 Rabinovici J, Barkai G, Reichman B, Serr DM, and Mashiach S. Internal podalic version with unruptured membranes for the second twin in transverse lie. *Obstetrics & Gynecology* 1988;**71**:428–430.

121 Drew JH, McKenzie J, Kelly E, and Beischer NA. Second twin: quality of survival if born by breech extraction following internal podalic version. *Australian and New Zealand Journal of Obstetrics and Gynaecology* 1991;**31**:111–114.

122 Roman AS, Fishman S, Fox N, Klauser C, Saltzman D, and Rebarber A. Maternal and neonatal outcomes after delayed-interval delivery of multifetal pregnancies. *American Journal of Perinatology* 2011;**28**:91–96.

123 Platt JS and Rosa C. Delayed interval delivery in multiple gestations. *Obstetrical and Gynecological Survey* 1999;**54**:343–348.

124 Zhang J, Hamilton B, Martin J, and Trumble A. Delayed interval delivery and infant survival: a population-based study. *American Journal of Obstetrics & Gynecology* 2004; **191**:470–476.

125 Oyelese Y, Ananth CV, Smulian JC, and Vintzileos AM. Delayed interval delivery in twin pregnancies in the United States: Impact on perinatal mortality and morbidity. *American Journal of Obstetrics & Gynecology* 2005;**192**:439–444.

126 Rosbergen M, Vogt HP, Baerts W *et al.* Long-term and short-term outcome after delayed-interval delivery in multi-fetal pregnancies. *European Journal of Obstetrics & Gynecology and Reproductive Biology* 2005;**122**:66–72.

127 Zhang J, Johnson CD, and Hoffman M. Cervical cerclage in delayed interval delivery in a multifetal pregnancy: a review of seven case series. *European Journal of Obstetrics & Gynecology and Reproductive Biology* 2003;**108**:126–130.

CHAPTER 11
Obstetrical emergencies

Christina S. Han and Christian M. Pettker
Department of Obstetrics, Gynecology, and Reproductive Sciences, Yale University School of Medicine, New Haven, CT, USA

11.1 Background

Obstetrical emergencies result in significant morbidity and mortality in mothers and fetuses worldwide. The World Health Organization (WHO) reported in 2011 that the rates of mothers dying from complications of pregnancy and childbirth declined by 34% between 1990 and 2008 [1]. However, each year 358,000 women still succumb to reproductive complications, with 99% occurring in developing countries. As such, the global community will likely fail to achieve the targeted decline of a 75% reduction in maternal mortality by the year 2015, set as Millennium Development Goal 5 by WHO. Similar regional discrepancies are seen in rates of perinatal and neonatal mortality.

The major obstetrical emergencies include postpartum hemorrhage, shoulder dystocia, cord prolapse, head entrapment, seizures, cardiac arrest, and perimortem cesarean delivery. Although risk factors exist for each type of emergency, the majority unfortunately cannot be predicted. In some cases, such as head entrapment or cardiac arrest, the low incidence rates contribute to provider unfamiliarity with management options and potentially catastrophic outcomes. Therefore, management of all obstetrical emergencies requires mitigation of the circumstances through understanding of the pathophysiology of pregnancy, optimization of management protocols, dedicated training drills, and timely multidisciplinary approaches.

11.2 Postpartum hemorrhage

11.2.1 Incidence and background

Postpartum hemorrhage (PPH) is a leading cause of maternal mortality worldwide, accounting for approximately one-quarter of maternal deaths each year [2].

Management of Labor and Delivery, Second Edition. Edited by George A. Macones.

Rates of PPH vary regionally, with a range from 1 in 1000 in developing countries to 1 in 100,000 in developed countries [3]. Although most maternal deaths occur in low-income regions, PPH incidence in high-resource countries is on the rise [4]. In the United States, PPH is the second leading cause of maternal mortality, behind thromboembolic disease.

No universally accepted definitions of PPH exist, but commonly used descriptions include estimated blood loss (EBL) greater than 500 mL for vaginal delivery, EBL greater than 1000 mL for cesarean delivery, hematocrit decrease of 10%, or the need for transfusion of blood or other blood products [3]. Postpartum hemorrhage can be categorized temporally into primary or secondary, with the former occurring within 24 hours of delivery and the latter between 24 hours and 6–12 weeks postpartum [5]. Primary PPH occurs in 4–6% of pregnancies, with approximately 80% attributed to uterine atony [6].

Obstetrical hemorrhage can be frank, such as intraoperative or vaginal bleeding, or concealed, as with postoperative or retroperitoneal bleeding. Signs and symptoms of hemorrhage include syncope, tachycardia, oliguria, shortness of breath, coagulopathy, and hypotension. Pain can also be a presenting symptom, especially in cases of vaginal hematoma or intraperitoneal collection.

11.2.2 Etiologies and risk factors

The causes of postpartum bleeding are categorized into four groups, colloquially known as the "four T's": tone, trauma, tissue, and thrombin. *Tone* refers to physiologic contraction of the smooth muscle fiber network in the uterine myometrium [3]. In the absence of postpartum uterine tone, whether induced by endogenous oxytocin release or exogenous oxytocin administration, the smooth muscle fibers are unable to constrict around the dilated uterine vasculature, resulting in continued and excessive bleeding from the raw endometrial surfaces. *Trauma* can occur at any point along the path of the birth canal, including uterine rupture and lacerations of the cervix, vagina, perineum, or uterine vessels. *Tissue* refers to complications involving the products of conception, such as placental abruption, retained placenta, invasive placentation, and molar pregnancies. Lastly, *thrombin* serves as the mnemonic for defects in the coagulation cascade, which may be inherited, acquired, or iatrogenic. These etiologies and risk factors of postpartum bleeding are summarized in Table 11.1.

Duration of the third stage of labor significantly influences the incidence of PPH, with rates of PPH progressively rising once the third stage exceeds 30 minutes, and reaching a plateau at 75 minutes [6]. Delivery characteristics that significantly prolong third stage after vaginal delivery include: preterm delivery (adjusted OR 3.81, 95% CI 2.89–5.02), delivery in a labor bed instead of a delivery room (adjusted OR 2.17, 95% CI 1.71–2.76), preeclampsia (adjusted OR 1.76, 1.17–2.67), augmented labor (adjusted OR 1.47, 95% CI 1.17–1.85), nulliparity (adjusted OR 1.45, 1.16–1.81), maternal age above 30 years (adjusted OR 1.36, 95% CI 1.09–1.70), delivery by midwife instead of physician

Table 11.1 Etiology and risk factors for postpartum hemorrhage.

Primary postpartum hemorrhage	• Uterine atony o Uterine fatigue (e.g. prolonged labor, prolonged augmentation of labor, grand multiparity, precipitous labor) o Medications (e.g. magnesium sulfate, calcium channel blockers, terbutaline) o Anatomy (e.g. fibroids) o Infection o Overdistention (e.g. polyhydramnios, multiple gestation, macrosomia) • Uterine inversion • Coagulation defect o Inherited (e.g. von Willebrand's disease) o Acquired (e.g. disseminated intravascular coagulation) o Iatrogenic (e.g. anticoagulants) • Retained placenta (e.g. invasive placentation, cord avulsion, succenturiate lobe)
Secondary postpartum hemorrhage	• Subinvolution of placental site • Retained products of conception • Infection • Coagulation defect

(adjusted OR 1.36, 95% CI 1.02–1.80), and history of previous termination (adjusted OR 1.35, 95% CI 1.09–1.67) [6]. Factors that were not associated with increased duration of third stage were previous cesarean delivery, duration of membrane rupture, use of regional anesthesia, infection, induction of labor, and prepregnancy weight.

11.2.3 Prevention

Primary prevention of PPH may decrease maternal morbidity and blood product requirements [7]. One such intervention is active management of the third stage of labor, defined by one or more maneuvers intended to effect timely placental delivery. These maneuvers include transabdominal uterine massage, prophylactic administration of uterotonic medication, early cord clamping, and controlled cord traction [8]. Active management of third stage of labor reduces the risk of postpartum bleeding in excess of 1000 mL (RR 0.34, 95% CI 0.14–0.87) and maternal hemoglobin less than 9 mg/dL (RR 0.50, 95% CI 0.38–0.83) [8]. However, these interventions can result in side effects such as increased pain, nausea, vomiting, and increased maternal diastolic blood pressure. Offspring effects include a decrease in birthweight, theorized to be due to lower blood volume from decreased placental-neonatal transfer when the cord is clamped early [8]. Furthermore, active management of the third stage of labor may preclude delayed cord clamping and its positive impact on neonatal hematocrit.

The benefits seen with active management of third stage of labor are attributed mostly to oxytocin administration, and not to cord traction or early clamping. Omission of controlled cord traction in a large multicenter randomized controlled trial involving more than 12,000 subjects in each arm demonstrated very little effect on the risk of severe hemorrhage [9].

Another systematic review focusing on early versus delayed cord clamping reported no difference in rates of maternal hemorrhage (RR 1.22, 95% CI 0.96–1.55) [10]. Delayed cord clamping improved neonatal hemoglobin by 2.17 g/dL (95% CI 0.28–4.06), but early cord clamping decreased the risk of polycythemia and hyperbilirubinemia and the need for phototherapy (RR 0.59, CI 0.38–0.92) [10]. The elevation in hemoglobin did not persist to six months of life, although ferritin levels did [10]. Currently, both expectant and active approaches are acceptable in the management of third stage of labor.

11.2.4 Management

Prompt recognition of PPH and utilization of a multidisciplinary team approach are integral parts of establishing a culture of patient safety in obstetrics [11]. As a result, many institutional, regional, national, and international organizations have established comprehensive maternal hemorrhage protocols to reduce morbidity and mortality secondary to PPH. Examples of such protocols include those provided by California Maternal Quality Care Collaborative [12], the American Congress of Obstetricians and Gynecologists (ACOG) [5], and the WHO [13].

Integral to each protocol is identification and reversal of the initial insult that precipitated bleeding, such as repair of laceration, correction of uterine atony, or evacuation of retained placenta. Given its simplicity and non-invasiveness, fundal massage is an appropriate first step to stimulate uterine contractions while assessing for alternate causes of bleeding. However, fundal massage does not appear to reduce hemorrhage in the absence of oxytocin [14]. Adequate lighting, leg positioning, tissue retraction, and exposure allows for thorough examination of the perineum, vagina, sulci, fornices, and cervix. Anesthesia may be necessary to enable adequate manual exploration of the lower uterine segment, particularly in patients with prior myometrial interruption, such as myomectomy or cesarean deliveries. Medical and surgical management options for management of PPH are listed in Table 11.2 [5]. Surgical management of obstetrical emergencies is reviewed in detail in Chapter 12. Maintenance of normothermia is also a less invasive measure that can be performed in the delivery room and reduces risk for coagulopathy.

Concurrent to the above interventions, correction of hypovolemia and anemia must be initiated in order to maintain intravascular volume and ensure adequate peripheral oxygen delivery. Two large-bore (14–18-gauge) intravenous lines should be placed, and a bladder catheter inserted for close monitoring of urine output. Large volume isotonic crystalloid (normal saline or Lactated Ringer's solution) is administered as first line for prevention of hypotension [15].

Table 11.2 Medical and surgical management of postpartum hemorrhage.

Management	Procedure	Comments
Medical	Oxytocin	IV (10–40 units in 1 L of saline or Lactated Ringer's) or IM (10 units)
	Methyl-ergonovine	IM (0.2 mg), every 2–4 hours; Contraindication: hypertension
	15-methyl-PGF-2a	IM (0.25 mg), every 15–90 minutes; Contraindication: asthma, hepatic, renal, cardiac disease
	Dinoprostone	Per vagina or rectum (20 mg), every 2 hours; Must be stored frozen and thawed prior to use. Contraindication: hypotension
	Misoprostol	Per rectum (800–1000 mcg)
Surgical	Uterine tamponade	Packing with gauze (may soak in thrombin 5000 units in 5 mL of sterile saline), Foley catheter (instill 60–80 mL), tamponade balloon (per product instructions)
	Uterine curettage	
	Uterine artery ligation	Bilateral, decreases pulse pressure
	B-Lynch suture	
	Hypogastric artery ligation	Less successful than previously thought, difficult technique
	Repair of uterine rupture	
	Repair of laceration	
	Uterine artery embolization	
	Hysterectomy	

Source: American College of Obstetricians and Gynecologists Practice Bulletin No. 76, 2006 [5]. Reproduced with permission from Lippincott Williams & Wilkins.

However, blood products are the mainstay for resuscitation and are necessary for reversal of blood loss anemia or coagulopathy. The delivery ratio of packed red blood cell (PRBC) to fresh frozen plasma (FFP) is important to prevent dilutional coagulopathy. Evidence from trauma literature suggests optimal outcomes with administration of 1 unit of FFP for every 1 to 2 units of PRBC, often referred to as a "massive transfusion protocol" [16,17]. The available types of blood products and expected benefits are listed in Table 11.3. Establishment of institutional massive transfusion protocols may help expedite delivery of blood products to the obstetrical unit under emergent conditions, although the exact components of these guidelines vary from institution to institution. At our institution, the massive transfusion protocol consists of prompt delivery of an initial set of 6 units of PRBC, 4 units of FFP, and 10 units of platelets. If needed, additional packages containing 10 units of PRBC, 10 units of FFP, 10 units of platelets,

Table 11.3 Blood product components.

Component	Contents	Indications	Volume (mL)	Shelf life	Expected effect
Packed red blood cells	Red cells, some plasma, few WBCs	Correct anemia	300	21 days	Increase HCT 3%/unit, Hgb 1 g/unit
Leukocyte-poor blood	RBCs, some plasma, few WBCs	Correct anemia, reduce febrile reactions	250	21–24 days	Increase HCT 3%/unit, Hgb 1 g/unit
Platelets	Platelets, some plasma, RBCs, few WBCs	Bleeding due to thrombocytopenia	50	5 days	Increase total platelet count 7500 μL/unit
Fresh frozen plasma	Plasma, clotting factors V, XI, XI	Treatment of coagulation disorders	250	Thawed: 2 hours; Frozen: 12 months	Increase total fibrinogen 7–10 mg/dL/unit
Cryoprecipitate	Fibrinogen, factors V, VIII, XIII, von Willebrand factor	Hemophilia A, von Willebrand disease, fibrinogen deficiency	40	Thawed: 4–6 hours	Increase total fibrinogen 10–15 mg/dL/unit

and 10 units of cryoprecipitate are delivered sequentially. Subsequent transfusions should also use this 1:1:1 ratio. In cases of intractable hemorrhage and coagulopathy, recombinant activated factor VII has been used successfully in obstetrics, although the use remains off-label. Risks of thrombosis, including myocardial infarction, and the high cost of this parenteral medication hinder its use, though in life-threatening situations this risk may be suitable.

Laboratory tests, including complete blood count and coagulation panel, should be obtained for baseline at the onset of event, and serially monitored during and after the insult. Hemodilution and equilibration may unmask anemia several hours following acute blood loss. Continued occult bleeding may also be identified with intractable decreases in hemoglobin and hematocrit. Continued maternal tachycardia, hypotension, or oliguria long after the acute event are harbingers of continued bleeding or inadequate resuscitation.

In patients who are hemodynamically stable, but are suspected to have a slow bleed or are at high risk of recurrent bleeding, percutaneous transcatheter embolization (PTE) of the uterine artery by interventional radiologists can be considered. Success rates for bilateral uterine artery devascularization in management of postpartum or postcesarean bleeding are 80–90% [18]. Benefits for the patient and the healthcare system include low complication rates, avoidance of further surgical risks, fertility preservation, and shorter hospitalizations [18]. Embolization may be favored for the stable patient who continues to bleed after a vaginal delivery, in whom atony and coagulopathy has been addressed. During the embolization procedure, diagnostic angiography with intravenous contrast is first performed to identify vascular anatomy and sources of extravasation. Occlusive agents are then deployed into the affected area. For the uterine artery, options include absorbable gelatin foam pledgets, coils, and glue. Alternative agents such as particles and microspheres are avoided secondary to the large diameter of the target vessel, and the risk of subsequent pulmonary embolization.

All appropriate team members should be mobilized as early in the process as possible, including obstetricians, nurses, anesthesiologists, interventional radiologists, laboratory personnel, and the blood bank. In some cases where hemorrhage is anticipated, such as with invasive placentation, the teams should be preemptively activated prior to delivery. Furthermore, when PPH is severe or complicated, subspecialists such as critical care providers and additional subspecialty surgeons are often necessary.

11.2.5 Complications and outcomes

Complications of PPH include hypovolemia, shock, coagulopathy, sepsis, need for surgery and/or hysterectomy, and maternal death. End-organ ischemia may be seen with severe anemia, including myocardial infarction, acute renal failure, cerebrovascular accident, and pituitary infarction. Treatments employed in management of PPH may also precipitate additional complications, such as fluid overload, transfusion reactions, dilutional coagulopathy, and complications associated with cesarean hysterectomy. In cases where fertility is retained, risk of recurrence in a subsequent pregnancy ranges from 10 to 28.4% [19,20].

In an analysis to determine preventability, an expert panel deemed a majority (54%) of cases of obstetric hemorrhage were potentially avoidable [21]. Overall preventability was not statistically different by level of hospital, and 88% were provider-related errors, in particular delay in diagnosis and treatment [21]. Given this, prompt recognition and response to hemorrhage may be as important as any single therapy or intervention. The United States Joint Commission on Accreditation of Healthcare Organizations recommends development and use of protocols and drills for responding to obstetrical hemorrhage to prevent such provider-related errors. Each institution and region should refine its local protocol by identifying and fixing systems problems that would cause near-misses [22]. Simulations, either *in situ* or simulation-center-based, may be helpful for practice and developing teamwork in these situations [23]. The development and implementation of these patient safety programs are described in Chapter 19.

11.3 Shoulder dystocia

11.3.1 Incidence

First described in literature in 1779 by Smellie [24], shoulder dystocia classically occurs during vaginal delivery when the fetal shoulders become impacted on the maternal bony structures in the pelvis [25]. The anterior shoulder may become wedged behind the maternal pubic symphysis, while the posterior shoulder may be unable to clear the sacral promontory. The biomechanical effects on the fetal neck and maternal pelvis result in the significant fetal and maternal adverse outcomes seen in complicated shoulder dystocia. Inability to deliver the infant during the shift from placental to pulmonary gas exchange can lead to the most critical injury of hypoxic-ischemic injury.

Shoulder dystocia is vaguely defined by the need for additional obstetric maneuvers to effect delivery of the impacted shoulder [25,26]. There is no accepted interval from delivery of the head to the delivery of the shoulder to define shoulder dystocia. In vaginal deliveries of fetuses in cephalic presentation, reported incidences of shoulder dystocia range from 0.24 to 2%, reflecting the subjective nature of the current definition [27–29].

11.3.2 Risk factors

Risk factors for shoulder dystocia include fetal macrosomia, maternal diabetes, and history of prior shoulder dystocia. Macrosomia is an independent risk factor for shoulder dystocia, though 40–50% of cases occur in neonates with weights < 4000 g [25]. Birthweight greater than 5000 g was reported in 0.9% of singleton pregnancies in the comprehensive national birth registry of Iceland, with an associated increase in risk of shoulder dystocia compared to birthweight less than 5000 g (OR 26.9, 9% CI: 11.1–65.1) [30]. A study of non-diabetic women reported shoulder dystocia in 5.2% of infants weighing 4000–4250 g, 9.1% of 4250–4500 g, 14.3% of 4500–4750 g, and 21.1% of 4750–5000 g [31]. This trend was mirrored but further elevated in diabetic pregnancies, with shoulder dystocia reported in 12.2% of infants weighing 4000–4250 g, 16.7% of 4250–4500 g, 27.3% of 4500–4750 g, and 34.8% of 4750–5000 g [31]. Furthermore, shoulder dystocia increased by approximately 35–45% in vacuum- or forceps-assisted vaginal deliveries. After controlling for confounders, an increased risk of shoulder dystocia was noted in diabetes (OR 1.7, $p = 0.0001$), assisted delivery (OR 1.9, $p = 0.0001$), and induction of labor (OR 1.3, $p = 0.0001$) [31].

Parity also plays a role in risk of shoulder dystocia. In a Norwegian study with 1.9 million deliveries, 75% of all shoulder dystocia cases occurred in deliveries of offspring weighing 4000 g or more, with pregnancies of higher parity at *increased* risk [27]. Compared to pregnancies producing offspring weighing 3000–3499 g, parous women with offspring greater than 5000 g were at significantly higher risk of shoulder dystocia (OR 246.4, 95% CI 205.4–295.5), while primiparous women with offspring greater than 5000 g showed increased, but less, risk (OR 135.7, 95% CI 111.6–165.1).

Rates of shoulder dystocia are further elevated in women who have experienced a prior delivery complicated by shoulder dystocia. In a large single-center retrospective analysis, the recurrence rate of shoulder dystocia was higher than the incidence in the general population (3.7% vs 0.7%, OR 7.36, 95% CI 3.68–4.23) [32]. Other characteristics associated with increased risk of shoulder dystocia include maternal obesity, multiparity, postterm gestation, previous history of a macrosomic birth (with or without shoulder dystocia), labor induction, and epidural anesthesia [25]. One factor that has been studied, but is *not* associated with shoulder dystocia, is a protracted labor, even in those with diabetes or macrosomia [33,34].

However, the presence of risk factors such as diabetes and macrosomia predict only 55% of cases with shoulder dystocia, with close to half of all cases occurring in maternal-fetal dyads without identifiable risk factors [35]. This unpredictability unfortunately renders this complication unpreventable in many cases.

11.3.3 Diagnosis

Diagnosis of shoulder dystocia is made clinically with inability to deliver the anterior shoulder upon routine gentle downward traction of the fetal head, requiring the use of additional obstetric maneuvers. An ominous sign that may indicate impaction of the anterior shoulder is retraction of the fetal head and neck against the perineum after each expulsive force, known as the "turtle sign" [25]. Although the provider's subjective determination is sufficient for diagnosis, an alternative objective definition based on duration of event has been proposed. Sixty seconds, or two standard deviations above the mean head-to-body delivery time, identified a group with higher risk of adverse outcomes [36].

Brachial plexus injury, a major complication of shoulder dystocia, is diagnosed in a newborn when the affected upper extremity remains flaccid while the passive range of motion is equal on both sides [37]. If both active and passive motions are equally restricted, injury to the proximal humeral epiphyses should be suspected.

11.3.4 Anatomy and biomechanics

The fetal bisacromial diameter, defined by the distance between the outermost points of the fetal shoulders, normally descends into the maternal pelvis at an oblique angle, the widest dimension in a gynecoid pelvis [38]. During external rotation of the fetal head, the fetal shoulders rotate to an anteroposterior alignment to allow for the anterior shoulder to slide under the pubic symphysis, followed sequentially by the posterior shoulder. Impaction of the anterior shoulder against the pubic symphysis or posterior shoulder against the sacral promontory can occur if the fetal shoulders remain in the anteroposterior alignment during initial descent, or both shoulders attempt to pass the bony structures simultaneously. Furthermore, excess fetal soft tissue, as often seen in macrosomia, can provide further friction against maternal tissue.

The brachial plexus is a network of somatic nerves arising from the ventral rami of spinal nerves C5 to T1 [39]. The trunks of the plexus traverse the posterior triangle of the neck and pass inferolaterally behind the clavicle into the axilla. This important plexus is responsible for motor innervation to muscles of the upper extremities (except the levator scapulae and trapezius) and cutaneous innervation to skin of the upper limb (except the axilla and an area supplied by the supraclavicular nerve). Repeated and forceful pressure on the fetal neck from either maternal expulsive forces or iatrogenic downward traction on the fetal head during an impaction event is thought to result in stretching injuries. However, brachial plexus injuries are also documented in cases of cesarean delivery, albeit at a lower rate than vaginal deliveries, demonstrating that all cases may not be attributable to delivery maneuvers [40].

11.3.5 Management and maneuvers

Given the unpredictability of shoulder dystocia, this obligate emergency requires prompt recognition, orderly step-wise management, and a multidisciplinary team approach to optimize outcomes. Management protocols are based mostly on expert opinion, as randomized controlled trials comparing maneuvers are sparse. Fetal demise cases, which present a higher risk for shoulder dystocia, can allow a team to practice maneuvers without risk of neonatal consequences. Simulation may also provide opportunities to practice skills/knowledge and teamwork, and has been shown to improve clinical outcomes [41,42].

The first steps in management of shoulder dystocia should be performed simultaneously. The diagnosis should be audibly announced to the delivery staff in an efficient and controlled fashion, and the patient should be informed of the need for additional maneuvers. Voluntary expulsive attempts from the mother should be temporarily halted. Ineffective and potentially damaging forces, such as forceful head traction (exceeding routine gentle pressure) and fundal pressure, should not be applied. If not already done, the patient should be repositioned to the bottom edge of the bed and the bladder drained.

While the provider is performing the above, the obstetrical nurse should promptly communicate the need for additional obstetricians, nursing staff, anesthesiologists, and pediatricians to the remainder of the obstetrical floor. The time of initial diagnosis should be documented in order to determine the head-to-body delivery interval.

The delivering provider should rapidly evaluate the maternal perineum to determine if adequate space is available for introduction of the provider's hands to perform additional maneuvers. Because shoulder dystocia is a disorder involving the bony structures, isolated release of soft tissue will not resolve the impaction. The risks of episiotomy, including increased maternal bleeding, pain, and pelvic floor trauma, should be weighed against the provider's need for additional space.

The least invasive maneuver is flexion and abduction of the maternal lower extremities, known by the eponymous McRoberts maneuver. This initial maneuver brings the thighs up to the lateral aspects of the maternal abdomen and requires two additional personnel to assist in optimal positioning of each leg. The movement straightens the lumbosacral lordosis that is exaggerated in pregnancy, and shifts the sacral promontory posteriorly to release the posterior shoulder.

The anterior pelvic rotation widens the dimensions of the pelvic inlet and laterally flexes the fetal spine toward the mother's anterior side, further enabling passage of the posterior shoulder. Maternal Valsalva maneuver can be reinitiated at this point in conjunction with the maneuver. In fact, this positioning may improve expulsive forces by increasing intrauterine pressure as well [43]. McRoberts position alleviated shoulder dystocia in 39.5–42% of cases, and was successful as the solitary maneuver in lower risk deliveries with lower birthweight, shorter duration of active phase, and shorter second stage of labor [44,45].

Simultaneously, a third assistant may apply suprapubic pressure. The most effective application is placement of the assistant's heel of the palm or fist in the mother's suprapubic region, in order to apply downward and lateral pressure to the posterior aspect of the fetal anterior shoulder. This movement drives the anterior shoulder out of the anteroposterior alignment into an oblique angle to release the impaction. The combination of McRoberts maneuver and suprapubic pressure yields a success rate of 58% [44].

The subsequent rotational maneuvers, Rubin and Woods' screw, are often used interchangeably or in combination, depending on provider preference. Classically, the Rubin maneuver consists of the provider placing a hand into the vaginal vault behind the posterior fetal shoulder followed by application of pressure to rotate the posterior shoulder anteriorly into an oblique alignment [46]. Alternatively, if the posterior shoulder is difficult to access, the maneuver can be adapted to the anterior shoulder, with similar pressure to move the anterior shoulder anteriorly toward the fetal face. The optimal provider hand to execute this maneuver is the hand on the same side as the fetal spine. For example, if the fetal spine is on the maternal left (with fetus facing maternal right), the provider's right hand will be placed behind the desired shoulder. Adequate analgesia via regional block is preferred, but may not always be available under emergent circumstances.

The Woods' screw maneuver is also performed with the provider's hand in the vaginal vault, but placed on the anterior aspect of the posterior shoulder, directly over the clavicle [47]. The pressure is directed posteriorly in order to "screw" the shoulder in a nut-into-bolt motion for 180 degrees. Simultaneously, the Rubin maneuver can be applied to the anterior shoulder to enhance the rotational torque. For the Woods' screw, the optimal provider hand is the hand opposite the fetal spine. For example, if the fetal spine is on the maternal left (with fetus facing maternal right), the left hand would be placed anterior to the posterior shoulder.

Delivery of the posterior arm, or the Barnum maneuver, is an alternative to the rotational maneuvers [48]. The provider introduces a hand into the posterior vaginal vault, but continues to advance it superiorly beyond the fetal shoulders to the fetal elbow. Pressure is applied to the antecubital fossa to flex the fetal elbow across the chest. The forearm is grasped, swept across the fetal chest, and extracted from the vaginal vault. Delivery of the posterior arm significantly reduces the presenting diameter and is almost always effective in relieving the impaction. If delivery of the posterior shoulder is unsuccessful in relieving the anterior impaction, the Rubin or Woods' screw maneuvers can be used to rotate the fetus 180 degrees, and the procedure repeated on the remaining contralateral shoulder. The greatest risk of this procedure is humeral fracture.

The Gaskin maneuver, introduced by the legendary midwife Ina May Gaskin, is also known as the "all-fours maneuver" [49]. The mother rotates from the supine position, as the description implies, onto her hands and knees in order to alter the effects of gravitational pull on the fetus. In this position, the posterior shoulder may be dislodged from the sacral promontory as the fetus and maternal abdomen drop toward the bed. Delivery is then performed in this position, with either gentle upward traction on the anterior shoulder or gentle downward traction on the posterior shoulder. The non-invasive nature of this maneuver, similar to the McRoberts maneuver and suprapubic pressure, is sometimes preferred in women without analgesia.

The above routine obstetrical maneuvers can be summarized using the "HELPERR" mnemonic, shown in Table 11.4 [50]. However, when delivery is unsuccessful after exhausting these maneuvers, final measure alternatives include intentional clavicular fracture, Zavanelli maneuver, symphysiotomy, and hysterotomy.

Clavicular fracture is performed by pulling the shaft of one clavicle anteriorly and outward. The action shortens the bisacromial diameter, but the significant force required can result in adjacent vascular, neurologic, and pulmonary damage, though the anterior and superior direction of the force aims to reduce this risk. Zavanelli maneuver is performed by replacement of the fetal head into the pelvis [51]. After administration of uterine relaxants, such as nitroglycerine

Table 11.4 "HELPERR" Mnemonic for management of shoulder dystocia.

H	**Help** – Request assistance from team, including mobilization of nursing anesthesia, obstetric, and pediatric personnel.
E	**Episiotomy** – Evaluation for episiotomy is necessary to determine if soft tissue may obstruct maneuverability during additional obstetric maneuvers.
L	**Legs** – Flexion and abduction of the maternal hips, known as McRobert's maneuver, can be effected by positioning the maternal thighs on the abdomen.
P	**Pressure** – Suprapubic pressure should be applied by an assistant during simultaneous gentle downward traction on the fetal neck. Pressure should be placed on the posterior aspect of the fetal anterior shoulder in a downward and lateral motion.
E	**Entry maneuvers** – Internal maneuvers, such as the Wood's and Rubin's maneuvers may be performed next.
R	**Remove the posterior arm** – Extraction of the posterior arm is performed by flexion at the elbow, followed by delivery of the forearm in a sweeping motion over the anterior chest wall.
R	**Roll** – Gaskin's maneuver involves rolling the patient into a hands-and-knees position.

or terbutaline, the provider reverses the sequence of actions previously taken by the fetus during the normal cardinal movements. The fetus is first rotated to an occiput anterior position to reverse restitution. The extended head is then reversed to its previously flexed position. The palm of the provider's dominant hand is used to replace the fetal head back into the vaginal vault, while the contralateral hand depresses the perineal soft tissue. After rapid placement of a bladder catheter and fetal scalp electrode, the patient is promptly transferred to the operating room for cesarean delivery. Reports of success of the Zavanelli maneuver are largely limited to case reports; the literature demonstrates a high rate of success, though this enthusiasm should be tempered by publication bias where adverse cases are probably not reported [52].

Symphysiotomy is an alternative when all other maneuvers have failed or cesarean delivery is not possible [53]. After infiltration of local anesthetic into the skin over the pubic symphysis, the urethra – with catheter *in situ* – is displaced laterally by the provider's index and middle fingers. The anterior and cephalad portion of the pubic symphysis cartilage is then incised with a scalpel blade to allow for separation of the pelvic bones. Repair of the symphysiotomy may require the expertise of urologic or orthopedic specialists. The mother should observe bed rest for approximately 2 days, and will require the use of crutches and possibly physiotherapy for pelvic instability.

Lastly, hysterotomy can be considered in catastrophic cases where Zavanelli or symphysiotomy are unsuccessful [54]. The posterior arm can be delivered through a low-transverse uterine incision with subsequent passage of the fetal hand to a vaginal assistant. The posterior arm is then delivered vaginally as previously described. The abdominal surgeon can then apply pressure to the anterior fetal shoulder in the same fashion as that applied via suprapubic pressure.

An integral component of management of shoulder dystocia is timely and accurate documentation of the sequence of events, maneuvers undertaken, and clinical outcomes. We recommend utilization of a standardized medical record form, which should be made readily available to the providers in a pre-printed or electronic format. A sample shoulder dystocia documentation form is shown in Figure 11.1.

11.3.6 Complications and outcomes

Shoulder dystocia can result in maternal and offspring complications. Infant injuries include fractures, brachial plexus injury, encephalopathy, and, ultimately, death. Maternal risks include postpartum hemorrhage, fourth-degree lacerations, and fistula formation.

Neonatal fractures may be an unintended result of internal maneuvers, such as humeral fracture during delivery of the posterior arm, or may be intentionally performed to decrease the bisacromial diameter, such as clavicular fracture. Clavicular fractures are reported in 1.7–9.5% of shoulder dystocia cases, while humeral fractures are found in 0.1–4.2% [55,56]. The majority of fractures resolve spontaneously without long-term sequelae [57].

SHOULDER DYSTOCIA DOCUMENTATION TOOL

Delivery Date: __________ Delivery Time: __________ Attending MD/CNM: ____________________

Assistant: ____________________

SELECTED PRENATAL INFORMATION

Gravida ______ Para ______

Diabetic: Yes ____ No ____ Gestational ______ Medical ______

Maternal weight: Estimated prepregnancy weight _______ Maternal height _______

Current weight _______ Total weight gain _______ lbs.

Obstetrical history: ☐ Prior shoulder dystocia ☐ Prior c/s for FTP

Gestational age on admission: _______ wks.

Estimated fetal weight on admission: ___________ ☐ clinical ☐ u/s u/s date ________

LABOR AND DELIVERY

Oxytocin used for: ☐ not used ☐ induction ☐ augmentation

Labor curve: Onset of active labor _____ Start of second stage _____

Delivery of head _____ Delivery of posterior shoulder _____

Delivery of body _____

Mode of delivery: ☐ Spontaneous

☐ Forceps Station at time applied _______ # pulls _____

☐ Vacuum Station at time applied _______ # pulls _____ # pop offs _____

Shoulder dystocia: Anterior shoulder: R L

Episiomy/laceration: 2nd 3rd 4th None

Maneuvers in order performed:

____

____

____

____

Comments: ______________________________

MD/CNM signature ______________________________

Date Completed __________ Time Completed __________

Figure 11.1 Sample form for documentation of shoulder dystocia events.

Brachial plexus injuries are reported in 3–16.8% of shoulder dystocia cases, but only 10% of these cases, or 1–2 of every 10,000 births, result in permanent sequelae [55,56]. Transient brachial plexus injury resolves with conservative physical therapy, with the majority experiencing normal function by 1 year of life. Of the permanent injuries, 80% involve the upper nerve roots (C5–C7), known as Erb–Duchenne palsy. The remainder of neurologic injuries involve the lower nerve roots (C8–T1), known as Klumpke palsy. Importantly, these injuries have also been reported after cesarean deliveries and normal spontaneous vaginal deliveries [58,59].

Hypoxic-ischemic encephalopathy has been reported in 0.3% of infants affected by shoulder dystocia. The fetal pH has been shown to decline at a rate of 0.04 units/minute between delivery of the head and trunk [60,61]. In one series, a head-to-shoulder interval threshold of 7 minutes or longer had a sensitivity and specificity of 67% and 74%, respectively, in predicting brain injury [61]. In another series, however, increasing head-to-body delivery interval was not correlated with pH, pCO2, or base deficit [62].

Postpartum hemorrhage is the most common maternal complication seen in shoulder dystocia, and affects 11% of cases [45]. Fourth-degree lacerations are also reported in 3.8% of cases [45]. Rates of episiotomy extension may be decreased by use of mediolateral episiotomies. Obstetrical fistulae may develop as a result of fourth-degree lacerations or, as can be seen in developing countries, with prolonged impaction causing maternal tissue ischemia. Management of these maternal complications is discussed elsewhere.

11.3.7 Prevention

Prophylactic cesarean delivery to prevent shoulder dystocia has been suggested in cases with risk factors, but this intervention has not been shown to be clinically or cost-effective [61]. If thresholds of 4000–4500 g estimated fetal weight by ultrasound are used for elective cesarean deliveries in non-diabetic women, a decision analysis estimates that 2345–3695 cesarean deliveries would need to be performed to prevent one permanent brachial plexus injury, with an associated additional cost of between $4.9 and $8.7 million annually [63]. ACOG recommends that although ultrasound estimation of fetal weight is imprecise, cesarean delivery may be considered for suspected fetal macrosomia with estimated fetal weights greater than 5000 g in women without diabetes and greater than 4500 g in women with diabetes [25].

Similarly, prophylactic induction of labor has not been shown to improve rates of brachial plexus palsy and may have unintended consequences on cesarean delivery rates. Institution of a protocol that recommended elective cesarean delivery for diabetic women with EFW greater than 4250 g or elective induction of labor for those with EFW greater than the 90th percentile (but less than 4250 g) in an institution resulted in a decrease in diagnosis of shoulder dystocia from 18.8 to 7.4% [64]. However, no improvement in rates of brachial plexus palsy was seen, with an increase in rate of cesarean delivery from 21.7 to 25.1% ($p < 0.04$) [64]. A retrospective study comparing induction of labor versus expectant management in patients with EFW > 90% also showed an increase in cesarean rates in the induced group without difference in shoulder dystocia rates [65].

Lastly, as noted previously, a woman with a history of shoulder dystocia is at elevated risk of recurrent shoulder dystocia. The true incidence of recurrence is difficult to estimate because many physicians and patients often choose not to undergo a repeat trial of labor [25]. ACOG currently recommends a thorough discussion of risks and benefits with the patient, with either mode of delivery as acceptable options.

The unpredictability of shoulder dystocia unfortunately renders this complication unpreventable in many cases. Management, therefore, should be geared at minimizing complications after diagnosis of shoulder dystocia. To optimize outcomes, the United States Joint Commission on Accreditation of Healthcare Organizations also recommends development and use of protocols and drills in preparation for shoulder dystocia [66].

11.4 Umbilical cord prolapse

11.4.1 Incidence and risk factors

Umbilical cord prolapse is a rare emergency occurring in only 0.14–0.62% of deliveries [67], but can have severe fetal consequences. Cord prolapse is defined by descent of the umbilical cord beyond the fetal presenting part and is diagnosed clinically with palpation of a pulsatile mass upon sterile digital examination or direct visualization of the umbilical cord. The cord may descend into the vagina beyond the fetal presenting part (45%), to the introitus (11%), or beyond the introitus (4%), resulting in umbilical cord compression [68]. Often, the diagnosis is made during a sudden fetal deceleration or bradycardia.

Risk factors for cord prolapse can be categorized into maternal, fetal, and iatrogenic factors. The primary maternal characteristic predisposing to cord prolapse is multiparity. Patients with cord prolapse are 1.6 times more likely to be multiparous, with an overall multiparity rate of 63–74% in umbilical cord cases [69,70]. The increased likelihood of rupture of membranes prior to engagement of fetal presenting part in multiparous women may account for this association. Rupture of membranes, both artificial or spontaneous, can cause the cord to slide past the fetal head during the evacuation of amniotic fluid.

Fetal risk factors for cord prolapse include malpresentation, prematurity, multiple gestation, polyhydramnios, and funic presentation. Although 50–63% of cord prolapses are seen in pregnancies in cephalic presentation [71], malpresented fetuses account for a disproportionate number of cases. Although breech and transverse presentations are only found in 3–4% [72] and 0.3% [73] of pregnancies at term, they contribute to 3.5% and 9.6% of cord prolapses, respectively [74]. Conversely, cord prolapse occurs in only 0.24% of cephalic presentations [74].

Prematurity is the most common factor in pregnancies complicated by malpresentation, and, therefore, premature fetuses are at increased risk of cord prolapse [73]. Even in cephalic presentations, the small size of the presenting part in premature fetuses allows for unobstructed passage of the cord. Similarly, the increased risk of cord prolapse in twin gestations arises from the risk of malpresentation and non-engaged presenting part in the second twin. The elevated levels of amniotic fluid in polyhydramnios also facilitate carriage of the cord beyond the unengaged fetal presenting part during the robust efflux of amniotic fluid.

Funic presentation, defined as the sonographic detection of umbilical cord below the fetal presenting part with intact membranes, is a harbinger of impending cord prolapse. Diagnosis of funic presentation can be made on antepartum ultrasound and is confirmed with color Doppler evaluation [75]. In some cases of antepartum cervical shortening, the umbilical cord can be seen protruding into the "hourglassing membranes" or cervical funnel [75]. A diagnosis of funic presentation is a contraindication for amniotomy and mandates planning for a cesarean delivery.

Iatrogenic factors that cause cord prolapse include active rupture of membranes, amnioinfusion, and insertion of internal monitoring devices. Each of these maneuvers duplicates the maternal or fetal risk factors that predispose to cord prolapse, by promoting rapid efflux of amniotic fluid, increasing the quantity of amniotic fluid, or manually elevating the fetal presenting part.

11.4.2 Management

The first sign of occult cord prolapse is often abrupt onset of fetal decelerations on cardiotocographic monitoring. All alternative causes of fetal decelerations or bradycardia should be considered in the differential diagnosis, and these are addressed elsewhere in this text. Once a cord is palpated and prolapse is diagnosed, the goal of management should be an expedited delivery to prevent fetal vascular compromise. As with many obstetrical emergencies, management protocols are based primarily on expert opinion, as the infrequent and emergent nature of this diagnosis render prospective randomized trials difficult.

Cesarean delivery is the preferred method of effecting delivery, and should be performed emergently unless vaginal delivery is imminent or cesarean delivery is not feasible. The diagnosing provider should immediately announce the diagnosis of cord prolapse to trigger mobilization of the delivering team, including obstetricians, anesthesiologists, nursing staff, and pediatricians.

While preparing for the cesarean delivery, temporizing measures should be attempted to decrease life-threatening external compressive forces on the umbilical cord. Oxytocin, if being administered, should be discontinued. The provider performing the initial vaginal examination should keep the examining hand within the vaginal vault in order to elevate the fetal presenting part. The cesarean delivery is then performed in an expedited manner, with the vaginal hand remaining in place until the fetal presenting part is elevated out of the maternal pelvis by the abdominal surgeons.

The patient can also be placed in Trendelenburg or hands-knees position to facilitate the movement of the fetus upwards and away from the maternal pelvis during transfer to the operating suite. Alternative methods of decreasing compression include retrograde bladder filling and tocolytic administration.

11.4.3 Prevention of complication

Prevention of cord prolapse complications begins with primary prevention, by avoidance of iatrogenic risk factors, or via secondary prevention, by early diagnosis and prompt intervention. Active rupture of membranes in a labor patient with an unengaged fetal head should be discouraged, unless necessary for access to place internal monitors. Similarly, placement of internal monitors and initiation of amnioinfusion should only be considered when indicated. In cases of polyhydramnios or unengaged head, rupture of membranes should be performed with a small-gauge needle or fetal scalp electrode, instead of the routine amniotomy hook device. Fundal pressure during amniotomy can help descend the fetal head into the pelvis.

11.4.4 Outcomes

Mechanical compression of the cord between the fetus and the maternal pelvic structures, such as the cervix or pubic symphysis, can lead to compromise of blood flow and fetal decelerations. Newborns that deliver after umbilical cord prolapse are at higher risk of lower Apgar score < 7 at 5 minutes compared to controls (6.3 vs 1.4%, $p = 0.002$) [70], with a perinatal mortality rate of 39–430 per 1000 cases [69,76]. Morbidity and mortality have significantly decreased over the past century as ability to perform expedited deliveries and neonatal resuscitation protocols have improved in industrialized countries.

The offspring outcome primarily depends on diagnosis-to-delivery interval, which hinges on the application of an efficient multidisciplinary approach. A large retrospective study from the United Kingdom showed that Apgar scores were better with a shorter diagnosis-to-delivery interval, but that a diagnosis-to-delivery interval of less than 30 minutes had little influence on Apgar scores at 1 and 5 minutes [77]. The risk of umbilical cord arterial pH < 7.1 increases after 10 minutes. Consequently, extramural cord prolapses have significantly higher rates of neonatal morbidity and mortality compared to those diagnosed in the hospital.

11.5 Head entrapment

11.5.1 Incidence and risk factors

Fetal head entrapment can result in significant fetal compromise, and the maneuvers to correct the emergency can result in maternal complications. The diagnosis is most often encountered in delivery of a fetus in breech presentation via either the vaginal or cesarean route. Fetuses with larger head-to-abdomen ratio, such as that seen in prematurity or congenital head and neck anomalies, are at significantly increased risk due to insufficient dilation of the cervix or hysterotomy opening by the fetal body prior to delivery of the head.

The increased risk of head entrapment for prematurity may be confined to extremely premature fetuses weighing 1000–1249 g, where an odds ratio of 6.4 (95% CI 1.6–26.1) has been reported [78]. In one study of 321 consecutive singleton breech deliveries from 28–36 weeks, head entrapment occurred in 7.7% of neonates delivering vaginally and 5.2% of neonates delivering by cesarean section [78].

11.5.2 Diagnosis

Diagnosis is made when routine maneuvers of a breech delivery, such as suprapubic pressure or Mauriceau–Smellie–Veit maneuvers, are unable to achieve delivery of the fetal head. These maneuvers and the use of Piper's forceps are described in Chapters 6 and 10.

11.5.3 Management

In most cases of vaginal breech deliveries, obstetricians, anesthesiologists, nursing staff, and pediatricians are all already mobilized and in the delivery room. Upon diagnosis of a head entrapment, a uterine relaxant should be administered to alleviate any lower uterine segment and cervical constriction. Medication options include terbutaline (0.25 mg intravenous or subcutaneous) or nitroglycerine (50–200 mg intravenous) [79].

If incomplete cervical dilation is suspected, particularly during delivery of a preterm fetus, cervical incisions can be made to expand the cervical os. Duhrssen incisions are performed in a chevron pattern with incisions at 2, 6, and 10 o'clock. This specific arrangement of the incisions avoids transection of the bilateral descending cervical branches of the uterine arteries. The cervix and cervicovaginal junction are identified using the operator's fingers, placed to protect the fetal head and neck soft tissue. Bandage scissors can provide further protection for the fetus. Complications of Duhrssen incisions include hemorrhage, urologic injury, need for hysterectomy, and future cervical insufficiency.

Failure to deliver the head after uterine relaxants and Duhrssen incisions can lead to significant morbidity for the fetus, given the obligate cord compression that occurs with head entrapment. Similar to shoulder dystocia, case reports of symphysiotomy and Zavanelli maneuver for resolution of head dystocia exist in catastrophic cases. These maneuvers are described under shoulder dystocia, and are associated with significant maternal and fetal morbidity.

11.5.4 Outcomes

Offspring complications related to head entrapment include hypoxemic-ischemic encephalopathy, spinal cord injury, soft tissue lacerations, and death [80]. Maternal complications are primarily related to the obstetric maneuvers required for breech delivery, such as lacerations, urologic injury, and hemorrhage.

11.6 Seizure

11.6.1 Differential diagnoses

Seizure in pregnancy can be secondary to an established seizure disorder or an obstetrical complication. Preexisting seizures may result from genetic predisposition, trauma, infection, fevers, tumors, hypoglycemia, strokes, congenital malformations, drug intoxication, or inborn errors of metabolism, or be idiopathic [81]. Recurrent seizures during pregnancy in women with known seizure disorder may arise from subtherapeutic levels of antiepileptic medications, non-compliance with medications, infection, trauma, or stress. Anticonvulsant levels decline as pregnancy progresses, even in the face of constant and, in some cases, increased dosages of medications [82]. This pharmacokinetic change is secondary to physiologic alterations in liver metabolism, renal clearance, protein binding, and volume of distribution [83].

The primary obstetrical complication presenting as new-onset seizures in pregnancy is eclampsia, defined by the presence of new-onset *grand mal* seizures in a pregnant woman above 20 weeks of gestation with preeclampsia [84]. Eclamptic seizures occur in approximately 2–3% and 0.6% of cases of severe preeclampsia and mild preeclampsia, respectively [85]. Incidence rates vary by region, with developed nations reporting 1.6–10 cases and developing nations reporting 6–157 cases per 100,000 deliveries [85].

In one study, most eclamptic seizures occurred despite antenatal care (70%) and within one week of the woman's last visit to a doctor or midwife (85%) [86]. Forty-four per cent of cases occurred postpartum, more than a third (38%) antepartum, and the remainder (18%) intrapartum. Antepartum eclampsia, which was more likely to occur preterm, was associated with a higher rate of maternal complications and a higher neonatal mortality. Risk factors for eclampsia are carried over from those predisposing to preeclampsia, such as underlying hypertension, diabetes, renal disease, extremes of maternal age, and nulliparity. Preeclampsia and hypertensive disorders of pregnancy are discussed in detail elsewhere in this text.

11.6.2 Management

The various underlying etiologies of seizure disorders demand differing management protocols. For this chapter on obstetrical emergencies, we will focus on the acute management of a seizing patient, instead of the antepartum management of preeclampsia or chronic management of seizure disorders.

Initial management of the pregnant seizing patient is identical to that of a non-pregnant patient, including evaluation of immediate safety of surroundings, protection of the patient from trauma, placement of patient in a lateral decubitus position, maintenance of a patent airway, and evaluation of maternal and fetal vital signs. As the first seizure often occurs without warning, these maneuvers are geared around prevention of further complications. Left lateral decubitus position serves two purposes: prevention of maternal aspiration and improvement of uteroplacental perfusion. Important maternal vital signs for immediate assessment include heart rate, blood pressure, respiratory rate, oxygenation, and fingerstick blood glucose. Supplemental oxygenation should be provided via face mask. Maternal hypertension should be treated, as hypertensive urgency and emergency may lead to maternal stroke. In the third trimester, cervical examination should also be documented secondary to association of eclamptic seizures with uterine tachysystole and rapid progression of labor [87].

Fetal vital signs include documentation of fetal heart rate for the pre-viable fetus, or continuous cardiotocographic monitoring of the viable fetus. Fetal heart rate decelerations and prolonged bradycardia are frequently seen in the setting of acute tonic-clonic seizures, due to maternal hypoventilation, uterine tachysystole, and shunting of maternal blood away from the splanchnic vasculature into the extremities [88]. In the absence of placental abruption, the bradycardia almost always resolves after cessation of seizure activity, and may be followed by a period of compensatory fetal tachycardia with loss of variability [87]. For this reason, immediate delivery is not always necessary.

Subsequent management, after a seizure, focuses on prevention of recurrent seizures, which occur in approximately 10% of cases [89]. When intravenous access is available, parenteral magnesium sulfate (typically 4–6 g over 15–30 minutes, followed by a 2 g/hr maintenance dose) is the first line for seizure prophylaxis in eclampsia. However, when intravenous access is difficult or when the seizure is extramural, intramuscular magnesium sulfate (5 g once every 4 hours) is also effective. Magnesium sulfate administration is preferred over traditional antiepileptic medications secondary to the findings of the Collaborative Eclampsia Trial [90]. Women receiving magnesium sulfate experienced 52% and 67% fewer recurrences in convulsions compared to women who received diazepam or phenytoin, respectively. Furthermore, magnesium sulfate administration in preterm infants may provide neuroprotection against cerebral palsy [91]. Specifics on magnesium dosage and monitoring are discussed separately.

When a patient on magnesium experiences recurrent seizures, magnesium sulfate can be readministered with an additional 2-g bolus intravenously. Failure of control thereafter should prompt initiation of alternative antiepileptic drugs and evaluation for other etiologies for seizure disorder. Diazepam (0.1–0.3 mg/kg or 5 mg IV over 60 seconds, with a maximum cumulative dose of 20 mg), lorazepam (0.02–0.03 mg/kg or 2–4 mg IV over 2–4 minutes), or phenobarbital (125 mg IV) are available options.

Determination of mode and timing of delivery are important components of management in eclampsia, since prolonged expectant management is contraindicated. During the acute seizure episode and associated fetal bradycardia, intrauterine resuscitation should be initiated instead of proceeding to emergent cesarean delivery. After maternal and fetal stabilization, the combination of cervical Bishop's score, fetal status, gestational age, and prior obstetrical history will allow the provider to determine whether induction or augmentation of labor can be attempted. The duration of induction, chance of successful vaginal delivery, and future fertility plans should all be factored into the provider and patient's decision-making process. Intrapartum and postpartum management of the preeclamptic patient, including fluid status and monitoring for signs of magnesium toxicity, is described elsewhere.

As with all obstetrical emergencies, a team approach is required for optimal outcomes. Anesthesiologists should be notified immediately upon diagnosis of eclampsia, given the high-risk maternal status and the possible need for cesarean delivery. To ensure team awareness, anesthesiologists should be notified of all antepartum or intrapartum preeclamptic patients upon admission to the hospital or initial diagnosis. Pediatricians should be notified of impending delivery. At periviable or premature gestational ages, neonatologists should be consulted on the institution-specific rates of perinatal morbidity and mortality. Nurse-to-patient ratios should be reorganized to allow for care and monitoring of the critical patient. Simulation specific to eclampsia management can improve knowledge and skills [92].

11.6.3 Outcomes

Maternal mortality has been reported in 1.8% of women experiencing eclampsia, with 35–70% of all women experiencing at least one major complication [86,89]. Maternal complications of eclampsia include disseminated intravascular coagulation, liver rupture, renal failure, transient blindness, cerebrovascular accident, urinary tract infections, lower respiratory tract infections, pulmonary edema, postpartum hemorrhage, or death [86]. Repeated seizure activity can lead to cerebral trauma, rhabdomyolysis, metabolic acidosis, aspiration pneumonia, or respiratory failure. Brain damage from cerebral hemorrhage or ischemia is the most common cause of death. Hemolysis, elevated liver enzymes, and low platelets (HELLP) syndrome develops in 10–20% of women with eclampsia.

Offspring complications include placental abruption, preterm delivery, hypoxic-ischemic injury, and perinatal death. The rate of stillbirths and neonatal deaths was 22.2/1000 and 34.1/1000, respectively [86]. As expected, complication rates are intimately associated with gestational age at delivery, and can drive mortality rates up to 23% at the lower limits of viability [93].

With subsequent pregnancies, the patient is not only at risk for recurrent preeclampsia, but also for eclampsia. In a group of 406 women with preeclampsia or eclampsia in their first pregnancies, recurrence rate of preeclampsia was 46.8% in a second pregnancy and 20.7% in subsequent pregnancies, compared to 7.6% and 7.7% in normotensive controls [94]. Rates of recurrent eclampsia are approximately 2% in a subsequent pregnancy [95]. Long-term sequelae include maternal hypertension, diabetes, and renal complications [95,96].

11.7 Cardiopulmonary arrest and perimortem cesarean delivery

11.7.1 Incidence and risk factors

Cardiac arrest during pregnancy is exceedingly rare, with estimated prevalence of 1/20,000 to 1/50,000 [97–99]. However, the increasing severity and frequency of maternal co-morbidities, the use of assisted reproductive technologies in older women who could not previously conceive, and the advances in surgical repair of congenital cardiac lesions, have contributed to rising prevalence rates.

Causes of terminal cardiopulmonary compromise can be divided into direct obstetrical causes and indirect causes. Direct obstetrical causes include hemorrhage (17%), peripartum cardiomyopathy (8%), preeclampsia-eclampsia (2.8%), and amniotic fluid embolism. Indirect causes include pulmonary embolism (29%), sepsis (13%), stroke (5%), anesthesia complications (2%), myocardial infarction, and trauma [99]. Toxicity from magnesium sulfate, a medication commonly used in seizure prophylaxis, fetal neuroprotection, and tocolysis, can also result in cardiopulmonary arrest.

Underlying maternal cardiac disease can be congenital, acquired, or other etiologies of cardiomyopathy. Advances in the surgical palliation and correction of congenital heart lesions have improved survival and increased the number of patients living into adulthood [100]. Current surgical mortality rates for congenital heart disease (CHD) are less than 5%, and it is estimated that within the next decade, as many as 1 in 150 young adults will have some form of CHD [100,101]. Therefore, the management of pregnant adults with CHD is increasingly relevant.

With the rise of cesarean delivery rates, complications arising from anesthesia are also increasing. The complications that may lead to cardiopulmonary arrest include airway-related catastrophes, local anesthetic toxicity, and aspiration. Anesthesia-related complications are the seventh leading cause of maternal death in the United States and the United Kingdom [102]. The majority of anesthesia-related deaths in pregnancy (82%) occur in the setting of cesarean delivery. The risk ratio of mortality for general anesthesia was 2.3 times that of regional anesthesia [102].

11.7.2 Management

Management of cardiopulmonary arrest in pregnancy differs from management of the non-pregnant patient secondary to the additional fetal concerns and physiologic changes of pregnancy. Due to the rarity of such events, no randomized controlled trials are available to evaluate the efficacy of the resuscitative measures listed below. The guidelines from routine Advanced Cardiac Life Support (ACLS) protocols have been modified to fit the maternal anatomy and physiology, with the overall tenet that the best hope of fetal survival is maternal survival [103].

Primary intervention in the patient who is critically ill or at significant risk of cardiac events should be prevention of cardiopulmonary arrest [103]. These interventions include administration of 100% oxygen and establishment of intravenous access above the diaphragm. Administration of fluid into a site in the groin or lower may be less effective secondary vascular compression from the gravid uterus. The patient should be placed into full left-lateral decubitus position to decrease aortocaval compression and allow for improved cardiac preload and output. Maternal hypotension, defined by a systolic blood pressure of < 100 mmHg or < 80% below baseline, should be reversed via administration of crystalloid or colloid solutions. These maneuvers increase placental perfusion and oxygenation. Reversible causes of critical illness should be diagnosed and treated to prevent further decompensation.

Once cardiac arrest is diagnosed, timing of resuscitation plays an integral role in outcome and prognosis. Continuing the theme of multidisciplinary approach in this chapter, the initial intervention should be initiation of the hospital-wide cardiopulmonary arrest code system, often known as "Code Blue." The predetermined code team is commonly designed for medical and surgical floors and does not include a delivery team. As such, obstetricians, appropriate nursing staff, surgical technicians, and pediatricians should also be immediately summoned, and, if the arrest is off the labor and delivery unit, a cesarean kit procured. The time of diagnosis should be clearly documented, given the time-sensitive nature of the interventions.

Cardiopulmonary resuscitation (CPR) is immediately initiated. ACLS protocols from the American Heart Association (AHA) previously focused on "ABCD," a mnemonic for airway, breathing, circulation, and defibrillation [104]. This sequence of the actions was changed 50 years later in 2010 to "CAB," to place an emphasis on circulation via chest compression before oxygenation [105]. Another "D" can be added to this mnemonic to include displacement of the gravid uterus in patients in the third trimester.

The airway remains of significant importance and concern in gravid patients, given the rapid rate of oxygen consumption and decreased functional residual capacity [103]. Airway edema from physiologic pregnancy changes or pathologic changes in preeclampsia and/or fluid overload can also render airway access difficult in the third trimester. In extreme cases, surgical airway may be required. One hundred per cent oxygen should be administered.

External chest compressions may be difficult in the left lateral position. A firm wedge or tilt board under the mother's right side can provide tilt and displacement, with a goal of greater than or equal to 30 degrees. Alternatively, when tilting is not possible, manual leftward displacement of the uterus with one or two hands may suffice [103]. In addition, chest compressions are best shifted upward on the sternum to account for the upward displacement of the maternal diaphragm in the third trimester. The exact anatomic location for ideal chest compression has not yet been specified.

In cases of ventricular arrhythmia, the AHA states that the use of an automatic external defibrillator (AED) is reasonable, although it is not well studied [103]. Physiological changes during pregnancy do not appear to affect transthoracic impedance or transmyocardial current [106]. The authors conclude that current energy requirements for adult defibrillation are appropriate for use during pregnancy. Fetal adverse outcomes from AED use have been reported, possibly due to transmission of electrical current through the amniotic fluid. These risks include fetal arrhythmia, burns, and death. Medications required during CPR, such as amiodarone, do not change in the gravid state. The benefits gained from maternal resuscitation far outweigh any risk associated with the medications and defibrillation.

During resuscitation, fetal estimated gestational age should be simultaneously determined, if not already known from prenatal care. Transabdominal palpation of uterine size can provide a rough estimate of gestational age in situations without rapid ultrasound capabilities. Fundal height in centimeters, measured from the most cephalad point of the pubic symphysis to the uterine fundus, is approximately equal to gestational age in weeks. An even more rudimentary estimate of potential fetal viability is a uterine fundus that is located more than 4 cm above the umbilicus. These external measurements can be misleading if uterine leiomyoma, morbid obesity, amniotic fluid abnormalities, or congenital abnormalities are present.

When portable bedside ultrasound is available, as is often the case in emergency rooms and labor and delivery, rapid sonographic evaluation of the fetus can be performed to determine potential fetal viability. In the third trimester, head circumference is the most accurate predictor of gestational age among the parameters measured in fetal biometry [107]. Signs of fetal maturity may be determined via evaluation of the bony epiphyses, although a trained sonographer is required. The femoral epiphyseal and proximal tibial ossification centers are well visualized by 32 and 35 weeks of gestational age, respectively [108,109].

If maternal resuscitation is unsuccessful by 4 minutes, perimortem cesarean delivery should begin. This action may improve both fetal and maternal outcomes. Several case reports of emergency cesarean section in maternal cardiac arrest indicate a return of spontaneous circulation or improvement in maternal hemodynamic status only after the uterine contents have been evacuated [103]. Redistribution of cardiac output and shunting of the blood supply away from the uterus may provide maternal benefit. As with the overarching principle of management of cardiac arrest in pregnancy, maternal survival gives the best chance for offspring survival.

The initiation of hysterotomy at 4 minutes after cessation of cardiac activity is to enable the "5-minute rule" in timing of delivery [103]. At greater than 24–25 weeks of gestation, the best survival rate for the offspring occurs when the infant is delivered no more than 5 minutes after the mother's heart stops beating. At gestational ages greater than 30 weeks, infant survival has been seen even when delivery occurred after 5–30 minutes from onset of maternal cardiac arrest. To enable a timely delivery, transport of the patient from the emergency department or labor room to operating room is not necessary. When summoned, the obstetrician should bring an emergency cesarean delivery kit and personnel to the location of the patient. Unfortunately, the reality remains that very few cases of perimortem cesarean delivery are completed within the recommended 5-minute period [98].

In futile cases where maternal prognosis is severely grim and the fetus remains viable, proceeding to an emergent cesarean delivery before the 4-minute cut-off may be beneficial to the offspring. After delivery of the fetus, if maternal resuscitation remains unsuccessful at 15 minutes, thoracotomy and direct cardiac massage should be considered as terminal measures by appropriately trained personnel. Cardiopulmonary bypass has also been reported [110].

Experts have emphasized the importance of preparation and training to minimize time-to-delivery intervals and optimize outcomes. Team planning should be done in collaboration with the obstetric, neonatal, emergency, anesthesiology, intensive care, and cardiac arrest services [103]. The AHA summary algorithm for cardiac arrest in pregnancy is shown in Figure 11.2. Simulation training has been shown to improve knowledge and skills related to response to a maternal arrest [111].

Lastly, the role of post-cardiac arrest care also requires a multidisciplinary approach to address the underlying etiology and any sequelae. One potential intervention is the application of hypothermia. Hypothermia can decrease the metabolic requirements of the mother and be protective. A case report of a woman who experienced cardiac arrest at 13 weeks and arrived at the hospital in a comatose state has been described [112]. Hypothermia was initiated for 24 hours after the acute event. Although the patient suffers from mild neurologic deficit, she delivered a healthy term infant without neurologic sequelae. It should be noted that fetal heart rate often decreases during hypothermia; this may be physiologic rather than representing a pathologic bradycardia or fetal distress, and other signs such as loss of variability or absence of accelerations can improve specificity. While hypothermia may also protect the fetus by lowering metabolic requirements, it also inhibits fetal gas exchange. Cooling is often associated with an increase in uterine tone.

11.7.3 Outcomes

Overall survival of cardiopulmonary arrest in pregnancy is below that of the non-pregnant patient, despite the inherently younger cohort compared to the general population. Reported survival rates range from 6.9 to 15% [98]. However, these statistics may reflect the poor compliance to the 5-minute rule.

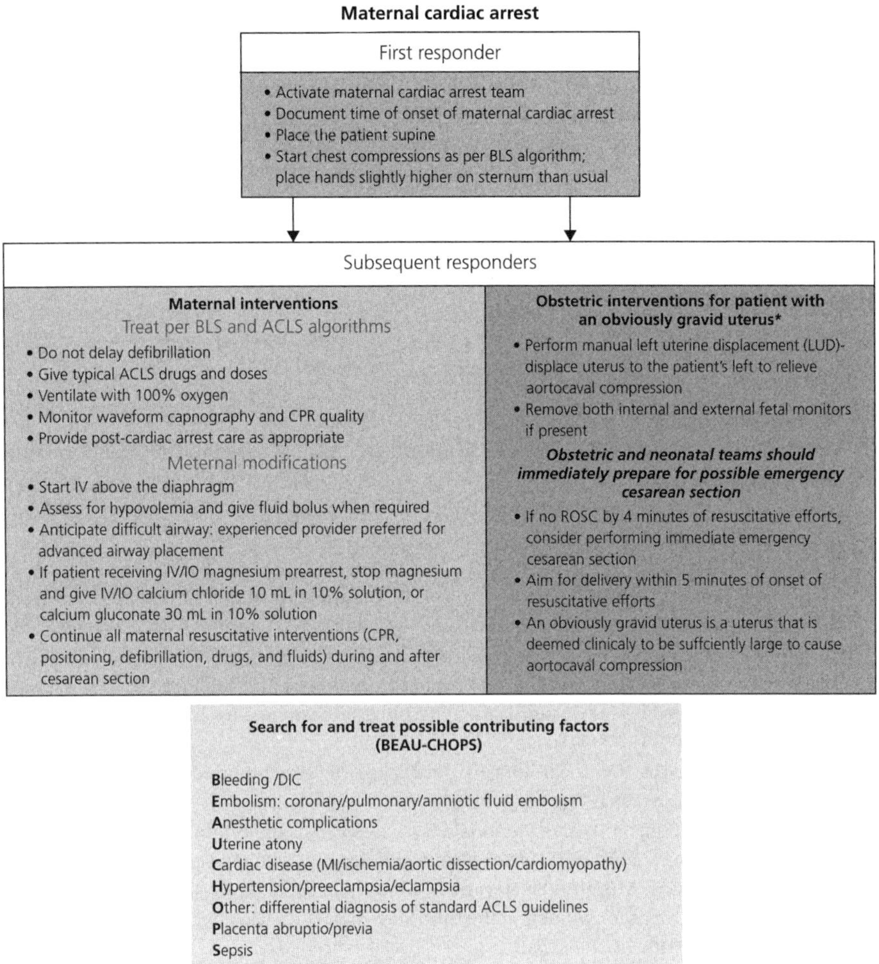

Figure 11.2 American Heart Association Maternal Cardiac Arrest algorithm. *Source*: Vanden Hoek *et al.*, 2003 [103]. Reproduced with permission from Lippincott Williams & Wilkins.

11.8 Summary

Although significant advances have been made in the understanding, prevention, and management of obstetrical emergencies, these events will continue to be a reality in the lives of obstetrical providers and our patients. Further adding fuel to the flames are the improved capabilities of assisted reproductive technologies, rapid rise of multifetal gestations, epidemic of maternal co-morbidities such as diabetes, and advances in surgical repair of congenital anomalies. Combined, these factors will shift our obstetrical population to an increasingly complicated demographic, increasing our risk for obstetrical emergencies.

Prompt recognition and response to each obstetrical emergency is the most important tenet for management. The unifying theme for each of the above obstetrical emergencies is the need for a multidisciplinary and structured team approach to the unpredictable events. Only by enhancing the team mentality and promoting a culture of patient safety can the obstetrical community achieve the desired reduction in mortality and morbidity rates.

References

1 Hogan MC, Foreman KJ, Naghavi M, Ahn SY, Wang M, Makela SM *et al.* Maternal mortality for 181 countries, 1980–2008: a systematic analysis of progress towards Millennium Development Goal 5. *Lancet* 2010;**375**(9726):1609–1623.

2 C. A. Antepartum and postpartum hemorrhage. AD MCL, editor. Boston: Harvard University Press, 1998.

3 Mousa HA and Alfirevic Z. Treatment for primary postpartum haemorrhage. *Cochrane Database of Systematic Reviews* 2003;(1):CD003249.

4 Knight M, Callaghan WM, Berg C, Alexander S, Bouvier-Colle MH, Ford JB *et al.* Trends in postpartum hemorrhage in high resource countries: a review and recommendations from the International Postpartum Hemorrhage Collaborative Group. *BMC Pregnancy and Childbirth* 2009;**9**:55.

5 American College of Obstetricians and Gynecologists Practice Bulletin No. 76 Clinical Management Guidelines for Obstetrician-Gynecologists: postpartum hemorrhage. *Obstetrics & Gynecology* 2006;**108**(4):1039–1047.

6 Combs CA and Laros RK Jr. Prolonged third stage of labor: morbidity and risk factors. *Obstetrics & Gynecology* 1991;**77**(6):863–867.

7 Prendiville WJ, Elbourne D, and McDonald S. Active versus expectant management in the third stage of labour. *Cochrane Database of Systematic Reviews* 2000;(**3**):CD000007.

8 Begley CM, Gyte GM, Murphy DJ, Devane D, McDonald SJ, and McGuire W. Active versus expectant management for women in the third stage of labour. *Cochrane Database of Systematic Reviews* 2010;(7):CD007412.

9 Gulmezoglu AM, Lumbiganon P, Landoulsi S, Widmer M, Abdel-Aleem H, Festin M *et al.* Active management of the third stage of labour with and without controlled cord traction: a randomised, controlled, non-inferiority trial. *Lancet* 2012;**379**(9827):1721–1727.

10 McDonald SJ and Middleton P. Effect of timing of umbilical cord clamping of term infants on maternal and neonatal outcomes. *Cochrane Database of Systematic Reviews* 2008;(2):CD004074.

11 Shields LE, Smalarz K, Reffigee L, Mugg S, Burdumy TJ, and Propst M. Comprehensive maternal hemorrhage protocols improve patient safety and reduce utilization of blood products. *American Journal of Obstetrics & Gynecology* 2011;**205**(4):368 e1–8.

12 OB Hemorrhage: Compendium of Best Practices. 2007; Available from: http://www.cmqcc.org/ob_hemorrhage/.

13 Gülmezoglu AM, Souza JP, Chou D, Mathai M, Hill S, Abalos E (eds). *WHO Guidelines for the Management of Postpartum Haemorrhage and Retained Placenta. WHO Technical Consultation on the Management of Postpartum Haemorrhage and Retained Placenta.* Geneva, Switzerland: World Health Organization, 2009.

14 Abdel-Aleem H, Singata M, Abdel-Aleem M, Mshweshwe N, Williams X, and Hofmeyr GJ. Uterine massage to reduce postpartum hemorrhage after vaginal delivery. *International Journal of Gynecology & Obstetrics* 2010;**111**(1):32–36.

15 Alam HB and Rhee P. New developments in fluid resuscitation. *Surgical Clinics of North America* 2007;**87**(1):55–72, vi.

16 Davenport R, Curry N, Manson J, De'Ath H, Coates A, Rourke C *et al.* Hemostatic effects of fresh frozen plasma may be maximal at red cell ratios of 1:2. *Journal of Trauma* 2011;**70**(1): 90–95; discussion 5–6.

17 Holcomb JB, Jenkins D, Rhee P, Johannigman J, Mahoney P, Mehta S *et al.* Damage control resuscitation: directly addressing the early coagulopathy of trauma. *Journal of Trauma* 2007;**62**(2):307–310.

18 Vedantham S, Goodwin SC, McLucas B, and Mohr G. Uterine artery embolization: an underused method of controlling pelvic hemorrhage. *American Journal of Obstetrics & Gynecology* 1997;**176**(4):938–948.

19 Ford JB, Algert CS, Kok C, Choy MA, and Roberts CL. Hospital data reporting on postpartum hemorrhage: under-estimates recurrence and over-estimates the contribution of uterine atony. *Maternal and Child Health Journal* 2011;**16**(7):1542–1548.

20 Hall MH, Halliwell R, and Carr-Hill R. Concomitant and repeated happenings of complications of the third stage of labour. *BJOG* 1985;**92**(7):732–738.

21 Della Torre M, Kilpatrick SJ, Hibbard JU, Simonson L, Scott S, Koch A *et al.* Assessing preventability for obstetric hemorrhage. *American Journal of Perinatology* 2011;**28**(10):753–760.

22 The Joint Commission. Sentinel Event Alert. *Preventing Maternal Death* 2010;**44**. Available from: http://www.jointcommission.org/assets/1/18/sea_44.pdf (accessed May 15, 2015).

23 Daniels K and Parness AJ. Development and use of mechanical devices for simulation of seizure and hemorrhage in obstetrical team training. *Simulation in Healthcare* 2008;**3**(1): 42–46.

24 Smellie W. A collection of cases and observation in midwifery to illustrate his former treatise or first volume on that subject. In: Cadell T and Nicol G (eds). London: W. Strahan, 1779: 446–448.

25 Sokol RJ and Blackwell SC. American College of Obstetricians and Gynecologists Practice Bulletin No. 40: Shoulder dystocia. *International Journal of Gynecology & Obstetrics* 2003;**80**(1):87–92.

26 Resnik R. Management of shoulder girdle dystocia. *Clinical Obstetrics and Gynecology* 1980;**23**(2):559–564.

27 Overland EA, Vatten LJ, and Eskild A. Risk of shoulder dystocia: associations with parity and offspring birthweight. A population study of 1,914,544 deliveries. *Acta Obstetricia et Gynecologica Scandinavica* 2012;**91**(4):483–488.

28 Baskett TF and Allen AC. Perinatal implications of shoulder dystocia. *Obstetrics & Gynecology* 1995;**86**(1):14–17.

29 Nocon JJ, McKenzie DK, Thomas LJ, and Hansell RS. Shoulder dystocia: an analysis of risks and obstetric maneuvers. *American Journal of Obstetrics & Gynecology* 1993;**168**(6 Pt 1): 1732–1737; discussion 7–9.

30 Vidarsdottir H, Geirsson RT, Hardardottir H, Valdimarsdottir U, and Dagbjartsson A. Obstetric and neonatal risks among extremely macrosomic babies and their mothers. *American Journal of Obstetrics & Gynecology* 2011;**204**(5):423 e1–6.

31 Nesbitt TS, Gilbert WM, and Herrchen B. Shoulder dystocia and associated risk factors with macrosomic infants born in California. *American Journal of Obstetrics & Gynecology* 1998;**179**(2):476–480.

32 Ouzounian JG, Gherman RB, Chauhan S, Battista LR, and Lee RH. Recurrent shoulder dystocia: analysis of incidence and risk factors. *American Journal of Perinatology* 2012;**29**(7):515–518.

33 McFarland M, Hod M, Piper JM, Xenakis EM, and Langer O. Are labor abnormalities more common in shoulder dystocia? *American Journal of Obstetrics & Gynecology* 1995;**173**(4):1211–1214.

34 Lurie S, Levy R, Ben-Arie A, and Hagay Z. Shoulder dystocia: could it be deduced from the labor partogram? *American Journal of Perinatology* 1995;**12**(1):61–62.
35 Acker DB, Sachs BP, and Friedman EA. Risk factors for shoulder dystocia. *Obstetrics & Gynecology* 1985;**66**(6):762–768.
36 Spong CY, Beall M, Rodrigues D, and Ross MG. An objective definition of shoulder dystocia: prolonged head-to-body delivery intervals and/or the use of ancillary obstetric maneuvers. *Obstetrics & Gynecology* 1995;**86**(3):433–436.
37 Kay SP. Obstetrical brachial palsy. *British Journal of Plastic Surgery* 1998;**51**(1):43–50.
38 Ouzounian JG and Goodwin TM. Shoulder dystocia. In: Goodwin TM, Montoro MN, Muderspach L, and Roy S (eds). *Management of Common Problems in Obstetrics and Gynecology*, 5th edn. Chichester: Wiley-Blackwell, 2010: 45.
39 Leonard RJ. The head and neck. In: Leonard RJ (ed.). *Human Gross Anatomy: An Outline Text*, 1st edn. Oxford University Press, 1995: 215.
40 Alexander JM, Leveno KJ, Hauth J, Landon MB, Thom E, Spong CY *et al.* Fetal injury associated with cesarean delivery. *Obstetrics & Gynecology* 2006;**108**(4):885–890.
41 Deering S, Poggi S, Macedonia C, Gherman R, and Satin AJ. Improving resident competency in the management of shoulder dystocia with simulation training. *Obstetrics & Gynecology* 2004;**103**(6):1224–1228.
42 Draycott TJ, Crofts JF, Ash JP, Wilson LV, Yard E, Sibanda T *et al.* Improving neonatal outcome through practical shoulder dystocia training. *Obstetrics & Gynecology* 2008;**112**(1):14–20.
43 Buhimschi CS, Buhimschi IA, Malinow A, and Weiner CP. Use of McRoberts' position during delivery and increase in pushing efficiency. *Lancet* 2001;**11;358**(9280):470–471.
44 McFarland MB, Langer O, Piper JM, and Berkus MD. Perinatal outcome and the type and number of maneuvers in shoulder dystocia. *International Journal of Gynecology & Obstetrics* 1996;**55**(3):219–224.
45 Gherman RB, Goodwin TM, Souter I, Neumann K, Ouzounian JG, and Paul RH. The McRoberts' maneuver for the alleviation of shoulder dystocia: how successful is it? *American Journal of Obstetrics & Gynecology* 1997;**176**(3):656–661.
46 Rubin A. Management of shoulder dystocia. *Journal of the American Medical Association* 1964;**14**;189:835–837.
47 Woods C. A principle of physics as applicable to shoulder delivery. *American Journal of Obstetrics & Gynecology* 1943;**45**:796–812.
48 Schwartz BC and Dixon DM. Shoulder dystocia. *Obstetrics & Gynecology* 1958;**11**(4):468–471.
49 Bruner JP, Drummond SB, Meenan AL, and Gaskin IM. All-fours maneuver for reducing shoulder dystocia during labor. *Journal of Reproductive Medicine* 1998;**43**(5):439–443.
50 Gobbo R and Baxley EG. Shoulder dystocia. In: *ALSO: advanced life support in obstetrics provider course syllabus*. American Academy of Family Physicians: Leawood, Kansas, 2000.
51 Sandberg EC. The Zavanelli maneuver: a potentially revolutionary method for the resolution of shoulder dystocia. *American Journal of Obstetrics & Gynecology* 1985;**152**(4):479–484.
52 Sandberg EC. The Zavanelli maneuver: 12 years of recorded experience. *Obstetrics & Gynecology* 1999;**93**(2):312–317.
53 Hartfield VJ. Symphysiotomy for shoulder dystocia. *American Journal of Obstetrics & Gynecology* 1986;**155**(1):228.
54 O'Shaughnessy MJ. Hysterotomy facilitation of the vaginal delivery of the posterior arm in a case of severe shoulder dystocia. *Obstetrics & Gynecology* 1998;**92**(4 Pt 2):693–695.
55 Hoffman MK, Bailit JL, Branch DW, Burkman RT, Van Veldhusien P, Lu L *et al.* A comparison of obstetric maneuvers for the acute management of shoulder dystocia. *Obstetrics & Gynecology* 2011;**117**(6):1272–1278.
56 Gherman RB, Chauhan S, Ouzounian JG, Lerner H, Gonik B, and Goodwin TM. Shoulder dystocia: the unpreventable obstetric emergency with empiric management guidelines. *American Journal of Obstetrics & Gynecology* 2006;**195**(3):657–672.

57 Hsu TY, Hung FC, Lu YJ, Ou CY, Roan CJ, Kung FT *et al.* Neonatal clavicular fracture: clinical analysis of incidence, predisposing factors, diagnosis, and outcome. *American Journal of Perinatology* 2002;**19**(1):17–21.
58 Paradiso G, Granana N, and Maza E. Prenatal brachial plexus paralysis. *Neurology* 1997;**49**(1):261–262.
59 Dunn DW and Engle WA. Brachial plexus palsy: intrauterine onset. *Pediatric Neurology* 1985;**1**(6):367–369.
60 Wood C, Ng KH, Hounslow D, and Benning H. Time – an important variable in normal delivery. *The Journal of Obstetrics and Gynaecology of the British Commonwealth* 1973;**80**(4):295–300.
61 Gherman RB. Shoulder dystocia: an evidence-based evaluation of the obstetric nightmare. *Clinical Obstetrics and Gynecology* 2002;**45**(2):345–362.
62 Ouzounian JG, Korst LM, Ahn MO, and Phelan JP. Shoulder dystocia and neonatal brain injury: significance of the head-shoulder interval. *American Journal of Obstetrics & Gynecology* 1998;**178**(1):S76.
63 Rouse DJ, Owen J, Goldenberg RL, and Cliver SP. The effectiveness and costs of elective cesarean delivery for fetal macrosomia diagnosed by ultrasound. *Journal of the American Medical Association* 1996;**276**(18):1480–1486.
64 Conway DL and Langer O. Elective delivery of infants with macrosomia in diabetic women: reduced shoulder dystocia versus increased cesarean deliveries. *American Journal of Obstetrics & Gynecology* 1998;**178**(5):922–925.
65 Combs CA, Singh NB, and Khoury JC. Elective induction versus spontaneous labor after sonographic diagnosis of fetal macrosomia. *Obstetrics & Gynecology* 1993;**81**(4):492–496.
66 Sentinel Event Alert Issue 30. Preventing infant death and injury during delivery. *Advances in Neonatal Care* 2004;**4**(4):180–181.
67 Koonings PP, Paul RH, and Campbell K. Umbilical cord prolapse. A contemporary look. *Journal of Reproductive Medicine* 1990;**35**(7):690–692.
68 Yla-Outinen A, Heinonen PK, and Tuimala R. Predisposing and risk factors of umbilical cord prolapse. *Acta Obstetricia et Gynecologica Scandinavica* 1985;**64**(7):567–570.
69 Uygur D, Kis S, Tuncer R, Ozcan FS, and Erkaya S. Risk factors and infant outcomes associated with umbilical cord prolapse. *International Journal of Gynecology & Obstetrics* 2002;**78**(2):127–130.
70 Dilbaz B, Ozturkoglu E, Dilbaz S, Ozturk N, Sivaslioglu AA, and Haberal A. Risk factors and perinatal outcomes associated with umbilical cord prolapse. *Archives of Gynecology and Obstetrics* 2006;**274**(2):104–107.
71 Clark DO, Copeland W, and Ullery JC. Prolapse of the umbilical cord. A study of 117 cases. *American Journal of Obstetrics & Gynecology* 1968;**101**(1):84–90.
72 Martin JA, Hamilton BE, Sutton PD, Ventura SJ, Menacker F, and Kirmeyer S. Births: final data for 2004. *National Vital Statistics Reports* 2006;**55**(1):1–101.
73 Gemer O and Segal S. Incidence and contribution of predisposing factors to transverse lie presentation. *International Journal of Gynecology & Obstetrics* 1994;**44**(3):219–221.
74 Barclay M. Umbilical cord prolapse and other cord accidents. In: Sciarra JJ (ed.) *Gynecology & Obstetrics*. Philadelphia, PA: Lippincott, 1989: 1.
75 Raga F, Osborne N, Ballester MJ, and Bonilla-Musoles F. Color flow Doppler: a useful instrument in the diagnosis of funic presentation. *Journal of the National Medical Association* 1996;**88**(2):94–96.
76 Katz Z, Shoham Z, Lancet M, Blickstein I, Mogilner BM, and Zalel Y. Management of labor with umbilical cord prolapse: a 5-year study. *Obstetrics & Gynecology* 1988; **72**(2):278–281.
77 Murphy DJ and MacKenzie IZ. The mortality and morbidity associated with umbilical cord prolapse. *BJOG* 1995;**102**(10):826–830.

78 Robertson PA, Foran CM, Croughan-Minihane MS, and Kilpatrick SJ. Head entrapment and neonatal outcome by mode of delivery in breech deliveries from 28 to 36 weeks of gestation. *American Journal of Obstetrics & Gynecology* 1996;**174**(6):1742–1747; discussion 7–9.
79 Dufour P, Vinatier D, and Puech F. The use of intravenous nitroglycerin for cervico-uterine relaxation: a review of the literature. *Archives of Gynecology and Obstetrics* 1997;**261**(1):1–7.
80 Vialle R, Pietin-Vialle C, Vinchon M, Dauger S, Ilharreborde B, and Glorion C. Birth-related spinal cord injuries: a multicentric review of nine cases. *Child's Nervous System* 2008;**24**(1): 79–85.
81 Schachter SC. Iatrogenic seizures. *Neurologic Clinics*. 1998;**16**(1):157–170.
82 Yerby MS, Friel PN, McCormick K, Koerner M, Van Allen M, Leavitt AM *et al.* Pharmacokinetics of anticonvulsants in pregnancy: alterations in plasma protein binding. *Epilepsy Research* 1990;**5**(3):223–228.
83 Chen SS, Perucca E, Lee JN, and Richens A. Serum protein binding and free concentration of phenytoin and phenobarbitone in pregnancy. *British Journal of Clinical Pharmacology* 1982;**13**(4):547–552.
84 American College of Obstetricians and Gynecologists Practice Bulletin No. 33: Diagnosis and management of preeclampsia and eclampsia. *Obstetrics & Gynecology* 2002;**99**(1):159–167.
85 Sibai BM. Magnesium sulfate prophylaxis in preeclampsia: lessons learned from recent trials. *American Journal of Obstetrics & Gynecology* 2004;**190**(6):1520–1526.
86 Douglas KA and Redman CW. Eclampsia in the United Kingdom. *BMJ* 1994;**309**(6966): 1395–1400.
87 Paul RH, Koh KS, and Bernstein SG. Changes in fetal heart rate-uterine contraction patterns associated with eclampsia. *American Journal of Obstetrics & Gynecology* 1978;**130**(2):165–169.
88 Costello DJ and Cole AJ. Treatment of acute seizures and status epilepticus. *Journal of Intensive Care Medicine* 2007;**22**(6):319–347.
89 Pritchard JA, Cunningham FG, and Pritchard SA. The Parkland Memorial Hospital protocol for treatment of eclampsia: evaluation of 245 cases. *American Journal of Obstetrics & Gynecology* 1984;**148**(7):951–963.
90 Which anticonvulsant for women with eclampsia? Evidence from the Collaborative Eclampsia Trial. *Lancet* 1995;**345**(8963):1455–1463.
91 Doyle LW, Crowther CA, Middleton P, Marret S, and Rouse D. Magnesium sulphate for women at risk of preterm birth for neuroprotection of the fetus. *Cochrane Database of Systematic Reviews* 2009;(**1**):CD004661.
92 Ellis D, Crofts JF, Hunt LP, Read M, Fox R, and James M. Hospital, simulation center, and teamwork training for eclampsia management: a randomized controlled trial. *Obstetrics & Gynecology* 2008;**111**(3):723–731.
93 Lopez-Llera M. Main clinical types and subtypes of eclampsia. *American Journal of Obstetrics & Gynecology* 1992;**166**(1 Pt 1):4–9.
94 Sibai BM, el-Nazer A, and Gonzalez-Ruiz A. Severe preeclampsia-eclampsia in young primigravid women: subsequent pregnancy outcome and remote prognosis. *American Journal of Obstetrics & Gynecology* 1986;**155**(5):1011–1016.
95 Chesley SC, Annitto JE, and Cosgrove RA. The remote prognosis of eclamptic women. Sixth periodic report. *American Journal of Obstetrics & Gynecology* 1976;**124**(5):446–459.
96 Sibai BM, Mercer B, and Sarinoglu C. Severe preeclampsia in the second trimester: recurrence risk and long-term prognosis. *American Journal of Obstetrics & Gynecology* 1991; **165**(5 Pt 1):1408–1412.
97 Cantwell R, Clutton-Brock T, Cooper G, Dawson A, Drife J, Garrod D *et al.* Saving mothers' lives: reviewing maternal deaths to make motherhood safer: 2006–2008. The eighth report of the confidential enquiries into maternal deaths in the United Kingdom. *BJOG* 2011; **118**(Suppl 1):1–203.

98 Dijkman A, Huisman CM, Smit M, Schutte JM, Zwart JJ, van Roosmalen JJ *et al.* Cardiac arrest in pregnancy: increasing use of perimortem caesarean section due to emergency skills training? *BJOG* 2010;**117**(3):282–287.

99 Suresh MS, LaToya Mason C, and Munnur U. Cardiopulmonary resuscitation and the parturient. *Best Practice & Research: Clinical Obstetrics & Gynaecology* 2010;**24**(3):383–400.

100 Ortman AJ. The pregnant patient with congenital heart disease. *Seminars in Cardiothoracic and Vascular Anesthesia* 2012;**16**:(4):220–234.

101 Warnes CA, Williams RG, Bashore TM, Child JS, Connolly HM, Dearani JA *et al.* ACC/AHA 2008 guidelines for the management of adults with congenital heart disease: executive summary. A report of the American College of Cardiology/American Heart Association Task Force on Practice Guidelines (writing committee to develop guidelines for the management of adults with congenital heart disease). *Circulation.* 2008;**118**(23):2395–2451.

102 Hawkins JL. Anesthesia-related maternal mortality. *Clinical Obstetrics and Gynecology* 2003;**46**(3):679–687.

103 Vanden Hoek TL, Morrison LJ, Shuster M, Donnino M, Sinz E, Lavonas EJ *et al.* Part 12: cardiac arrest in special situations: 2010 American Heart Association guidelines for cardiopulmonary resuscitation and emergency cardiovascular care. *Circulation.* 2010; **122**(18 Suppl. 3):S829–S861.

104 Cooper JA and Cooper JM. New strategies for cardiopulmonary resuscitation. *Current Treatment Options in Cardiovascular Medicine* 2008;**10**(1):49–58.

105 Field JM, Hazinski MF, Sayre MR, Chameides L, Schexnayder SM, Hemphill R *et al.* Part 1: executive summary: 2010 American Heart Association guidelines for cardiopulmonary resuscitation and emergency cardiovascular care. *Circulation* 2010;**122**(18 Suppl. 3): S640–S656.

106 Nanson J, Elcock D, Williams M, and Deakin CD. Do physiological changes in pregnancy change defibrillation energy requirements? *British Journal of Anaesthesia* 2001;**87**(2):237–239.

107 Chervenak FA, Skupski DW, Romero R, Myers MK, Smith-Levitin M, Rosenwaks Z *et al.* How accurate is fetal biometry in the assessment of fetal age? *American Journal of Obstetrics & Gynecology* 1998;**178**(4):678–687.

108 Mahony BS, Callen PW, and Filly RA. The distal femoral epiphyseal ossification center in the assessment of third-trimester menstrual age: sonographic identification and measurement. *Radiology* 1985;**155**(1):201–204.

109 Chinn DH, Bolding DB, Callen PW, Gross BH, and Filly RA. Ultrasonographic identification of fetal lower extremity epiphyseal ossification centers. *Radiology* 1983;**147**(3):815–818.

110 Marty AT, Hilton FL, Spear RK, and Greyson B. Postcesarean pulmonary embolism, sustained cardiopulmonary resuscitation, embolectomy, and near-death experience. *Obstetrics & Gynecology* 2005;**106**(5 Pt 2):1153–1155.

111 Fisher N, Eisen LA, Bayya JV, Dulu A, Bernstein PS, Merkatz IR *et al.* Improved performance of maternal-fetal medicine staff after maternal cardiac arrest simulation-based training. *American Journal of Obstetrics & Gynecology* 2011;**205**(3):239 e1–5.

112 Rittenberger JC, Kelly E, Jang D, Greer K, and Heffner A. Successful outcome utilizing hypothermia after cardiac arrest in pregnancy: a case report. *Critical Care Medicine* 2008; **36**(4):1354–1356.

CHAPTER 12
Surgical management of obstetrical emergencies

Laurie S. Swaim and Gary A. Dildy, III
Department of Obstetrics and Gynecology, Baylor College of Medicine and Texas Children's Hospital, Houston, TX, USA

12.1 Introduction

Obstetrical hemorrhage is the leading cause of maternal morbidity and mortality worldwide, accounting for 140,000 maternal deaths per annum [1]. Postpartum hemorrhage (PPH) is a leading cause of maternal mortality in both industrialized and developing countries [2,3]. Primary PPH, defined as that which occurs within the first 24 hours post-delivery, occurs in up to 5% of all deliveries [4].

Various definitions of PPH have been proposed in an attempt to prompt recognition of clinically significant estimated blood loss (EBL). One longstanding definition of PPH is an EBL > 500 mL for vaginal delivery and > 1000 mL after cesarean [1]. These definitions have limited clinical utility, as quantification of blood loss is inaccurate (usually underestimated) and the degree of hemorrhage may not be reflected in hemoglobin concentration changes during the acute phases of hemorrhage. Furthermore, underlying medical conditions (e.g. cardiopulmonary disease, preexisting anemia) will affect an individual's capacity to adapt to acute blood loss. One key to recognizing significant maternal hemorrhage lies within basic physiologic parameters, the vital signs. Patients may experience tachycardia and lightheadedness after a blood loss of 10–15%, whereas a loss of 15–25% of maternal blood volume is evidenced by weakness, tachycardia, and mild hypotension. Losses of greater than 25% are associated with hypotension, pallor, confusion, lethargy, and oliguria [1].

Decisions regarding management of PPH must be made rapidly and succinctly. While the patient's wishes for future childbearing should be taken into account, the ultimate goal is to save the life of the patient in the manner associated with the least morbidity. Severe hemorrhage and hypovolemia may require massive transfusion and fluid resuscitation, resulting in disseminated intravascular coagulation

Management of Labor and Delivery, Second Edition. Edited by George A. Macones.

(DIC), renal failure, adult respiratory distress syndrome, and pituitary necrosis. While fertility-sparing procedures are available, the provider must rely on sound clinical judgment while making decisions regarding the management of patients with postpartum hemorrhage, which in some cases may include proceeding directly to hysterectomy.

Uterine atony is the most common cause of postpartum uterine hemorrhage, accounting for more than 75% of all cases. Medical management of uterine atony with uterotonic medications is usually curative. When medical management fails to adequately treat bleeding after vaginal delivery, direct endometrial compression is most commonly undertaken as the next step. However, when uterine bleeding does not respond to conservative measures, judicious use of surgical treatment can be lifesaving. These surgical techniques have also been successfully employed in cases of postpartum hemorrhage secondary to placenta previa and suspected accreta.

12.2 Uterine tamponade and packing

Not long ago, uterine packing with materials such as gauze rolls was thought to increase the risk of infection and concealed hemorrhage and it began to fall out of favor in the latter half of the twentieth century [5]. Indeed, the 1990 the American College of Obstetricians and Gynecologists (ACOG) technical bulletin stated that the technique of uterine packing had been abandoned [6]. However, a renewed interest in this technique has brought uterine tamponade to the forefront of modern postpartum uterine hemorrhage management, using various inflatable intrauterine catheter devices. Intrauterine packing may impede hemorrhage by several theoretic mechanisms including direct compression of vascular sinuses, alteration of uterine shape, and effects on uterine vascular flow [5,7]. The ease of placement, availability, and minimal risk make balloon tamponade an ideal early intervention in the management of postpartum hemorrhage after vaginal delivery. Uterine tamponade techniques may also be applied after cesarean delivery. In 2001, Bakri reported success with a silicone balloon for uterine tamponade in five patients with suspected low-lying placenta, or placenta previa. Two of these women also had preoperative balloon hypogastric artery ligation [8] (Figure 12.1).

Retrospective studies of uterine packing have noted success rates of 77–100%; however, low patient numbers limit the generalizability of these studies [5,9]. Recently, Ge *et al.* reviewed the outcomes of 70 women with postpartum hemorrhage associated with placenta previa treated with uterine packing. The technique was hysterectomy sparing in 93% [10]. The Scottish Confidential Audit of severe maternal morbidity reported a success rate of 78% (50 of 64 women) after balloon tamponade [11]. In a retrospective review, prevention of hysterectomy was noted in 90% (18 of 20 women) after balloon placement.

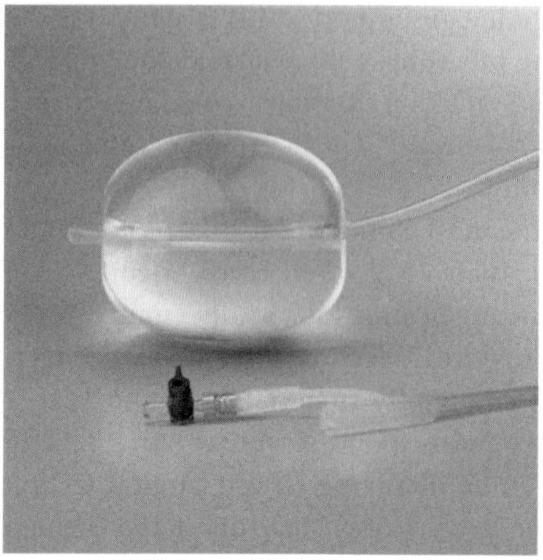

Figure 12.1 Bakri Balloon for uterine tamponade. *Source*: Cook Medical. Reproduced with permission of Cook Medical, Bloomington, IN.

The success was 100% (11 women) when the etiology of the postpartum hemorrhage was atony [12]. Tamponade, if successful only when the balloon is inflated, may be considered for transport or as an interim measure during resuscitation or before uterine arterial embolization or surgery. If uterine tamponade does not result in immediate and substantial decrement in bleeding, surgical intervention is required.

The entire uterus must be tightly packed, and many instruments have been created for such purposes (e.g. Holmes packer, Broadhead packer, Torpin packer, and uterine packing forceps); however, these devices are not likely going to be available at most hospitals. Balloon tamponade with an inflatable catheter has several theoretical advantages over gauze packing, including easier insertion, less risk for uterine perforation, and, with a smooth contour, decreased friction and re-bleeding at removal. Various balloon devices have been used or created specifically for postpartum hemorrhage, including the Foley catheter, Sengstaken–Blakemore tube, Rusch® urologic balloon (Rusch Urologics, Morrissville, NC), Bakri Postpartum Balloon® (Cook Medical, Spencer, IN), condom catheter, and the BT-Cath® (Utah Medical Products Inc, Midvale, UT).

The Belfort–Dildy Obstetrical Tamponade System, trade-named ebb® (Glenveigh Medical, Chattanooga, TN) is a more recently developed catheter for uterine tamponade. (Figure 12.2) The sterile single-use dual-balloon tamponade catheter trade-named ebb, also referred to as the Belfort–Dildy Obstetrical Tamponade System® (BD-OTS), features an upper uterine balloon (maximum recommended fill volume 750 mL) and a lower vaginal balloon (maximum recommended fill volume 300 mL). These are filled by attaching an intravenous fluid bag to the in-line "spike" and manually filling the balloon by squeezing the intravenous bag until tamponade is achieved. The balloons can be moved

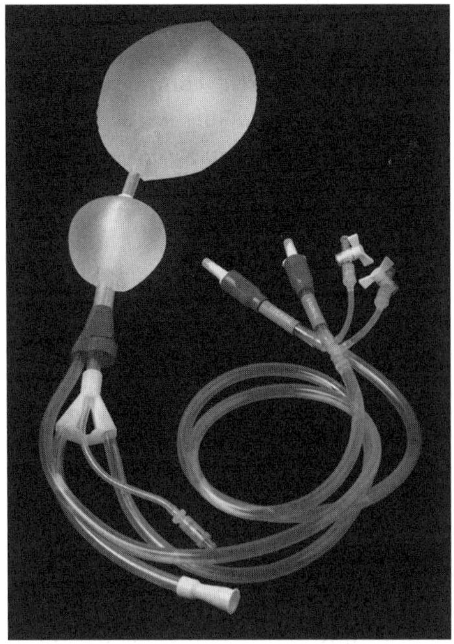

Figure 12.2 Glenveigh Belfort-Dildy Obstetric Tamponade System (ebb™). *Source*: Glenveigh Medical. Reproduced with permission of Glenveigh Medical, Chattanooga, TN.

independently of each other to properly accommodate maternal anatomy. Fundal irrigation can be performed through a third port situated above the uterine balloon, and a central drain enables monitoring of fundal blood loss. The balloon can be deflated in an independent fashion.

In order to place a single-balloon uterine tamponade device, moisten the balloon, grasp the anterior cervix with a ring forceps, and introduce the empty balloon to the fundus. The manufacturers generally recommend placement under ultrasound guidance [13]. After appropriate placement, the balloon is then inflated with sterile isotonic fluid until it is snug in the fundus. Too much liquid will force the balloon downward and through the cervix. This position may be beneficial when the majority of the bleeding is from the lower uterine segment, but may be difficult to keep in place. Furthermore, for maximum benefit and appropriate placement, the entire balloon must be above the external cervical os [13]. After correct placement of the balloon, vaginal packing gauze is moistened with lubricating jelly and placed in the vagina. A urometer is attached to record output from the port distal to the balloon. The bladder is drained with an indwelling urinary catheter. It is our practice to mark the skin at the top of the uterine fundus with a permanent marker so that any significant concealed bleeding may be recognized by a rising uterine fundus. Flushing the outflow tubing with saline may dislodge clots that may form in the outflow tubing. Patients should remain on an acute care unit where vital signs and urine output can be monitored hourly. Venous thromboembolism prophylaxis in the form of compression stockings or sequential compression devices should be placed. Recommendations for the duration of the compression balloon vary from 4–6 to a maximum of 24 hours [11,13,14]. While some advocate gradual, sequential balloon deflation, this step is likely unnecessary. The vaginal balloon of the Belfort–Dildy Obstetrical Tamponade System has been found to help anchor the uterine balloon in place, thus eliminating the need for vaginal packing to maintain intrauterine placement.

12.3 Uterine compression sutures

B-Lynch originally described a uterine compression suture (UCS) in 1997 as a method of treatment for uterine atony at the time of cesarean [15]. While originally developed for the treatment of uterine atony, uterine compression sutures have been successfully used in cases of placenta previa and suspected placenta accreta. Several modifications of the uterine compression suture have been reported since 1997, most with reasonable success. Success rates, complication rates, and fertility rates are inexact because the majority of data arise from case reports or small case series. Furthermore, the degree of obstetric hemorrhage and the timing of the intervention differ between studies. The success of the B-Lynch suture for controlling postpartum hemorrhage has been reported to be 86% [16]. Review of pooled reports showed that hysterectomy was avoided in 82 of 88 women (95%) after placement of the B-Lynch suture [17]. The use of uterine compression suture for postpartum hemorrhage has been reported in over 1800 women [18]. Nanda published the largest single series of patients treated with the Hayman modification of the B-Lynch suture, in which 45 of 48 women (94%) were successfully managed, and all 30 available for follow-up experienced regular menses. Six of the women subsequently delivered term neonates [19]. This impressive success rate may be due to selection bias or bias related to surgeon experience, as a more recent population-based study of women in the UK found that of 211 women treated with uterine compression suture for PPH, 25% required hysterectomy [20]. Risk factors for hysterectomy included maternal age greater than 35 years, delay of compression suture placement of 2–6 hours postpartum, multiparity, and vaginal delivery [20]. Decisions to perform hysterectomy may be made more liberally in multiparous and older women, thus affecting study results. Forty of 539 women(7%) required hysterectomy after compression sutures or uterine artery ligation for uterine atony, placenta previa, or lacerations in recent retrospective review from Argentina [21]. French researchers have shown that the failure rate of UCS with uterine artery ligation is 15 times greater in women with placenta accreta as compared to women with postpartum hemorrhage unrelated to accreta [22]. In their extensive review, Matsubara *et al.* conclude that current studies are not rigorous enough to support the use of one type of UCS over another [23]. The ease of placement combined with the overall good success has prompted the Royal College of Obstetricians and Gynaecologists to suggest posting a laminated diagram of the uterine "brace" suture in the operating room [14].

Return of regular menses is reportedly common (98.5%; 66/67) following UCS [17,19,24,25]. Post procedure pregnancy rates are difficult to determine, as most authors have not followed patients over long periods of time, and patients' desire for and attempts at childbearing are difficult to determine. However, successful pregnancy has been reported after UCS placement [16]. Examination of the uterus at the time of subsequent cesarean or delayed hysterosalpingogram or hysteroscopy has revealed normal endometrial cavities [19,24] as well as the presence of uterine synechiae [26].

Myometrial ischemia has been reported after uterine compression sutures [27]. Concerns have been raised regarding the risk of postoperative infection when compression sutures traverse the endometrial cavity. Baskett reported an incidence of postoperative endomyometritis of 36% in 22 women after UCS [16], and a case of pyometra after UCS [28] has been published. However, the majority of case series do not describe significant infection rates. The etiology of postoperative infection in these patients is likely multifactorial, and may not be categorically blamed on the presence of the UCS itself. Not enough data exist for recommendations regarding antibiotic prophylaxis in this setting.

12.4 Uterine compression suture technique

Uterine compression sutures are appealing because they can be performed rapidly, little surgical skill is required, and injury to vascular structures and adjacent organs is unlikely. Furthermore, special equipment is not required, as any *absorbable suture* may be used. Lithotomy position facilitates visual assessment of vaginal bleeding during the procedure.

B-Lynch described a test procedure whereby the uterus is manually compressed posteriorly to anteriorly in order to determine if the amount of vaginal bleeding has diminished. The initial suture is placed anteriorly inferior to the hysterotomy into the endometrial space (serosal to endometrial), then brought toward the fundus and threaded through the anterior uterine wall (from endometrial surface, through myometrial and serosal) a few centimeters above the incision, the suture is then pulled over the fundus, and the same needle passed posteriorly at the level of the ipsilateral uterosacral ligament (serosal through myometrium and endometrium). The same suture is then placed a few centimeters lateral at the same level through the myometrium posteriorly (endometrial to serosal) at the level of the uterosacral ligament on the opposite side. The suture is pulled over the fundus (posterior to anterior), passed

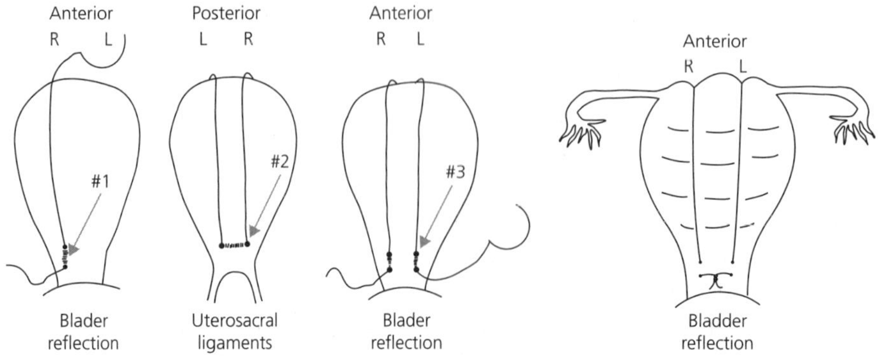

Figure 12.3 Drawing of the B-Lynch uterine compression suture.

through the myometrium (serosal to endometrial) a few centimeters above to the uterine incision, and then passed again (endometrial to serosal) a few centimeters below the incision lateral to the first puncture in the uterus. The suture is then tied in the midline after closure of the hysteroromy (Figure 12.3).

The Hayman modification obviates the need for a hysterotomy: sutures are passed full thickness anterior to posterior and tied (like suspenders). A cervicoisthmic suture is also described in conjunction with the fundal compression stitch after cesarean. This has been suggested in cases of significant lower uterine segment or cervical bleeding [29]. This technique has been described as simple, easy to learn, and less time consuming than the B-Lynch [30]. The Cho UCS results in obliteration of the uterine cavity as catgut on a straight needle is passed through and through the uterine fundus anterior to posterior, and posterior to anterior a few centimeters laterally. The same suture is reintroduced 2–3 cm inferiorly and a square is formed. A series of these sutures are placed and they may be placed at various uterine sites depending on the areas of heaviest bleeding. The authors contend that the use of the straight needle and multiple sutures make this technique easier than the B-Lynch suture, as well as more successful as multiple areas of the uterus are sutured [24]. The Cho technique was found to be an effective means of preventing hysterectomy in a retrospective review of Argentinian women with postpartum hemorrhage [21]. Hackethal has suggested multiple U-shaped sutures.0 Vicryl XLH (straightened) is passed through and through anterior to posterior and posterior to anterior 2–4 cm laterally and tied. Multiple sutures may be placed where needed [17]. Other modifications have included the Matsubara–Yano, which consists of three longitudinal and two transverse sutures, the Meydanli, which is similar to the B-Lynch but involves anchoring of the fundal portion of the suture in the myometrium, the Marasinghe, which also involves anchoring of the suture to the fundus, and the Huissoud technique, which combines UAL with a fundal suture as well as a cerclage like UCS [24,25,31,32].

12.5 Uterine artery ligation

First described in 1952 by Waters, the uterine artery ligation (UAL) decreases uterine blood flow via the main branch of the uterine artery in order to control postpartum hemorrhage [33]. O'Leary reported a personal success rate of approximately 96% [34]. When performing UAL, 2–3 cm of myometrium should be included in the suture. Traction on the uterine fundus medially, and on the round ligament and fallopian tube laterally, will in most cases allow adequate exposure of the uterine vascular bundle. Dissection of the vesico-uterine fold and mobilization of the bladder inferiorly will often be required for the correct placement of the UAL suture. Care must be taken to avoid incorporation of the bladder and ureter. A delayed absorbable suture on a CTX needle (or similar large needle) is passed 2–3 cm medial to the uterine vessels 2–3 cm below the uterine incision (or similar location if vaginal delivery), and threaded through an avascular portion of the broad ligament lateral to the uterine vessels and secured. The procedure is repeated on the contralateral side. Immediate examination of the patient in lithotomy is preferred to assess the amount of vaginal bleeding. The most common cause of failure is incomplete ligation. Return to normal menses and successful pregnancy have been reported after UAL.

12.6 Combination procedures for uterine preservation

A retrospective review of 56 women with postpartum hemorrhage after cesarean evaluated the success of bilateral UAL, followed by UCS (Cho technique). Forty-three of 56 (76%) women required UCS after UAL, which was successful in 88% [22]. However, in 1994 AbdRabbo reported a 75% success rate for bilateral UAL in 103 women with postpartum hemorrhage prospectively managed with stepwise uterine devascularization [35].

Yoong *et al.* described their success of a combination of uterine tamponade and compression suture, or "uterine sandwich," in 11 women with postpartum hemorrhage due to atony and placenta previa. No hysterectomies were required after the placement of a Bakri Balloon followed by either the B-Lynch or Hayman technique. The presence of the balloon "tail" is proposed to prevent the development of theoretic cervical stenosis and all women subsequently developed regular menses [36].

12.7 Hypogastric artery ligation

In 1964 Burchell described ligation of the internal iliac (hypogastric) artery for the treatment of obstetric hemorrhage [37]. Utilization of this technique has decreased over time, which may in part be related to the popularity, simplicity, and success of uterine compression sutures and devices designed specifically for uterine tamponade. With waning utilization of hypogastric artery ligation, current trainees in obstetrics may not gain enough experience with hypogastric artery ligation to reliably include the technique in their armamentarium against postpartum hemorrhage. Fear of injury to hypogastric vessels and adjacent structures may also contribute to the rarity of this procedure. Both the American Congress of Obstetricians and Gynecologists and the Royal College of Obstetricians and Gynaecologists recognize the difficulty of the procedure and the need for expertise before this procedure is undertaken [1,14].

Nevertheless, bilateral hypogastric artery ligation has been shown to markedly decrease pulse pressure and therefore pelvic hemorrhage [37]. Bilateral hypogastric artery ligation has been associated with decreased pelvic hemorrhage in cases of uterine atony, placenta accreta, and cervical laceration, with reported success rates of approximately 40–60% [38–40].

The technique of hypogastric artery ligation involves entry into the retroperitoneum and palpation of the bifurcation of the common iliac artery. The anatomy is revealed using blunt dissection, and the ureter identified and retracted medially. Isolation of the hypogastric artery is performed working with a blunt instrument or right angle clamp, taking care to avoid laceration of the underlying adjacent hypogastric vein. A silk suture is passed around the artery 3 cm or more distal to the bifurcation to avoid the posterior division; the artery is doubly ligated, and not transected. Femoral and dorsalis pedis pulses should be palpated before and immediately after the procedure to ensure proper placement of the suture.

12.8 Peripartum hysterectomy

Peripartum hysterectomy is required as a lifesaving measure in approximately 0.8/1000 deliveries in the US [41–43]. Cesarean delivery (and its accompanying co-morbidities) is the single the greatest risk factor for peripartum hysterectomy. These co-morbidities include abnormal placentation (e.g. placenta accreta) and uterine rupture. In an extensive review, Rossi reported that two-thirds of 845 patients who required postpartum hysterectomy had previous uterine surgery, 84% of which were cesarean [41]. In the same analysis, 73% of peripartum hysterectomies were performed immediately after cesarean delivery. The most common indication for peripartum hysterectomy was placenta accreta (38%), followed by uterine atony (29%), uterine rupture (12%), "bleeding" (9%), and placenta previa (7%). Similarly, a case control study of 896 cases of peripartum hysterectomy revealed that the incidence increased from 0.25/1000 deliveries in 1987 to 8.2/1000 in 2006; the odds ratio for peripartum hysterectomy in this study was 7.9 in women with a prior cesarean delivery [42]. Prospective observational data as well as retrospective review have supported this finding. Shellhaas *et al.* found a slight decline in the rate of cesarean hysterectomy (0.5%) in contrast to other studies; their prospective observation revealed that 82% of 71 women who required a peripartum hysterectomy for placenta accreta had a prior history of cesarean delivery [44]. In a cross-sectional study of peripartum hysterectomy reported through the National Inpatient Sample, Bateman *et al.* also reported that the incidence of peripartum hysterectomy increased 23% between 1994 and 2007, and that this increase was due directly to or from consequences associated with cesarean delivery [45]. Studies regarding the influence of multifetal gestation as a risk factor for peripartum hysterectomy have produced conflicting results [42,46]. Expanding pelvic hematoma, complications of abruptio placentae, and uterine inversion may also be indications for emergency hysterectomy [47].

Maternal transfusion rates associated with peripartum hysterectomy are reported to range between 44 and 84% [41,42,48]. While fertility-sparing interventions are frequently performed in the face of postpartum hemorrhage, these techniques have been associated with an increased need for blood products, and decreased postoperative hemoglobin concentrations in women ultimately treated with peripartum hysterectomy [49]. Complications from peripartum hysterectomy are unfortunately common. DIC affected 22% of 519 women who underwent peripartum hysterectomy [41]. The incidence of intraoperative injury is approximately 3–5%, and the urinary tract is the most commonly involved organ system [48,42]. Subtotal (supracervical) hysterectomy has been suggested as a means to avoid urinary tract injury. However, Rossi *et al.* found no difference in morbidity between women after subtotal versus total abdominal hysterectomy [41]. The decision to perform subtotal versus total hysterectomy can be individualized; however, total hysterectomy is often required to control cervical bleeding. Postoperative morbidity, including urinary tract infection, fever, cuff cellulitis, and pneumonia, has been reported with a frequency of 5–26% [41,42,48]. Approximately 5% of women will require reoperation secondary to persistent hemorrhage or adjacent organ injury [41]. Literature review and case control series reveal a maternal death rate of 1.6–2.6% [41,42].

In cases where peripartum hysterectomy is expected, for example suspected placenta percreta, informed consent for surgical management should be obtained prior to hospital admission. The consent is valid throughout the entire "episode" of pregnancy and can be scanned into the electronic medical record.

A coordinated multidisciplinary effort is the cornerstone of successful management of postpartum hemorrhage. The obstetrician should communicate with the nursing staff and coordinate care with the multidisciplinary team, which will include the anesthesiologist and often the transfusion service pathologist, who will be critical in effecting massive transfusion protocol components. Aggressive fluid and blood product resuscitation should begin early in the course of postpartum hemorrhage. One review found that women undergoing cesarean hysterectomy associated with abnormal placentation require, on the average, a transfusion of more than 6 units of blood [50].

Intraoperative cell salvage in obstetrics has not been rigorously studied; however, with more than 800 procedures reported without any case of resultant amniotic fluid embolism, this technique should be considered, if available, for managing severe PPH [51].

Recent massive transfusion experience in combat and in civilian trauma centers has evolved massive transfusion protocols toward more proactive administration of packed red blood cells (PRBC), fresh frozen plasma (FFP), and platelets (PLT). In the face of massive hemorrhage, outcome is improved when a ratio of PRBC: FFP is 1:1 [52]. These practices have been extrapolated to obstetrics as well as other fields of medicine. The California Maternal Quality Care Collaborative (CMQCC) obstetrical hemorrhage tool kit recommends transfusion ratios (PRBC: FFP: PLT apheresis pack) of 6:4:1 for initial PPH with conversion to a ratio of 4:4:1 in the face of continued PPH [53].

If not already done, an indwelling urinary catheter with urometer should be inserted, and a sequential compression device (SCD) placed. Use of an indwelling three-way Foley catheter enables easy backfilling of the bladder if necessary.

Improved abdominal wall relaxation may be an operative benefit of general anesthesia, and facilitates packing of the bowel into the upper abdomen. Anesthesiologists however, may prefer to use an indwelling epidural catheter for this procedure; however adequate anesthesia may not be possible if upper abdominal packing is required.

The patient may be placed in the lithotomy or supine position. The advantages of lithotomy are easier access to the operative field for more than two members of the surgical team, and to the urethra in the event cystoscopy is needed. Position change for patients undergoing hysterectomy after cesarean is not suggested. A vertical abdominal incision is suggested by ACOG, and provides optimal visualization of the pelvis [1]. This becomes exceedingly important in women in whom significant pelvic adhesion or placenta percreta is suspected. However, PPH may be performed through either a transverse or a vertical abdominal incision, and is most often performed through a transverse incision when postpartum hemorrhage is encountered after cesarean. After adequate anesthesia, the patient is placed in Trendelenburg to facilitate bowel mobilization and packing. Placement of a self-retaining retractor takes but a few minutes, and can markedly improve visualization of the operative field. Depending on the physical characteristics of the patient, a Balfour retractor with the upper arm and associated malleable or the Bookwalter retractor are useful options. In the event of hysterectomy for uterine hemorrhage unrelated to placenta percreta, the technique is not dissimilar to that of a hysterectomy performed for non-emergent indications. The surgeon must recognize, however, that the pedicles are larger and more vascular as compared to a non-puerperal patient. The hysterectomy is performed in a stepwise and prompt manner. Rapid closure of the hysterotomy site in a patient delivered by cesarean can decrease blood loss, and improve visualization. This may be accomplished with towel clips; however, a quick running locking closure of the uterine incision using a large non-braided suture takes a similar amount of time, and leaves fewer instruments on the field. Uterine traction may be performed manually; however, in our experience, incorporation of the utero-ovarian ligament, the fallopian tube, and the round ligament with Kocher clamps at the bilateral cornu of the uterus aids in traction and prevents back-bleeding as these structures are transected. At this point the surgeon may choose to proceed in the traditional manner of "clamp, cut, tie" by securing each pedicle with a size O delayed absorbable suture, or the "clamp, cut, drop" method, whereby the clamps are "dropped" and secured in reverse order after the uterine vessels are clamped [48,54]. Surgeons at our institution often perform this portion of the procedure with the handheld bipolar vessel sealing device LigaSure (Covidien, Mansfield, MA). A meta-analysis of studies of various surgical procedures comparing bipolar vessel sealing technology with more traditional methods of hemostasis found that the use of the device was associated with a statistically significant decrease in operative time [55]. This method has not been studied in postpartum hysterectomy, and caution should be used when securing large vascular pedicles, which are often encountered during peripartum surgical procedures. Some surgeons prefer to doubly clamp these large dilated vascular pedicles. The hypertrophic and sometimes edematous tissues of the uterus and parametrium tend to sheer and tear, therefore clamp manipulation must be kept to a minimum. The dissection of the vesicouterine space is best performed sharply. However, such dissection may lead to profuse hemorrhage and/or urinary tract injury in the setting of placenta percreta. Intentional cystotomy has been suggested, with resection of the infiltrated portion of the posterior bladder wall [23]. Meticulous attention to tissue planes decreases the incidence of cystotomy, although in some instances of placenta percreta this complication is unavoidable. Clamp placement can be challenging due to the dilated cervix: the delineation of the myometrium and lateral tissues is more difficult to "feel" with the clamp. It is for this reason that clamps must be placed at right angles to the cervix when securing the uterine vessels. Once the uterus has been devascularized to the level of the uterine vessels, sequential pedicles of the cardinal ligament are taken with heavy (i.e. Ballantyne) clamps to the level of the external cervical os when performing a total hysterectomy. Identification of the external os may be challenging, as this area is not easily palpable in some women, especially after complete cervical dilation. An easy method for finding the external os is to create a vertical incision over the midline of the cervix. One finger is introduced and palpates the anterior cervix until the external os is reached. A ring forceps may be placed on the edge of the cervix if desired. Haeney clamps are then easily placed in lateral positions under the cervix, and the specimen excised. The vaginal angles are secured with interrupted delayed absorbable suture. The vaginal cuff is a common site of postoperative bleeding, which may be quite brisk. Closure of the cuff may proceed with interrupted figure-of-8 or running-locking sutures, taking care to include the posterior and anterior vaginal mucosa. Ureteral identification ideally takes place prior to securing the uterine vascular pedicle. This may be performed by entering the retroperitoneum, or by visualization and palpation through the peritoneum.

The use of dedicated multidisciplinary teams at tertiary care centers for the management of placenta accreta is associated with decreased volume of transfused blood products and decreased incidence of reoperation [56]. Attempts should be made to identify and transfer patients with potential placenta percreta to a tertiary care center. However, prenatal care and access is not universal, thus the obstetrician may be faced with a patient with a placenta percreta in the absence of appropriate support. If the patient and baby are stable, closure of the abdomen until appropriate consultants are available or transfer to a tertiary care facility may be considered.

Pelvic packing has been used with success for patients with intractable post-hysterectomy hemorrhage [57]. Recombinant factor VIIa has also been used in more than 2000 women with a purported success rate of 75–80% in the setting of postpartum hemorrhage [58,59]. Thromboembolic sequelae have been associated with the use of recombinant FVIIa.

12.9 Retained placenta

Risk factors for retained placental fragments include previous uterine surgery, history of uterine infection, and accessory placental lobes. Retained placental fragments can be associated with immediate or delayed postpartum hemorrhage. When faced with immediate or primary postpartum hemorrhage, consideration of retained placenta must be considered. Bimanual examination of the uterine cavity frequently reveals palpable placental fragments; however, all placental tissue will not be recognized in this manner. Abnormal bleeding in the setting of a third stage of labor that lasts more than 30 minutes, or the need for manual removal of the placenta, should raise the suspicion of abnormally adherent placental tissue [60]. Furthermore, during placental inspection, one should make an attempt to identify all cotyledons. Vessels that end abruptly in the amniotic membranes should alert the attendant of a possible succenturiate placental lobe.

Ultrasound has been suggested as an adjunct to clinical diagnosis of retained products of conception (POC) in the acute setting [60], and ACOG has suggested that ultrasound be undertaken prior to intrauterine instrumentation [1]. In their study evaluating uterine ultrasound and retained POC, Lousquy *et al.* found that 90% of women with postpartum bleeding and a negative ultrasound were successfully managed by medical means [61]. However, uterine curettage should not be withheld in the event that ultrasonography is not rapidly available. Furthermore, the accuracy of ultrasound for identification of retained placenta is limited. Following placental delivery, histologic and gross identification of placenta obtained by curettage immediately after evaluation of the uterus by ultrasound has revealed a positive and negative predictive value of 58 and 87%, respectively [62]. The ACOG practice bulletin also suggests that ultrasound guidance for curettage may make the removal of retained tissue easier and decrease the risk of perforation [1].

Evacuation of postpartum placental fragments may be accomplished in the delivery room or in the operating room (OR). The anesthesia staff should be alerted regarding all patients with postpartum hemorrhage, and should be on hand to provide assistance with resuscitation as well as adequate pain control. A ring forceps can be applied to the anterior lip of the cervix. The use of a hand to guide the curette into the fundus may be a useful maneuver to avoid posterior perforation. The curette is swept over the endometrium in the direction from the fundus to the cervix and repositioned until the entire cavity has been evaluated and the endometrium has a "gritty" feel. A large (i.e. 16-mm diameter) plastic cannula with suction is sometimes employed, and curettage carried out in a similar fashion to first trimester curettage. Continued bleeding after curettage should prompt an immediate consideration of and treatment for placenta accreta, other causes of PPH, and coagulopathy.

There is insufficient data regarding the role of prophylactic antibiotics in this setting. Prophylactic antibiotics are not universally recommended in the setting of manual placental removal [63]. The decision to administer prophylactic antibiotics should be made on an individual basis. Reported post-curettage complications include uterine perforation, endomyometritis and uterine synechiae.

12.10 Obstetric laceration

Evidence that the routine use of episiotomy is directly related to third- and fourth-degree obstetric lacerations has resulted in recommendations to avoid episiotomy in most situations [64]. Even with restricted use of episiotomy, severe lacerations to the lower genital tract may be a consequence of vaginal delivery, especially those associated with fetal macrosomia, nulliparity, and operative vaginal delivery [65,66]. Continued vaginal bleeding after vaginal delivery should raise the possibility of cervical or vaginal laceration. The Consortium on Safe Labor (CSL) analyzed data from 536 women with cervical lacerations after vaginal delivery. These women represented 0.8% of the cohort of more than 71,000 patients in the study. Identified risk factors for cervical laceration have included cervical cerclage, precipitous labor, vacuum assisted delivery [67] and induction of labour [68,69]. Of these, cervical cerclage is consistently reported as a significant risk factor for postpartum cervical laceration, and is associated with a 3.7- to 12.7-fold increased risk for primigravidae and multiparas, respectively [69].

Minor cervical lacerations are common and usually do not require intervention. Significant bleeding requires repair of the cervical laceration. Laceration repair is accomplished with a delayed absorbable suture, which is placed in a running locked fashion to effect hemostasis and restore normal anatomy. As in all obstetric laceration repairs, adequate visualization is needed to secure the apex of the incision and complete an anatomic approximation. Genital tract lacerations may be fraught with brisk bleeding. In these instances, the use of a Yankauer suction device facilitates visualization.

12.11 Acute postpartum hematoma

Most obstetric postpartum hematomas develop within 24 hours after delivery. A retrospective review published in 1996 reported an incidence of 1/526 vaginal deliveries [70]. The mode of delivery often predicts the location of the hematoma: those developing below the levator plate more commonly present after vaginal delivery, whereas those identified above the levators are more commonly associated with cesarean delivery [71]. Expanding pelvic, labial, and perineal hematomas are emergent situations.

Risk factors implicated in the development of post-delivery pelvic hematoma include episiotomy, coagulopathy, operative vaginal delivery, nulliparity, and fetal macrosomia. However, pelvic hematomas may develop without risk factors or visible laceration [72]. The lower genital tract is richly vascularized with multiple anastomoses. Increased blood flow during pregnancy, and the forces of labor and expulsion, can result in vascular shearing and concealed bleeding. Bleeding dissects along anatomic planes and in soft-tissue spaces until limited by fascia and membranous surfaces. Therefore, infralevator hematomas spread laterally and may involve the ischiorectal fossa. Posterior triangle hematomas will not cross the midline at the perineal body. Supralevator hematomas are less common than infralevator, and dissect laterally and retroperitoneally. Hematomas that are the result of uterine artery tears may displace the uterus laterally and are frequently associated with hemodynamic instability of the patient. Expansion of the vulvar hematoma is limited by anterior and posterior triangle boundaries, thus bleeding dissects under the skin resulting in visible distention, ecchymosis, and pain [72]. Patients with puerperal hematomas often complain of pain greater than anticipated for the visible laceration and repair, and significant rectal discomfort and pressure is a common symptom.

Recommendations for management of pelvic hematomas are largely based on expert opinion. Close observation and analgesia are acceptable for non-expanding hematomas measuring less than 3–5 cm [71,72]. Patients should be monitored for evidence of hemodynamic instability with frequent assessment of vital signs, urine output, and laboratory evaluation, including studies to assess hemoglobin as well as coagulation parameters. Venous thromboembolism (VTE) prophylaxis in the form of sequential compression devices should be placed on the non-ambulatory parturient. Intervention is indicated if the hematoma is expanding, the patient is unstable, or the mass is large. While embolization of pelvic hematomas has been reported [73–75], the majority of postpartum hematomas are managed surgically. Endovascular catheter embolization may be considered in cases refractory to surgical management. Evacuation of pelvic hematoma is best performed in the operating room where adequate lighting, instrumentation, and anesthesia may be provided. Preparations for transfusion should be made, and the massive transfusion protocol triggered if necessary. The vulvar or vaginal hematoma is incised, clots manually evacuated, the cavity inspected, and attempt made to identify the bleeding vessel(s). If identified, the bleeding vessel is ligated; however, more frequently a specific bleeding vessel is not clear, and the space is closed with interrupted delayed absorbable suture. The technique is similar for vulvar and vaginal hematomas; however, care must be taken to avoid incorporation of bowel or ureters when taking wide suture bites during vaginal hematoma repair. Whiteside described the use of fibrin sealant for hemostasis during hematoma repair in a postpartum patient when friable tissue precluded adequate tissue purchase for repair [76]. After evacuation and repair, a vaginal pack may be placed in patients with a non-vulvar hematoma. Administration of broad-spectrum antibiotics has been recommended in the setting of evacuated hematoma [71], although no data exist to support or refute this recommendation. Closed system drainage has been advocated; however, too little information exists to make a firm recommendation [70]. Supralevator retroperitoneal hematomas may be associated with life-threatening hemorrhage. The presence of an obstetrician familiar with retroperitoneal hematoma management is suggested, as hypogastric artery ligation may be required. The use of retroperitoneal packing has been described in the orthopedic literature [77], and may be considered in the event of intractable hemorrhage due to postpartum pelvic hematoma.

12.12 Emergency cesarean

Cesarean delivery remains one of the most common surgical procedures performed in the US. The percentage of women delivered by cesarean in the US is currently around 34% [78]. In 2006, Bloom *et al.* reported an emergency caesarean rate of approximately 24% of more than 11,000 cesarean deliveries [79]. Indications for emergent cesarean delivery include umbilical cord prolapse, Category III and some Category II fetal heart rate (FHR) patterns, abruptio placentae, suspected uterine rupture, and placenta previa with hemorrhage. While a decision-to-incision interval of 30 minutes has been historically supported, this recommendation has been called into question, as a number of studies have not identified an increase in adverse neonatal outcomes when this time frame is increased [79–82]. The recent ACOG practice bulletin notes that the evidence for a 30-minute decision-to-incision interval is lacking [83]. Nonetheless, a cesarean delivery for emergent indications should be performed in a safe and clinically appropriate time frame.

The technique for emergent cesarean differs from non-emergent cesarean with respect to the rapidity of the surgical movements, but not the surgical steps performed. Preparation for such an operation requires swift and deft teamwork. Nomenclature used to define emergent versus urgent and non-urgent cesarean deliveries should be created and routinely reviewed with all individuals who may be involved in the care of women in labor and delivery. With an emergency rate as high as 24% of all cesareans, a rapid yet calm and orderly procedure should be the expectation. A chaotic approach whereby "all hands on deck" are alerted and rush to assist can result in inefficiency, disjointed communication, and enhanced patient anxiety. Unit-wide drills should be integrated into practice such that each individual present in the OR is aware of their assigned task. Clerks and staff should be well versed in the communication algorithm such that the appropriate individuals, including personnel experienced in neonatal resuscitation, are alerted. Well-meaning staff presenting to "lend a hand" leave their patients unattended, and can contribute to disorganization and confound efforts of the care team.

It is prudent to perform a rapid bedside ultrasound for fetal cardiac activity when a woman presents to the hospital with fetal bradycardia. This may avoid emergent cesarean in the event that the fetal bradycardia is associated with an arrhythmia, or if the bradycardia represents maternal pulse in the setting of fetal demise.

Once an indication for emergent cesarean delivery is diagnosed, uterotonic medications should be discontinued, use of a uterine relaxant medication such as terbutaline may be considered, and fetal intrauterine resuscitation measures such as maternal hyper-oxygenation and position change may be performed if needed. Intravenous fluid bolus may also be administered, and can potentially blunt maternal hypotension during epidural bolus for surgical level.

Anesthetic considerations include the severity of the FHR abnormality, the presence of an existing regional anesthetic, and maternal co-morbidities (e.g. preeclampsia), anatomy, and body habitus. When an epidural is in place, a "top off" is the preferred method of most anesthesiology attendants, and if a level suitable for surgery can be achieved in a matter of minutes, this method avoids the potential morbidity of intubation and general anesthesia. Per the Royal College of Anaesthetists compendium, at least 85% of "emergency" cesareans should be under regional anesthesia and only 3% of women with a regional anesthetic should require conversion to general [84]. Decisions regarding the rapid placement of regional anesthesia and general anesthesia are individualized depending on the clinical scenario. Local anesthetic infiltration has been used for emergency cesarean in the morbidly obese and those who are not good candidates for regional or general anesthesia [85].

Once in the operating room, an indwelling urinary catheter and sequential compression devices for the prevention of VTE should be placed. Prophylactic antibiotics are administered. Surgical site infection is increased after emergency versus non-emergent cesarean deliveries [86]. There are no data evaluating antibiotic regimens specific to emergency cesarean, thus Surgical Care Improvement Project (SCIP) recommendations for routine cesarean should be followed. Similarly, there are no data regarding the abdominal prep for emergent cesarean and the risk of infection. While hair clipping is often performed for non-emergent cesareans, this step is best skipped in the face of profound fetal bradycardia or maternal hemorrhage. Chlorhexidine paint has been shown to be superior to Betadine (Purdue Products, Stamford, CT) for the prevention of surgical site infection after cesarean delivery [87]; however, the need to wait a full 3 minutes after application makes its use impractical in the setting of emergency cesarean. In individual scenarios the clinician may judge the effect of 3 additional minutes on fetal or maternal outcome to be negligible and proceed with chlorhexidine.

The majority of US surgeons enter the abdomen through a Pfannensteil incision during an emergent cesarean. A randomized trial comparing Joel-Cohen and Pfannensteil incisions revealed that the delivery time was 50 seconds greater in the Pfannensteil group, but there was no difference in fetal outcome [88]. Similarly, when comparing Pfannensteil to vertical incision in 3525 emergency cesareans, Wylie *et al.* found that the use of the Pfannensteil increased time to delivery by 1 minute during primary cesareans, and 2 minutes during repeat cesareans, as compared to the vertical incision, without an increase in neonatal morbidity [89]. The Cochrane collaborative recommend the Joel-Cohen incision for *routine* cesarean, citing improved clinical benefits including decreased operative time, decreased postoperative fever and pain medication use, and decreased blood loss [87]. While no recommendations were made regarding incision type for emergency cesarean, the Cochrane review found an overall weighted mean difference of 3.84 minutes less for incision-to-delivery time when comparing the Joel-Cohen to other incision types [87].

Regardless of incision choice, care must be taken to avoid fetal injury. Accidental fetal lacerations have been reported in 0.7–1.9% [90] of cesarean deliveries; however, they are more common during emergency procedures [91]. Dessole described a fetal laceration rate of 3% with an odds ratio of 1.7 with emergency cesarean in a retrospective cohort study of more than 3000 women delivering by cesarean [92]. Breech presentation may also be a risk factor [90].

While the Pfannensteil incision is slightly curved and positioned 3 cm above the symphysis pubis, the creation of a straight, transverse incision 3 cm below the anterior superior iliac spine begins the Joel-Cohen technique. The Joel-Cohen is continued as follows: the subcutaneous tissues are opened in the middle 3 cm of the incision, and the fascia is opened in this space. Observational studies show no difference in wound complications when comparing electrocautery and scalpel [93]. It is not necessary to change scalpels after skin incision. The remaining intact subcutaneous tissues and fascia are extended bluntly to the full extent of the skin incision, and the rectus muscles and peritoneum are also split bluntly. Traction is placed on the peritoneum to create a space large enough to deliver the fetus. A transverse incision is then created on the uterus and manually extended laterally.

Blunt entry into the peritoneum may decrease the risk of injury to bowel and other organs, but blunt and sharp peritoneal entry techniques have not been compared for speed or related injury. Incision of the visceroperitoneum and creation of a bladder flap results in increased operative time and blood loss [94]. A small transverse uterine incision created sharply and manually extended in the caudal and cranial direction is suggested [95]. Placental delivery and uterine and anterior abdominal wall closure proceeds as per non-emergent cesarean.

12.13 Perimortem cesarean

Most physicians are inexperienced with perimortem cesarean delivery, as the incidence of cardiac arrest during pregnancy is low (approximately 1/30,000 pregnancies) [96]. No trials exist to guide the physician, thus guidelines are based on case series and expert opinion. Fetal status prior to the arrest and gestational age are factors affecting fetal outcome, which are not fully described in most reports of perimortem cesarean. It has been noted that published case series are biased given that an unknown number of perimortem cesareans are performed and not reported in the literature. Even today, many states do not have maternal mortality review boards, thus state and national data regarding maternal and fetal outcome after perimortem cesarean may be inaccurate.

Relief of aortocaval compression by the gravid uterus may improve maternal cardiac output by as much as 25–30% [97]. In 1986, Katz suggested the "4-minute rule" after review of 61 cases in which time from maternal death to delivery was noted. Seventy percent of newborns survived when delivery was accomplished less than 5 minutes from the onset of arrest [98]. Reports of intact maternal and fetal survival after perimortem cesarean performed at intervals greater than 4 minutes have prompted reminders that the "4-minute rule" is not absolute [97]. Finegold *et al.* reported an instance of maternal and neonatal survival after a maternal-cardiac-arrest-to-delivery interval of 15 minutes [99]. In a 2005 literature review, Katz *et al.* reported that out of 24 cases of surviving newborns delivered by perimortem cesarean, more than half were delivered after 5 minutes, and almost one-third were delivered 15 minutes after the onset of cardiac arrest [100]. Time intervals for non-surviving infants from arrest to delivery were not recorded. Improved maternal resuscitation has also been documented after evacuation of the gravid uterus [100]. However, a retrospective cohort study of maternal and neonatal outcomes after perimortem cesarean before and after an emergency skills training course in the Netherlands found that while the number of perimortem cesarean deliveries increased, maternal case fatality was greater in the cesarean group (67% vs 83%). However, of the 12 women delivered by perimortem cesarean, none were performed within 5 minutes due to transportation or other issues. Four of these women experienced arrest outside of the hospital [101].

Although some reports highlight the possibility of maternal and newborn survival at arrest-to-delivery intervals greater than 5 minutes, delay will not result in improved outcome for the mother or the fetus. Perimortem cesarean should be undertaken in the third trimester in the event that CPR does not immediately restore a sustained pulse. Women with pre-viable fetuses pose a more difficult problem. It has been suggested that evacuation of a second trimester uterus may enhance CPR efforts, but the reader is cautioned that this is based on opinion alone.

Ultrasound to assess FHR utilizes precious time and will not improve outcome. Delivery serves the purpose of improving both maternal and fetal chances for survival.

CPR is performed in the same fashion during pregnancy as for the non-pregnant individual. Lateral displacement of the uterus improves maternal cardiac output; however, maximum force attained when CPR is performed with the patient in the lateral versus supine position is reduced by almost two-thirds [97]. The Cardiff wedge was developed to achieve the optimal degree of tilt for relief of aortocaval compression and maximal CPR force [102]. However, high-quality chest compressions are best achieved when a patient is supine, and supine lateral displacement of the uterus has been shown to be as effective as lateral tilt in reduction of uterine aortocaval compression. This has led some to suggest lateral uterine displacement as a substitute for a wedge in the setting of CPR [103].

The technique of the cesarean is similar to that of the emergent cesarean, with the following caveats: the patient should not be moved – neonatology and neonatal resuscitation equipment are much easier to transport than a pregnant adult with CPR in progress; CPR should continue throughout the surgery; one scalpel should be used for the entire procedure, and the most experienced attendant should perform the cesarean. After delivery of the fetus and placenta, the uterus and the fascia are closed in the usual fashion. Subcutaneous fat closure is unnecessary and skin closure may be completed after termination of the code.

12.14 Conclusion

The practitioner of obstetrics depends upon a broad array of medical, obstetrical, and surgical skills in daily clinical practice. Surgical intervention may be relatively simple and routine (e.g. primary cesarean delivery), but may also require more challenging emergency procedures (e.g. peripartum hysterectomy), which are less often and unpredictably called upon. These procedures should be familiar tools in the obstetrician's armamentarium to correct life-threatening complications, which may affect both high-risk and low-risk parturients.

References

1 American College of Obstetricians and Gynecologists Practice Bulletin No. 76, Clinical Management Guidelines for Obstetrician-Gynecologists: postpartum hemorrhage. *Obstetrics & Gynecology* 2006;**108**(4):1039–1047.
2 *National Vital Statistics Reports* 2012;**61**(6):1039–1047.
3 Control, D.o.H.a.H.S.C.f.D., Maternal Health Epidemiology, Reproductive Health Epidimiology Series. 2003. Module 2: 10.
4 Jacobs AJ. Overview of Postpartum Hemorrhage. *UpToDate* 2012.
5 Maier RC. Control of postpartum hemorrhage with uterine packing. *American Journal of Obstetrics & Gynecology* 1993;**169**(2 Pt 1):317–321, discussion 321–323.
6 American College of Obstetricians and Gynecologists Technical Bulletin No. 143: Diagnosis and management of postpartum hemorrhage. *International Journal of Gynecology & Obstetrics* 1991;**36**(2):159–163.
7 Rath W, Hackethal A, and Bohlmann MK. Second-line treatment of postpartum haemorrhage (PPH). *Archives of Gynecology and Obstetrics* 2012;**286**(3):549–561.
8 Bakri YN, Amri A, and Abdul Jabbar F. Tamponade-balloon for obstetrical bleeding. *International Journal of Gynecology & Obstetrics* 2001;**74**(2):139–142.
9 Hsu S *et al.* Use of packing in obstetric hemorrhage of uterine origin. *Journal of Reproductive Medicine* 2003;**48**(2):69–71.
10 Ge J *et al.* Uterine packing during cesarean section in the management of intractable hemorrhage in central placenta previa. *Archives of Gynecology and Obstetrics* 2012;**285**(2):285–289.
11 Gynecology, R.C.o.O.a., Confidenial Enquiry into Maternal and Child Health. Why Mothers Die 2000–2002. Sixth Report on Confidential Enquiries into Maternal Deaths in the United Kingdom. RCOG Press, 2003.
12 Dabelea V, Schultze PM, and McDuffie RS Jr. Intrauterine balloon tamponade in the management of postpartum hemorrhage. *American Journal of Perinatology* 2007;**24**(6):359–364.
13 cook medical website
14 Prevention and Management of Postpartum Haemorrhage. Royal College of Obstetricians and Gynaecologists, 2009. Green-top Guideline No. 52: 1–24.
15 B-Lynch C *et al.* The B-Lynch surgical technique for the control of massive postpartum haemorrhage: an alternative to hysterectomy? Five cases reported. *BJOG* 1997;**104**(3):372–375.
16 Baskett TF. Uterine compression sutures for postpartum hemorrhage: efficacy, morbidity, and subsequent pregnancy. *Obstetrics & Gynecology* 2007;**110**(1):68–71.
17 Hackethal A *et al.* Uterine compression U-sutures in primary postpartum hemorrhage after cesarean section: fertility preservation with a simple and effective technique. *Human Reproduction* 2008;**23**(1):74–79.
18 Koh E, Devendra K, and Tan LK. B-Lynch suture for the treatment of uterine atony. *Singapore Medical Journal* 2009;**50**(7):693–697.
19 Nanda S, and Singhal SR. Hayman uterine compression stitch for arresting atonic postpartum hemorrhage: 5 years experience. *Taiwanese Journal of Obstetrics and Gynecology* 2011;**50**(2):179–181.

20 Kayem G *et al.* Uterine compression sutures for the management of severe postpartum hemorrhage. *Obstetrics & Gynecology* 2011;**117**(1):14–20.
21 Palacios-Jaraquemada JM. Efficacy of surgical techniques to control obstetric hemorrhage: analysis of 539 cases. *Acta Obstetricia et Gynecologica Scandinavica* 2011;**90**(9):1036–1042.
22 Blanc J *et al.* Is uterine-sparing surgical management of persistent postpartum hemorrhage truly a fertility-sparing technique? *Fertility and Sterility* 2011;**95**(8):2503–2506.
23 Matsubara S *et al.* Uterine compression sutures for postpartum hemorrhage: an overview. *Acta Obstetricia et Gynecologica Scandinavica* 2013;**92**(4):378–385.
24 Cho JH, Jun HS, and Lee CN. Hemostatic suturing technique for uterine bleeding during cesarean delivery. *Obstetrics & Gynecology* 2000;**96**(1):129–131.
25 Meydanli MM *et al.* Meydanli compression suture: new surgical procedure for postpartum hemorrhage due to uterine atony associated with abnormal placental adherence. *Journal of Obstetrics and Gynaecology Research* 2008;**34**(6):964–970.
26 Amorim-Costa C *et al.* Uterine compression sutures for postpartum hemorrhage: is routine postoperative cavity evaluation needed? *Acta Obstetricia et Gynecologica Scandinavica* 2011;**90**(7):701–706.
27 Joshi VM and Shrivastava M. Partial ischemic necrosis of the uterus following a uterine brace compression suture. *BJOG* 2004;**111**(3):279–280.
28 Ochoa M, Allaire AD, and Stitely ML. Pyometria after hemostatic square suture technique. *Obstetrics & Gynecology* 2002;**99**(3):506–509.
29 Hayman RG, Arulkumaran S, and Steer PJ. Uterine compression sutures: surgical management of postpartum hemorrhage. *Obstetrics & Gynecology* 2002;**99**(3):502–506.
30 Ghezzi F *et al.* The Hayman technique: a simple method to treat postpartum haemorrhage. *BJOG* 2007;**114**(3):362–365.
31 Huissoud C *et al.* A stitch in time: layers of circular sutures can staunch postpartum hemorrhage. *American Journal of Obstetrics & Gynecology* 2012;**206**(2):177 e1–2.
32 Marasinghe JP and Condous G. Uterine compression sutures for post-partum bleeding with atony; modification of the B-Lynch suture. *Australian and New Zealand Journal of Obstetrics and Gynaecology* 2009;**49**(1):67–70.
33 Waters EG. Medical and surgical treatment for parturitional hemorrhage. *Journal of the Medical Association of the State of Alabama* 1952;**22**(4):95–99.
34 O'Leary JA. Uterine artery ligation in the control of postcesarean hemorrhage. *Journal of Reproductive Medicine* 1995;**40**(3):189–193.
35 AbdRabbo SA. Stepwise uterine devascularization: a novel technique for management of uncontrolled postpartum hemorrhage with preservation of the uterus. *American Journal of Obstetrics & Gynecology* 1994;**171**(3):694–700.
36 Yoong W *et al.* Application of uterine compression suture in association with intrauterine balloon tamponade ('uterine sandwich') for postpartum hemorrhage. *Acta Obstetricia et Gynecologica Scandinavica* 2012;**91**(1):147–151.
37 Burchell RC. Physiology of internal iliac artery ligation. *Journal of Obstetrics and Gynaecology of the British Commonwealth* 1968;**75**:642–651.
38 Clark SL *et al.* Hypogastric artery ligation for obstetric hemorrhage. *Obstetrics & Gynecology* 1985;**66**(3):353–356.
39 Evans S and McShane P. The efficacy of internal iliac artery ligation in obstetric hemorrhage. *Surgery, Gynecology & Obstetrics* 1985;**160**(3):250–253.
40 Joshi VM *et al.* Internal iliac artery ligation for arresting postpartum haemorrhage. *BJOG* 2007;**114**(3):356–361.
41 Rossi AC, Lee RH, and Chmait RH. Emergency postpartum hysterectomy for uncontrolled postpartum bleeding: a systematic review. *Obstetrics & Gynecology* 2010;**115**(3):637–644.
42 Bodelon C *et al.* Factors associated with peripartum hysterectomy. *Obstetrics & Gynecology* 2009;**114**(1):115–123.

43 Whiteman MK *et al.* Incidence and determinants of peripartum hysterectomy. *Obstetrics & Gynecology* 2006;**108**(6):1486–1492.
44 Shellhaas CS *et al.* The frequency and complication rates of hysterectomy accompanying cesarean delivery. *Obstetrics & Gynecology* 2009;**114**(2 Pt 1):224–229.
45 Bateman BT *et al.* Peripartum hysterectomy in the United States: nationwide 14-year experience. *American Journal of Obstetrics & Gynecology* 2012;**206**(1):63 e1–8.
46 Francois K *et al.* Is peripartum hysterectomy more common in multiple gestations? *Obstetrics & Gynecology* 2005;**105**(6):1369–1372.
47 Hankins GD (ed.). *Operative Obstetrics*, 1st edn. Appelton & Lange: Norwalk, CT. 1995, 336.
48 Plauche WC. Cesarean hysterectomy: indications, technique, and complications. *Clinical Obstetrics and Gynecology* 1986;**29**(2):318–328.
49 Awan N, Bennett MJ, and Walters WA. Emergency peripartum hysterectomy: a 10-year review at the Royal Hospital for Women, Sydney. *Australian and New Zealand Journal of Obstetrics and Gynaecology* 2011;**51**(3):210–215.
50 Zelop CM *et al.* Emergency peripartum hysterectomy. *American Journal of Obstetrics & Gynecology* 1993;**168**(5):1443–1448.
51 Liumbruno GM, Liumbruno C, and Rafanelli D. Intraoperative cell salvage in obstetrics: is it a real therapeutic option? *Transfusion* 2011;**51**(10):2244–2256.
52 Holcomb JB *et al.* Increased plasma and platelet to red blood cell ratios improves outcome in 466 massively transfused civilian trauma patients. *Annals of Surgery* 2008;**248**(3):447–458.
53 C.M.Q.C.C.C.H.T., Obstetric Hemorrhage Care Guidelines, 2009. 1–4.
54 Wright JD *et al.* Peripartum hysterectomy. *Obstetrics & Gynecology* 2010;**116**(2 Pt 1):429–434.
55 Macario A *et al.* Operative time and other outcomes of the electrothermal bipolar vessel sealing system (LigaSure) versus other methods for surgical hemostasis: a meta-analysis. *Surgical Innovation* 2008;**15**(4):284–291.
56 Eller AG *et al.* Maternal morbidity in cases of placenta accreta managed by a multidisciplinary care team compared with standard obstetric care. *Obstetrics & Gynecology* 2011;**117**(2 Pt 1): 331–337.
57 Dildy GA, III. Postpartum hemorrhage: new management options. *Clinical Obstetrics and Gynecology* 2002;**45**(2):330–344.
58 Alfirevic Z *et al.* Use of recombinant activated factor VII in primary postpartum hemorrhage: the Northern European registry 2000–2004. *Obstetrics & Gynecology* 2007;**110**(6): 1270–1278.
59 Phillips LE *et al.* Recombinant activated factor VII in obstetric hemorrhage: experiences from the Australian and New Zealand Haemostasis Registry. *Anesthesia & Analgesia* 2009;**109**(6): 1908–1915.
60 Porreco RP and Stettler RW. Surgical remedies for postpartum hemorrhage. *Clinical Obstetrics and Gynecology* 2010;**53**(1):182–195.
61 Lousquy R *et al.* Routine use of abdominopelvic ultrasonography in severe postpartum hemorrhage: retrospective evaluation in 125 patients. *American Journal of Obstetrics & Gynecology* 2011;**204**(3):232 e1–6.
62 Carlan SJ *et al.* Appearance of the uterus by ultrasound immediately after placental delivery with pathologic correlation. *Journal of Clinical Ultrasound* 1997;**25**(6):301–308.
63 American College of Obstetricians and Gynecologists Practice Bulletin No. 120: Use of prophylactic antibiotics in labor and delivery. *Obstetrics & Gynecology* 2011;**117**(6):1472–1483.
64 American College of Obstetricians and Gynecologists Practice Bulletin No. 71 Clinical Management Guidelines for Obstetrician-Gynecologists: Episiotomy. *Obstetrics & Gynecology* 2006;**107**(4):957–962.
65 Hudelist G *et al.* Factors predicting severe perineal trauma during childbirth: role of forceps delivery routinely combined with mediolateral episiotomy. *American Journal of Obstetrics & Gynecology* 2005;**192**(3):875–881.

66 Angioli R *et al.* Severe perineal lacerations during vaginal delivery: the University of Miami experience. *American Journal of Obstetrics & Gynecology* 2000;**182**(5):1083–1085.

67 Melamed N *et al.* Intrapartum cervical lacerations: characteristics, risk factors, and effects on subsequent pregnancies. *American Journal of Obstetrics & Gynecology* 2009;**200**(4):388 e1–4.

68 Parikh R, Brotzman S, and Anasti JN. Cervical lacerations: some surprising facts. *American Journal of Obstetrics & Gynecology* 2007;**196**(5):e17–18.

69 Landy HJ *et al.* Characteristics associated with severe perineal and cervical lacerations during vaginal delivery. *Obstetrics & Gynecology* 2011;**117**(3):627–635.

70 Zahn CM, Hankins GD, and Yeomans ER. Vulvovaginal hematomas complicating delivery. Rationale for drainage of the hematoma cavity. *Journal of Reproductive Medicine* 1996;**41**(8): 569–574.

71 You WB and Zahn CM. Postpartum hemorrhage: abnormally adherent placenta, uterine inversion, and puerperal hematomas. *Clinical Obstetrics and Gynecology* 2006;**49**(1):184–197.

72 Mirza FG and Gaddipati S. Obstetric emergencies. *Seminars in Perinatology* 2009;**33**:97–103.

73 Fargeaudou Y *et al.* Severe primary postpartum hemorrhage due to genital tract laceration after operative vaginal delivery: successful treatment with transcatheter arterial embolization. *European Radiology* 2009;**19**(9):2197–2203.

74 Villella J *et al.* Postpartum angiographic embolization for vulvovaginal hematoma. A report of two cases. *Journal of Reproductive Medicine* 2001;**46**(1):65–67.

75 Heffner LJ *et al.* Primary management of postpartum vulvovaginal hematomas by angiographic embolization. *American Journal of Perinatology* 1985;**2**(3):204–207.

76 Whiteside JL, Asif RB, and Novello RJ. Fibrin sealant for management of complicated obstetric lacerations. *Obstetrics & Gynecology* 2010;**115**(2 Pt 2):403–404.

77 Smith WR *et al.* Retroperitoneal packing as a resuscitation technique for hemodynamically unstable patients with pelvic fractures: report of two representative cases and a description of technique. *Journal of Trauma* 2005;**59**(6):1510–1514.

78 Healthgrades 2012: Trends in Women's Health in American Hospitals Report 2012. Healthgrades Inc. 2012.

79 Bloom SL *et al.* Decision-to-incision times and maternal and infant outcomes. *Obstetrics & Gynecology* 2006;**108**(1):6–11.

80 MacKenzie IZ and Cooke I. What is a reasonable time from decision-to-delivery by caesarean section? Evidence from 415 deliveries. *BJOG* 2002;**109**(5):498–504.

81 Holcroft CJ *et al.* Cord gas analysis, decision-to-delivery interval, and the 30-minute rule for emergency cesareans. *Journal of Perinatology* 2005;**25**(4):229–235.

82 Hillemanns P *et al.* Crash emergency cesarean section: decision-to-delivery interval under 30 min and its effect on Apgar and umbilical artery pH. *Archives of Gynecology and Obstetrics* 2005;**273**(3):161–165.

83 American College of Obstetricians and Gynecologists Practice Bulletin No. 116: Management of intrapartum fetal heart rate tracings. *Obstetrics & Gynecology* 2010;**116**(5):1232–1240.

84 Royal College of Anaesthetists. Raising the standard: a compendium of audit recipes. London: RCoA, 2012.

85 Gautam PL, Kathuria S, and Kaul TK. Infiltration block for caesarean section in a morbidly obese parturient. *Acta Anaesthesiologica Scandinavica* 1999;**43**(5):580–581.

86 Ghuman M *et al.* Post-caesarean section surgical site infection: rate and risk factors. *New Zealand Medical Journal* 2011;**124**(1339):32–36.

87 Hofmeyr GJ *et al.* Techniques for caesarean section. *Cochrane Database of Systematic Reviews* 2008;(**1**):CD004662.

88 Franchi M *et al.* Joel-Cohen or Pfannenstiel incision at cesarean delivery: does it make a difference? *Acta Obstetricia et Gynecologica Scandinavica* 2002;**81**(11):1040–1046.

89 Wylie BJ *et al.* Comparison of transverse and vertical skin incision for emergency cesarean delivery. *Obstetrics & Gynecology* 2010;**115**(6):1134–1140.

90 Smith JF, Hernandez C, and Wax JR. Fetal laceration injury at cesarean delivery. *Obstetrics & Gynecology* 1997;**90**(3):344–346.

91 Alexander JM *et al.* Fetal injury associated with cesarean delivery. *Obstetrics & Gynecology* 2006;**108**(4):885–890.

92 Dessole S *et al.* Accidental fetal lacerations during cesarean delivery: experience in an Italian level III university hospital. *American Journal of Obstetrics & Gynecology* 2004;**191**(5): 1673–1677.

93 Berghella V. Cesarean Delivery: Technique. *UpToDate* 2013.

94 Hohlagschwandtner M *et al.* Is the formation of a bladder flap at cesarean necessary? A randomized trial. *Obstetrics & Gynecology* 2001;**98**(6):1089–1092.

95 Dahlke JD *et al.* Evidence-based surgery for cesarean delivery: an updated systematic review. *American Journal of Obstetrics & Gynecology* 2013;**209**(4):294–306.

96 Murphy N, R.S.D.J., Eisinger SH editors., Maternal resuscitation and trauma. Advanced Life Support in Obstetrics (ALSO) provider course syllabus. Leawood (KS): American Academy of Family Physicians, 2000: 1–25.

97 Mallampalli A, Powner DJ, and Gardner MO. Cardiopulmonary resuscitation and somatic support of the pregnant patient. *Critical Care Clinics* 2004;**20**(4):747–761, x.

98 Katz VL, Dotters DJ, and Droegemueller W. Perimortem cesarean delivery. *Obstetrics & Gynecology* 1986;**68**(4):571–576.

99 Finegold H *et al.* Successful resuscitation after maternal cardiac arrest by immediate cesarean section in the labor room. *Anesthesiology* 2002;**96**(5):1278.

100 Katz V, Balderston K, and DeFreest M. Perimortem cesarean delivery: were our assumptions correct? *American Journal of Obstetrics & Gynecology* 2005;**192**(6):1916–1920, discussion 1920–1921.

101 Dijkman A *et al.* Cardiac arrest in pregnancy: increasing use of perimortem caesarean section due to emergency skills training? *BJOG* 2010;**117**(3):282–287.

102 Rees GA and Willis BA. Resuscitation in late pregnancy. *Anaesthesia* 1988;**43**(5):347–349.

103 Jeejeebhoy FM *et al.* Management of cardiac arrest in pregnancy: a systematic review. *Resuscitation* 2011;**82**(7):801–80.

CHAPTER 13
Maternal disorders affecting labor and delivery

Audrey Merriam[1] and Anthony Sciscione[2]
[1] *Division of Maternal-Fetal Medicine, Department of Obstetrics and Gynecology, Columbia University, New York, NY, USA*
[2] *Department of Obstetrics and Gynecology, Christiana Hospital, Newark, DE, USA*

13.1 Hypertensive disorders of pregnancy

Blood pressure in normotensive pregnant women is dynamic, varying throughout the day and over the course of the pregnancy. The normal circadian fluctuations seen in nonpregnancy patients are also seen in the pregnant population, with daily blood pressures being lowest in the morning and peaking during the late afternoon and evening [1]. Over the course of pregnancy, diastolic blood pressure reaches its nadir around 18–22 weeks of gestation. Conversely, systolic blood pressure gradually demonstrates a slight increase throughout gestation [2]. In labor, blood pressure can transiently increase up to35 mmHg systolic and 25 mmHg diastolic [3]. Hypertensive disorders are becoming increasingly common in pregnancy, primarily because of the increase in the number of patients with chronic hypertension who become pregnant. Chronic hypertension is present in 5% of pregnant women, and approximately 20% of women with chronic hypertension will develop superimposed preeclampsia (this rate varies depending on the severity of the hypertension) [4,5]. The rate of preeclampsia in patients without preexisting hypertension is approximately 5–8% [4].

13.2 Gestational hypertension

The term "gestational hypertension" has replaced "pregnancy-induced hypertension" and is the most common cause of elevated blood pressure during pregnancy, affecting 6–17% of nulliparous mothers and 2–4% of multiparous women [6]. To make the diagnosis, a woman must have an elevated blood pressure after the 20th week

Management of Labor and Delivery, Second Edition. Edited by George A. Macones.

of gestation without proteinuria or other laboratory abnormalities. Elevated blood pressure during pregnancy is defined as a systolic blood pressure greater than or equal to 140 mmHg or a diastolic blood pressure greater than or equal to 90 mmHg [6]. Women diagnosed with gestational hypertension do not have a history of elevated blood pressure prior to the 20th week of gestation and their blood pressure normalizes within the first 12 weeks of the postpartum period [7]. The risk of progression of gestational hypertension to preeclampsia is gestational age dependent, with a risk of approximately 50% when gestational hypertension is diagnosed at less than 30 weeks of gestation and decreasing with the development of gestational hypertension at later gestational ages [6,8].

Patients with gestational hypertension that is well controlled, with or without medications, can typically have induction of labor or a cesarean delivery at 37 weeks of gestation. Development of gestational hypertension after 37 weeks of gestation is an indication for delivery without expectant management [5]. Women who develop new-onset hypertension with persistent blood pressures in the severe range (≥160 mmHg systolic or ≥ 110 mmHg diastolic) in the absence of proteinuria or severe features should still receive magnesium sulfate therapy during delivery and the immediate postpartum period for the prevention of eclampsia (see below for further discussion of magnesium sulfate therapy). There is no contraindication to intravenous analgesia, epidural anesthesia, or spinal anesthesia in the case of cesarean delivery. Continuous blood pressure monitoring and close observation is necessary in these patients during delivery and in the immediate postpartum period to determine if there are any sustained elevations from baseline blood pressure or development of symptoms of preeclampsia. Sustained elevations in blood pressure should prompt further investigation including laboratory investigation into whether the patient has developed preeclampsia.

13.3 Chronic hypertension/superimposed preeclampsia

The number of women who have chronic hypertension is increasing and, while the prevalence varies by population, the American College of Obstetrics and Gynecology (ACOG) estimated approximately 5% of pregnant women have the diagnosis [5]. Chronic hypertension is defined as elevated blood pressure prior to pregnancy, diagnosed in pregnancy prior to 20 weeks of gestation or retrospectively when elevated blood pressure noted after 20 weeks of gestation persists longer than 12 weeks postpartum [9]. This can be classified as mild or severe chronic hypertension (see Table 13.1).

Identification of chronic hypertension in pregnancy is important so that a potential strategy can be implemented to help decrease potential pregnancy

Table 13.1 Systolic and diastolic blood pressure criteria for diagnosis of mild and severe chronic hypertension.

Mild chronic hypertension	Systolic BP 140–159 mmHg *or* Diastolic BP 90–109 mmHg
Severe chronic hypertension	Systolic BP ≥ 160 mmHg *or* Diastolic BP ≥110 mmHg

Table 13.2 Recommended gestational age for delivery for women with chronic hypertensive disease in pregnancy.

Condition	Delivery time (weeks)
Well-controlled chronic hypertension on or off antihypertensive medication	37–38
Severe chronic hypertension and/or difficult-to-control hypertension	36–37

complications. The risk of maternal mortality, cerebrovascular accidents, pulmonary edema, placental abruption, stillbirth, small-for-gestational-age infants and perinatal mortality are elevated in women with chronic hypertension compared to normotensive women [10,11]. These increased risks appear to be further increased when chronic hypertension is poorly controlled, with high risk being associated with higher blood pressure (> 160 / > 100) and the presence of end-organ disease. The likelihood of preterm birth and delivery via cesarean section is also increased in women with chronic hypertension, which is important when counseling women [9].

Management of chronic hypertension in labor does not differ greatly from that of the normotensive woman. In general, induction of labor is recommended and, although there are no randomized control trials evaluating the best time for delivery, the following recommendations have been made based on expert opinion (see Table 13.2) [12].

Cesarean delivery is only recommended for obstetric indications, although it is important to counsel these women on the slight increased risk of cesarean delivery due to chronic hypertension. There are no contraindications to any form of labor analgesia or anesthesia.

Development of superimposed preeclampsia is an important consideration for pregnant women with chronic hypertension. Initial evaluation of pregnant women with chronic hypertension should include a baseline 24-hour urine collection for total protein, creatinine clearance, electrocardiography, and ophthalmologic exam. Patients with superimposed preeclampsia can present with new-onset proteinuria or increased proteinuria from baseline, abnormal renal or liver function tests, hematologic abnormalities, or severe features of preeclampsia (i.e. headache, right upper quadrant pain, increased baseline blood pressure, vision changes). Uric acid levels may be increased in women with chronic hypertension; there is evidence to suggest this may precede other laboratory abnormalities in patients with chronic hypertension who develop superimposed preeclampsia [13].

Women who develop superimposed preeclampsia should be managed in a similar way to those who develop preeclampsia during pregnancy. Those women with superimposed preeclampsia without severe features (discussed later in this chapter) should undergo delivery at 37 weeks of gestation. For women with chronic hypertension who develop severe features of preeclampsia, delivery should occur at 34 weeks of gestation or when criteria are met for severe features beyond 34 weeks of gestation [5].

13.4 Preeclampsia

Preeclampsia is a hypertensive disorder of pregnancy that is defined by elevated blood pressure and proteinuria or other laboratory / physical exam findings. Preeclampsia can be with or without severe features depending on the patient's symptoms and blood pressure readings.

The standard definition of mild preeclampsia has been a systolic blood pressure ≥ 140 mmHg or a diastolic blood pressure ≥ 90 mmHg that occurs after 20 weeks of gestation with accompanying proteinuria of ≥ 0.3 grams of protein in a 24-hour period [14]. A 24-hour urine collection should be obtained regardless of proteinuria present on dipstick evaluation or random protein/creatinine urine spot test, unless delivery is imminent [15]. These patients must have

Table 13.3 Diagnostic criteria for preeclampsia and preeclampsia with severe features.

Preeclampsia	Systolic blood pressure ≥ 140 mmHg *or* diastolic blood pressure ≥ 90 mmHg after 20 weeks of gestation on two occasions 4 hours apart Proteinuria ≥ 0.3 grams in a 24-hour period; protein/creatinine ratio ≥ 0.3; dipstick of 1+ protein
Preeclampsia with severe features	Systolic blood pressure ≥ 160 mmHg *or* diastolic blood pressure ≥ 110 mmHg on two occasions 4 hours apart unless antihypertensive medication is initiated prior to 4 hours Cerebral or visual disturbances Pulmonary edema Epigastric or right upper quadrant pain unresponsive to medication Impaired liver function (liver function enzymes twice the normal limit) Thrombocytopenia (<100,000/microliter) Progressive renal insufficiency (creatinine > 1.1 mg/dL or a doubling of the serum creatinine)

Table 13.4 Maternal and fetal indications for delivery in patients with severe preeclampsia.

Variable	Indication
Maternal	Persistent severe headache or visual changes; eclampsia
	Shortness of breath or chest tightness +/− rales and pulse oximetry < 94% on room air or pulmonary edema
	Epigastric / right upper quadrant pain with AST or ALT > 2 times the upper limits of normal
	Uncontrolled severe hypertension, despite maximum doses of antihypertensive agents
	Oliguria (<500 mL/24hr) or a serum creatinine level of ≥ 1.5 mg/dL
	Persistent platelet count < 100,000/mm^3
	Suspected placental abruption, progressive labor +/− rupture of membranes
Fetal	Persistent severe oligohydramnios (AFI < 5 cm)
	Repetitive late or variable fetal heart rate decelerations
	Persistent biophysical profile ≤ 4 (evaluations 6 hours apart)
	Umbilical artery Doppler imaging with reverse diastolic blood flow
	Fetal death

previously normal blood pressure and have at least two elevated blood pressure readings approximately 4 hours apart. The disease prevalence is estimated at 5–8% of pregnant women (see table 13.3).

Delivery of women with preeclampsia is recommended at 37 weeks of gestation or whenever the woman meets criteria for diagnosis of preeclampsia past 37 weeks of gestation [6]. Development of preeclampsia prior to 37 weeks of gestation can be expectantly managed in the inpatient setting or in the outpatient setting, if the patient is reliable. Other indications for delivery include the following: possible placental abruption; ≥ 34 weeks of gestation with labor; preterm premature rupture of membranes or fetal growth restriction; and abnormal maternal or fetal testing [6].

Delivery of women with preeclampsia with severe features is recommended at 34 weeks of gestation or whenever the patient develops severe preeclampsia if greater than 34 weeks of gestation. Criteria for expectant management of patients prior to 34 weeks of gestation are not as clear. However, if the clinical picture changes and any of the conditions in Table 13.4 are met then the patient should be delivered.

Some patients, while requiring delivery before 34 weeks of gestation, can delay delivery for antenatal steroid administration with close monitoring for worsening status: amniotic fluid index < 5, ultrasound demonstrated estimated fetal weight less than the fifth percentile, reversed umbilical artery end-diastolic flow, labor, or rupture of membranes [16]. Patients and providers opting for this management strategy should do so only in facilities where there are adequate maternal and neonatal intensive care resources.

A third category of hypertensive disorders of pregnancy that requires attention in this section is HELLP syndrome, which is defined as hemolysis, elevated liver enzymes and low platelets with or without hypertension. While up to 20% of women with severe preeclampsia may develop HELLP syndrome not all patients with HELLP develop hypertension, and of those that do approximately 30% can have mild range blood pressure [17]. Thrombocytopenia and coagulopathies are more pronounced in patients with HELLP compared to patients solely with preeclampsia. There should be close, serial monitoring with complete blood counts, coagulation panels, and fibrinogen levels. At Christiana Care Health System we customarily follow these laboratories every 6–8 hours until the clinical situation changes and repeat based on worsening or improvement clinically. Platelet counts < 100,000/μL are more concerning for development of coagulopathies [18]. In general, the need for platelet transfusions is rare and not recommended unless the platelet count is < 20,000/μL or until the patient experiences spontaneous bleeding, as the platelets will be consumed in the coagulopathy [19]. Fibrinogen levels < 100 mg/dL should be replaced with fresh frozen plasma and cryoprecipitate. The use of these for replacement therapies is based on need for other coagulation factors and volume (see Table 13.5).

Red blood cell transfusion should be considered for severe anemia < 7 mg/dL. In general, one unit of packed red blood cells will raise hemoglobin. Once a patient has become coagulopathic, it is critical to have a team approach, including maternal-fetal medicine specialists, anesthesiology, critical care specialists, and hematology. If these specialist services are not available then transfer to a tertiary care facility should be strongly considered.

Patients diagnosed with HELLP require immediately delivery as laboratory abnormalities are only expected to worsen, placing the pregnancy and the mother at increased risk [20]. Patients in spontaneous labor can be allowed to continue with vaginal delivery as long as fetal tracing remains reassuring and the mother is medically stable. Patients preterm and/or remote for delivery should have consideration for delivery via cesarean [21,22].

13.5 Management of preeclampsia in labor

13.5.1 Preeclampsia without severe features

The goals of managing women with preeclampsia without severe features (previously known as mild preeclampsia) in labor are as follows: (1) identification of severe features indicating progression of disease, (2) prevention of maternal complications, and (3) detection of fetal heart rate abnormalities. Whether a patient is known to have preeclampsia prior to induction of labor or they present with elevated blood pressure for the first time, a baseline set of laboratory studies should be obtained, including a complete blood count, liver function studies, and renal function studies with the potential of a coagulation

Table 13.5 The content, volume, and indications for blood product replacement in the case of severe hemorrhage or coagulopathy.

Product	Contents	Volume (mL)	Effect	Indication
Packed red blood cells	Red blood cells Few white blood cells Some plasma	300 (leukocyte poor 250)	Increase hematocrit 3%/unit, hemoglobin 1g/unit	Anemia (leukocyte poor decreases febrile reactions)
Platelets	Platelets Some plasma Red blood cells Few white blood cells	50	Increase total platelet by 7500μL/unit	Bleeding due to thrombocytopenia
Fresh frozen plasma	Plasma Clotting factors V, XI, XII	250	Increase fibrinogen by 10–15%/unit	Treat coagulation disorders
Cryoprecipitate	Fibrinogen Factors V, VIII, XIII, von Willebrand factor	40	Increase fibrinogen by 10–15mg/dL/unit	Fibrinogen deficiency von Willebrand disease Hemophilia A

panel [4]. There are no set guidelines for when to repeat these labs during labor; at Christiana Care Health System, if the initial values are normal the labs do not necessarily need to be repeated unless the clinical picture changes. If the initial laboratory values are markedly abnormal then they should be repeated at 6- to 8-hour intervals or if the clinical picture changes. Patients should be repeatedly asked during labor if they are having any new-onset symptoms or changes in symptoms (i.e. headache, scotomata, blurry vision, and right upper quadrant pain) [23]. Development of neurologic symptoms, pulmonary edema, or laboratory values suggesting severe features should alter the patient's management to that of a patient with preeclampsia with severe features.

While there are no randomized trials looking at the optimal mode of delivery for women with preeclampsia or gestational hypertension without severe range blood pressure, induction of labor with continuous fetal monitoring should be attempted if there are no contraindications [6]. In general, cesarean delivery should be reserved for obstetric indications such as non-reassuring fetal heart tracing, arrest of dilation, or arrest of descent.

All patients in labor should have blood pressure taken serially; however, this is especially true for patients with preeclampsia. At our institution for patients with gestational hypertension without severe range blood pressure and preeclampsia without severe features we record blood pressure readings every 30–60 minutes, and more frequently if severe range blood pressure is noted.

Table 13.6 Subsets of oliguria (I–III), the associated hemodynamic findings, and recommended treatments.

Group	Cardiac output	Pulmonary capillary wedge pressure	Systemic vascular resistance	Treatment
I	Increased	Low	Increased	IV fluid
II	Normal/increased	Normal/increased	Normal	Afterload/preload reduction (dopamine)
III	Decreased	Elevated	Increased	Afterload reduction and fluid restriction (diuretics)

Source: Clark *et al.*, 1986 [26]. Reproduced with permission of Elsevier.

Blood pressure during labor is expected to rise secondary to pain and the increased physical activity from pushing. Sustained elevations of blood pressure into the severe range should still be concerning and the management of such will be discussed below. Patients who have had their blood pressure controlled on oral anti-hypertensive medication prior to delivery should continue all such medication in labor to the best of their ability as this will help prevent severe range blood pressure requiring more intensive management [6].

Preeclampsia is a state of intravascular fluid depletion secondary to vessel endothelial dysfunction leading to third-spacing of fluids with a resultant increase in oncotic pressure, hemoconcentration, and edema. These pathophysiologic changes in preeclamptic patients can make fluid management particularly challenging. Intravenous fluid replacement during labor needs to be closely monitored and should be used to compensate for the intravascular fluid depletion, insensible losses, and expected intravascular depletion from bleeding after delivery. Patients with preeclampsia in labor should have a Foley catheter placed to adequately asses urine output and intake, and output should be closely monitored and recorded [24]. Fluid replacement with crystalloid solutions (i.e. normal saline or Lactated Ringers) should occur at a rate of around 125 mL/hr. Patients should be monitored for adequate urine output. Urine output of less than 20–30 ml/hr for 2 hours, or more accurately < 0.5 mL/kg/h, is considered oliguria. Any oliguria or anuria should not be treated with a diuretic as these patients are intravascularly depleted and it will only worsen the intravascular depletion. Since most patients with oliguria have intravascular depletion, fluid boluses of 500–1000 mL can be used to a maximum of 2 liters if the patient does not have a history of heart failure or is not currently in pulmonary edema [25]. If that does not result in a resolution in oliguria than renal vasospasm or heart failure need to be considered. Clark *et al.* developed subsets of oliguria in hemodynamically complicated patients, which are defined below along with recommended treatments [26]. Patients who develop pulmonary edema should be considered to have preeclampsia with severe features, and expeditious delivery should be considered.

Management of maternal pain from labor should be managed per patient request during labor in consultation with an anesthesiologist. There is no evidence to suggest that the type of labor anesthesia or analgesia used, or the use of magnesium sulfate seizure prophylaxis, alters the mode of delivery [27]. Intravenous opioid administration and epidural anesthesia are both effective and acceptable methods for pain management during labor in patients with gestational hypertension without severe range blood pressure and preeclampsia without severe features [28,29].

Patients with preeclampsia without severe features do not seem to be at the same risk of adverse maternal outcomes as patients with severe features. Two randomized placebo control trials, with a total of 357 women with preeclampsia without severe features, evaluated the effectiveness of magnesium sulfate in prevention of disease progression. Neither trial had an instance of eclampsia and the trials overall were small [27,30]. Larger trials are needed to further evaluate the risk–benefit ratio of using magnesium sulfate in patients with preeclampsia without severe features, but currently in Delaware we do not use magnesium sulfate for seizure prevention in patients with preeclampsia without severe features, as recommended by Sibai [6].

13.5.2 Preeclampsia with severe features

The goals of managing patients with preeclampsia with severe features or gestational hypertension with persistent severe range blood pressure are the same as those of managing patients with preeclampsia without severe features, but more intensive blood pressure management, increased patient surveillance, and use of magnesium sulfate for seizure prophylaxis is generally required. Initial evaluation of patients with known or suspected preeclampsia with severe features should include serial blood pressure measurements occurring every 15 minutes. Initial blood pressures that are ≥ 160 mmHg systolic or ≥ 110 mmHg diastolic for more than 15 minutes are considered a hypertensive emergency and require immediate treatment [31]. Patients with blood pressure in the severe range (≥ 160/≥ 110 mmHg) are at increased risk of cerebral infarction, cerebral hemorrhage, and seizure [32,33]. The goal is not to normalize the blood pressure in these patients as that may result in insufficient placental perfusion resulting in a compromise in fetal status, but rather blood pressure should be lowered to 140–160/90–100 mmHg. In addition to fetal complications of persistently elevated blood pressure, maternal risk of cerebrovascular accidents is also increased. Blood pressure monitoring can be performed with non-invasive monitoring for most patients; however, there are indications that

Table 13.7 Indications for invasive monitoring of maternal status in preeclampsia.

Indications
Pulmonary edema unresponsive to conventional treatment or of uncertain etiology
Persistent oliguria despite aggressive volume expansion
Induction of general anesthesia in hemodynamically unstable patients
Medical complications that would otherwise necessitate invasive monitoring

may necessitate invasive hemodynamic monitoring [34]. Consultation of a maternal-fetal medicine specialist or critical care specialist should be considered if invasive monitoring of blood pressure is required.

Although there are no randomized control trials evaluating the best antihypertensive treatment, at Christiana Care Health System we use either IV labetalol or IV hydralazine for first-line management in patients with severe range blood pressure as per ACOG guidelines (see Figure 13.1) [31].

Both hydralazine and labetalol have a long track record of use in pregnant women and appear safe and effective. Hydralazine acts directly on arteriolar smooth muscle to cause vasodilation and can cause maternal hypotension. Hydralazine is traditionally administered intravenously with a starting dose of 5 mg and a maximum dose of 40 mg. There is the potential for severe maternal hypotension with the use of IV hydralazine [31]. Labetalol is an alpha and beta adrenergic antagonist with slightly more effect on beta receptors than alpha. Potential side effects of labetalol use include neonatal bradycardia and should be avoided in women with asthma or heart failure. Labetalol is given in increments

1. Notify physician if systolic BP measurement is greater than or equal to 160 mm Hg or if diastolic BP measurement is greater than or equal to 110 mm Hg.
2. Institute fetal surveillance if undelivered and fetus is viable.
3. Administer labetalol (20 mg IV over 2 minutes).
4. Repeat BP measurement in 10 minutes and record results.
5. If either BP threshold is still exceeded, administer labetalol (40 mg IV over 2 minutes). If BP is below threshold, continue to monitor BP closely.
6. Repeat BP measurement in 10 minutes and record results.
7. If either BP threshold is still exceeded, administer labetalol (80 mg IV over 2 minutes). If BP is below threshold, continue to monitor BP closely.
8. Repeat BP measurement in 10 minutes and record results.
9. If either BP threshold is still exceeded, administer hydralazine (10 mg IV over 2 minutes). If BP is below threshold, continue to monitor BP closely.
10. Repeat BP measurement in 20 minutes and record results.
11. If either BP threshold is still exceeded, obtain emergency consultation from maternal–fetal medicine, internal medicine, anesthesia, or critical care specialists.
12. Give additional antihypertensive medication per specific order.
13. Once the aforementioned BP thresholds are achieved, repeat BP measurement every 10 minutes for 1 hour, then every 15 minutes for 1 hour, then every 30 minutes for 1 hour, and then every hour for 4 hours.
14. Institute additional BP timing per specific order.

1. Notify physician if systolic BP is greater than or equal to 160 mm Hg or if diastolic BP is greater than or equal to 110 mm Hg.
2. Institute fetal surveillance if undelivered and fetus is viable.
3. Administer hydralazine (5 mg or 10 mg IV over 2 minutes).
4. Repeat BP measurement in 20 minutes and record results.
5. If either BP threshold is still exceeded, administer hydralazine (10 mg IV over 2 minutes). If BP is below threshold, continue to monitor BP closely.
6. Repeat BP measurement in 20 minutes and record results.
7. If either BP threshold is still exceeded, administer labetalol (20 mg IV over 2 minutes). If BP is below threshold, continue to monitor BP closely.
8. Repeat BP measurement in 10 minutes and record results.
9. If either BP threshold is still exceeded, administer labetalol (40 mg IV over 2 minutes) and obtain emergency consultation from maternal–fetal medicine, internal medicine, anesthesia, or critical care specialists.
10. Give additional antihypertensive medication per specific order.
11. Once the aforementioned BP thresholds are achieved, repeat BP measurement every 10 minutes for 1 hour, then every 15 minutes for 1 hour, then every 30 minutes for 1 hour, and then every hour for 4 hours.
12. Institute additional BP timing per specific order.

Figure 13.1 Recommendations from the American College of Obstetricians and Gynecologists for the use of intravenous labetalol and hydralazine in the management of severe range blood pressure. *Source:* Committee Opinion No. 514: Emergent Therapy for Acute-Onset, Severe Hypertension with Preeclampsia or Eclampsia. [31].

every hour with a maximum dose in a 24-hour period of 300 mg. In the event that the patient does not have IV access, oral labetalol can be used. The recommended initial dose is 200 mg, which can be repeated every 30 minutes until the goal blood pressure range is reached. The maximum dose in a 24-hour period for oral labetalol is 2400 mg.

There are second-line antihypertensive agents that can be used for blood pressure management if hydralazine and labetalol are not available or are contraindicated in a particular patient, or if the first-line agents have not been effective in decreasing a patient's blood pressure. The following agents should be used in consultation with a maternal-fetal medicine subspecialist, anesthesiologist, or critical care specialist. Labetalol can be given by continuous infusion pump as well as can nicardipine. Nifedipine is a calcium channel blocker and should be used in patients also receiving magnesium sulfate for seizure prophylaxis as there is a theoretical risk of severe hypotension and cardiovascular collapse secondary to exaggerated hypotensive response [35]. Sodium nitroprusside, a vasodilator, at an initial dose of 0.25 μg/kg/min, can be used but only for the shortest time possible as there are concerns about cyanide and thiocyanate toxicity leading to methemoglobinemia for the mother and fetus as well as the potential for increased intracranial pressure and worsening of cerebral edema in the mother [36].

In addition to the close blood pressure monitoring required by these patients, their laboratory abnormalities and symptomatology also require close monitoring. Laboratory assessment should occur upon presentation in labor, prior to induction of labor or cesarean section. Assessment should include a complete blood count for hemoglobin and platelet levels, liver function tests, renal function tests, urinalysis, blood type and screen, fibrinogen level and coagulation panel [37–39]. Patients should also be frequently asked about development of new symptoms or changes in symptoms, as noted above.

Patients with preeclampsia with severe features, either by blood pressure or symptom criteria, or women with gestational hypertension with severe range blood pressure, are at increased risk for seizures and the development of eclampsia. Magnesium sulfate is the drug of choice for seizure prevention in patients with severe preeclampsia and should be used in labor for all patients with severe preeclampsia who do not have contraindications to magnesium administration (i.e. myasthenia gravis) [40]. Magnesium sulfate has been proven to be more effective than placebo in randomized control trials in seizure prevention. In one trial with 10,110 patients from 33 different countries, magnesium sulfate was found to decrease the risk of eclampsia by 58%, and decrease maternal mortality (RR 0.55) with no increase in neonatal mortality [41]. Magnesium sulfate has also been compared to phenytoin for effectiveness in seizure prevention. A Cochrane review showed magnesium sulfate to be superior to phenytoin in seizure prevention and there was a trend toward decreased maternal mortality with magnesium sulfate use. Infants from mothers treated with magnesium sulfate had fewer NICU admissions [42]. Another Cochrane review comparing magnesium sulfate to diazepam showed the former to be superior in prevention of seizure and maternal mortality [43].

Magnesium sulfate is administered intravenously and is given as follows: initial bolus of 4 g over as little as 5 minutes followed by 2 g/hr [44]. In situations where magnesium cannot be continuously administered intravenously an intramuscular regimen can be given as follows: 4-g intravenous dose plus a 10-g intramuscular loading dose followed by a 5-g intramuscular dose every 4 hours [45]. In general, for patients with preeclampsia with severe features or patients with gestational hypertension with severe range blood pressure, magnesium sulfate is continued for 24 hours postpartum; however, there has only been one study showing adverse effects when discontinuing magnesium sulfate in < 24 hours postpartum, and the magnesium sulfate was discontinued after the onset of maternal diuresis (>100 mL/h for 2 consecutive hours) [46]. Signs of magnesium toxicity should be monitored for during administration and include decreased or absent deep tendon reflexes, shortness of breath secondary to decreased respiratory drive, somnolence, double vision, nausea, and slurred speech. If patients exhibit these symptoms magnesium sulfate levels should be drawn and magnesium sulfate infusion should be stopped while awaiting results. There is no evidence that titrating magnesium to a specific serum level is effective but, in general, levels between 4 and 7 mg/dL are considered therapeutic [47]. Toxicity from magnesium can appear between 9 and 12 mg/dL and if this level is reached there should be consideration to stop the infusion [48]. Other considerations for a slower magnesium sulfate infusion rate (1 g/hr) include patients with renal impairment, defined as having a creatinine level greater than 1.4 mg/dL, which was shown in the Magpie trial to be effective at seizure prevention. Serum magnesium levels should be closely monitored in patients with severe renal impairment. At serum magnesium levels at or above 13 mg/dL cardiac arrest and respiratory depression can occur [48]. Treatment for this severe complication includes stopping the magnesium infusion, respiratory support with intubation if needed, cardiac monitoring, and administration of calcium gluconate (10 mL of a 10% solution intravenously over 2 minutes) [49].

Due to intravascular depletion, fluid management follows the same guidelines as preeclampsia without severe features. All patients should have a Foley catheter placed and strict monitoring of fluid intake and output. Crystalloid administration should occur at the same rate as used in mild preeclampsia. Oliguria can be treated with fluid boluses if necessary if the patient does not have a history of heart failure and is not exhibiting signs of pulmonary edema. Women with the diagnosis of preeclampsia with severe features are at an increased risk of pulmonary edema (2.9% incidence), and development of pulmonary edema in a patient with mild preeclampsia changes the diagnosis to preeclampsia with severe features [50]. Pulmonary edema can be delayed and occur during the postpartum diuresis, so patients' respiratory distress in the postpartum period should be evaluated for pulmonary edema. In a case series by Sibai *et al.* 70% of the cases of pulmonary edema occurred in the postpartum period [50]. Diagnosis of pulmonary edema is clinical and includes shortness of breath, rales on lung auscultation, and low pulse oximetry readings. An arterial blood gas performed on patients with pulmonary edema will often demonstrate a P_{02} of < 70 mmHg on room air. While a chest X ray should be performed to confirm the diagnosis of pulmonary edema, treatment is warranted based on a high clinical suspicion. Treatment of pulmonary edema includes supplemental oxygen administration, continuous pulse oximetry, Foley catheter placement if not already done, continued monitoring of fluid intake and output, and decreasing intravenous fluid administration and diuresis. Patients should be intubated if needed, recognizing that once treatment ensues resolution is usually rapid. Diuresis with furosemide is considered first time therapy. Intravenous furosemide administration of 10–40 mg over 1–2 minutes should result in diuresis within 1 hour. If no diuresis is seen an 80 mg IV dose can be given [51].

Mode of delivery for patients with preeclampsia with severe features and gestational hypertension with severe range blood pressure should be via induction of labor with continuous fetal monitoring when possible. Cesarean delivery is generally reserved for patients who have contraindications to induction of labor, failed induction of labor, or another obstetrical indication for cesarean delivery (i.e. non-reassuring fetal heart tracing, arrest of dilation or descent, placental abruption with non-reassuring fetal heart rate changes). Preeclampsia with severe features alone is not an indication for cesarean delivery but these patients are at increased risk of requiring a cesarean delivery if they develop severe features early in gestation that cannot be expectantly managed or if they have uncontrolled blood pressures or development of seizures during induction of labor. Additionally, patients who are < 32 weeks of gestation with an unripe cervix that require delivery should be delivered via cesarean section as the success of induction of labor is likely to be small [16]. In these cases, mothers should be made as medically stable as possible before proceeding with cesarean delivery. There is also no preferred method of anesthesia for patients with severe preeclampsia. Patients can use intravenous opioid administration or epidural anesthesia as they desire for vaginal delivery [52,53]. Spinal anesthesia is preferred for cesarean delivery. This is especially true in patients with extremely elevated blood pressures that are difficult to control because induction of general anesthesia and intubation may result in further elevation of blood pressures that can lead to intravascular hemorrhage or vasospasm, which may lead cerebral vascular accident [52]. However, spinal anesthesia and cesarean delivery may be contraindicated in women who have severe thrombocytopenia or a coagulopathy. If possible, patients with platelet count < 50,000/μL should undergo induction of labor to minimize bleeding at cesarean delivery. When the platelet count is < 50,000/μL and cesarean delivery cannot be avoided transfusion of platelets should occur before skin incision is made to avoid potential complications from a coagulopathy. The risk for hematoma formation in these patients is elevated, and delayed skin closure and increased duration of pressure dressing placement should be considered. While it has been recommended that spinal anesthesia or epidural not be administered with platelet counts < 100,000/μL, small case series have shown a low rate of hematoma formation (1.8%) with use of spinal or epidural anesthesia with platelet counts between 50,000 and 100,000/μL; however, in patients with platelet counts above this the risk of hematoma formation is much lower (0.0004%) [54,55]. Patients requiring a cesarean delivery with platelet counts less than this will likely require general anesthesia. Patients undergoing induction of labor with low platelet counts should have an epidural catheter placed early, in anticipation that their platelet count may drop below 100,000/μL during labor. The epidural infusion does not have to be started or even used at all during labor, but this allows the patient the freedom to consider the use of epidural anesthesia [28,29].

13.6 Eclampsia

Eclampsia is defined as the occurrence of seizures in a woman with preeclampsia that cannot be attributed to any other causes. There is no blood pressure criteria required to diagnose a woman with eclampsia. The majority of patients will report at least one symptom but this may present before or after the onset of the seizure and can include headache (83%), visual changes (45%), hyperreflexia (80%), edema (60%), or right upper quadrant/epigastric pain (20%) [56]. The seizure can occur in the antepartum, intrapartum, or postpartum period, with the majority occurring in the antepartum period and up to 48 hours postpartum [57]. While, the maternal mortality rate associated with eclampsia has decreased significantly in developed countries (0–1.8%) it remains at 15% in developing countries. Other complications associated with eclampsia include placental abruption, disseminated intravascular coagulopathy, pulmonary edema, acute renal failure, aspiration pneumonia, and cardiopulmonary arrest. Perinatal mortality remains at 7–15% due to the reasons listed above [58,59].

Initial management of an eclamptic seizure should include securing the patient's airway, preventing aspiration by placing the patient in the lateral decubitus position, and protecting the mother (i.e. padding side rails, lowering the patient to the floor if seated). Most eclamptic seizures last only a few minutes; however, once the patient's airway is secured and she is stable, steps should be made to stop the seizure and prevent further seizures by beginning magnesium sulfate therapy. Oxygen supplementation via face mask should be started if it has not already been so. Magnesium sulfate is the preferred method for seizure treatment and prevention in eclamptic patients and is superior to phenytoin and diazepam even in these patients [42,43]. The initial magnesium sulfate bolus should be 4–6 g followed by a maintenance dose of 2 g/hr. Again, there is no specified therapeutic range and magnesium levels do not need to be followed in these patients unless magnesium toxicity is suspected. Up to 10% of eclamptic patients will have a second seizure. A second seizure after the initial magnesium sulfate bolus while the patient is receiving the maintenance dose should be treated with a bolus of 2 g IV push over 3–5 minutes. No more than 8 g of magnesium sulfate should be given at the onset of treatment [51]. Subsequent seizures after the second magnesium sulfate bolus should be treated with sodium amobarbital, a short-acting barbiturate, which is given in a dose of 250 mg IV over 3–5 minutes. If the seizures are ongoing, IV thiopental sodium and diazepam can be used as alternative therapies; however, diazepam should be used with caution because it can increase the risk of maternal and neonatal respiratory depression.

After the seizure activity has been controlled it is important to monitor the fetus and the maternal blood pressure. It is common for the fetus to have a non-reassuring fetal heart rate during a maternal seizure and it should not be acted on due to maternal instability and the self-limited nature of eclamptic seizures; for this reason it is not advisable to try to perform fetal monitoring during an eclamptic seizure. Maternal blood pressure should be maintained at 140–160/90–100 mmHg in order to avoid perfusion pressures that would be too low for maternal cerebral vasculature and placental vasculature. Medications for blood pressure control are the same as for any woman with severe range blood pressure (i.e. labetalol and hydralazine). Continuous fetal monitoring is important after an eclamptic seizure. Increased uterine tone may be noted for up to 10 minutes after the cessation of the seizure. Fetal heart rate abnormalities including bradycardia, minimal variability, late decelerations, or tachycardia can be seen [60]. In general, one should not act on these changes immediately as the fetus needs time to recover from the maternal hypoxemia and acidosis that occurred during the seizure and the mother should be made stable before acting on the fetal tracing; however, if the mother is stable and the bradycardia and/or late decelerations persist beyond 10–15 minutes, then the patient should be taken for emergency cesarean delivery.

In general, eclampsia does not necessitate cesarean delivery but it does require delivery regardless of gestational age [61]. Patients already in labor who are recovered from the seizure and stable may be allowed to proceed with vaginal delivery. Induction of labor may also be undertaken in patients with a favorable cervix if they are stable after the seizure. Success rates for induction of labor after eclamptic seizure have been reported to be as high as 80% [38]. Magnesium sulfate therapy does not appear to decrease the rate of vaginal delivery or the duration of labor [27]. Patients remote from term, with an unfavorable cervix, or who have other contraindications to induction of labor or vaginal delivery will require a cesarean section for a safe delivery. The same principals for maternal pain control that apply to patients with preeclampsia with severe features apply to patients with eclampsia. Any anesthesia method may be used unless the patient has a coagulopathy or severe thrombocytopenia (platelet count < 100,000/μL). General anesthesia further increases the aspiration risk in eclamptic patients, and airway edema may further complicate intubation. Patients with severe range blood pressure undergoing general anesthesia induction should have close blood pressure monitoring, and induction will cause a further increase in blood pressure.

13.7 Cardiac disease

Advances in early identification and treatment of cardiac disease, structural and non-structural, have resulted in a significant increase in the number of women with cardiac disease reaching childbearing age. These women, it is hoped, have been counseled extensively about the risks of pregnancy for the mother and fetus before they become pregnant. Once pregnant, depending on the etiology, complexity, and extent of the disease, these patients should have a team approach to pregnancy besides there obstetrician/gynecologist, including maternal-fetal medicine, cardiology, genetics, and anesthesiology. In general, these women should be transferred to a tertiary care center for care as early as feasible.

Multiple cardiovascular alterations take place as a result of pregnancy. Plasma volume begins increasing early in gestation to a maximum of 45% above baseline, in addition to increases in red blood cell mass of 20–30% [62]. However, as plasma volume has a greater increase this leads to the physiologic anemia of pregnancy. Structural changes in the heart include increases in left ventricle muscle mass as well as left atrial diameter [63]. Cardiac output also begins to increase in the first trimester to a maximum of 30–50% above prepregnant values, and to cause this change, stroke volume and heart rate must also increase [64]. These changes in cardiac output and stoke volume increase again during labor, by approximately 10–30% and 20%, respectively. The second stage of labor results in cardiac output increasing even further, by around 50% [65]. These changes are not as profound if the patient receives epidural or spinal analgesia or is placed in the left lateral decubitus position [66].

13.7.1 New York Heart Association classification

One of the most important predictors of pregnancy outcomes for women with preexisting cardiac disease is the patients' New York Heart Association (NYHA) classification prior to pregnancy Table 13.8. This classification system grades the extent of heart failure in patients with heart disease. It classifies patients on their functional status while performing normal levels of daily physical activity and while at rest.

A point system has also been established by Sui *et al.* to assess the rate of maternal cardiac events given certain signs and symptoms. One point is assigned for each of the following: NYHA > II or cyanosis, prior arrhythmia, myocardial dysfunction, left heart obstruction, or prior cardiac events. For women with

Table 13.8 New York Heart Association classification of heart failure by patient symptoms.

Class	Description
Class I (mild)	No limitations of physical activity.
Class II (mild)	Slight limitation of physical activity. Ordinary physical activity precipitates symptoms, no symptoms at rest.
Class III (moderate)	Less than normal physical activity precipitates symptoms that cause moderate limitations in activity. Comfortable at rest.
Class IV (severe)	Patients have symptoms at rest and marked discomfort with physical activity.

Source: Roeder *et al.*, 2011 [67]. Reproduced with permission of Lippencott Williams & Wilkinns.

either a 0, 1 or > 1 score at the time of pregnancy the associated risk of cardiac event was 3%, 30%, and 66%, respectively. This system plus the NYHA classification should be used when counseling women with a history of cardiac disease about their risk of cardiac event in pregnancy [68].

For women with certain lesions it is advisable that they undergo consultation prior to conception for the best possible pregnancy outcome. These lesions include: large atrial septal defect / ventricular septal defect with mild to moderate pulmonary hypertension, patent ductus arteriosus with mild to moderate pulmonary hypertension, severe coarctation of the aorta, severe mitral stenosis or regurgitation, severe aortic stenosis or regurgitation, and Tetralogy of Fallot. There are also a few preexisting cardiac disease processes for which pregnancy should be contraindicated and these include: dilated cardiomyopathy or left ventricular dysfunction with an ejection fraction < 40%, severe pulmonary hypertension, and Marfan syndrome with an aortic root > 4cm diameter [69].

13.7.2 Endocarditis prophylaxis guidelines

Endocarditis prophylaxis is rarely needed during vaginal delivery or cesarean delivery. Recent statements from the American Heart Association and American College of Cardiology recommend endocarditis prophylaxis in the following situations: cyanotic heart disease, prosthetic valves or both for both uncomplicated vaginal and cesarean deliveries. For patients who are not already receiving either antibiotics for prevention of GBS disease of the newborn or prophylactic antibiotics prior to cesarean delivery, intravenous antibiotics should be administered 30–60 minutes prior to delivery [70]. Patients diagnosed with chorioamnionitis or pyelonephritis also do not require additional antibiotic coverage on top of what they are already receiving.

13.7.3 Mitral stenosis

Mitral stenosis can be either acquired or congenital. The most common cause of mitral stenosis in the world is rheumatic heart disease; however, this is exceedingly uncommon in the developed world. Findings common with rheumatic

Table 13.9 Maternal cardiac disease and risk stratification during pregnancy.

Low Maternal and Fetal Risks	High Maternal and Fetal Risks	High Maternal Risk
Asymptomatic aortic stenosis with low mean outflow gradient (<50 mmHg) and normal LV systolic function.	Sever aortic stenosis with or without symptoms.	Ejection fraction < 40%.
Aortic regurgitation, NYHA Class I or II with normal LV function.	Aortic regurgitation, NYHA class III or IV.	Previous heart failure.
Mitral regurgitation, NYHA Class I or II, with normal LV function.	Mitral stenosis, NYHA class II, III, or IV.	Previous stroke or transient ischemic attack.
Mitral valve prolapse with no to moderate mitral regurgitation, normal LV function.	Aortic or mitral valve disease with pulmonary hypertension.	
Mild to moderate mitral stenosis, no pulmonary hypertension.	Aortic or mitral valve disease with LV dysfunction.	
Mild to moderate pulmonary valve stenosis.	Maternal cyanosis.	
	Reduced function status, NYHA class III or IV.	

Source: Roeder *et al.*, 2011 [67]. Reproduced with permission of Lippencott Williams & Wilkins.

heart disease include enlarged left atrium and right ventricle, diastolic murmur, pulmonary hypertension, and narrowed mitral valve. Since pregnancy results in increased blood volume, heart rate and cardiac output patients with rheumatic heart disease can experience an increase in left atrial pressure that leads to pulmonary congestion. Symptoms associated with pulmonary congestion include exertional dyspnea, orthopnea, paroxysmal nocturnal dyspnea, and pulmonary edema. These women are also at increased risk for infective endocarditis and atrial tachyarrhythmias during pregnancy. Approximately 20% of patients will experience an atrial tachyarrhythmia and more than 60% will have symptoms of pulmonary edema. The highest maternal mortality risk is present during the third trimester and the immediate postpartum period [67].

Patients who do not undergo percutaneous balloon or open surgical valvuloplasty prior to pregnancy should be followed closely during the antenatal period. Co-management with a cardiologist and maternal-fetal medicine specialist is advised. Pregnant women with mitral stenosis typically require activity restriction and salt restriction. Patients who develop pulmonary edema can be treated with diuretics, primarily furosemide. There is an increased risk of pulmonary edema during labor and especially during the immediate postpartum period due to fluid

Table 13.10 Indications for endocarditis prophylaxis in the pregnant patient during labor and delivery.

Cardiac conditions with high risk of endocarditis in the presence of bacteremia
Prosthetic valve or prosthetic material used for valve repair.
Patients with previous infective endocarditis.
Patients with congenital heart disease (CHD):
– Unrepaired cyanotic CHD.
– Completely repaired CHD repaired with prosthetic material during the first 6 months after the procedure.
– Repaired CHD with residual defects at the site or adjacent to the site of the prosthetic patch.
Cardiac transplant recipients with valve regurgitation due to structurally abnormal valve.

Source: Practice Bulletin No. 120: Use of Prophylactic Antibiotics in Labor and Delivery [88]. Reproduced with permission of Lippencott Williams & Wilkins.

shifts. Intravenous fluids and urine output should be closely monitored. Placing a Foley catheter is recommended for more accurate measurements. Intravenous fluid rates should be approximately 75 ml/hr so as not to increase the patient's risk for pulmonary edema. Monitoring during labor with a pulmonary arterial catheter is preferred, allowing for more judicious fluid management, especially in patients with moderate to severe disease. Frank pulmonary edema rarely occurs with pulmonary wedge pressures < 28–30 mmHg, and optimal pre-delivery wedge pressure is ≤ 14 mmHg to prevent the increase in pulmonary wedge pressures seen with the fluid shifts in the immediate postpartum period [71,72]. Laboring in the left lateral decubitus position is preferred. If acute pulmonary edema occurs, either prior to labor or during labor, sedation to decrease the heart rate allowing for increased cardiac filling, diuretic treatment, and prompt delivery, typically via cesarean section, should occur [73].

Because there is a decreased filling time with tachycardia there should be a concerted effort to prevent its occurrence. Beta-blockers or calcium channel blockers can be used to lower maternal heart rate and are generally recommended with maternal heart rates > 100 beats per minute. Tachycardia leads to decreased cardiac output due to decreased diastolic filling time, which can compromise fetal well-being. Esmolol (500 mcg/kg IV loading dose over 1 minute then continuous infusion as needed in 50 mcg/kg/min increments every 4 minutes up to 300 mcg/kg/min) is the preferred beta-blocker in labor because it is short acting; however, propranolol (1–3 mg IV every 4 hours or 10–30 mg orally 3–4 times a day) can be used for longer term control in the antepartum period. Diltiazem (0.25 mg/kg as IV bolus or 5–10 mghr as a continuous infusion increasing up to 15 mg/hr for up to 24 hours) is the preferred calcium channel blocker for short-term control [72]. Atrial tachyarrhythmias are more likely to occur in the presence of tachycardia. If an atrial tachyarrhythmia does occur patients should receive anticoagulation (with heparin or low-molecular weight

Table 13.11 Recommended antibiotic prophylaxis regimens for prevention of bacterial endocarditis for women during labor and delivery.

Treatment	Antibiotic	Regimen (administer 30–60 minutes prior to delivery)
Intravenous therapy	Ampicillin OR	2 g IV
	Cefazolin or ceftriaxone	1 g IV
Allergy to penicillin or ampicillin	Cefazolin or ceftriaxone OR	1 g IV
	Clindamycin	600 mg IV
Oral	Amoxicillin	2 g
	* Vancomycin can be used if enterococcus is a concern	

Source: Practice Bulletin No. 120: Use of Prophylactic Antibiotics in Labor and Delivery [88]. Reproduced with permission of Lippencott Williams & Wilkins.

heparin, further discussed below) and an anti-arrhythmic agent such as digitalis (0.25 mg IV every 2 hours up to 1.5mg as a loading dose then 0.125–0.25 mg IV or 0.125–0.375 mg orally daily) [67].

Percutaneous balloon mitral valvuloplasty may be indicated during pregnancy for symptoms of atrial tachyarrhythmia and pulmonary edema that do not respond to typical medical management. More than 100 patients have undergone this procedure during pregnancy without increases in maternal or fetal mortality and it appears safer than the previously preferred open mitral commissurotomy [74]. Lead shielding should be used during the procedure if fluoroscopy is used; however, cases have been successfully performed with transesophageal echocardiography, which eliminates the radiation exposure to the fetus. Potential complications include cardiac tamponade, maternal arrhythmia, transient uterine contractions, and systemic thromboembolism [75].

Preferred mode of delivery depends on the severity of the lesion. As discussed above, patients with acute, severe pulmonary edema should undergo cesarean section. In addition, patients with severe mitral stenosis should undergo cesarean section under general anesthesia to prevent the fluid shifts that can occur with spinal anesthesia [71]. If a labor floor cannot accommodate monitoring with a pulmonary arterial catheter, cesarean delivery under general anesthesia may also be safer for the patient. Barring these situations, vaginal deliveries with either epidural or combined spinal/epidural are safe for most patients with mitral stenosis [67]. Continuous cardiac monitoring and pulse oximetry should be used during labor in addition to monitoring with a pulmonary arterial catheter as mentioned above. Use of mid-forceps to shorten the second stage of labor should be used for standard obstetric indications or if Valsalva results in dangerously low drops in preload [67,76]. Patients with moderate to severe disease typically require monitoring for 12–24 hours in an intensive care setting postpartum.

13.7.4 Cardiomyopathy

Peripartum cardiomyopathy is defined as development of cardiomyopathy (EF < 45%) in the last month of pregnancy or the first 5 months postpartum in a women without previous cardiac disease. This diagnosis can be made only after exclusion of other causes of cardiac failure [77]. The incidence in the United States is approximately 1 in 3000–4000 live births, with a peak in the second month postpartum. There is also an increased incidence among older women, multiparous women, African Americans, and those whose pregnancies were complicated by multiples and hypertensive disorders of pregnancy [78]. Patients report increasing fatigue, dyspnea, and edema. On exam there is evidence of heart failure including rales and jugular venous distension. Work-up for suspected cardiomyopathy should include chest X ray (infiltrates and blunted costophrenic angles), electrocardiogram (LV and atrial dilation), CBC, CMP, BNP, and echocardiogram.

Treatment for women with cardiomyopathy includes beta-blockers, diuretics, and afterload reducers. Oxygen and sodium restriction should also be utilized. Beta-blockers should be withheld until improvement in acute heart failure. The type of afterload reducer depends on whether the patient is antepartum or postpartum. In the antepartum period hydralazine is the preferred therapy whereas in the postpartum period angiotensin-converting enzyme inhibitors (ACE-I) and angiotensin II receptor blockers (ARBs) can be used. If the patient is still symptomatic despite maximum therapy on the above listed drugs, or has an atrial arrhythmia associated with the cardiomyopathy, digoxin may be used at doses of 0.375–0.5 mg/day [78]. In patients with decreased ejection fractions (<35%) anticoagulation should be considered to prevent intracardiac thrombosis. Either heparin products or warfarin may be used, depending on whether the patient is in the antepartum or postpartum period. For severely ill women, inotropes, vasopressors, and aldosterone antagonists can be added but should only be done in consult with a cardiologist or critical care specialist.

The mode of delivery for patients with peripartum cardiomyopathy is determined by obstetric indications and maternal functional status. For most patients, a vaginal delivery can be achieved when the mother receives appropriate medical management and has well compensated cardiac function [79]. Vaginal delivery allows for decreased blood loss, lower risk of postoperative infection, and greater hemodynamic stability. Continuous pulse oximetry and cardiac monitoring should be utilized during labor. Slow administration of epidural anesthesia provides pain control, minimizes tachycardia and hypertension secondary to pain response, and decreases preload and afterload to help accommodate volume from uterine autotransfusion after delivery [67]. Cesarean delivery should be reserved for obstetric indications and can be performed using spinal or general anesthesia. Patients typically require a pulmonary arterial catheter for invasive monitoring during labor and delivery [71].

An important note with peripartum cardiomyopathy is its tendency to recur. Up to one-third of patients will continue to have depressed left ventricular (LV) function or require a heart transplant at 1 year post diagnosis. Initial degree of LV dysfunction does not predict long-term outcome [75]. Those who have had a return to normal cardiac size and normal LV function can expect 11–14% mortality in subsequent pregnancies, but those with persistent cardiomyopathy have upwards of 40–80% mortality with a subsequent pregnancy. Patients with persistent cardiomyopathy or depressed LV function should be counseled against subsequent pregnancies [76,77]. Patients should be counseled early, preferably preconception, about these risks.

13.7.5 Pulmonary hypertension

Pulmonary hypertension is a disease process classically defined as a chronic elevation of mean pulmonary artery pressure (>25 mmHg at rest or > 30 mmHg with exercise) and low pulmonary capillary wedge pressure (<12 mmHg) diagnosed using right heart catheterization. Newer definitions from the World Health Organization include a systolic pulmonary artery pressure > 40 mmHg that can be diagnosed with echocardiography. Of note, an echocardiogram done during pregnancy may not truly be able to diagnosis pulmonary hypertension as echocardiograms done for this purpose are not generally accurate and can over- or underdiagnose the condition; however, cardiac catheterization, which is another method of assessing pulmonary hypertension, carries substantially more risk and should be avoided if possible in pregnancy [80]. Primary pulmonary hypertension is a contraindication to pregnancy as maternal mortality is approximately 50%, with most maternal deaths occurring during labor and the immediate postpartum period [81].

Patients with pulmonary hypertension will have symptoms of right heart failure and volume overload including pulmonary edema, dyspnea, and peripheral edema. Work-up is ideally done prior to conception but can include the following: CMP, CBC, BNP, electrocardiogram (right axis deviation, right ventricular hypertrophy, right ventricular strain, or right atrial enlargement), chest X ray (enlargement of central pulmonary arteries with peripheral tapering), echocardiography (tricuspid regurgitation, right ventricular and atrial enlargement, paradoxic motion of the intraventricular septum, reduction in LV size), and right heart catheterization (elevated pulmonary artery pressures and normal pulmonary capillary wedge pressure) [80]. Maternal hemoglobin should be maintained > 20 g/dL and P_aO_2 should be maintained > 70 mmHg [82,83].

Treatment in the antepartum period should be accomplished with consultation with a cardiologist and a maternal-fetal medicine specialist. Diuretics (furosemide) are used to treat the edema but the patient should be monitored for electrolyte abnormalities. Supplemental oxygen is required in most patients during pregnancy, especially as the gestation increases. Calcium channel blockers can be very effective in symptom improvement in 25–30% of patients, and those that respond favorably have an improved 5-year survival rate [84]. Other therapeutic options include ACE-inhibitors (in the postpartum period), adenosine, and anticoagulants (EF < 35%). Vasodilators are a relatively new addition to treatment but have proven to be very important in management of patients with pulmonary hypertension. Continuous infusion epoprosentol has been shown to lower pulmonary vascular resistance and improve right ventricular function [85]. Aerosolized iloprost and nitric oxide have also been shown to lower pulmonary artery pressure. Sildenafil is a new class of medication that has shown promise and can be used in pregnant patients [86].

Management of patients during labor involves intensive management. Patients should have placement of a pulmonary arterial catheter for more intensive monitoring of fluid status, continuous cardiac monitoring, and pulse oximetry [87]. Patients with pulmonary hypertension cannot tolerate hypotension well, so fluid management is very important. A Foley catheter should be placed to closely monitor fluid output and intravenous normal saline should be run as 125 ml/hr with fluid boluses used as needed (i.e. prior to epidural initiation). Endocarditis prophylaxis should be administered in patients with primary pulmonary hypertension 30–60 minutes prior to delivery [88]. Extreme caution should be taken to avoid hypotension with epidural administration, and slow initiation of epidural anesthesia or combined epidural/spinal anesthesia should be undertaken. General anesthesia should be avoided if possible due to increased pulmonary artery pressure and potential for alkalosis due to low P_aCO_2. Blood loss post-delivery should also be closely monitored as patients cannot tolerate large volumes of blood loss. Method of delivery should be vaginal delivery, with cesarean delivery being reserved for obstetric indications. Previous reviews of the literature have shown higher mortality with cesarean delivery versus vaginal delivery (63% vs 37%) and this may be a result of the higher blood loss and increased reduction in preload [87]. Patients should be monitored for hypercarbia, hypoxia, and acidosis, and pain, anxiety, and stress should be kept at a minimum as these can precipitate the above symptoms. Monitoring central venous pressure through a pulmonary arterial catheter can warn of impending right ventricular dysfunction in labor. Intrapartum inotropic therapy or pulmonary vasodilatory therapy may be required and require cardiology consultation. Patients should have an assisted second stage delivery with application of mid-forceps to decrease the amount of Valsalva needed during delivery as this will decrease preload.

The immediate postpartum period also requires close monitoring due to the fluid shifts and increases in pulmonary vascular resistance that occur. Oxytocin should be infused slowly after placental delivery because large boluses can be fatal in hemodynamically unstable therapy [89]. Anticoagulation should be started in the postpartum period if not previously given. Monitoring in a critical care unit for a minimum of 24 hours postpartum with typical postpartum hospital stay of at least 1 week is recommended.

13.8 Pulmonary disease

One of the most important physiologic adaptions in pregnancy is that of the maternal respiratory system. Upward displacement of the diaphragm as the uterus and fetus grow causes a decrease in functional residual capacity, decreased expiratory reserve volume, and decreased residual volume. The increased circulating levels of progesterone result in smooth muscle relaxation and outward displacement of the ribs. Maternal tidal volume increases, as does minute ventilation [90,91]. The respiration rate does not change during pregnancy and a persistent respiration rate > 20 should prompt a search for a cause. Pregnancy is a state of a mild respiratory alkalosis, with an arterial pH of 7.44, a bicarbonate level of 22 mE1/L, and a carbon dioxide level that slowly decreases to a nadir of 28–31 mmHg at term [92]. This normal respiratory alkalosis is important to keep in mind when reviewing blood gases of pregnant patients for abnormalities because typical values reported by laboratories are for a normal adult and pregnant women can be in respiratory distress despite having normal lab values of a non-pregnant adult. It is also important to remember that, due to the increased maternal oxygen consumption (as oxygen is shunted to the fetus and due to an increased basal metabolic rate) and decreased function residual capacity, any respiratory pathology can result in earlier maternal decompensation.

13.8.1 Pulmonary embolism

Pregnancy is a hypercoagulable state with an increase in plasma concentration of coagulation factors (fibrinogen, Factors VII, VIII, IX, X, XII, and von Willebrand factor) and a decrease in the activity of protein S, an anticoagulant factor [93]. The risk of venous thromboembolism (VTE) in pregnancy is increased sixfold, with further increases after cesarean delivery and situations requiring prolonged bed rest [94]. Personal history of VTE, presence of a thrombophilia, obesity, tobacco use, and hypertension further increase the probability of VTE during pregnancy and the postpartum period [11].

The presentation of a pulmonary embolism (PE) in pregnancy is variable and can be particularly difficult to identify. Symptoms that may be reported by a pregnant patient can include acute chest pain, shortness of breath, palpitations, and dizziness [95]. There is no one symptom that is diagnostic for a PE in pregnancy so clinical suspicion should be broad. Expert opinion suggests that any pregnant woman presenting with the report of acute onset of chest pain receive a computed tomographic pulmonary angiogram, or CTPA [96]. There are many benefits of a CTPA compared to other imaging studies of the lungs. A chest radiograph is rarely diagnostic of a PE and patients undergoing a chest radiograph for evaluation of a PE will likely require a subsequent study, which increases the amount of radiation the patient and the fetus are exposed to [96]. Ventilation-perfusion scans (VQ scans) require the injection and inhalation of radiolabeled isotopes, resulting in higher fetal exposure to radiation when compared to CTPA (0.11–0.22 mGy versus 0.003–0.08 mGy) [97]. However, the overall radiation dose with any test is very low with the risk of leukemogenesis estimated at 1/16,000 fetuses with exposure to 1 mGy of radiation [98]. Definitive diagnose of PE are significantly morc frequent with CTPA compared to VQ scans, more accurately diagnosing nonembolic causes of patients' symptoms than VQ scans. The false-negative rate for spiral computed tomographic scanners is approximately 5% [99,100]. Magnetic resonance arteriography (MRA) is a newer technology for evaluating the pulmonary vasculature. Benefits include the lack of any radiation; however, studies have not examined its accuracy in pregnant patients and it is a more time-consuming test than a CTPA. Although contrast pulmonary arteriography is considered the gold standard, the invasive nature of the procedure, with associated risks, exposure to iodinated contrast material, and level of radiation (0.5 mGy brachial vein route), in the presence of other accurate tests make it a prohibitive test during pregnancy [101].

Supplemental tests that may be performed on pregnant patients with a suspected PE include electrocardiogram, echocardiography, and arterial blood gas (ABG). An electrocardiogram is a quick, simple test to perform on patients presenting with chest pain, shortness of breath, and/or palpitations; however, "classic" electrocardiogram changes associated with PEs are typically only seen with massive PEs and are not universal (i.e. S_1 T_3 T_3 pattern, right bundle branch block, or right axis deviation) [102]. Furthermore, there are no reliable changes in pregnant patients with PE and the physiologic changes of pregnancy can produce abnormal electrocardiogram results. Echocardiography may be useful as it can demonstrate a dilated, hypokinetic right ventricle and tricuspid regurgitation, which are suggestive of PE, but optimal screening requires transesophageal echocardiography, which is technically more challenging than traditional echocardiography [108]. As previously mentioned, ABG results in pregnancy demonstrate a respiratory alkalosis, which is considered normal. ABGs done on non-pregnant, healthy patients with PE often fail to demonstrate low P_{O2} values that are seen in older patients with PE. P_{O2} levels are even higher in pregnant patients, which is likely to lead to false-negative results [109]. It is recommended that a pregnant patient being evaluated for PE with a $PaO_2 < 85$ mmHg should receive anticoagulation while diagnostic tests for PE are performed [51].

Treatment for pregnant patients who develop VTE requires prolonged use of anticoagulation therapy and this should continue into the immediate postpartum period. Therapeutic levels of anticoagulation should be used during pregnancy once PE has been diagnosed and then continue at prophylactic levels for up to 6 weeks postpartum. The mainstay of initial VTE therapy has been unfractionated heparin. Heparin products are considered safe during pregnancy and they do not cross the placenta. Initial dosing of unfractionated heparin should be weight based and be administered intravenously while the patient is an inpatient. Intravenous therapy is required for 5 days, with longer duration (7–10 days) for larger PE [105]. Upon discharge, unfractionated heparin can be administered subcutaneously twice daily. Unfractionated heparin therapy should be followed with aPTT levels. Goal levels during pregnancy are 1.5–2.5. Platelet counts also require monitoring during the first 2 weeks of heparin therapy due to the small possibility of developing heparin-induced thrombocytopenia (see below). Prophylactic dosing can begin after 4 months of therapeutic treatment and continue through 6 weeks postpartum [106]. Prophylactic dosing of unfractionated heparin consists of 5000 U subcutaneously twice daily and is increased by 2500 U in the second and third trimesters [106]. Benefits of using unfractionated heparin include ease of rapid reversal with protamine sulfate and long history of safe use and efficacy documented in pregnancy. Potential risks of using unfractionated heparin include bruising at injection sites and development of heparin-induced thrombocytopenia, unpredictable dose response, and bleeding complications. The main advantage is cost when compared to the newer low-molecular-weight heparins (LMWH).

LMWH has largely replaced the use of unfractionated heparin in the pregnant and non-pregnant population and has become the first line of therapy in both groups at Christiana Hospital. While, there are no studies looking at the effectiveness in the pregnant population, the studies from the non-pregnant population show that LMWH has fewer complications and a greater reduction in thrombus size compared to unfractionated heparin [107]. There are two LMWH agents approved for use, enoxaparin (1 mg/kg subcutaneously twice daily) and tinzaparin (175 IU/kg subcutaneously once daily). Dalteparin is a third agent that has been used off-label for VTE treatment (100 U/kg twice daily). During therapeutic treatment with LMWH it is recommended to monitor anti-Xa activity, with a goal of 0.5–1.0 IU/mL 4 hours after injection. Prophylactic dosing is not weight based for LMWH (enoxaparin 40 mg subcutaneously twice daily and dalteparin 5000 U subcutaneously once daily) [106]. Monitoring for an appropriate prophylactic LMWH dose anti-Xa level is controversial and if undertaken the goal is 0.6–1.2 mL 4 hours after injection [108]. Therapeutic treatment with LMWH for VTE should also be continued for 4 months during pregnancy and then transitioned to prophylactic doses continuing until 6 weeks postpartum [109]. Benefits of using LMWH include lower risk of heparin-induced thrombocytopenia, more predictable dosing effect, and fewer major hemorrhages and deaths. Both heparin products can result in bone mineral loss but the effect is less when using LMWH [110,111].

There are many other conditions during pregnancy that necessitate the use of anticoagulation, both therapeutic and prophylactic. Patients with thrombophilias with and without a history of VTE, a history of VTE that was estrogen related, and a history of VTE without a thrombophilia all require some form of anticoagulation [108]. The recommendation for therapeutic or prophylactic dosing, as well as whether treatment is required in the antepartum period, postpartum period, or both, depends on the patient's history (see Figure 13.2 and Figure 13.3) [108].

Clinicalscenario	Antepartum management	Postpartum management
Low-risk thrombophilia without previous VTE.	Surveillance without anticoagulation therapy.	Surveillance without anticoagulation therapy or postpartum anticoagulation therapy if the patient has additional risks factors.
Low-risk thrombophilia with a first-degree relative with a history of VTE.	Surveillance without anticoagulation therapy.	Postpartum anticoagulation therapy or intermediate-dose LMWH/UFH.
Low-risk thrombophilia with a single previous episode of VTE–not receiving long-term anticoagulation therapy.	Prophylactic or intermediate-dose LMWH/UFH or surveillance without anticoagulation therapy.	Postpartum anticoagulation therapy or intermediate-dose LMWH/UFH.
High-risk thrombophilia without previous VTE.	Surveillance without anticoagulation therapy or prophylactic LMWH or UFH.	Postpartum anticoagulation therapy.
High-risk thrombophilia with a single previous episode of VTE or first-degree relative with a history of VTE-not receiving long-term anticoagulation therapy.	Prophylactic, intermediate dose, or adjusted-dose LMWH/UFH regimen.	Postpartum anticoagulation therapy or intermediate or adjusted-dose LMWH/UFH for 6 weeks (therapy level should be at least as high as antepartum treatment).
No thrombophilia with previous single episode of VTE associated with transient risk factor that is no longer present–excludes pregnancy- or estrogen-relate drisk factor.	Surveillance without anticoagulation therapy.	Postpartum anticoagulation therapy.
No thrombophilia with previous single episode of VTE associated with transient risk factor that was pregnancy- or estrogen-related.	Prophylactic-dose LMWH or UFH.	Postpartum anticoagulation therapy.
No thrombophilia with previous single episode of VTE without an associated risk factor (idiopathic)–not receiving long-term anticoagulation therapy.	Prophylactic-dose LMWH or UFH.	Postpartum anticoagulation therapy.
Thrombophilia or no thrombophilia with two or more episodes of VTE–not receiving long-term anticoagulation therapy.	Prophylactic or therapeutic-dose LMWH or prophylactic or therapeutic-dose UFH.	Postpartum anticoagulation therapy or therapeutic-dose LMWH/UFH for 6 weeks.
Thrombophilia or no thrombophilia with two or more episodes of VTE–receiving long-term anticoagulation therapy.	Therapeutic-dose LMWH or UFH.	Resumption of long-term anticoagulation therapy.

Figure 13.2 Recommendations for anticoagulation prophylaxis or treatment during the antepartum and postpartum period for women with a history of VTE or inherited thrombophilia from the American College of Obstetricians and Gynecologists. Low-risk thrombophilias include factor V Leiden heterozygous, prothrombin mutation heterozygous, and protein C or S deficiency. High risk thrombophilias include antithrombin deficiency, double heterozygous prothrombin mutation and factor V Leiden, factor V Leiden homozygous, and prothrombin mutation heterozygous. *Source*: American College of Obstetricians and Gynecologists Practice Bulletin No. 138. Thromboembolism in Pregnancy. ACOG: Washington, DC. 2013. Reproduced with permission of Lippencott Williams & Wilkins.)

Management of anticoagulation around the time of delivery requires the obstetrician to balance effective anticoagulation with the patient's desire for pain relief during labor and delivery. Patients who have been receiving anticoagulation

Management type	Dosage
Prophylactic LMWH	Enoxaparin, 40 mg SC once daily Dalteparin, 5000 units SC once daily Tinzaparin, 4500 units SC once daily
Therapeutic LMWH (also referred to as weight-adjusted, full-treatment dose)	Enoxaparin, 1 mg/kg every 12 hours Dalteparin, 200 units/kg once daily Tinzaparin, 175 units/kg once daily Dalteparin, 100 units/kg every 12 hours Target anti-Xa level 0.6–1.0
Minidose prophylactic UFH	UFH, 5000 units SC every 12 hours
Prophylactic UFH	UFH, 5000–10000 units SC every 12hours UFH, 5000–7500 units SC every 12 hours in first trimester UFH, 7500–10000 units SC every 12 hours in the second trimester UFH,10000 units SC every 12 hours in the third trimester,unless the aPTT is elevated
Therapeutic UFH (Also referred to as weight-adjusted, full-treatment dose)	UFH, 10,000 units or more SC every 12 hours in doses adjusted to target aPTT in the therapeutic range (1.5–2.5, 6 hours after injection)
Postpartum anticoagulation	Prophylactic LMWH/UFH for 4–6 weeks or Vitamin K antagonists for 4–6 weeks with a target INR of 2.0–3.0, with initial UFH or LMWH therapy overlap until the INR is 2.0 or more for 2 days

Figure 13.3 Prophylactic and therapeutic anticoagulation doses for the antepartum and postpartum periods from the American College of Obstetricians and Gynecologists. *Source*: American College of Obstetricians and Gynecologists Practice Bulletin No. 138. Thromboembolism in Pregnancy. ACOG: Washington, DC. 2013. Reproduced with permission of Lippencott Williams & Wilkins.)

during the antepartum period, either prophylactic or therapeutic, should be switched to unfractionated heparin around 36–37 weeks of gestation due to the possibility of spontaneous labor beyond this point [106]. Unfractionated heparin around the time of delivery is desirable because protamine is available as a reversal agent and it has a shorter half-life [112]. Patients can safely deliver 4–6 hours after the last dose of prophylactic unfractionated heparin administration. Patients who are on unfractionated heparin who deliver before 4–6 hours from their last heparin dose or experience bleeding require rapid reversal with protamine. Protamine is administered by IV infusion starting at < 20 mg/min with no more than 50 mg/10 minutes [113]. Small repeated infusions of protamine are generally required when heparin is administered subcutaneously. Patients can safely receive spinal or epidural anesthesia when they are on prophylactic doses of unfractionated heparin (5000 U subcutaneously twice daily). Patients on therapeutic doses of heparin should have their aPTT checked before induction of anesthesia to assure the level is not too high. Patients who have been on prophylactic LMWH prior to delivery can receive neuraxial anesthesia 10–12 hours from the last dose or 24 hours from the last therapeutic dose [114]. All patients who have been receiving anticoagulation therapy during the antenatal period should have pneumatic compression boots placed during delivery, for either cesarean delivery or vaginal delivery. Resumption of either LMWH or unfractionated heparin after delivery should not be started sooner than 4–6 hours after vaginal delivery and 6–12 hours after cesarean delivery [106]. If the patient received an epidural for pain control during labor and is restarting therapeutic doses of anticoagulation it may be safer to wait 12 hours after removal of the epidural [114].

Warfarin is considered contraindicated during pregnancy because of known teratogenicity; however, many patients are bridged to warfarin in the postpartum period as it is an oral medication, is easier to administer, and likely has a higher compliance. Initial warfarin dosing should be 5 mg for 2 days with subsequent doses being determined by monitoring the international normalized ratio (INR). Patients being transitioned to warfarin must be maintained on LMWH or unfractionated heparin until the INR is in the therapeutic range (2–3) for 2 consecutive days to ensure that patient dose not experience paradoxical thrombosis and skin necrosis. Duration of anticoagulation therapy in the postpartum period depends on the condition for which the woman was receiving anticoagulation therapy [106]. Patients who are receiving anticoagulation for a VTE that occurred during pregnancy should receive anticoagulation for at least 6 weeks postpartum and up to 6 months postpartum depending on when the VTE occurred during the antepartum period and for how long the patient has been receiving treatment already [115]. Warfarin is safe in the postpartum period and can be used for mothers who are breastfeeding [116,117]. Vitamin K can be used for patients with elevated INRs, orally if there is no associated bleeding and by subcutaneous dosing if the patient is experiencing bleeding complications. Fresh frozen plasma can be used in cases of severe hemorrhage.

Second-line therapies for VTE are reserved for patients with special considerations. Fondaparinux is a synthetic heparin pentasaccharide that can be used in patients who have heparin-induced thrombocytopenia type 2. Weight-based, subcutaneous, once-daily dosing is used for treatment. This drug is considered class B in pregnancy and has been successfully used in a small number of pregnancies [118,119]. Thrombolytic therapies have been used in some pregnant women. Concerns for use in the antenatal period are due to the risk of abruption and puerperal hemorrhage. There is a small risk of maternal and fetal mortality associated with this treatment and it should be reserved for patients who have failed with heparin therapy, with large PE causing hemodynamic instability.

Pregnant patients begun expeditiously on appropriate treatment for VTE experience a very low mortality rate [108]. The mortality rate increases with hemodynamic instability, typically seen with larger PE, and for patients with delayed diagnosis and treatment of PE [108]. Patients with known thrombophilias, history of VTE, or strong family history of VTE should be seen in consultation to see if they require antepartum anticoagulation.

Although rare, inferior vena cava (IVC) filter placement is indicated in conditions where recurrent thromboembolism occurs despite adequate anticoagulation or when anticoagulation is contraindicated, such as after a delivery complicated by severe hemorrhage. Preliminary experience appears reassuring with the use of a vena cava filter in pregnancy [120].

13.9 Renal disease

13.9.1 Normal renal disease

Demands and resultant adaptive physiologic changes occur in the renal system of pregnant women. Renal plasma flow increases by up to 80% during the mid-second trimester before falling to 50% above prepregnancy values by the third trimester [121]. Glomerular filtration rate (GFR) also increases in pregnancy to a peak of about 50% above prepregnancy values at the end of the third trimester. This increase in GFR leads to decreased serum creatinine and urea concentrations [122]. Serum creatinine levels fall during pregnancy in each trimester with mean levels of 0.7, 0.6, and 0.5 mg/dL in the first, second, and third trimesters, respectively. Urea concentrations also decrease but not in the same linear fashion [123]. Due to this expected decrease in creatinine, creatinine levels around normal non-pregnant values, especially in the third trimester, should be considered abnormal. Overall, there is a net increase in sodium and potassium during pregnancy, primarily due to increased reabsorption [124,125]. There is increased glucose excretion in pregnancy as a result of impaired reabsorption such that low levels of glycosuria are not uncommon in pregnancy [126].

13.9.2 Chronic renal disease

Chronic renal disease is a relatively uncommon finding in pregnant patients because of the associated reduced fertility rates and increased rates of early spontaneous abortion. In addition, many women with severe renal impairment are often beyond childbearing age [127]. Disease prevalence is estimated to be between 0.03 and 0.12% of pregnant women [128].

Pregnancy outcomes with chronic renal disease vary greatly depending on the patient's stage of renal dysfunction. Chronic kidney disease (CKD) is classified into five stages based on the patient's GFR. Patients with mild disease (CKD stage 1 and 2) have a lower risk of adverse pregnancy outcomes compared to patients with higher disease stages. Patients with mild disease have a GFR of > 60 mL/min and a serum creatinine of 0.9–1.4 mg/dL. While there are increased risks for intrauterine growth restriction (IUGR), preterm delivery, and preeclampsia in women with mild CKD during labor and delivery, care does not differ from that for patients without renal disease [129]. Patients may experience some worsening of their renal function during gestation due to the increased demand placed on the kidneys from the increased plasma volume, but this has not been shown to persist after delivery and there does not appear to be any adverse effect of pregnancy on long-term maternal renal outcomes [130].

Patients with moderate to severe CKD (stages 3–5) have much poorer reproductive outcomes compared to patients with mild disease. Due to the small number of patients who fall into this category, most of the data on outcomes on these patients come from small, observational, retrospective studies [113]. Patients in this category have a GFR of < 60 mL/min and a serum creatinine of > 1.4 mg/dL. When discussing risks for pregnancy in this population it is important to further break down baseline serum creatinine. Almost 50% of patients with a baseline serum creatinine of 1.4 mg/dL or greater can expect a worsening of renal function during pregnancy, with half of these patients having persistent deteriorated function postpartum [131]. As many as 65% of patients with a baseline creatinine of > 2 mg/dL experience a decline in renal function during pregnancy, nearly all have persistent deteriorated renal function, and 35% progress to end-stage renal disease [132,133].

Worsening renal function in pregnancy is not uncommon in patients with renal disease and in some cases may lead to the need for dialysis in patients who previously did not require this intervention. Indications for dialysis in the pregnant population are similar to those for the non-pregnant population. Indications include severe metabolic acidosis, creatinine and/or urea build-up (>5–7 mg/dL and > 60–8 mg/dL, respectively), electrolyte imbalances (particularly hyperkalemia), and volume overload causing congestive heart failure or pulmonary edema [128]. Regardless of whether dialysis was begun before or during pregnancy, two types are available: hemodialysis and peritoneal dialysis. Hemodialysis uses vascular access for extracorporeal treatment, whereas peritoneal dialysis uses a surgically placed peritoneal catheter that is left in the peritoneal cavity. Both types have risks and benefits but have similar fetal survival rates. Hemodialysis can be easier to initiate when a patient is already pregnant, but peritoneal dialysis catheters have been reported to be placed as late as at 29 weeks of gestation [134]. Hemodialysis does require the use of anticoagulation and typically results in a more severe anemia than peritoneal dialysis. Peritoneal dialysis allows for the steady-state removal or urea and results in fewer episodes of hypotension (and placental insufficiency) due to the easier fluid removal and less fluid fluctuation [135,136]. The disadvantages to peritoneal dialysis are: peritonitis, which is rare, possible laceration of enlarged uterine vessels during later gestation, and the need to stop dialysis if a cesarean delivery is indicated to allow for wound healing and to prevent peritoneal dialysate leaking [137,138]. Restarting peritoneal dialysis after delivery should begin with small volumes and gradually increase as needed. It is useful to remember that, regardless of the dialysis type, the time spent dialyzing increases the further a patient gets in gestation.

Patients with renal disease are at an increased risk for maternal anemia, preeclampsia, IUGR, and preterm delivery. The physiologic anemia of pregnancy is worsened by the deficiency in erythropoietin due to kidney disease and the suppression of bone marrow due to uremia. Fortunately, recombinant erythropoietin can be used in pregnancy with little complication [139]. Blood transfusions and iron supplementation should also be used as necessary. The risk of preeclampsia increases with the severity of CKD, and patients with a creatinine of > 2 mg/dL have up to a 60% risk of developing preeclampsia during pregnancy. Preeclampsia in a patient with chronic renal disease should be managed the same as in a patient without renal disease. Because the incidence of IUGR also increases with increasing CKD stage, patients with chronic renal disease should be monitored by ultrasound and patients with severe IUGR (< fifth percentile) may necessitate preterm delivery. The incidence of preterm delivery is > 95% when the patient's creatinine is > 2 mg/dL [129,132]. However, even patients with stage 1 or 2 CKD have an incidence of preterm delivery of 30% [140].

While the use of tocolytics to prevent preterm birth remains controversial. Magnesium sulfate, calcium channel blockers (nifedipine) and indomethacin have all been used safely for tocolysis in women with chronic renal disease [141]. Magnesium sulfate infusion, whether for tocolysis or for seizure prophylaxis for preeclampsia, typically has to be decreased to 1 mg/hr in patients with kidney disease, and magnesium levels should be checked frequently in this population, with a goal of 5–7 mg/dL [51]. The use of MgSO4 for neuroprotection is becoming more common; however, in women with renal insufficiency the proper dosing or level to see a potential benefit is unclear. Those patients who necessitate preterm delivery due to non-reassuring fetal testing or preterm labor or premature preterm rupture of membranes should be allowed to have a trial of vaginal delivery or induction or labor. There is no difference in the mode of delivery for patients with chronic renal disease regardless of whether they are on dialysis or not. During labor patients should have extremely close monitoring of fluid balance. Patients should also be receiving close blood pressure monitoring due to the increased risk of preeclampsia. Patients can opt for any type of pain relief during labor, although if an epidural or spinal is utilized there should be consideration to slow initiation of anesthesia to avoid fluid shifts that the patient may not be able to compensate for and that may result in prolonged uteroplacental insufficiency. Cesarean delivery should be reserved for obstetric indications. As stated above, peritoneal dialysis will have to be held to allow for healing of the abdominal wall and hemodialysis can be utilized in the interim [138,142].

Patients who have a renal transplant require intense monitoring during the antepartum period just like other renal disease patients. These patients are also at risk for hypertensive complications of pregnancy, IUGR, anemia, and preterm delivery. In addition, their immunosuppressive regimen requires close monitoring by a multidisciplinary team. That being said, 90% of pregnant women who have a renal transplant and make it past the first trimester succeed in having a live born infant [143]. Mode of delivery in these patients should not be influenced by the presence of the transplant, and cesarean delivery should be reserved for obstetric reasons. The typical lower-uterine segment approach for cesarean delivery is usually reasonable but care should be taken during the surgery because the pelvis is the frequent location of transplanted kidneys and scarring can make identification of normal anatomic structures difficult.

13.10 Diabetes

13.10.1 Normal changes in pregnancy

Pregnancy is a state of maternal insulin resistance. This metabolic alteration leads to hyperinsulinemia and fasting hypoglycemia. These changes allow a constant supply of nutrients to reach the growing fetus. Insulin resistance is brought about by the pregnancy-related hormone human placental lactogen. After delivery, this hormone rapidly decreases causing insulin and glucose levels to return to their normal, nonpregnancy state. Despite these physiologic changes in glucose metabolism in pregnancy, most women should be able to compensate appropriately without developing hyperglycemia. Those women who develop persistent hyperglycemia during pregnancy are at increased risk for adverse maternal and fetal outcomes. Women with gestational diabetes require increased surveillance during

Table 13.12 White's classification of diabetes.

White class	Age at onset or duration	Complications
A	Any	Diagnosed in pregnancy no vascular disease
B	≥20 years old at diagnosis OR < 10 years duration	No vascular disease
C	10–19 years old at diagnosis OR 10–19 years duration	No vascular disease
D	<10 years old at diagnosis OR ≥ 20 years duration	Background retinopathy only or hypertension
E		Calcification of pelvic arteries (no longer used)
F		Nephropathy (>500 mg of proteinuria per day)
H		Artherosclerotic heart disease
R		Proliferative retinopathy of vitreous hemorrhage
T		After renal transplantation

pregnancy. Those with preexisting diabetes (type 1 and type 2), 8.8% of women over 20, also require increased surveillance during pregnancy to ensure euglycemia and good pregnancy outcomes [144].

13.10.2 Gestational diabetes

Gestational diabetes (GDM) has been defined by the American Diabetes Association as diabetes diagnosed during pregnancy that is not clearly overt diabetes [145]. This definition includes women who may have some level of insulin resistance outside of pregnancy but have not been previously diagnosed as having diabetes. Eighty-five percent of the reported cases of diabetes in pregnancy are due to GDM [146,147]. GDM affects 3–9% of pregnant women. Screening for GDM should take place between 24 and 28 weeks of gestation for all pregnant women; however, patients with certain risk factors (obesity, strong family history of diabetes, history of GDM) should be screened as soon as they present for prenatal care [148,149]. The current guidelines for screening for GDM in the United States involves a 1-hour glucose tolerance test, and those patients who have elevated 1-hour glucose levels go on to a 3-hour glucose tolerance test. Current cutoff values for having patients proceed with a 3-hour glucose tolerance test vary across the United States. Cutoff values of 130 mg/dL for the 1-hr screening test result in a sensitivity of nearly 100% and increase the percentage of patients requiring a 3-hour test to 23%. Alternatively, if a cutoff value of 140 mg/dL is used for the 1-hour screening test the sensitivity will be 90% and 14% of patients will require the 3-hour diagnostic test [149]. If patients have two out of four glucose levels elevated on the 3-hour test then they are considered to have GDM.

Pregnancies complicated by GDM are at risk for adverse maternal and fetal outcomes. The presence of GDM increases maternal risks for cesarean delivery, shoulder dystocia, hypertensive disorders of pregnancy (gestational hypertension and preeclampsia), increased weight gain during pregnancy, polyhydramnios, and higher likelihood of induction of labor [147]. Infants born to mothers with GDM

Table 13.13 Carpenter–Coustan blood glucose cutoffs for the 100-gram glucose test in pregnancy. Two or more values elevated above the cutoffs are used to diagnose the patient with gestational diabetes.

Status	Plasma or Serum Glucose Level Carpenter/Coustan Conversion	
	mg/dL	mmol/L
Fasting	95	5.3
One hour	180	10.0
Two hours	155	8.6
Three hours	140	7.8

Table 13.14 Duration and onset of action for various types of insulin used in pregnancy.

Insulin type	Time to peak action (hr)	Total duration of action (hr)	Additional information
Lispro (Humalog®)	1–2	4–5	Onset within 10 min of injection; do not delay meal.
Aspart (Novolog®)	1–2	4–5	Onset within 10 min of injection; do not delay meal.
Regular insulin	2–4	6–8	Onset within 30 min; give 20–30 minutes prior to eating.
NPH	5–7	13–18	Intermediate-acting; control risk of 3AM hypoglycemia.
Glargine (Lantus®)	No peak	24	Prolonged flat action; limited pregnancy experience.

are at increased risk of neonatal hypoglycemia, hyperbilirubinemia, polycythemia, large for gestational age, and birth trauma.

Patients initially diagnosed with GDM should undergo counseling on a diabetic diet and be instructed on home monitoring of blood sugars, which typically involves checking fasting and postprandial blood sugars during the remainder of their pregnancy. Patients who can maintain adequate glycemic control, typically defined as a fasting glucose of 90–99 mg/dL and 1-hour postprandial glucose of < 140 mg/dL or a 2-hour postprandial glucose of 120–127 mg/dL, on diet alone are classified as A1 diabetics [148].

Patients compliant with the diabetic diet who consistently have blood glucose values outside expected ranges require some type of glycemic control with medication and are considered A2 diabetics. Adequate glycemic control in patients with GDM decreases the risks of large-for-gestational age infants, birth weight > 4000 g, shoulder dystocia, cesarean delivery, and hypertensive disorders of pregnancy [147]. There is no one preferred treatment for patients with GDM requiring treatment with more than diet. Glyburide is a second-generation sulfonylurea that was shown in 2000 to be comparable to insulin for glucose control in GDM with no increase in fetal macrosomia [150]. Typical dosing for glyburide is begun at 2.5 mg daily and can be increased to 20 mg daily and given in divided doses. Although glyburide is still considered a pregnancy category C drug by the Food and Drug Administration (FDA), reports of fetal anomalies have been largely anecdotal. Metformin, a biguanide, is another oral hypoglycemic agent that has been studied for use during pregnancy. Most information on drug safety with metformin comes from use in type 2 diabetics and patients with polycystic ovarian syndrome using metformin for ovulation induction, and it is considered an FDA pregnancy category B drug even though it readily crosses the placenta. Dosing typically starts with 500 mg daily and is increased slowly (due to gastrointestinal side effects) to a maximum dose of 2000 mg daily. When metformin was compared to insulin there were no differences in neonatal hypoglycemia, respiratory distress, need for phototherapy, birth trauma, and prematurity; however, a recent randomized control trial showed that metformin was not as effective as glyburide and resulted in a failure rate 2.1 times higher than glyburide [151,152]. Insulin therapy has been the preferred medication for glucose control for women with GDM for many years. The type of insulin used (long acting versus short acting) and the dosing schedule vary with patients and where their individual elevated glucose readings fall.

Patients with well controlled GDM (controlled by diet or medication) are not at increased risk for stillbirth and in general do not require induction of labor prior to 39 weeks of gestation [153]. Timing delivery between 39 and 40 weeks allows for adequate fetal lung development, which is delayed in pregnancies complicated by diabetes, but decreases the risk of fetal macrosomia and birth trauma related to macrosomia. After 40 weeks of gestation the benefits of conservative management are less than the potential fetal risks from induction of labor. Although macrosomia can still be a concern in this population even prior to 39 weeks of gestation, ultrasound estimates of fetal weights come with a margin of error. One study reported that only 50% of the infants predicted to be ≥ 4500 g were within 10% of this estimated weight at delivery [154]. Despite this margin of error with ultrasound, given the risks of shoulder dystocia and birth trauma associated when the estimated fetal weight (EFW) is > 4500 g, elective cesarean delivery can be considered according to ACOG [155]. When the EFW is between 4000 and 4500 g, the patient's history, clinical pelvimetry, and fetal abdominal circumference should be taken into consideration when deciding between vaginal and cesarean delivery. Patients with GDM do not have any special anesthesia considerations in labor.

Blood glucose management during labor is extremely important to prevent neonatal hypoglycemia upon delivery. Patients on long-acting insulin therapy should not take their long-acting insulin on the day of labor induction or cesarean delivery [153]. Glucose levels should be obtained on arrival to labor and delivery. Care should be taken to ensure patients with GDM do not receive intravenous fluids containing dextrose. There are no set criteria for blood glucose monitoring intrapartum but these patients should have their blood glucose periodically checked with frequency increasing to every 1–2 hours when the patient is in the active stage of labor. ACOG recommends that patients with persistent blood glucose elevations > 110–120 mg/dL require insulin therapy during labor; however, the majority of women with well controlled GDM do not require use of insulin during labor [153]. Use of insulin drips during labor will be discussed further below. Patients presenting for a cesarean delivery with an initial blood glucose > 140 mg/dL should receive some type of insulin therapy before delivery. Postpartum, patients with GDM should have their blood glucose monitored in a similar fashion to antepartum while in the hospital to ensure a return to a euglycemic state while off medical therapy and diet restrictions. Due to the fact that 35–60% of patients will develop type 2 diabetes within 10 years, these patients require long-term follow-up, starting with a 2-hour glucose tolerance test approximately 6–8 weeks postpartum [148].

13.10.3 Preexisting diabetes

Patients with diabetes prior to pregnancy comprise a much smaller percentage of diabetes in pregnancy compared to GDM. This group includes patients with type 1 diabetes (autoimmune destruction of pancreatic β-cells) and type 2 diabetes (loss of balance between insulin sensitivity and insulin response). Patients with preexisting diabetes are at even more risk for adverse pregnancy outcomes than patients with GDM. These patients may have preexisting renal disease, hypertension, or heart disease, making pregnancy more risky. In addition, these patients are at increased risk of preeclampsia, cesarean delivery, congenital anomalies, miscarriages, fetal growth abnormalities (IUGR and macrosomia), stillbirth, fetal cardiac anomalies, and neonatal respiratory distress, in addition to the same complications that can affect patients with GDM. These patients require much more intensive antenatal monitoring compared to patients without diabetes, including an increase in office visits, serial sonograms for fetal growth, fetal echocardiography, and testing for fetal well-being.

Ideally, patients with preexisting diabetes will have an endocrinologist or maternal-fetal medicine specialist who has been managing their diabetes and ensuring optimal glycemic control prior to pregnancy. Patients should be instructed to switch their blood glucose monitoring schedule to fasting and 1 hour postprandial. The same parameters for glucose control apply as listed above. Strict glucose control is important to decrease the risks of pregnancy complications and diabetic ketoacidosis (discussed further below). Additionally, patients desiring conception should ideally have their diabetes controlled with a medication proven to be safe for use during pregnancy (i.e. insulin, glyburide, or metformin). The dosing parameters for glyburide and metformin are the same as listed above. Patients, particularly type 1 diabetics, need to be vigilant about monitoring blood sugars, being aware of symptoms of hypoglycemia and hyperglycemia and reporting these to their obstetrician and/or endocrinologist. Patients familiar with carbohydrate counting can continue to do so but the ratio of insulin to grams of carbohydrate typically needs to be adjusted (first trimester 1:15, second trimester 1:10 to 1:6, third trimester 1:6 to 1:2). Patients who are very strict about their diet and monitoring carbohydrate intake have better outcomes when using carbohydrate counting to help dose their insulin [113]. Finally, patients who have been using an insulin pump for diabetic control prior to pregnancy can continue use antenatally. Two small cohort studies showed no difference in glycemic control, perinatal outcome, macrosomia, and cesarean delivery rates in patients using insulin pumps compared to standard insulin administration [156,157]. Benefits of insulin pump use include continuous, programmable infusion with changing basal rates depending on the time of day and no need for needles, syringes, or medication vials. Downfalls of pump therapy include the possibility of insulin pump malfunction, abscess formation, and unexpected poor uptake from injection site. Use of an insulin pump requires a knowledgeable and committed patient with co-management with endocrinology. As pregnancy progresses, insulin and hypoglycemic agents needs increase due to the relative insulin resistance encountered by pregnancy, regardless of the type of diabetes the patient has.

During labor, glucose management becomes particularly important, not just to prevent neonatal hypoglycemia but to prevent hypoglycemia or hyperglycemia in the mother, which could lead to a potentially dangerous situation such as diabetic ketoacidosis. Patients controlled on oral hypoglycemic agents should not take their morning dose of medication on the day of planned cesarean delivery or induction of labor. Blood glucose monitoring during labor follows the same general guidelines for type 2 diabetics as for gestational diabetics. Blood glucose levels should be monitored periodically in labor with frequency of monitoring increasing to every 1–2 hours in the active phase of labor. Blood glucose goals should be < 110–120 mg/dL [157]. Type 2 diabetics with acceptable blood glucose during labor can receive normal saline for IV fluids. If a patient's blood glucose drops below 70 mg/dL their IV fluids should be switched to a solution containing 5% dextrose and their blood sugars should be monitored every hour [158].

Patients who are continually at or above blood glucose of 110–120 mg/dL require an insulin drip during labor. Additionally, all type 1 diabetics require an insulin drip during labor as their body does not produce insulin. Use of insulin drips in labor requires IV fluids that contain 5% dextrose and initial IV infusion rate should be 100 mL/hr. The combined use of glucose and insulin maintains the maternal blood glucose in a more narrow range and reduces the incidence of neonatal hypoglycemia [159]. The insulin drip should contain regular insulin and dosing depends on the patient's measured blood glucose. Patients should have their blood glucose monitored hourly while they are on an insulin drip. If a facility cannot do an insulin drip, an intermittent subcutaneous injection method is possible. Patients should take half of their normal insulin dose in the morning before induction of labor or cesarean delivery. Intravenous fluids containing 5% dextrose at 100 mL/hr are used throughout labor. Maternal blood sugars are checked hourly and regular insulin is administered at doses between 2 and 5 units to maintain maternal blood sugars in the target range [113]. Postpartum insulin requirements rapidly decrease and patients' insulin and oral hypoglycemic regimens should be decreased appropriately to avoid hypoglycemia. Patients can also go back to checking blood sugars as they did prior to conception.

Timing of delivery for patients with preexisting diabetes should be a balance between decreasing neonatal morbidity and mortality and maximizing the chance for a vaginal delivery. In general, delivery before 38 weeks without other indication is generally not recommended as fetal lung maturity is delayed in diabetic pregnancies, especially those that have had less than good control. Indications for delivery at < 38 weeks of gestation include non-reassuring fetal assessment, evidence of fetal growth arrest, decline in fetal growth rate with decreased amniotic fluid, preeclampsia, or failing maternal renal function. A study by Kios *et al.* showed that expectant management of patients with class B diabetes beyond 38 weeks did not alter the cesarean delivery rate but did increase the percentage of infants with shoulder dystocia and large for gestational age [160]. Patients with diabetes should be allowed a trial of labor if there are no obstetric indications. The same ACOG recommendations for elective cesarean delivery of a suspected macrosomic infant apply to patients with pregestational diabetes (see above) [158]. There are no contraindications to IV analgesia, epidural, spinal, or general anesthesia in patients with preexisting diabetes.

13.10.4 Diabetic ketoacidosis

Diabetic ketoacidosis (DKA) is a serious metabolic complication and can be seen in any type of diabetic in pregnancy but is most frequently observed in in type 1 diabetics. While the risk of maternal death from DKA is currently < 1%, fetal loss rates remain as high as 10–25% [161,162]. Risk factors for development of DKA during pregnancy include accelerated starvation, dehydration, decreased caloric intake (secondary to nausea), decreased buffering capacity (pregnancy is a state of compensated respiratory alkalosis), stress, patient non-compliance, and presence of insulin antagonists.

Patients in DKA will present with feelings of malaise, emesis, weakness, polyuria, polydipsia, tachypnea, and dehydration. Kusmal respirations and a fruity odor on the patient's breath (due to the presence of acetone) may also be noticed. Patients with pregnancies complicated by diabetes presenting with any of these symptoms should have their blood glucose checked immediately; however, the glucose level alone should not be used to rule a patient in or out for DKA. In a report by Cullen, four out of 11 patients presented in DKA with an initial glucose < 200 mg/dL [163]. Initial laboratory work-up, besides a serum glucose, for patients suspected of DKA should include electrolytes, serum osmolality, creatinine, BUN, urinalysis, arterial blood gas, lactic acid, CBC, and serum acetone and plasma β-hydroxybutyric acid if possible. A pH < 7.4 should cause concern as pregnancy is normally a state of compensated respiratory alkalosis. Also concerning is an anion gap of > 12. Serum potassium may appear falsely elevated at first as acidosis causes extracellular movement of potassium ions, but one should keep in mind that DKA is typically associated with hypokalemia.

If clinical suspicion is high for DKA, treatment should be initiated while waiting for laboratory results to return. Since fluid management is imperative in the management of pregnant patients with DKA, patients should have IV access obtained and fluid boluses of isotonic saline should be started immediately. After two 1-liter boluses over 1 hour the fluid rate can be decreased to 250 ml/hr. A Foley catheter should be placed to adequately monitor the patient's fluid

Table 13.15 Management of fluid and metabolic derangements associated with diabetic ketoacidosis in pregnancy.

Maternal assessment	• Arterial blood gas • Oxygen saturation monitoring • Urine culture • Chest X ray and/or blood cultures if indicated
Insulin therapy	• Regular insulin • Loading dose: 0.2–0.4 units/kg • Maintenance 2–10 units/hr • If serum glucose does not decrease by 50 mg/dl in the first hour, then double the infusion rate • When serum glucose 200 mg/dl decrease the infusion rate to 0.05 units/kg/hr • Maintain serum glucose in 150–200 mg/dl range
Fluid management	• Place Foley catheter • Goal urine output > 50 cc/hr • Initial IV fluids: normal saline at 1 liter/hr x2 hours • 500–1000 ml/hr for the next 2–4 hours • 250 ml/hr until 80% replaced • Goal 4–6 liters replaced in first 12 hours • When serum glucose is 200–250 mg/dl concert to D5 ½ normal saline
Potassium management	• K < 3.3 mEq/L then infuse 15–20 mEq/hr • K > 5.3 mEq/L repeat assessment every 2 hours until < 5.3 mEq/L • K 3.3–5.3 mEq/L add 20–30 mEq to each liter of IV fluid to maintain K in the range of 4–5 mEq/L
Bicarbonate management	• No replacement if maternal pH > 7.1 • pH < 7.1 add 1 ampule (44 mEq) in 1 liter of ½ normal saline

balance. Insulin therapy should be started as soon as possible. Subcutaneous therapy can be used if immediately available and intravenous therapy is not. Treatment should be started with an insulin bolus (10–15 units either intravenous or subcutaneously) and then given at a continuous rate of 0.1 units/kg/hr. Serum glucose should be monitored hourly and continuous infusion rate should be increased if there is no significant drop in glucose in the first hour of treatment. Insulin therapy will predictably drive potassium ions intracellularly, so if the initial potassium level is < 3.3 mEq/L then a potassium infusion (10 mEq/hr) should be administered prior to giving insulin. Serum potassium levels should be monitored every 1–2 hours and replaced as needed. In general, patients should have repeat ABG and electrolytes drawn every 1–2 hours to monitor the acidosis and electrolyte disturbances. Other laboratory values can be repeated as necessary. Replacement of bicarbonate is an area of controversy in pregnant patients with DKA. In general there is a limited amount of data on bicarbonate administration when pH is < 7.0; however, the limited studies that exist fail to demonstrate a difference in outcome [164,165]. Due to the small amount of data, bicarbonate (one ampule = 44 mEq) administration is recommended when pH is < 7 or bicarbonate level is < 5. Fetal monitoring should be started in patients with viable pregnancies. However, fetal distress is not uncommon in patients with DKA; this is due to vasoconstriction and dehydration in the mother and hyperglycemia and osmotic diuresis in the fetus. The acidotic maternal pH will also result in an acidotic fetal pH. Despite any non-reassuring features of the fetal heart tracing, every effort should be made to correct the DKA before proceeding to delivery. Correcting DKA will often improve the fetal tracing and allow for pregnancy prolongation [166]. If the fetal heart tracing does not improve with correction of DKA or if there are other obstetric indications then delivery should occur.

13.11 Neurologic disorders

13.11.1 Seizure disorders

Seizure disorders are the second most common neurologic problem seen during pregnancy, the first being migraines. The cause of new-onset seizures during pregnancy must be investigated and can include epilepsy, eclampsia, electrolyte disturbances, vascular malformation, hemorrhage, intracranial mass, substance abuse or withdrawal, and infection. In general, patients with new-onset seizures should have a careful history taken including questions about symptoms of infection, preceding headache, substance abuse, medication adherence, vision disturbances, and family and past medical history. Laboratory investigation to consider includes CBC, CMP, magnesium, calcium, and phosphorous, urine drug screen, and CT of the head.

Epilepsy is a predisposition to recurrent seizures based on dysfunction of the central nervous system and has a prevalence of 5–10/1000 in the developed world [167]. This prevalence is not any different in reproductive-aged women. Pregnancy does not have a predictable effect on seizure frequency. Previous studies report that approximately 25% of women had decreased seizure frequency, 25% had increased seizure frequency, and 50% had no change [168].

Epilepsy can adversely affect pregnancy outcomes. There has been a consistently higher stillbirth rate reported among epileptics, likely related to the acidosis and hypoxemia that occur during seizures. Neonatal deaths are also increased in this population but the exact reason is not known. The increase may be related to increased incidence of congenital malformations, preterm delivery, and seizures. Increases in preterm delivery, preeclampsia, and hemorrhage have been reported inconsistently in pregnant women with epilepsy [169,170].

Management of antiepileptic drugs can be one of the more challenging parts of managing epilepsy during pregnancy. All antiepileptic drugs have some level of folic acid antagonism, which increases the risks of neural tube defects, heart defects, and cleft lip and palate in fetuses [171]. Despite this fact, discontinuation of these medications during gestation is not recommended and all pregnant

Table 13.16 Clinical presentation and diagnostic work-up for various neurologic conditions commonly seen in pregnancy.

Condition	Clinical presentation	Diagnostic work-up
Brain tumor	Most likely to become symptomatic in the first trimester. Rare.	Papilledema prominent with supratentorial tumors.
Intracranial hemorrhage	Sudden, severe headache or loss of consciousness.	Arteriovenous malformations more likely in younger, non-hypertensive patients. Aneurysms are more likely in older, parous, hypertensive patients.
Cerebral venous thrombosis	Fluctuating deficits and/or consciousness.	More common in late pregnancy and postpartum.
Gestational epilepsy	Variable. Very rare.	Diagnosis of exclusion.
Eclampsia	Preceded by general headache, visual disturbances, and/or abdominal pain.	Associated with hypertension, proteinuria, and other symptoms and laboratory abnormalities (elevated liver function studies, decreased platelets).
Pseudoseizures	Atypical physical findings (unresponsiveness without movement, asynchronous extremity movement, geotropic eye movements).	

patients with a known seizure disorder should be receiving additional folic acid supplementation of at least 4 mg/day starting prior to conception; however, the actual supplement dose needed in this population is not truly known [172]. Due to the increased maternal blood volume and hepatic metabolism associated with pregnancy, there is a decrease in the total amount of antiepileptic medication circulating in pregnant women [169]. Drug levels should be monitored in these patients and adjusted as needed. Because blood volume fluctuates during the postpartum period, drug levels should be monitored and adjusted as needed. Co-management with the patient's neurologist is an important part of the management of antiepileptic medications.

There are multiple antiepileptics that can be used to manage seizure disorders during pregnancy. Valproic acid is one medication that is discouraged due to its higher risk of neural tube defects compared to other medications. Other commonly used medications include carbamazepine, Dilantin, Neurontin, ethosuximide, phenytoin, and phenobarbital [51]. These medications come with their own side effects, including congenital malformations (phenytoin, phenobarbital, and carbamazepine), neonatal withdrawal (phenobarbital), cardiac malformations, and potential coagulopathy [171]. The coagulopathy has not been shown consistently and as most infants now receive vitamin K injections at birth the bleeding

Table 13.17 Dosages of commonly used antiepileptic drugs in pregnancy.

Drug	Dose
Carbamazepine	Starting dose 200 mg BID Max dose 1600 mg/d
Dilantin	Starting dose 100 mg TID Max dose 600 mg/d
Neurontin	Starting dose 300 mg TID Max dose 1800 mg/d
Ethosuximide	Starting dose 500 mg/d Max dose 1.5 g/d
Phenytoin	Starting dose 100 mg TID Max dose 600 mg/d
Phenobarbital	Starting dose 50–100 mg ID or TID Max dose 400 mg/d

tendency is usually mitigated [173]. Patients should be continued on their antiepileptic medications during labor to prevent seizures during labor.

Patients with well controlled seizure disorders do not require induction of labor and most patients in this group can have successful vaginal deliveries. There is a subset of patients for whom cesarean delivery should be considered and that includes patients with seizures during labor, patients with poor seizure control, patients with neurologic or mental deficits that prohibit following commands for pushing during labor, and patients with other obstetric indications [174]. As with eclamptic seizures during labor, the mother should be stabilized before proceeding with cesarean delivery and efforts should be made to correct non-reassuring fetal heart tracings related to seizures before making the decision to proceed with cesarean delivery. Patients should receive an anesthesia consult prior to labor. In general, patients can have IV analgesia, epidural, or spinal anesthesia as required as there is no evidence of adverse effects on seizure frequency with their use.

13.11.2 Status epilepticus

Status epilepticus is a rare complication of epilepsy in pregnant patients but is a medical emergency and should be distinguished from eclampsia. Occurrence is $< 1\%$ of all pregnant patients with epilepsy and is defined as a state in which seizures occur without full recovery in-between or when a seizure lasts more than 30 minutes. Unlike eclamptic seizures, these may not be self-limited and can result in significant maternal and fetal mortality related to hypoxia and acidosis. Gaining control of the seizure as soon as possible is of the utmost importance because the longer the seizure activity continues the more difficult it is to halt the seizures and the higher the fetal and maternal mortality.

The first step when a patient is noted to be having a seizure during pregnancy, regardless of whether or not the patient is in status epilepticus, should be

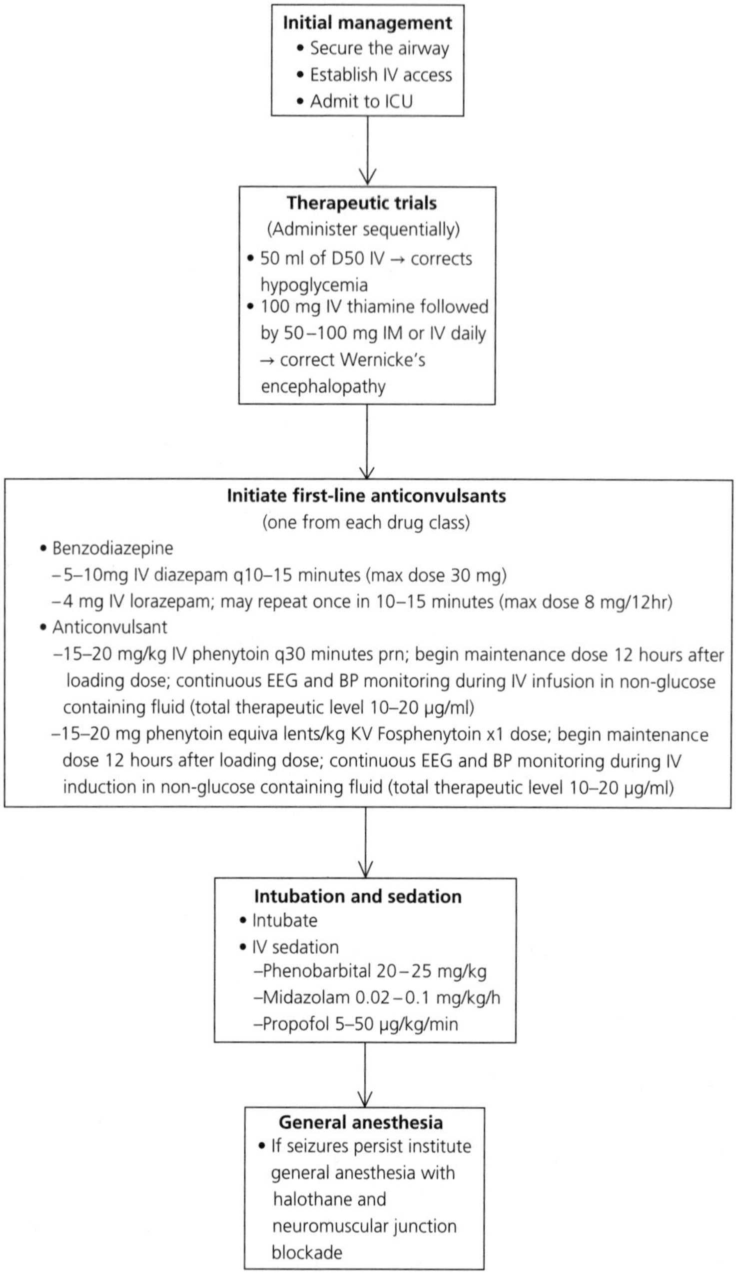

Figure 13.4 Flowchart for management of status epilepticus in a pregnant patient.

to secure a maternal airway, and oxygen should be administered as necessary as judged by pulse oximetry (see Figure 13.4). Intubation should be used if necessary. Intravenous access should be obtained if the patient does not already have IV access and care should be taken to protect the mother from injury (lowering the patient to the floor, bedrail pads). Laboratory studies should be obtained but should not prevent treatment initiation. Laboratory studies should include a CBC, electrolytes, calcium, glucose, phosphorus, UDS, arterial blood gas, and levels of anticonvulsant drugs if appropriate. Fetal well-being should be assessed with fetal heart rate monitoring when of a viable gestational age.

Once eclampsia has been ruled out, initial treatment of seizure activity in pregnancy should include administration of a glucose bolus and thiamine. These two agents are administered simultaneously to diagnose and treat hypoglycemia and Wernicke's encephalopathy, respectively, and regardless of the etiology these will not worsen the patient's condition. The next agent to add if the patient is still seizing is IV lorazepam or diazepam, which can be repeated at 10- to 15-minute intervals as needed. An anticonvulsant, such as phenytoin or fosphenytoin, should be administered next. Persistent seizure activity at this point should result in sedation and intubation of the patient. Sedation can be accomplished with phenobarbital, or with general anesthetic if seizure activity persists through the phenobarbital. Continuous electroencephalographic (EEG) monitoring with neurologist supervision should occur at this point [175,176].

Many physiologic changes can accompany status epilepticus. Hypertension, maternal tachycardia, and cardiac arrhythmias can be seen in addition to fetal tachycardia. Non-reassuring fetal heart tracings can be seen as well. Hyperthermia can result from vigorous, continuous muscle activation. Lactic acidosis can also result for the same reason.

13.11.3 Cerebrovascular accidents

Although rare, cerebrovascular accidents (CVA) or strokes account for almost 15% of maternal deaths. Risk of thrombotic CVA increases during pregnancy (12–13x) regardless of other risk factors a patient may possess [177]. Other risk factors include African American ethnicity, maternal age > 35, hypertension, heart disease, thrombophilia, sickle cell disease, anemia, thrombocytopenia, lupus, blood transfusion, obesity, diabetes, substance abuse, and migraine headaches [178]. Between 8 and 15% of patients who suffer a stroke during pregnancy die and another 10% are discharged to some sort of assisted living facility [179]. CVAs can be the result of vessel occlusion or hemorrhage and the cause must be sought out to ensure correct treatment. Treatment requires co-management with critical care specialists, neurologists, and potentially neurosurgeons. While this chapter focuses on management of CVAs during labor it should be noted that only around 10% of CVAs occur during the antepartum period, 40% immediately around labor and delivery, and the majority, 50%, in the postpartum period [179].

Symptoms of stroke in a pregnant patient are similar to those of a non-pregnant patient (one-sided weakness, altered gait, altered speech, loss of consciousness, confusion, visual disturbances). This patient population may also experience transient ischemic attacks that precede a major thrombotic event. Initial work-up of these patients should include CBC, erythrocyte sedimentation rate, electrolytes, coagulation studies (PTT and aPTT) and electrocardiogram. Cranial CT is also vitally important to distinguish hemorrhagic from thrombotic stroke. Pregnancy should not deter obtaining a CT when the suspicion is high and shielding of the abdomen can be accomplished to decrease radiation dose to the fetus (<1 milirad exposure). If the CT does not show evidence of a hemorrhage then the patient should receive an MRI/MRA/MRV to evaluate for thrombotic events [180,181]. There is no radiation involved in the procedure and it is considered generally safe in pregnancy. While iodinated CT contrast can be used in pregnancy (class B) the gadolinium used for MRI contrast should be avoided as it crosses the placenta and has unknown fetal effects. If suspicion is high for an arterial thrombotic event then the patient should be begun on anticoagulation therapy as soon as hemorrhagic event has been ruled out.

Anticoagulation with therapeutic dosing of IV heparin is the preferred initial treatment. The patient can then be maintained on subcutaneous heparin. Studies have not been done evaluating the effectiveness of fixed, therapeutic-dose low-molecular heparin but it may be a suitable alternative. Alternative treatment with thrombolytic agents, such as tissue plasminogen activator (tPA) has been used in some cases successfully. Treatment with tPA should be begun within 3 hours of symptom onset at a dose of 0.9 mg/kg (maximum dose 90 mg). The first 10% is given as a bolus with the rest following as a continuous infusion over 1 hour [182]. Multiple case reports and one case series with 28 patients exist for patients receiving tPA in pregnancy. In the case series, thrombolysis was successful in 25 of the 28 patients, two patients had subsequent death (7%), and two cases of pregnancy loss were directly attributed to tPA administration. Of note, this case series included patients receiving tPA for indications other than CVA [183]. Hemorrhagic complications are more likely in the first few days after administration and this treatment should not be used close to delivery or in the immediate postpartum period due to bleeding risks. Warfarin may be used in the postpartum period to maintain anticoagulation.

Delivery method for patients with thrombotic arterial occlusive events depends on how much time there is between injury and delivery. Patients with remote events that are under maintenance anticoagulation and have no neurologic deficit can typically undergo a vaginal delivery unless obstetric indications exist that necessitate a cesarean delivery. Patients with neurologic deficits that impair pushing may require delivery via cesarean section. Also, patients who have acute thrombotic events during labor should be stabilized as best as possible before undergoing an emergent cesarean delivery so appropriate work-up and treatment can be started as soon as possible. Anticoagulation should be managed as discussed above.

Patients with venous thrombotic events can also be seen during pregnancy. Thrombosis of the cerebral veins and sinuses occurs more often in females and usually occurs later in gestation or during the immediate postpartum [184]. Symptoms of cerebral venous occlusion can be similar to arterial occlusion but more often include persistent headache and seizures. A low-grade fever may also be noted. The symptoms are generally more insidious in onset, resulting in an average time from symptom onset to diagnosis of 7 days [185]. CT and MRI are used in diagnosis and the same laboratory work should be performed as for arterial thrombotic events. The CT will look normal, with venous occlusion just as with arterial, and MRI should show a hyperintense signal from the thrombosed area. Venous occlusions can result in increase in intracranial pressure more so than arterial occlusion, so papilledema may be seen in addition to increased cerebrospinal fluid pressure if a lumbar puncture is performed [184]. Thrombosis of superior sagittal sinus is particularly common in pregnant patients [198]. Risk factors for venous thrombosis include inherited and acquired thrombophilias (including pregnancy alone), sickle cell disease, and direct mechanical cause (i.e. head injury, lumbar puncture) [186]. Anticoagulant treatment for venous thrombosis follows the same guidelines as for arterial thrombosis, and tPA should be used with the same caution [187]. Patients with venous thrombosis may also require anticonvulsants to control seizures, if they occur, and agents to control cerebral edema, such as dexamethasone and mannitol. Patients with events remote from delivery can usually undergo a vaginal delivery, with assisted second stage if needed due to continued increased intracranial pressure at baseline. Patients with thrombosis close to delivery or during labor should usually undergo a cesarean delivery to prohibit increases in intracranial pressure.

13.11.4 Cerebral aneurysm

Aneurysms are a saccular dilation of a blood vessel, typically located at the angle of bifurcation. The true incidence of cerebral aneurysms is likely underestimated as the majority (95%) are asymptomatic and can easily go undetected. Locations from most to least common are internal carotid, anterior communicating/anterior cerebral artery, posterior communicating artery, and vertebral/basilar artery. Rupture rate for asymptomatic aneurysms is 1–2% per year with preceding activities involving those that can increase intracranial pressure (including emotional strain, heavy lifting, coughing, coitus, urination, and defecation). Rupture rates for symptomatic aneurysms are higher at 6% [188].

Optimal management of patients with aneurysms should involve co-management with a neurologist, neurosurgeon, or both. Ideally, patients with known aneurysms will have had surgery (embolization, clipping, or coils) to obliterate the aneurysm. Patients who have had treatment for cerebral aneurysms can have a spontaneous vaginal delivery, with cesarean delivery being reserved for obstetric indications. These patients can also safely have epidural or spinal anesthesia as desired [189].

Patients with known aneurysms that are found during pregnancy or have not been treated prior to pregnancy present a larger concern. Aneurysms can be successfully treated during pregnancy with coils or clips, both of which have been shown to decrease maternal mortality. The use of coils via intravascular delivery has been performed successfully in pregnancy and may be preferred as it is less invasive compared to open clipping [190,191]. Mode of delivery in these patients varies. Some physicians recommend elective cesarean delivery due to the fear of increased intracranial pressure with Valsalva during vaginal delivery; however, there are studies showing no increase in intracranial hemorrhage with untreated aneurysms in vaginal delivery compared to cesarean delivery [191,193]. The lower hemorrhage risk occurs due to cerebral autoregulatory changes that may provide compensatory relief in otherwise healthy patients. Epidural anesthesia can further decrease intracranial pressure increases during vaginal delivery [193].

Due to the fact that the vast majority of cerebral aneurysms are asymptomatic, it is very possible that a pregnant patient may present with intracranial bleeding as the first indication of the aneurysm's presence. Mortality from aneurysms increases drastically once bleeding occurs and those that survive often have lasting neurologic deficit [194]. Symptoms from intracerebral hemorrhage are not altered by pregnancy and include primarily headache (subarachnoid hemorrhage (SAH) – sudden-onset, intracerebral hemorrhage – slower onset) and can also include loss of memory and/or focus, nausea and vomiting, hypertension, loss of consciousness, and seizures [195]. Of note, intracerebral hemorrhage can occur from other processes, including hypertension, drug use (i.e. cocaine), trauma, arteriovascular malformations, and bleeding diatheses [196]. Aneurysmal bleeding typically results in subarachnoid hemorrhage and occurs in 20–30/100,000 pregnancies [197]. The risk of bleeding increases as pregnancy progresses, likely due to the increase in blood volume. Maternal mortality approaches one-third of patients and fetal mortality approaches 25% in patients with aneurysms. The patient's neurologic condition upon presentation is an important indicator of overall outcome [189].

Diagnosis of SAH due to ruptured aneurysm should include a CT of the head, which will identify the type of intracerebral hemorrhage with great accuracy. Fetal exposure to radiation can be decreased with shielding and typically results in 2 mrad of exposure [198]. A lumbar puncture can be used as a follow-up test if the CT is normal but the clinical suspicion of SAH remains high. Cerebrospinal fluid will be bloody and not clear throughout the procedure. Laboratory studies should include a work-up for preeclampsia (electrolytes, LFTs, creatinine), coagulation studies, CBC, and UDS. Patients should also receive an emergent neurology or neurosurgery consult with presumption of ruptured cerebral aneurysm. Continuous fetal monitoring should be utilized in patients with viable pregnancies. Blood pressure control is critical in these patients. Other considerations include hyperosmotic agents to lower intracranial pressure (i.e. mannitol) and agents to help prevent cerebral vasospasm [198]. Nimodipine is the most commonly used agent to prevent cerebral vasospasm in SAH and has been used safely in pregnancy, as demonstrated in studies of patients with preeclampsia/eclampsia [199,200]. Early aneurysm repair (48–72 hours after rupture) improves long-term survival.

Clipping and intravascular coil placement have both been used successfully [193]. No trials currently exist comparing coiling and clipping in pregnant patients.

Delivery indications in patients presenting with aneurysm rupture depend largely on gestational age. Patients below viability at their presenting institution should be treated with the focus on the treatment of the bleeding aneurysm. Patients with viable gestations who are not in labor should also have their treatment focused on their aneurysm [201]. Patients who present in labor or who have aneurysmal rupture during labor should undergo an emergent cesarean delivery before treatment for the aneurysm begins [202]. Cesarean delivery should also be used for patients with poor neurologic status after aneurysm rupture (i.e. unable to follow commands for pushing) and for those patients who go into labor after aneurysm repair or rupture in the preceding 2 months. Epidural anesthesia is considered acceptable for patients remote from aneurysm rupture with aneurysmal repair [202].

13.11.5 Myasthenia gravis

Myasthenia gravis (MG) is an autoimmune disorder affecting neurotransmitters on skeletal muscle resulting in weakness and easy fatigability. Patients with MG have an IgG antibody against the nicotinic acetylcholine receptors at the neuromuscular junction. Diagnosis is typically made prior to pregnancy and is established by injection of edrophonium chloride with ensuing muscle weakness [203]. The incidence is 14–20/100,000 people and occurs more often in females. Treatment of MG involves anticholinesterases (typically pyridostigmine), steroids, intravenous immunoglobulins, and plasmapheresis. Thymectomy may also be used to treat MG [204].

Pregnancy's influence on MG varies. One study showed improved symptoms during pregnancy in patients on therapy in 39%, with no change in symptoms in 42%, and worsening symptoms in 19% [205]. Maternal risks during pregnancy include myasthenic crisis, respiratory failure, and, rarely, death. Fetal effects include neonatal myasthenia (poor cry, respiratory difficulties, weak suckling), which occurs in 10–15% of infants born to mothers with MG. There is no correlation between disease severity and presence of neonatal MG. Treatment is with anticholinesterase drugs and symptoms typically resolve by 6 weeks of life [206].

During labor, patients who have been controlled on pyridostigmine should continue to receive their medication. Pyridostigmine can be administered via the intramuscular or intravenous route at 1/30th the patient's oral dose, if necessary [204]. Overtreatment can result in a cholinergic crisis (salivation, diaphoresis, diarrhea, miosis, abdominal cramps). Muscle weakness may occur with under- or overtreatment.

Patients who have been on chronic steroids (20 mg of prednisone daily for 3 or more weeks) prior to delivery should receive stress dose steroids to prevent adrenal crisis. During labor 100 mg hydrocortisone IV every 8 hours should be used. Patients undergoing a cesarean delivery should have 100 mg hydrocortisone IV prior to the start of the procedure. Postpartum patients should receive 50 mg hydrocortisone IV every 8 hours for 24 hours with a taper afterwards back to their normal daily dose [206].

Certain medications should be used with caution in patients with MG. Magnesium sulfate is contraindicated in patients with MG even if they develop preeclampsia/eclampsia, as it can worsen muscle weakness and precipitate and myasthenic crisis [204]. Alternative antiseizure medications should be used in these patients (phenytoin). Narcotics, barbiturates, and inhaled anesthetics can also precipitate a crisis or cause more respiratory depression than seen in a patient without MG [207].

Mode of delivery and choice of anesthesia are not affected by the presence of MG but anesthesia should be involved in the care early in these women. Epidural and spinal anesthesia is preferred to general anesthesia, as mentioned above. Patients should have a trial of labor as the uterine smooth muscle is not affected by the IgG antibodies. Prolonged activation of skeletal muscle during pushing may lead to fatigue, and assisted second stage with vacuum or forceps may be necessary. Cesarean delivery is reserved for obstetric indications [207].

13.11.6 Multiple sclerosis

Multiple sclerosis (MS) is a disorder that involves demyelination in the central nervous system at various sites and varying times. There are two courses to the disease: relapsing and remitting and chronic disease. In the former case, patients have great variation in the types and timing of exacerbations, with either complete or partial remission of symptoms in-between exacerbations. This type does result in increasing disability over many years. The later disease course has a slow, progressive course without remission periods. Women are affected more often than men. Disease symptoms can include diplopia, speech and gait abnormalities, and sensory disturbances. Physical findings include cerebellar ataxia, hyperreflexia, spasticity, and lower extremity weakness [208].

Treatment of the disease during symptom flares includes corticosteroids. Baclofen and dantrolene are used to treat painful spasms of the lower extremities in patients with more advanced disease [209]. Interferon beta-1a is a newer therapy used to treat some patients with MS. A recent small case series of patients treated with this drug had 32 patients with fetal exposure during pregnancy and resulted in 20 full-term, healthy infants, one preterm delivery, eight spontaneous abortions, one case of hydrocephalus, and one intrauterine fetal demise. There were not statistically significant differences from the patients not treated with interferon beta-1a [210]. No treatment is required during remission periods and therapy is primarily supportive. Patients with urinary retention are prone to bladder infections, and prophylactic antibiotic treatment may be required, especially during pregnancy. Patients with lower extremity symptoms may require ambulatory aids and should be counseled on falls during pregnancy.

Disease in pregnancy usually follows a predictable course. Most patients experience a remission during gestation with an increased tendency toward exacerbations in the postpartum period (up to 3–6 months). This is thought to be due to the exogenous increase in corticosteroids during pregnancy that helps to suppress symptoms. After delivery, corticosteroid levels drop abruptly resulting in MS flares [211,212].

Patients with MS should be allowed to have a vaginal delivery. The one exception may be patients with severe spasticity of the lower extremities, which can prohibit pushing in second stage of labor [213]. Patients with mild to moderate spasticity who have been on baclofen for treatment may continue this treatment intrapartum. Patients who were on chronic steroids immediately prior to delivery should be given stress dose steroids as discussed above. There is no contraindication to epidural or spinal anesthesia in these patients. Epidural anesthesia during labor may help to improve lower extremity spasticity in some patients. Cesarean delivery should be reserved for obstetric indications only [209,213].

13.12 Infections

13.12.1 Human immunodeficiency virus

Human immunodeficiency virus (HIV) is an infection caused by an RNA virus that has two strains, 1 and 2. Type 1 is more prevalent in the United States and throughout the world, and type 2 is more common in sub-Saharan Africa. While once a fatal diagnosis, with the advent of antiretrovirals people are living longer and having successful pregnancies. One of the most important points related to pregnancy is the decrease in maternal-fetal transmission accomplished in recent years. HIV screening with enzyme immunoassay (EIA) should be part of routine prenatal testing and in high-risk patients should be repeated again during the third trimester. Diagnosis prior to labor is essential to decrease maternal-fetal transmission. Positive results on the EIA should prompt the physician to send a Western blot confirmatory test; in most cases this is reflexive [214].

Risk factors for acquisition of the disease include multiple sexual partners, receptive anal intercourse, unprotected intercourse, concurrent STDs (particularly those with ulcer formation), sexual contact with an uncircumcised male, and bleeding during intercourse [215]. Transmission from receiving of blood products, organ donation, and artificial insemination is extremely rare [215]. The natural course of HIV progresses from the acute retroviral illness to the latent phase over a matter of weeks. During the latent phase viral loads tend to be low and patients may not know they are infected. Over a period of years the disease progresses to a symptomatic phase and eventually to acquired immunodeficiency syndrome (AIDS).

Patients diagnosed with HIV should have their CD4 counts and viral loads followed to monitor disease progression. The recommendation for non-pregnant women is to begin antiretroviral treatment when the CD4 count is < 350 mm/^{3}

Table 13.18 Recommended treatments for opportunistic infections in AIDs patients.

Condition	Treatment
Pneumocystis carinii pneumonia	TMP-SMX 1 DS tab daily indefinitely.
Toxoplasmosis encephalitis	TMP-SMX 1 DS tab daily indefinitely.
Tuberculosis	INH 300 mg daily plus pyridoxine 50 mg daily for 1 year.
Disseminated Mycobacterium avium complex (MAC)	Azithromycin 1200 mg weekly.
Cryptococcosis	Routine prophylaxis not needed; patients with previous treatment for acute infection require fluconazole 200 mg daily indefinitely.

Source: Kaplan *et al.*, 1995 [219].

or when the viral load is > 30,000–55,000 copies/mL, depending on the assay used. In pregnant patients the threshold for treatment is much lower as mother-to-fetus transmission rates are linked to viral loads and start increasing before 55,000 copies/mL is reached. Viral loads > 1000 copies/mL are shown to increase transmission rates especially in vaginal deliveries [214]. Without any treatment the risk of transmission is around 25%, but with appropriate azidothymidine therapy it can be reduced to 2% [216,217]. It is important to counsel HIV positive pregnant women on the importance of adherence to antiretroviral regimens during pregnancy as non-compliance increases the chances for the virus to become resistant, making treatment later for the mother and child increasingly difficult. In addition to viral load, other factors that affect transmission include history of a previously affected infant, severe maternal disease, preterm delivery, intrapartum blood exposure, rupture of membranes > 4 h, invasive antepartum procedures, chorioamnionitis, and concurrent STDs [218]. Additional testing that should be performed in pregnant patients with HIV, if not recently performed, includes STD screening, testing for hepatitis B and C, PPD to test for TB, toxoplasmosis, and cytomegalovirus. Patients at risk of opportunistic infections based on CD4 counts should receive all appropriate prophylaxis.

Treatment with highly active antiretroviral therapy (HAART) is the most important intervention to decrease maternal-fetal transmission [215]. Zidovudine was the first agent shown to decrease transmission rates and should be used whenever possible. Current dosing for adults is 200 mg three times daily or 300 mg twice daily [217]. The initial trial showed a decrease in transmission from 26 to 8% with zidovudine alone [216]. Multidrug therapy has been shown to decrease transmission rates to < 2%. The combination of zidovudine (300 mg) plus lamivudine (150 mg), also known as Combivir (ViiV Healthcare, Middlesex, UK), twice daily, and ritonavir (400 mg) plus lopinarvir (100 mg), also known as Kaletra (AbbVie, Chicago, IL), twice daily, is the current recommended treatment in pregnancy. A failure to decrease viral load within 12–16 weeks should prompt investigation into viral resistance [217]. Other drug regimens exist and can be used if viral resistance or patient allergy prevents use of Combivir and Kaletra. Antiretrovirals that should definitely not be used in pregnancy include efavirenz (teratogenic), hydroxyurea (teratogenic), and the combination of stavudine and didanosine (fatal lactic acidosis) [217].

Method of delivery is dependent on viral load at the time of delivery. Patients with viral load levels < 1000 copies/mL can be allowed to have a vaginal delivery; however, patients with viral loads > 1000 copies/mL despite adequate response to antiretroviral therapy should be offered a cesarean delivery at 38 weeks to decrease the chance of spontaneous labor and rupture of membranes, which increases the risk of vertical transmission. All patients should receive IV zidovudine regardless of cesarean or vaginal delivery. Patients undergoing vaginal delivery should have a bolus dose of 2 mg/kg over 1 hour then 1 mg/kg/hr until delivery. Those scheduled for cesarean delivery should receive zidovudine 2 mg/kg over an hour 4 hours prior to surgery [220–222]. Alternative regimens exist if zidovudine is not an option in labor. Patients who present in labor without known HIV status should have rapid testing performed. If rapid results return positive the patient should be counseled that a cesarean delivery and zidovudine prophylaxis prior to delivery will decrease vertical transmission [214,223]. Infants delivered to seropositive mothers are treated with antiretroviral agents for at least the first 6 weeks postpartum to further decrease transmission rates. Antiretrovirals in the mother may be discontinued after delivery if she does not meet non-pregnant criteria for the use of antiretrovirals [217].

13.12.2 Herpes simplex virus

Herpes simplex virus (HSV) is typically a relatively mild disease in mothers but when transmitted vertically can cause severe infections in neonates involving the central nervous system, skin, and mucous membranes. HSV infection in the newborn can be lethal. There are two types of HSV, 1 and 2. Classically HSV type 1 was more frequently associated with infection of the mouth and HSV type 2 was more often associated with genital infection; however, HSV 1 is accounting for increasing numbers of primary genital herpes outbreaks and type does not affect management in pregnancy [224].

HSV can clinically present in three ways: first episode with primary genital herpes (no antibodies present, symptoms lasting 3–6 weeks), first episode with non-primary genital herpes (antibodies present, symptoms present 1–2 weeks), and recurrent genital herpes (symptoms 1–2 weeks with milder symptoms). This distinction is important because the rates of vertical transmission are highest in primary infection when maternal antibodies are not present to provide some passive immunity to the fetus. Symptoms of genital HSV infection include painful vesicular lesions with or without tender inguinal adenopathy and fever. Testing when lesions are present involves viral culture from unroofed vesicles. This is the gold standard test and is most sensitive within the first 48–72 hours of lesions

Table 13.19 Recommend doses of antiviral medications for herpes in pregnancy.

Indication	Acyclovir	Valacyclovir
Primary or first-episode infection	400 mg orally, three times daily, for 7–10* days	1 g orally, twice daily, for 7–10* days
Symptomatic recurrent episode	400 mg orally, three times daily, for 5 days or 800 mg orally, twice daily, for 5 days	500 mg orally, twice daily, for 3 days or 1 g orally, daily, for 5 days
Daily suppression	400 mg orally, three times daily, from 36 weeks estimated gestational age until delivery	500 mg orally, twice daily, from 36 weeks estimated gestational age until delivery
Service or disseminated disease	5–10 mg/kg, intravenously, every 8 hours for 2–7 days, then oral therapy for primary infection to complete 10 days	

* Treatment may be extended if healing is incomplete after 10 days.

Adapted from Sexually transmitted diseases treatment guidelines, 2006 (published erratum appears in *MMWR Recommendations and Reports* 2006;55:997). Centers for Disease Control and Prevention. *MMWR Recommendations and Reports* 2006;55(RR-11):1–94.

appearing. Tzanck smear is much less sensitive and cannot differentiate between HSV 1 and 2 [225]. PCR to detect HSV is also available and useful because it involves serum, and lesions do not have to be present; however, routine serologic testing for HSV in pregnant women is controversial and has not been shown to be cost-effective [226,227].

Neonatal infection is acquired primarily through exposure to an infected lower maternal genital tract. The risk is considerably higher with primary infection compared to recurrent infections and with infections that occur closer to delivery compared to those that occur earlier in gestation [248]. Transplacental congenital infection is exceedingly rare and is thought to be the result of maternal viremia.

All mothers with known HSV history should be offered prophylaxis at 36 weeks of gestation. Acyclovir 400 mg three times daily or valacyclovir 500 mg twice daily are the current prophylactic recommendations [229]. Prophylaxis is recommended for all women known to be seropositive for HSV (even if there is no history of outbreaks) because asymptomatic viral shedding can occur in all women and daily prophylactic treatment has been shown to decrease viral shedding [228]. When patients with a history of HSV present in labor they should have a thorough external genital exam as well as a speculum exam to evaluate for HSV lesions. Patients should also be asked about any prodromal symptoms. Patients with prodromal symptoms or with HSV lesions seen on exam should have cesarean delivery. Patients without lesions or prodromal HSV symptoms can proceed with vaginal delivery. Treatment for primary or recurrent outbreaks is shown in Table 13.19 [229]. Supportive measures such as oral analgesics and topical anesthetics can also be used during HSV outbreaks. Patients with oral HSV at the time of delivery should be cautioned not to touch their infant until the lesions have become encrusted.

References

1 Herminda RC, Ayala DR, Mojon A *et al.* Blood pressure patterns in normal pregnancy, gestational hypertension and preeclampsia. *Hypertension* 2000;**36**:149–158.

2 Gaillard R, Bakker R, Willemsen SP *et al.* Blood pressure tracking during pregnancy and the risk of gestational hypertensive disorders: the generation R study. *European Heart Journal* 2011;**32**:3088–2097.

3 Robinson SC, Dunlop W, Boys RJ *et al.* Cardiac output during labor. *BMJ* 1987;**295**:1169.

4 American College of Obstetrics and Gynecology Taskforce on Hypertension in Pregnancy. *Hypertension in Pregnancy*. Washington, DC: ACOG, 2013.

5 American College of Obstetrics and Gynecology Practice Bulletin No. 125: Chronic Hypertension in Pregnancy. Washington, DC: ACOG, 2012.

6 Sibai BM. Diagnosis and management of gestational hypertension and preeclampsia. *Obstetrics & Gynecology* 2003;**102**:181–192.

7 Report of the National High Blood Pressure Education Program Working Group on High Blood Pressure in Pregnancy. *American Journal of Obstetrics & Gynecology* 2000;**183**:S1–S22.

8 Saudan P, Brown MA, Buddle ML, and Jones M. Does gestational hypertension become pre-eclampsia? *British Journal of Obstetrics and Gynaecology* 1998;**105**:1177–1184.

9 Sibai BM. Chronic hypertension in pregnancy. *Obstetrics & Gynecology* 2002;**100**:369–377.

10 Rey E and Couturier A. The prognosis of pregnancy in women with chronic hypertension. *American Journal of Obstetrics & Gynecology* 1994;**171**:410–416.

11 McCowan LM, Buist RG, North RA, and Gamble G. Perinatal morbidity in chronic hypertension. *British Journal of Obstetrics and Gynaecology* 1996;**103**:123–129.

12 Spong CY, Mercer BM, D'Alton M *et al.* Timing of indicated late-preterm and early term birth. *Obstetrics & Gynecology* 2011;**118**:323–333.

13 Hawkins TL-A, Roberts JM, Mangos GJ *et al.* Plasma uric acid remains a marker of poor outcome in hypertensive pregnancy: a retrospective cohort study. *British Journal of Obstetrics and Gynaecology* 2012;**119**:484–492.

14 Vigil De-Gracia P, Montufar-Rudea C, and Ruiz J. Expectant management of severe preeclampsia and preeclampsia superimposed on chronic hypertension between 24 and 34 weeks' gestation. *European Journal of Obstetrics & Gynecology and Reproductive Biology* 2003;**107**:24–27.

15 Meyer NL, Mercer BM, Friedman SA, and Sibai BM. Urinary dipstick protein: a poor predictor of absent or severe proteinuria. *European Journal of Obstetrics & Gynecology and Reproductive Biology* 1994;**170**(Pt 1)137–141.

16 Sibai BM and Barton JR. Expectant management of severe preeclampsia remote from term: patient selection, treatment and delivery indications. *European Journal of Obstetrics & Gynecology and Reproductive Biology* 2007;**196**:514 e1–e9.

17 Egerman RS and Sibai BM. HELLP syndrome. *Clinical Obstetrics and Gynecology* 1999;**42**:381–389.

18 Romero R, Mazor M, Lockwood DJ *et al.* Clinical significance, prevalence and natural history of thrombocytopenia in pregnancy-induced hypertension. *American Journal of Perinatology* 1989;**6**:32–38.
19 Katz VL, Thorp JM Jr, Rozas L, and Bowes WA Jr. The natural history of thrombocytopenia associated with preeclampsia. *American Journal of Obstetrics & Gynecology* 1990;**163**:1142–1143.
20 Sibai DM, Taslimi MM, El-Nazer A *et al.* Maternal-perinatal outcome associated with the syndrome of hemolysis, elevated liver enzymes and low platelets in severe preelampsia-eclampsia. *American Journal of Obstetrics & Gynecology* 1986;**155**:501–509.
21 Schlenzig C, Maurer S, Coppelt M, Ulm K, and Kolben M. Postpartum curettage in patients with HELLP-syndrome does not result in accelerated recovery. *European Journal of Obstetrics & Gynecology and Reproductive Biology* 2000;**91**:25–28.
22 Magann EF and Martin JNJ. Twelve steps to optimal management of HELLP Syndrome. *Clinical Obstetrics and Gynecology* 1999;**42**:532–550.
23 Gifford R, August P, Cunningham G *et al. The National High Blood Pressure Education Program Working Group on High Blood Pressure in Pregnancy.* Bethesda, MD: National Institutes of Health and National Heart, Lung and Blood Institute 2000.
24 Lee W, Gonik B, and Cotton DB. Urinary diagnostic indices in preeclampsia-associated oliguria: correlation with invasive hemodynamic monitoring. *American Journal of Obstetrics & Gynecology* 1987;**156**:100–103.
25 Sibai BM, Ramadan MK, Usta L *et al.* Maternal morbidity and mortality in 442 pregnancies with hemolysis, elevated liver enzymes and low platelets (HELLP syndrome). *American Journal of Obstetrics & Gynecology* 1993;**169**:1000–1006.
26 Clark SL, Greenspoon JS, Aldahl D, and Phelan JP. Severe preeclampsia with persistent oliguria: management of hemodynamic subsets. *American Journal of Obstetrics & Gynecology* 1986;**154**:490–494.
27 Whitlin AG, Friedman SA, and Sibai BM. The effect of magnesium sulfate therapy on the duration of labor in women with mild preeclampsia at term: A randomized, double-blind, placebo-controlled trial. *American Journal of Obstetrics & Gynecology* 1997;**176**:623–627.
28 Graham C and Goldstein A. Epidural analgesia and cardiac output in severe preeclamptics. *Anesthesia* 1980;**35**:709–712.
29 Gutsche B. The experts' opinion: is epidural block for labor and delivery and for cesarean section a safe form of analgesia is severe preeclampsia or eclampsia? *Survey of Anesthesiology* 1986;**30**:304–311.
30 Livington JC, Livingston LW, Ramsey R, Mabie BC, and Sibai BM. Magnesium sulfate in women with mild preeclampsia: a randomized controlled trial. *Obstetrics & Gynecology* 2003;**101**:217–220.
31 American College of Obstetricians and Gynecologists Committee Opinion No. 514. Emergent Therapy for Acute-Onset, Severe Hypertension with Preeclampsia or Eclampsia. Washington, DC: ACOG, 2011.
32 Martin JN Jr, Thigpen BD, Moore RC, Rose CH, Cushman J, and May W. Stroke and severe preeclampsia and eclampsia: a paradigm shift focusing on systolic blood pressure. *Obstetrics & Gynecology* 2005;**105**:246–254.
33 Centre for Maternal and Child Enquiries (CMACE). Saving mothers' lives: reviewing maternal deaths to make motherhood safer: 2006–08. The eighth report on confidential enquiries into maternal deaths in the United Kingdom. *BJOG* 2011;**118** (Suppl. 1):1–203.
34 Pritchard JA, Cunningham FG, and Pritchard SA. The parkland memorial hospital protocol for the treatment of eclampsia: evaluation of 245 cases. *American Journal of Obstetrics & Gynecology* 1984;**148**:951–963.
35 Waisman GD, Mayorga LM, Camera MI *et al.* Magnesium plus nifedipine: potentiation of hypotensive effect in preeclampsia? *American Journal of Obstetrics & Gynecology* 1988;**159**:308–309.

36 Pasch T, Schulz V, and Hoppelshauser G. Nictroprusside-induced formation of cyanide and its detoxification with thiosulfate during deliberate hypotension. *Journal of Cardiovascular Pharmacology* 1983;**5**:77–85.

37 Chelsey LC. Diagnosis of preeclampsia. *Obstetrics & Gynecology* 1985;**65**:423–425.

38 Pritchard JA, Cunningham FG, and Mason RA, Coagulation changes in preeclampsia: their frequency and pathogenesis. *American Journal of Obstetrics & Gynecology* 1976;**124**:855–864.

39 Weinstein L. Preeclampsia/eclampsia with hemolysis, elevated liver enzymes and thrombocytopenia. *Obstetrics & Gynecology* 1985;**66**:657–660.

40 Shelley WC and Gutsche BB. Magnesium and seizure control. *American Journal of Obstetrics & Gynecology* 1980;**136**:146–147.

41 Altman D, Carroli G, Duley L *et al.* Do women with pre-eclampsia, and their babies, benefit from magnesium sulphate? The Magpie Trial: a randomized placebo-controlled trial. *Lancet* 2002;**359**:1877–1890.

42 Duley L, Henderson Smart DJ, and Chou D. Magnesium sulphate versus phenytoin for eclampsia. *Cochrane Database of Systematic Reviews* 2010;(**10**):CD000128.

43 Duley L and Henderson-Smart D. Magnesium sulphate versus diazepam for eclampsia. *Cochrane Database of Systematic Reviews* 2000;(**2**):CD000127.

44 Sibai BM, Graham JM, and McCubbin JH. A comparison of intravenous and intramuscular magnesium sulfate regimens in preeclampsia. *American Journal of Obstetrics & Gynecology* 1984;**150**:728–733.

45 Pritchard JA. The use of magnesium iron in the management of exlamptogenic toxemias. *Surgery, Gynecology & Obstetrics* 1955;**100**:131–140.

46 Fontenot MT, Lewis DF, Frederick JB *et al.* A prospective randomized trial of magnesium sulfate in severe preeclampsia: use of diuresis as a clinical parameter to determine the duration of postpartum therapy. *American Journal of Obstetrics & Gynecology* 2005;**1952**:1788–1793.

47 Pritchard JA, MacDonald OC, and Grant NF. In: Pritchard JA and MacDonald PC (eds) *Hypertensive Disorders in Pregnancy Williams' Obstetrics*, 17th edn. Appleton-Century-Crofts: Norwalk, CT, 1985: 525.

48 Chelsey LC. Parenteral magnesium sulfate and the distribution, plasma levels and excretion of magnesium. *American Journal of Obstetrics & Gynecology* 1979;**133**:1–7.

49 American College of Obstetricians and Gynecologists Technical Bulletin No. 219: Hypertension in pregnancy. Washington, DC: American College of Obstetricians and Gynecologists, 1996.

50 Sibai, DM, Mabie BC, Harvey CJ, and Gonzalez AR. Pulmonary edema in severe preeclampsia-eclampsia: analysis of thirty-seven consecutive cases. *American Journal of Obstetrics & Gynecology* 1987;**156**:1174–1179.

51 Belfort M, Saade G, Foley M, Ohelan J, and Dildy G (eds). *Critical Care Obstetrics*, 5th edn. Chichester: Wiley-Blackwell, 2010.

52 Hodgkinson R, Husain FJ, and Hayashi RH. Systemic and pulmonary blood pressure during cesarean section in parturients with gestational hypertension. *Canadian Journal of Anesthesia* 1980;**27**:389–394.

53 Ramons-Santos E, Devoe LD, Wakefiled ML, Sherline DM, and Metheny WP. The effects of epidural anesthesia on the Doppler velocimetry of umbilical and uterine arteries in normal and hypertensive patients during active term labor. *Obstetrics & Gynecology* 1991;**77**:20–26.

54 Frenk V, Camann W, and Shankar KB. Regional anesthesia in parturients with low platelet counts. *Canadian Journal of Anesthesia* 2005;**114**. DOI 10.1007/BF03018594.

55 van Veen JJ, Nokes TJ, and Makris M. The risk of spinal hematoma following neuraxial anesthesia or lumbar puncture in thrombocytopenic individuals. *British Journal of Hematology* 2009;**148**:15–25.

56 Sibai BM, Lipshitz J, Anderson GD, and Dilts PV Jr. Reassessment of intravenous MgSO4 therapy in preeclampsia-eclampsia. *Obstetrics & Gynecology* 1981;**57**;199–202.

57 Lubarsky SL, Barton JR, Friedman SA *et al.* Late postpartum eclampsia revisited. *Obstetrics & Gynecology* 1994;**83**:502–505.
58 Sibai BM. Diagnosis, prevention and management of eclampsia. *Obstetrics & Gynecology* 2005;**105**:402–410
59 Douglas KA and Redman CWG. Eclampsia in the United Kingdom. *BMJ* 1994;**309**:1395–1399.
60 Paul RH, Koh KS, and Vernstein SG. Changes in fetal heart rate: uterine contraction patterns associated with eclampsia. *American Journal of Obstetrics & Gynecology* 1978;**130**:165.
61 Cunningham FG and Gant NF. Management of eclampsia. *Seminars in Perinatology* 1994;**18**:103–113.
62 Pritchard JA. Changes in the blood volume during pregnancy and delivery. *Anesthesiology* 1965;**26**:393.
63 Vered Z, Poler SM, Bigson P *et al.* Noninvasive detection of the morphologic and hemodynamic changes during normal pregnancy. *Clinical Cardiology* 1991;**14**:327.
64 Robson SC, Hunter S, Boys RJ *et al.* Serial study of factors influencing changes in cardiac output during human pregnancy. *American Journal of Physiology* 1989;**256**:H1060.
65 Robson SC, Dunlop W, Boys RJ *et al.* Cardiac output during labor. *BMJ* 1987;**295**:1169.
66 Adams JQ and Alexandar AM. Alterations in cardiovascular physiology during labor. *Obstetrics & Gynecology* 1958;**12**:542.
67 Roeder HA, Kuller JA, Barker PCA and James AH. Maternal valvular heart disease in pregnancy. *Obstetrical and Gynecological Survey* 2011;**66**:561–571.
68 Siu SC, Sermer M, Colman JM *et al.* Prospective multicenter study of pregnancy outcomes in women with heart disease. *Circulation* 2001;**96**:2789.
69 Sui SC, Sermer M, Harrison DA *et al.* Risk and predictors for pregnancy-related complications in women with heart disease. *Circulation* 1997;**96**:2789–2794.
70 Warnes CA, Williams RG, Bashore TM, Child JS, Connolly HM, and Dearani JA. ACC/AHA 2008 guidelines for the management of adults with congenital heart disease. A report of the American College of Cardiology/American Heart Association Task Force on Practice Guidelines (writing committee to develop guidelines on the management of adults with congenital heart disease) *Journal of the American College of Cardiology* 2008;**52**:143–263.
71 Clark SL, Horenstein JM, Phelan JP *et al.* Experience with the pulmonary artery catheter in obstetrics and gynecology. *American Journal of Obstetrics & Gynecology* 1985;**152**:374–378.
72 Clark SL, Phelan JP, Greenspoon J *et al.* Labor and delivery in the presence of mitral stenosis: central hemodynamic observations. *American Journal of Obstetrics & Gynecology* 1985;**152**:984–988.
73 Elkayam U, Bitar F. and Valvular heart disease and pregnancy. Part I: native valves. *Journal of the American College of Cardiology* 2005;**46**:223.
74 de Souza JAM, Martinex EE, Ambrose JA *et al.* Percutaneous balloon mitral valvuloplasty in comparison with open mitral valve commissurotomy for mitral stenosis during pregnancy *Journal of the American College of Cardiology* 2001;**37**:900.
75 Iung B, Cormier B, Elias J *et al.* Usefulness of percutaneous balloon commissurotomy for mitral stenosis during pregnancy. *American Journal of Cardiology* 1994;**73**:98–400.
76 American College of Obstetricians and Gynecologists Technical Bulletin No. 196. Operative Vaginal Delivery. Washington, DC: ACOG, 1994.
77 Ro A and Frishman WH. Peripartum cardiomyopathy. *Cardiology in Review* 2006;**14**:35–42.
78 Veille JC. Peripartum cardiomyopathies: a review. *American Journal of Obstetrics & Gynecology* 1984;**148**:805–818.
79 Durack DT. Prevention of infective endocarditis. *New England Journal of Medicine* 1995;**332**:38.
80 Penning S, Robinson KD, Major CA, and Garite TJ. A comparison of echocardiography and pulmonary artery catheterization for evaluation of pulmonary artery pressures in pregnancy patients with suspected pulmonary hypertension. *American Journal of Obstetrics & Gynecology* 2001;**184**:1568–1570.

81 Easterling TR, Ralph DD, and Schmucker BC. Pulmonary hypertension in pregnancy: treatment with pulmonary vasodilators. *Obstetrics & Gynecology* 1999;**93**:494–498.
82 Presbitero P, Somerville J, Stone S *et al.* Pregnancy in cyanotic congenital heart disease. Outcome of mother and fetus. *Circulation* 1994;**89**:2673–2676.
83 Sobrevilla LA, Cassinelli MT, Carcelen A *et al.* Human fetal and maternal oxygen tension and acid-base status during delivery at high altitude. *American Journal of Obstetrics & Gynecology* 1971;**111**:1111–1118.
84 Weiss BM, Zemp L, Seifert B, and Hess OM. Outcome of pulmonary vascular disease in pregnancy: a systematic overview from 1978 through 1996. *Journal of the American College of Cardiology* 1998;**31**:1650–1657.
85 Shapriro SM, Oudiz RJ, Cao T *et al.* Primary pulmonary hypertension: improved long-term effects and survival with continuous intravenous epoprostenol infusion. *Journal of the American College of Cardiology* 1997;**30**:343–349.
86 Sitbon O, Brenot F, Denjean A *et al.* Inhaled nitric oxide as a screening vasodilator agent in primary pulmonary hypertension: a dose-response study and comparison with prostacyclin. *American Journal of Respiratory and Critical Care Medicine* 1995;**151**:384–389.
87 Midwall J, Jaffin H, Herman MV *et al.* Shunt flow and pulmonary hemodynamics during labor and delivery in the Eisenmenger syndrome. *American Journal of Cardiology* 1978;**42**:299–303.
88 American College of Obstetricians and Gynecologists Practice Bulletin No. 120: Use of Prophylactic Antibiotics in Labor and Delivery. Washington, DC: ACOG, 2011.
89 Thomas JS, Koh SH, and Cooper GM. Haemodynamic effects of oxytocin given as i.v. bolus or infusion on women undergoing caesarean section. *Journal of Anesthesia* 2007;**98**:116–119.
90 Awe RJ, Nicortra MB, Newson TD *et al.* Arterial oxygenation and alveolar-arterial gradients in term pregnancy. *Obstetrics & Gynecology* 1979;**53**:182.
91 Crapo A. Normal cardiopulmonary physiology during pregnancy. *Clinical Obstetrics and Gynaecology* 1996;**39**:3–16.
92 McAuliffe f, Kameta N, Costello J *et al.* Respiratory function in singleton and twin pregnancy. *BJOG* 2002;**109**:765–768.
93 Breeme KA. Haemostatic changes in pregnancy. *Best Practice & Research Clinical Haematology* 2003;**16**:153–168.
94 Pomp ER, Lenselink AM, Rosendaal FR, and Doggen CJ. Pregnancy, the postpartum period and prothrombotic defects: risk of venous thrombosis in the MEGA study. *Journal of Thrombosis and Haemostasis* 2008;**6**:632–637.
95 Scarsbrook AF and Gleeson FV. Investigating suspected pulmonary embolism in pregnancy. *BMJ* 2007;**334**:418–419.
96 Clark SL and Hankins GDV. Preventing maternal death: 10 clinical diamonds. *Obstetrics & Gynecology* 2012;**119**:360–364.
97 Winer-Muram HT, Boone JM, Brown HL *et al.* Pulmonary embolism in pregnant patients: fetal radiation dose with helical CT. *Radiology* 2002;**224**:487–492.
98 National Council on Radiation Protection and Measurements. *Medical Radiation Exposure of Pregnant and Potentially Pregnant Women*. Bethesda, MD: National Council on Radiation Protection and Measurements, 1977.
99 Diffin D, Leyendecker JR, Johnson SP *et al.* Effect of anatomic distribution of pulmonary emboli on interobserver agreement in the interpretation of pulmonary angiography. *American Journal of Roantgenology* 1998;**171**:1085–1089.
100 Schaerfer-Prokop C and Prokop M. CTPA for the diagnosis of acute pulmonary embolism during pregnancy. *European Radiology* 2008;**18**:2705–2708.
101 Brent RL. The effect of embryonic and fetal exposure to x-ray, microwaves, and ultrasound: counseling the pregnant and non-pregnant patient about these risks. *Seminars in Oncology* 1989;**16**:347–368.

102 The Urokinase Pulmonary Embolism Trial: A national cooperative study. *Circulation* 1973;**47**(Suppl. 2):1–108.

103 Come PC. Echocardiographic evaluation of pulmonary embolism and its response to therapeutic interventions. *Chest* 1991;**101**:151s–162s.

104 Green RM, Meyer TJ Dunn M, and Glassroth J. Pulmonary embolism in younger adults. *Chest* 1992;**101**:1507–1511.

105 Tapson VF, Carroll BA, Dacidson BL *et al.* The diagnostic approach to acute venous thromboembolism: clinical practice guideline. American Thoracic Society. *American Journal of Respiratory and Critical Care Medicine* 1999;**160**:1043–1066.

106 American College of Obstetricians and Gynecologists Practice Bulletin No. 123: Thromboembolism in Pregnancy. Washington, DC: ACOG, 2011.

107 Dongen C, Belt A, Prins M, and Lensing A. Fixed dose subcutaneous low molecular weight heparins versus adjusted dose unfractionated heparin for venous thromboembolism. *Cochrane Database of Systematic Reviews* 2004;**4**:CD001100.

108 Bates SM, Greer IA, Pabinger I, Sofaer S, and Hirsh J. Venous thromboembolism, thrombophilia, antithrombotic therapy, and pregnancy: American College of Chest Physicians evidence-based clinical practice guidelines. 8th edn. American College of Chest Physicians. *Chest* 2008;**133**:844–86S.

109 Bates SM, Greer IA, Hirsh J, and Finsberg JS. Use of antithrombotic agents during pregnancy. The seventh ACCP conference on antithrombotic and thrombolytic therapy. *Chest* 2004;**126**:627S–644S.

110 Fausett MB, Vogtlander M, Lee RM *et al.* Heparin-induced thrombocytopenia is rare in pregnancy. *American Journal of Obstetrics & Gynecology* 2001;**185**:148–152.

111 Lepercq J, Conard J, Corel-Derlon A *et al.* Venous thromboembolism during pregnancy: a retrospective study of enoxaparin safety in 624 pregnancies. *BJOG* 2001;**108**:1134–1140.

112 Fejgin MD and Lourwood DL. Low molecular weight heparins and their use in the obstetrics and gynecology. *Obstetrical and Gynecological Survey* 1994;**49**:424–431.

113 Creasy RK, Resnik R, Iams JD, Lockwood CJ, and Moore TR (eds). *Creasy & Resnick's Maternal-Fetal Medicine*, 6th edn. Philadelphia, PA: Saunders Elsevier, 2009

114 Horlocker TT, Wedel DJ, Rowlingson JC, and Enneking FK. Executive summary: regional anesthesia in the patient receiving antithrombotic or thrombolytic therapy: American Society of Regional Anesthesia and Pain Medicine evidence-based guideline. *Regional Anesthesia and Pain Medicine* 2010;**35**:102–105.

115 James AH. Prevention and management of venous thromboembolism in pregnancy. *American Journal of Medicine* 2007;**120**(Suppl. 2):S26–34.

116 Orme ML, Lewis PJ, de Swiet M, Serlin MJ, Sibeon R, Baty JD *et al.* May mothers given warfarin breast-feed their infants? *BMJ* 1977;**1**:1564–1565.

117 McKenna R, Cole ER, and Vasan U. Is warfarin sodium contraindicated in the lactating mother? *Journal of Pediatrics* 1983;**103**:325–327.

118 Buller HR, Davidson BL, Decousus H *et al.* Matisse Investigators. Fondaparinux or enoxaparin for the initial treatment of symptomatic deep venous thrombosis: a randomized trial. *Annals of Internal Medicine* 2004;**140**:867–873.

119 Dempfle CE. Minor transplacental passage of fondaparinux in vivo. *New England Journal of Medicine* 2004;**350**:1914–1915.

120 Gupta S. Inferior vena cava filter use in pregnancy: preliminary experience. *BJOG* 2008;**115**:785–788.

121 Dunlop W. Serial changes in renal hemodynamics during normal human pregnancy. *BJOG* 1981;**88**:1.

122 Davison JM and Dunlop W. Changes in renal hemodynamics and tubular function induced by normal human pregnancy. *Seminars in Nephrology* 1984;**4**:198.

123 Davison JM and Dunlop W. Renal hemodynamics and tubular function in normal human pregnancy. *Kidney International* 1980;**18**:152.

124 Barron WM and Lindheimer MD. Renal sodium and water handling in pregnancy. *Obstetrics and Gynecology Annual* 1984;**13**:35–69.

125 Garland HO and Green R. Miropuncture study of changes in glomerular filtration and ion and water handling in the rat kidney during pregnancy. *Journal of Physiology* (Lond) 1982;**329**:389.

126 Bishop JHV and Green R. Effects of pregnancy on glucose reabsorption by the proximal convoluted tubule in the rat. *Journal of Physiology* (Lond) 1981;**319**:271.

127 Hladunewich M, Hercz AE, Keunen J, Chan C, and Pierratos A. Pregnancy in end stage renal disease. *Seminars in Dialysis* 2011;**24**:634–639.

128 Ramin SM, Vidaeff AC, Yeomans ER, and Gilstrap LC. Chronic renal disease in pregnancy. *Obstetrics & Gynecology* 2006;**108**:1531–1539.

129 Fischer MJ, Lehnerz SD. Hebert JR, and Parikh CR. Kidney disease is an independent risk factor for adverse fetal and maternal outcomes in pregnancy. *American Journal of Kidney Diseases* 2004;**43**:415–423.

130 Jungers P, Houillier P, Forget D *et al.* Influence of pregnancy on the course of primary chronic glomerulonephritis. *Lancet* 1995;**346**.1122–1124.

131 Davison JM and Lindheimer MD. Pregnancy and chronic kidney disease. *Seminars in Nephrology* 2001;**31**:86–99.

132 Jones DC and Hayslett JP. Outcome of pregnancy in women with moderate or severe renal insufficiency. *New England Journal of Medicine* 1996;**335**:226.

133 Epstein FH. Pregnancy and renal disease, *New England Journal of Medicine* 1996;**335**:277.

134 Reddy SS and Holley JL. Management of the pregnant chronic dialysis patient. *Advances in Chronic Kidney Disease* 2007;**14**:146–155.

135 Jakobi P, Ohel G, Szylman P, Levit A, Lewin M, and Paldi E. Continuous ambulatory peritoneal dialysis as the primary approach in the management of severe renal insufficiency in pregnancy. *Obstetrics & Gynecology* 1992;**79**:808–810.

136 Changs H, Miller Ma, and Bruns FJ. Tidal peritoneal dialysis during pregnancy improves clearance and abdominal symptoms. *Peritoneal Dialysis International* 2002;**22**:272–274.

137 Hou SH. Pregnancy and birth control in CAPD patients. *Advances in Peritoneal Dialysis* 1993;**9**:173–176.

138 Hou SH. Pregnancy in continuous ambulatory peritoneal dialysis (CAPD) patients. *Peritoneal Dialysis International* 1990;**10**:201–204.

139 Hou SH. Frequency and outcome of pregnancy in women on dialysis. *American Journal of Kidney Diseases* 1994;**23**:60–63.

140 Bar J, Ben –Rafael Z, Padoa A *et al.* Prediction of pregnancy outcome in subgroups of women with renal disease. *Clinical Nephrology* 2000;**53**:437–444.

141 Reister F, Reister B, Heyl W *et al.* Dialysis and pregnancy – a case report and review of the literature. *Renal Failure* 1999;**21**:533–539.

142 Redrow M, Lazaro C, Elliot J *et al.* Dialysis in the management of pregnant patents with renal insufficiency. *Medicine* 1988;**67**:199–208.

143 Davison JM and Baylis C. Pregnancy in patients with underlying renal disease. In: Davison AM, Cameron JC, Grunfeld JP, Ponticelli C *et al.* (eds) *Oxford Textbook of Clinical Nephrology*. Oxford: Oxford University Press, 2005: 2243.

144 Ferrara A, Kahn HS, Quesenberry CP *et al.* An increase in the incidence of gestational diabetes mellitus: northern California, 1991–2000. *Obstetrics & Gynecology* 2004;**103**:526–533.

145 American Diabetes Association. Standard of medical care in diabetes 2011. *Diabetes Care* 2011;**34**(Suppl. 1):S11–S61.

146 Gabbe SG and Graves CR. Management of diabetes mellitus complicating pregnancy. *Obstetrics & Gynecology* 2003;**102**:857–868.

147 Landon MB, Spong CY, Thom E *et al.* A multicenter, randomized trial of treatment for mild gestational diabetes. *New England Journal of Medicine* 2009; **361**(14):1339–1348.

148 Metzger BE, Buchanan TA, Coustan DR *et al.* Summary and recommendations of the fifth international workshop-conference on gestational diabetes mellitus. *Diabetes Care* 2007;**30**(Suppl. 2):S251–S260.

149 Coustan DE, Nelson C, Carpentern NW, Carr SR, Rotondo L, and Widness JA. Maternal age and screening for gestational diabetes: a population-based study. *Obstetrics & Gynecology* 1989;**73**:557–561.

150 Langer O, Conway DL, Berkus MD, and Gonzales O. A comparison of glyburide and insulin in women with gestational diabetes mellitus. *New England Journal of Medicine* 2000;**343**:1134–1138.

151 Rowan JA, Hague WM, Gao W, Battin MR, and Moore MP, MiG Trial investigators. Metformin versus insulin for treatment of gestational diabetes. *New England Journal of Medicine* 2008;**358**:2003–2015.

152 Moore LE, Clokey D, Rappaport VJ, and Curet LB. Metformin compared with glyburide in gestational diabetes: randomized control trials. *Obstetrics & Gynecology* 2010;**115**:55–59.

153 Hawkins JS, Casey BM, Lo JY *et al.* Weekly compared with daily blood glucose monitoring in women with diet treated gestational diabetes. *Obstetrics & Gynecology* 2009;**113**:1307–1312.

154 Benacerraf BR, Gelman, R, and Frigoletto FD Jr. Sonographically estimated fetal weights accuracy and limitation, *American Journal of Obstetrics & Gynecology* 1988;**159**:1118–1121.

155 American College of Obstetricians and Gynecologists Practice Bulletin No. 137: Gestational Diabetes. Washington, DC: ACOG, 2013.

156 Hieronimus S, Cupelli C, Bongain A *et al.* Pregnancy in type 1 diabetes: insulin pump versus intensified conventional therapy. *Gynécologie Obstétrique & Fertilité* 2005;**33**(6):398–394.

157 Lapolla A, Dalfra MG, Masin M *et al.* Analysis of outcome of pregnancy in type 1 diabetics treated with insulin pump of conventional insulin therapy. *Acta Diabetologica* 2003;**40**:143–149.

158 American College of Obstetricians and Gynecologists Practice Bulletin No. 60: Pregestational Diabetes Mellitus. Washington, DC: ACOG, 2005.

159 Balsells M, Corcoy R, Adelantado JM *et al.* Gestational diabetes mellitus: metabolic control during labour. *Diabetes, Nutrition & Metabolism* 2000;**12**:257.

160 Kios SL, Henry OA, Montoro M, Buchanan TA, and Mestman JH. Insulin-requiring diabetes in pregnancy: a randomized trial of active induction of labor and expectant management. *American Journal of Obstetrics & Gynecology* 1993;**169**:611–615.

161 Drury MI, Greene AT, and Stronge JM. Pregnancy complicated by clinical diabetes mellitus: a study of 600 pregnancies. *Obstetrics & Gynecology* 1977;**49**:519–522.

162 Montoro MN, Myers VP, Mestman, JH *et al.* Outcome of pregnancy in diabetic ketoacidosis. *American Journal of Perinatology* 1991;**10**:17–20.

163 Cullen MT, Reece EA, Homko CJ, and Sivan E. The changing presentations of diabetic ketoacidosis during pregnancy. *American Journal of Perinatology* 1996;**13**:449–451.

164 Kirabchi A, Umpierez G, Murphy M, and Barret E. Management of hyperglycemic crises in patients with diabetes. *Diabetes Care* 2001;**24**:131–153.

165 Viallon A, Zeni, F, Lafond P *et al.* Does bicarbonate therapy improve the management of severe diabetic ketoacidosis? *Critical Care Medicine* 1999;**27**:2690–2693.

166 Takahashi Y, lawabata I , Shinohara A, and Tamaya T, Transient fetal blood flow redistribution induced by maternal diabetic ketoacidosis diagnosed Doppler ultrasonography. *Prenatal Diagnosis* 2000;**20**:524–525.

167 Hauser AW, Annegers JF, and Hurland LT. Incidence of epilepsy and unprovoked seizures in Rochester, Minnesota, 1935–84. *Epilepsia* 1993;**34**:453–468.

168 Engel J and Perley T. Pregnancy and the mother. In: *Epilepsy: A Comprehensive Textbook.* Lippincott: Philadelphia, PA, 1998: 2029–2030.

169 Yerby MS. Pregnancy and epilepsy. *Epilepsia* 1991;**32** (Suppl. 6):S51.
170 Teramo K, Hiilesmaa CK, Bardy A *et al.* Fetal heart rate during a maternal grand mal epileptic seizure. *Journal of Perinatal Medicine* 1979;**7**:3.
171 Kelly TE. Teratogenicity of anticonvulsant drugs: Review of the literature. *American Journal of Medical Genetics* 1984;**19**:413–434.
172 MRC Vitamin Study Research Group. Prevention of neural tube defects: results of the Medical Research Council Vitamin Study. *Lancet* 1991;**338**:131–137.
173 Choulika S, Grabowski E, and Holmes LB. Is antenatal vitamin K prophylaxis needed for pregnant women taking anticonvulsants? *American Journal of Obstetrics & Gynecology* 2004;**190**:882–883.
174 Hiilesmaa VK. Pregnancy and birth in women with epilepsy. *Neurology* 1992;**42**(Suppl. 5):8.
175 Shaner DM, McCurdy SA, Herring MO, and Gabor AJ. Treatment of status epilepticus: a prospective comparison of diazepam and phenytoin versus phenobarbital and optional phenytoin. *Neurology* 1988;**38**:202.
176 Marik PE and Varon J. The management of status epilepticus. *Chest* 2004;**126**:582–591.
177 Weibers DO. Ischemic cerebrovascular complications of pregnancy. *Archives of Neurology* 1985;**42**:1106.
178 Ros HS, Lichtenstein P Bellocco R, Petersson G and Cnattingius S. Pulmonary embolism and stroke in relation to pregnancy: how can high-risk women be identified? *American Journal of Obstetrics & Gynecology* 2002;**186**:198–203.
179 James AH, Bushnell CD, Jamison MG, and Myers ER. Incidence and risk factors for stroke in pregnancy and the puerperium. *Obstetrics & Gynecology* 2006;**106**:509–516.
180 Schwartz RB. Neuroradiographic imaging: techniques and safety considerations. *Advances in Neurology* 2002;**90**:1–8.
181 American College of Obstetricians and Gynecologists Committee Opinion No. 299. Guidelines for Diagnostic Imaging During Pregnancy. Washington, DC: ACOG, 2004.
182 Wiese KM, Talkad A. Matthews M, and Wang D. Intravenous recombinant tissue plasminogen activator in a pregnant woman with cardioembolic stroke. *Stroke* 2006;**37**: 2168–2169.
183 Leonhardt G and Gauld C. Thrombolytic therapy in pregnancy. *Journal of Thrombosis and Thrombolysis* 2006;**21**:271–276.
184 Stam J. Thrombosis of the cerebral veins and sinuses. *New England Journal of Medicine* 2005;**352**:1791–1798.
185 Wilterdink JL and Easton JD. Cerebral ischemia. In: Devinsky O, Feldmann E, Hainline B (eds). *Neurological Complications of Pregnancy.* New York: Raven Press, 1–11.
186 Cantu C and Barinagarrementeria F. Cerebral venous thrombosis associated with pregnancy and the puerperium: review of 67 cases. *Stroke* 1993;**24**:1880–1884.
187 Einhaupl KM, Villringer A, Meister W *et al.* Heparin treatment in sinus venous thrombosis. *Lancet* 1991;**338**:597.
188 Barrow DL and Reisner A. Natural history of intracranial aneurysms and vascular malformations *Clinical Neurosurgery* 1993;**40**:3–39.
189 Stoodley MA, Macdonald RL, and Weir BK. Pregnancy and intracranial aneurysms. *Neurosurgery Clinics of North America* 1998;**9**:549.
190 Piotin M, de Souza Filho CB, Kothimbakam R, and Moret J. Endovascular treatment of acutely ruptured intracranial aneurysms in pregnancy. *American Journal of Obstetrics & Gynecology* 2001;**185**:1261–1262.
191 Brilstra EH, Rinkel GJE, van Rooij WJJ *et al.* Treatment of intracranial aneurysms by embolization with coils: a systematic review. *Stroke* 1999;**30**:470–476.
192 Robinson JL, Hall C, and Sedzimir CB. Arteriovenous malformations, aneurysms and pregnancy. *Journal of Neurosurgery* 1974;**41**:63.

193 Meyers PM, Halluch VV, Malek AM *et al.* Endovascular treatment of cerebral artery aneurysms during pregnancy: report of three cases. *American Journal of Neuroradiology* 2000;**21**:1306–1311.
194 Tidswell P, Dias PS, Sagar HJ *et al.* Cognitive outcome after aneurysm rupture: relationship to aneurysm site and perioperative complications. *Neurology* 1995;**45**:875.
195 Schievnik W. Intracranial aneurysms. *New England Journal of Medicine* 1997;**336**:28–40.
196 Jaigobin C and Silver FL. Stroke and pregnancy. *Stroke* 2000;**31**:2984–2951.
197 Mas JL and Lamy C. Stroke in pregnancy and the puerperium. *Journal of Neurology* 1998;**24**:305–313.
198 Sibai BM and Coppage KH. Diagnosis and management of women with stroke during pregnancy/postpartum. *Clinics in Perinatology* 2004;**31**:853–868.
199 Al-Yamany M and Wallace MC. Management of cerebral vasospasm on patients with aneurysmal subarachnoid hemorrhage. *Intensive Care Medicine* 1999;**25**:1463–1466.
200 Belfort MA, Saade GR, Yared M *et al.* Change in estimated cerebral perfusion pressure after treatment with nimodipine or magnesium sulfate in patients with preeclampsia. *American Journal of Obstetrics & Gynecology* 1999;**181**:402–407.
201 Bendok BR, Getch CC, Malisch TW *et al.* Treatment of aneurysmal subarachnoid hemorrhage. *Seminars in Neurology* 1998;**18**:521–531.
202 Sloan MA and Stern BL. Cerebrovascular disease in pregnancy. *Current Treatment Options in Neurology* 2003;**4**:391–407.
203 Mitchell PJ and Bebbingtom M. Myasthenia gravis in pregnancy. *Obstetrics & Gynecology* 1992;**80**:178–181.
204 Catanzarite VA, McHargue AM, Sandberg EC, and Dyson DC. Respiratory arrest during therapy for premature labor in a patient with myasthenia gravis. *Obstetrics & Gynecology* 1984;**64**:819–821.
205 Plauche WC. Myasthenia gravis in pregnancy: an update. *American Journal of Obstetrics & Gynecology* 1979;**135**:691–697.
206 Batocchi AP, Majolini L, Evoli A *et al.* Course and treatment of myasthenia gravis during pregnancy. *Neurology* 1999;**52**:447.
207 Hoff JM, Dalveit AK, and Gilhus NE. Myasthenia gravis: consequences for pregnancy, delivery and the newborn. *Neurology* 2003;**61**:1362.
208 Signore C, Spong CY, Krotoski D, Shinowara NL, Blackwell SC. Pregnancy in women with physical disabilities. *Obstetrics & Gynecology* 2011;**117**:935–947.
209 Ferrero S, Pretta S, and Ragni N. Multiple sclerosis: management issues during pregnancy. *European Journal of Obstetrics & Gynecology and Reproductive Biology* 2004;**115**:3–9.
210 Sandberg-Wollheim M, Frank D, Goodwin TM *et al.* Pregnancy outcomes during treatment with interferon beta-1a in patients with multiple sclerosis. *Neurology* 2005;**65**:802–806.
211 Confavreux C, Hutchinson M, Hours MM, Cortinovis-Tourniaire P, Moreau T, the Pregnancy in Multiple Sclerosis Group. Rate of pregnancy-related relapse in multiple sclerosis. *New England Journal of Medicine* 1998;**339**:285–291.
212 Birk K and Rudick R. Pregnancy and multiple sclerosis. *Archives of Neurology* 1986;**43**:719.
213 Dahl J, Myhr K, Daltveit AK *et al.* Pregnancy, delivery and birth outcome in women with multiple sclerosis. *Neurology* 2005;**65**:1961.
214 Minkoff HL. Human immunodeficiency virus infection in pregnancy. *Seminars in Perinatology* 1998;**22**:293–308.
215 Minkoff H and Augenbraun M. Antiretroviral therapy for pregnant women. *American Journal of Obstetrics & Gynecology* 1997;**176**:478–489.
216 Connor EM, Sperling RS, Gelber R *et al.* Reduction of maternal infant transmission of human immunodeficiency virus type 1 with zidovudine treatment. *New England Journal of Medicine* 1994;**331**:1173–1180.
217 Minkoff H and O'Sullivan MJ. The case for rapid HIV testing during labor. *Journal of the American Medical Association* 1998;**279**:1743–1744.

218 Temmerman M, Chomba EN, Ndinya-Achola J, Plummer FA, and Piot P. Maternal human immunodeficiency virus-1 infection and pregnancy outcome. *Obstetrics & Gynecology* 1994;**83**:495–501.

219 Kaplan JE, Masur H, and Holmes KK. USPHS/IDSA guidelines for the prevention of opportunistic infections in persons infected with human immunodeficiency virus: a summary. Centers for Disease Control. *Morbidity and Mortality Weekly Report* 1995; **44**:1–34.

220 American College of Obstetricians and Gynecologists Educational Bulletin No. 232. Human Immunodeficiency Virus Infection in Pregnancy. Washington, DC: ACOG, 1997.

221 American College of Obstetricians and Gynecologists Committee Opinion 234. Schedule Cesarean Delivery and the Prevention of Vertical Transmission of HIV Infection. Washington, DC: ACOG, 2000.

222 The International Perinatal HIV group. The mode of delivery and the risk of vertical transmission of human immunodeficiency virus type 1. *New England Journal of Medicine* 1999;**340**:977–987.

223 Watts DH. Management of human immunodeficiency virus infection in pregnancy. *New England Journal of Medicine* 2002;**346**:1879–1891.

224 Brown ZA, Selke S, Zeh J *et al.* The acquisition of herpes simplex virus during pregnancy. *New England Journal of Medicine* 1997;**337**:509.

225 Nahass GT, Goldstein BA, Zhu WY *et al.* Comparison of Tzank smear, viral culture and DNA diagnostic methods in detection of herpes simplex and varicella zoster infection. *Journal of the American Medical Association* 1992;**268**:2541.

226 Baker D, Brown Z, Holier LM *et al.* Cost-effectiveness of herpes simplex virus type 2 serologic testing and antiviral therapy in pregnancy. *American Journal of Obstetrics & Gynecology* 2004;**191**:2074.

227 Thung, SF and Grobman WA. The cost-effectiveness of routine antenatal screening for maternal herpes simplex virus 1 and 2 antibodies. *American Journal of Obstetrics & Gynecology* 2005;**192**:483.

228 Brown ZA, Wald A, Ashley-Morrow R *et al.* Effect of serological status and cesarean delivery on transmission rates of herpes simplex virus from mother to infant. *Journal of the American Medical Association* 2003;**289**:203.

229 American College of Obstetricians and Gynecologists Practice Bulletin No. 82: Management of Herpes in Pregnancy. Washington, DC: ACOG, 2007.

CHAPTER 14

Fetal disorders affecting labor and delivery

Audrey Merriam[1] and Anthony Sciscione[2]
[1] *Division of Maternal-Fetal Medicine, Department of Obstetrics and Gynecology, Columbia University, New York, NY, USA*
[2] *Department of Obstetrics and Gynecology, Christiana Hospital, Newark, DE, USA*

In addition to maternal conditions that warrant special consideration in the peripartum period, there are also a number of important fetal conditions. This chapter highlights a number of fetal disorders that may influence management on labor and delivery.

14.1 Growth disturbances

14.1.1 Intrauterine growth restriction

Intrauterine growth restriction (IUGR) is commonly defined as a birth weight less than the 10th percentile due to a pathologic cause at a given gestational age. IUGR is different from the term small for gestational age (SGA), which describes fetuses that have a weight below the 10th percentile but no pathologic cause. Near 70% of SGA infants are constitutionally small due to reasons such as ethnicity and maternal body mass index [1]. IUGR can be further divided into symmetric – head and abdomen are decreased in size proportionately – and asymmetric – abdominal size is proportionally smaller when compared to head growth. Between 70 and 80% of cases are asymmetric and 20–30% are symmetric [1]. There are multiple risk factors for IUGR, which are beyond the scope of this chapter but are listed in Table 14.1 [1].

Delivery considerations for IUGR depend first on gestational age. Infants that are diagnosed as being IUGR, symmetric or asymmetric, are most often delivered if the gestational age is greater than 37 weeks. Recent evidence has shown decreased NICU admissions with delivery at 38 weeks or greater, so if antenatal testing is reassuring some pregnancies with IUGR may be able to be expectantly managed until 38 weeks of gestation [2]. Determining the need for delivery

Management of Labor and Delivery, Second Edition. Edited by George A. Macones.

Table 14.1 Various maternal, fetal, and placental factors leading to intrauterine growth restriction of the fetus.

Fetal factors	Placental factors	Maternal factors
Chromosomal anomalies – Trisomy 13, 18, 21 – Monosomy (45, XO) – Deletions – Uniparental disomy – Confined placental mosaicism	Abnormal trophoblastic invasion	Genetic/constitutional (race)
Congenital malformations – Absence of fetal pancreas – Anencephaly – Diaphragmatic hernia – Omphalocele – Gastroschisis – Renal agenesis / dysplasia – Multiple malformations	Multiple placental infarctions (chronic abruption)	Nutrition/starvation – Inflammatory bowel disease – Ileojejunal bypass – Chronic pancreatitis – Low prepregnancy weight – Poor pregnancy weight gain, second and third trimester
Multiple gestations – Monochorionic twins – One fetus with malformations – Twin-to-twin transfusion – Discordant twins – Triplets	Umbilical-placental vascular anomalies	Hypoxic – Severe lung disease – Cyanotic heart disease – Sickle cell anemia
	Abnormal cord insertion (velamentous cord insertion)	Vascular – Chronic hypertension – Preeclampsia – Collagen vascular disease – Type I diabetes mellitus
	Placenta previa	Renal – Glomerulonephritis – Lipoid nephritis – Arteriolar nephrosclerosis – Renal transplantation
	Circumvallate placenta	Antiphospholipid antibodies
	Chorioangiomata	Environmental and drugs – High altitude – Emotional stress – Physical stress – Cigarette smoking – Alcohol abuse – Substance abuse (heroin, cocaine) – Therapeutic drugs (antimetabolites, anticonvulsants, anticoagulants) – Poor obstetric history (previous stillbirths, recurrent aborters, previous growth restricted infant, previous preterm births)

Source: Lin & Santolaya-Forgas, 1998 [1]. Reproduced with permission of Lippencott Williams & Wilkins.

most commonly depends on the results of antenatal surveillance, which usually occurs at regular intervals, with the frequency depending on the overall clinical picture. Infants meeting criteria for IUGR should receive antenatal testing, usually consisting of Doppler indices of blood flow to and in the fetus, and usually a biophysical profile or modified biophysical profile. Fetuses with reassuring antenatal testing that are less than 34 weeks of gestation are often best followed in utero with serial antenatal testing [3–5]. Determining what to do in pregnancies between 34 and 37 weeks can be difficult and there is no consensus. It is known that the outcome of IUGR infants is predominantly determined by gestational age at delivery [6]. Knowing this, it may be reasonable to expectantly manage infants between 34 and 37 weeks unless fetal lung maturity is confirmed or there are signs of impending fetal compromise. The Growth Restriction Intervention Trial (GRIT) trial showed no clinically significant differences in cognition, language, motor performance, and behavior at 2 years of age between immediate and delayed delivery of infants with IUGR at 24–30 and 31–36 weeks of gestation [7]. The decision to deliver an IUGR fetus is often difficult and usually it is performed in consultation with a maternal-fetal medicine specialist who weighs the fetal Doppler and antenatal testing results with the gestational age when considering delivery.

Pregnancies complicated by IUGR do not necessarily require delivery via cesarean section. Induction of labor and vaginal delivery are reasonable to attempt, and cesarean delivery should be performed for obstetric indications. Continuous fetal monitoring during labor is very important in these pregnancies as there is increased risk for abnormal fetal heart tracings secondary to oligohydramnios and or placental insufficiency. Delivery should be at a facility with neonatology available [3].

14.1.2 Macrosomia/fetal overgrowth

Fetal macrosomia is defined as a birth weight greater than or equal to the 90th percentile based on gestational age standards. The etiologies of macrosomia vary and can be due to constitutional factors (maternal age, parity, and maternal weight gain), uncontrolled diabetes, or genetic conditions that cause fetal overgrowth [8]. As a result of the varied causes of fetal macrosomia, management of the pregnancy varies with the suspected cause. Basic steps include ensuring correct dating, testing for maternal diabetes, and performing a detailed anatomy ultrasound looking for other congenital anomalies. Assuming the dating is correct and diabetes has been ruled out, genetic studies, such as amniocentesis and chorionic villus sampling, may be offered [9].

Delivery decisions for the macrosomic infant can be difficult due to ultrasound measurements having a 10–20% error in measurement [10]. Complications related to vaginal delivery of the macrosomic infant include prolonged first stage of labor, increased cesarean section rate, and increased blood loss [11]. In infants diagnosed with macrosomia due to maternal diabetes there is an increased risk of birth trauma to the mother and fetus [10]. These adverse outcomes have not been consistently seen in nondiabetic mothers [12]. However, given the risks of shoulder dystocia and birth trauma associated when the estimated fetal weight (EFW) is > 4500 g an elective cesarean delivery can be considered according to the American Congress of Obstetricians and Gynecologists [10]. When the EFW is between 4000 and 4500 g the patient's history, clinical pelvimetry, and fetal abdominal circumference should be taken into consideration when deciding between vaginal and cesarean delivery. In patients where vaginal delivery is attempted, close attention should be paid to the labor curve as deviations from this can signal cephalopelvic disproportion and need for cesarean delivery. Practitioners should also be prepared for a shoulder dystocia at delivery and to move through necessary steps to reduce a shoulder dystocia [13].

14.2 Hemophilia

There are two different types of hemophilia: hemophilia A, caused by deficiency of factor VIII, and hemophilia B, caused by deficiency of factor XI. Both conditions have an X-linked inheritance pattern, so having an affected mother is rare. So in the heterozygous female symptoms are typically mild if present at all. Male infants are of particular concern because 50% of male infants born to a heterozygous mother will be affected. Carrier detection can be achieved prenatally using factor VIII and XI gene mutation analysis or linkage analysis on amniotic fluid [14]. A more risky procedure using cordocentesis can be performed but is reserved for non-diagnostic genetic testing due to the increased risks associated with the procedure [15].

Although one might suspect that infants with a confirmed diagnoses of hemophilia would have an increased risk of bleeding during a vaginal delivery, cesarean delivery does not appear to significantly decrease the risk of fetal intracranial and extracranial hemorrhage [16]. Vaginal delivery is safe for fetuses affected with hemophilia. Fetal scalp electrodes, forceps and vacuum delivery, and circumcision should be avoided in infants with hemophilia [17]. For mothers affected with hemophilia, their levels of factor VIII or IX should be checked periodically during gestation and at time of delivery. If levels are noted to be < 50 IU/dL recombinant factor products should be given as the risk of bleeding is increased below this level [16]. Recombinant factor products should also be considered if there is bleeding at delivery [18]. Additionally, DDAVP can be helpful in women with hemophilia A but not B. Women with hemophilia can safely have spinal or epidural anesthesia if factor levels are at > 50 IU/dL [19].

14.3 Skeletal dysplasias

14.3.1 Achondroplasia

Achondroplasia is a form of dwarfism that results in shortened limbs and is one of the most common skeletal dysplasias. Incidence is estimated to be about 1 in 26,000 live births and more than 80% of the cases are due to spontaneous mutations [20,21]. Prenatal diagnosis cannot be accomplished until the second trimester and is most often diagnosed by shortening of the long bones between 21 and 27 weeks of gestation [22].

For pregnancies where the fetus is suspected of having achondroplasia there are no special considerations for delivery. Patients can undergo a vaginal delivery with cesarean delivery reserved for obstetric indications. The majority of infants also do not require NICU admission. Macrosomia can be an issue for fetuses with achondroplasia and management of macrosomia is discussed above.

For pregnant women affected with achondroplasia there are special considerations at delivery. All of these women should have cesarean delivery due to the likely presence of pelvic contractures in the mother causing cephalopelvic disproportion [23,24]. Spinal and epidural anesthesia have been used safely with these patients for delivery [25,26].

14.3.2 Osteogenesis imperfecta

Osteogenesis imperfecta (OI) is a heterogeneous disorder characterized by bone fragility and low bone mass. There are multiple subtypes and the severity and symptoms depend on the subtype present [27]. The majority of cases are type II and type III. The types, severity, and mode of inheritance are listed in Table 14.2. Identification of affected fetuses can be performed in utero based on sonographic findings. The classic findings are the presence of in utero fractures with callus formation at the site of healing. Skull abnormalities, shortened long bones, and small chest circumference can also be seen [28]. Attempts should be made to diagnose the type of OI as soon as it is suspected so patients can be made aware of the poor prognosis if types II or III are suspected.

Mode of delivery can be particularly worrisome for obstetricians. A review of 167 pregnancies with confirmed OI was done by Cubert *et al.* in 2001 [29]. Of these, no increase in fracture rates was noted with vaginal delivery for nonlethal forms of OI and there was no prolongation survival noted with cesarean delivery of infants with lethal forms of OI. Cesarean deliveries were performed primarily for obstetric indications rather than for fear of fracture risk. Of note, 37% of the infants were in the breech presentation at term and had a cesarean delivery for this indication alone [29]. The authors of that paper recommend that cesarean delivery be reserved for obstetric indications for fetuses diagnosed with OI; however, this remains controversial.

Table 14.2 Features of osteogenesis imperfecta by type.

Type	Mode of inheritance	Severity
I	Autosomal dominant	Mild
II	Autosomal dominant/autosomal recessive	Lethal
III	Autosomal dominant	Severe
IV	Autosomal dominant	Mild to moderate
V	Autosomal dominant	Moderate
VI	Autosomal recessive	Moderate
VII	Autosomal recessive	Moderate
VIII	Autosomal recessive	Lethal/severe
IX	Autosomal recessive	Lethal/severe
X	Autosomal recessive	Lethal/severe
XI	Autosomal recessive	Severe

Mothers affected with OI also present a challenge for delivery. Spontaneous uterine rupture during attempted vaginal delivery has been reported in multiple patients with OI; however, not all of these cases were catastrophic and some went unnoticed until cesarean delivery for other obstetric indications [30–33]. Increased bleeding risk due to dysfunction platelet aggregation has also been reported in women with OI type I [34]. Vaginal delivery can be attempted in these patients; however, consideration of past fractures and injuries should be taken into account as position for pushing may be an issue for some patients. When attempting a vaginal delivery, continuous fetal monitoring should be utilized and any non-reassuring fetal heart tracing, loss of fetal station, or severe abdominal pain should be concerns for uterine rupture and prompt delivery via cesarean section.

14.4 Genetic abnormalities

Trisomies are the result of an extra copy of a chromosome, either whole or translocated onto another chromosome. Trisomy 21 is the most common trisomy and occurs at a prevalence of 13.65/10,000 live births in the United States [35]. Patients with suspected Trisomy 21 based on ultrasound findings or other antenatal screening should be offered an amniocentesis, CVS, or free fetal DNA in maternal serum testing for a definitive diagnosis. If a diagnosis of Trisomy 21 is confirmed, further testing for cardiac and other anatomic defects should take place if the parents desire to continue the pregnancy; this is so as to better counsel the parents on outcomes and to prepare them for delivery. There is no preferred delivery method for Trisomy 21 infants. Vaginal delivery should be attempted, with cesarean delivery reserved for obstetric indications. Discussions about continuous fetal monitoring and cesarean delivery for non-reassuring fetal status should take place prior to delivery. If the parents desire full intervention then delivery should take place at a tertiary care center with neonatology and pediatric specialists available.

Trisomy 18 and 13 are distinct genetic diseases and are the second and third most common forms of trisomy. Trisomy 18 has an incidence of 1 in 3000–7000 live births, and Trisomy 13 is found in 1 in 5000 live births [36–38]. Abnormalities of both disorders have characteristic ultrasound findings. Trisomy 18 typically presents with IUGR, rocker-bottom feet, clenched hands, cardiac defects, omphalocele, single umbilical artery, and renal anomalies [39,40]. Trisomy 13 is associated with holoprosencephaly, hypotelorism, cleft lip and/or palate, cardiac defects, increased nuchal lucency, polydactyly, and microcephaly [41,42]. Both of these trisomies are uniformly lethal and often result in intrauterine fetal demise or loss. Efforts should be made to confirm diagnosis via CVS, amniocentesis, or free fetal DNA prior to 24 weeks of gestation so parents have the option to terminate the pregnancy [43,44]. Patients who opt to continue the pregnancy to term do not need to deliver in a tertiary care center. Discussions about continuous fetal monitoring in labor and emergent cesarean section for fetal distress should be discussed with the parents prior to delivery. Neither condition requires delivery via cesarean section nor in fact should cesarean section be encouraged as it increases maternal risk for no apparent fetal benefit [45].

14.5 Cardiac defects

Multiple different cardiac defects can be detected in the newborn and they all have varying degrees of severity. We will not discuss each entity separately but will list preferred delivery method and special considerations in Table 14.3.

14.6 Abdominal wall defects

14.6.1 Omphalocele

Omphaloceles are defects in the ventral abdominal wall that are lacking abdominal muscles, fascia, and skin. There is a membrane consisting of peritoneum and amnion that covers the protruding abdominal contents in which the umbilical cord inserts. Incidence ranges from 1 in 4000–7000 live births [46]. Incidence is higher when stillbirths are combined, reflecting the increased risk of intrauterine fetal demise. Elevated MSAFP levels may be the first clue to the presence of an abdominal wall defect and should prompt a targeted sonogram to determine the cause. The incidence of finding associated fetal anomalies is as high as 30% and careful assessment of the rest of the fetus should be performed. Because the incidence of cardiac defects can be particularly high, fetal echocardiography is recommended [47]. The incidence of pulmonary hypertension and hypoplasia is

Table 14.3 Considerations and recommended mode of delivery for fetal congenital heart defects.

Cardiac defect	Preferred delivery method	Special considerations
Tachyarrhythmias	Vaginal delivery	– Intrapartum monitoring may not be reliable in supraventricular tachycardia – If hydrops is present deliver expeditiously via cesarean section – Treat mother with digoxin for supraventricular tachycardia
Bradyarrhythmias	Signs of cardiac decompensation – cesarean section No signs of cardiac decompensation – vaginal delivery	
Atrial septal defects	Vaginal delivery	Large defects or associated with other anomalies, recommend delivery at a tertiary care center
Ventricular septal defects	Vaginal delivery	Large defects or associated with other anomalies, recommend delivery at a tertiary care center
Atrioventricular canal defect	Vaginal delivery Cesarean section if significant hydrops	– Strong association with Trisomy 21, consider karyotype – Prenatal consultation with pediatric cardiology – Deliver at center with on-site pediatric cardiology team – Worse outcome with early delivery
Ebstein anomaly	Vaginal delivery	– Delivery in a tertiary care center – If hydrops, consider cesarean section and early delivery
Hypoplastic right ventricle	Vaginal delivery	– Prenatal consultation with pediatric cardiology – Worse outcome with small tricuspid valve or no tricuspid regurgitation – Delivery in a tertiary care center with pediatric cardiologist and cardiothoracic surgeon
Hypoplastic left ventricle	Vaginal delivery	– Worse prognosis with hydrops – Delivery in a tertiary care center with pediatric cardiologist and cardiothoracic surgeon
Pulmonary stenosis and atresia	Vaginal delivery	– Delivery in a tertiary care center with pediatric cardiologist
Aortic stenosis	Vaginal delivery Cesarean delivery if critical stenosis	– Delivery in a tertiary care center with pediatric cardiologist and cardiothoracic surgeon – Unclear if early delivery changes prognosis when hydrops present

(continued)

Table 14.3 (*continued*)

Cardiac defect	Preferred delivery method	Special considerations
Coarctation of the aorta	Vaginal delivery	– Consider karyotype, strong association with genetic abnormalities – Delivery in a tertiary care center with pediatric cardiologist
Tetralogy of Fallot	Vaginal delivery	– Consider karyotype, strong association with genetic abnormalities – Poor prognosis when hydrops present, unclear if early delivery needed – Delivery in a tertiary care center with pediatric cardiologist and cardiothoracic surgeon
Double outlet right ventricle	Vaginal delivery	– Consider karyotype, strong association with genetic abnormalities (Trisomy 13 and 18) – Unclear if early delivery changes prognosis when hydrops present – Delivery in a tertiary care center with pediatric cardiologist and cardiothoracic surgeon
Truncus arteriosus	Vaginal delivery	– Delivery in a tertiary care center with pediatric cardiologist and cardiothoracic surgeon – Await spontaneous labor – Unclear if early delivery changes prognosis when hydrops present
Transposition of great arteries	Vaginal delivery	– Delivery in a tertiary care center with pediatric cardiologist and cardiothoracic surgeon – Pre-delivery echocardiography to evaluate for immediate balloon atrioseptostomy; if amenable to surgery discuss delivery method and timing with pediatric team – Unclear if early delivery changes prognosis when hydrops present
Cardiomyopathy	Vaginal delivery	– Rule out dysrhythmias – Dilated cardiomyopathy – screen for anti-Ro and anti-La antibodies – Rule out maternal infections and diabetes
Intracardiac tumors	Vaginal delivery	– Early delivery if compromising cardiac function – Treat mother with digoxin for supraventricular tachycardia – Genetic consult to evaluate for tuberous sclerosis

increased in these infants and neonatology should be present at delivery in anticipation of such complications [48].

Delivery of infants with omphalocele should occur at hospitals with neonatologists and availability of pediatric surgery. Efforts should be made to transport the mother to such a hospital prior to delivery. The defect should have application of a moist sterile wrapping upon delivery. Mode of delivery has been debated for years in the literature and remains controversial. The most recent retrospective reviews do not show improved survival or difference in neonatal morbidity with vaginal delivery compared to infants born via cesarean section [49–51]. Additionally, Lewis *et al.* showed that labor prior to delivery via cesarean section did not adversely affect neonatal outcome [51]. Giant omphaloceles, most often defined as when the majority of the fetal liver is present in the defect, were not included in the aforementioned studies and despite that lack of a proven benefit these fetuses are often delivered by cesarean to prevent membrane rupture and liver trauma. While some institutions may still advocate for cesarean delivery due to timing and coordination with the pediatric surgeons and neonatology team, for most omphaloceles vaginal delivery is safe and does not appear to increase neonatal morbidity or mortality; cesarean delivery should be reserved for obstetric indications.

14.6.2 Gastroschisis

Gastroschisis is an abdominal wall defect in which the defect is to the right of a normally placed umbilical cord; because there is no membrane covering the abdominal contents they are exposed to the amniotic fluid which may adversely affect the intestines. The prevalence of gastroschisis appears to be increasing in both developed and developing countries [51]. Current rates in the United States range from 0.006–0.089/1000 live births [53]. Young maternal age and cigarette smoking have been associated with the occurrence of gastroschisis [54]. Due to the anterior abdominal wall defect, elevated MSAFP levels are seen [55]. Despite increasing ultrasound image quality, detection of abdominal wall defects is still not 100% and may be due to size of the defect, sonographer experience, or equipment [56].

Just as with omphalocele, mode of delivery is still a subject of debate. Patients should be delivered at institutions with neonatology present and access to pediatric surgeons. Also, it has been shown that timing of delivery is important. Likely due to the adverse effects on the bowel, infants delivered prior to 36 weeks show less inflammatory reaction around the bowel at delivery but have longer hospital stays and longer time to enteral feeding than infants delivered at > 36 weeks of gestation [57]. Outcomes of infants do not seem to be affected by labor or rupture of membranes [51,58]. Comparing outcomes for vaginal versus cesarean delivery is difficult due to the presence of confounding factors. The stillbirth rate appears high in fetuses with gastroschisis, especially later in gestation [49]. Currently, there is no evidence advocating for cesarean delivery over vaginal delivery. Patients undergoing vaginal delivery should have continuous fetal monitoring, and cesarean delivery should be performed for obstetric indications as necessary [53].

14.7 Myelomeningocele

Myelomeningoceles are an open spinal cord defect, not covered by skin, that protrudes dorsally as a result of abnormal neural tube fusion. Incidence varies with ethnic and geographic differences. The use of MSAFP for screening for neural tube defects has decreased the incidence of myelomeningoceles from 1.5 to 4.5/1000 live births prior up to 1980 to 0.5–1/1000 live births after 1980 [59]. Other risk factors, such as maternal diabetes, heart disease, lung disease, and use of certain drugs (anticonvulsants, sulfonamides), have been correlated with neural tube defects. Screening for myelomeningocele is done with MSAFP and those above 2–2.5 multiples of the median are considered abnormal, although sonography appears more accurate [53]. Ultrasound findings consistent with myelomeningocele include small biparietal diameter, small head circumference, "lemon sign," cerebellar abnormality ("banana sign"), lateral ventriculomegaly, Chiari II abnormalities, meningocele sac, myelomeningocele sac, and splaying or dorsal vertebral elements [60,61]. Fetal MRI can help further define the level of myelomeningocele and help in counseling about prognosis [62].

Route of delivery is controversial, but the majority of studies do not show any neurologic benefit to cesarean delivery versus vaginal delivery for fetuses with myelomeningocele [63]. These recommendations have been further refined to say elective cesarean delivery should be performed when the fetus demonstrates knee and ankle movement and the myelomeningocele sac protrudes beyond the back. Cesarean delivery is not indicated for fetuses with known chromosomal anomalies that are potentially lethal or if there is no knee of ankle movement noted in the fetus [64]. In certain areas of the country fetal surgery may be available to repair neural tube defects while the fetus is still in utero. The Management of Myelomeningocele Study (MOMS) trial showed that infants that underwent closure of myelomeningocele in utero were less likely to need a ventricular shunt and had fewer incidents of Chiari malformation and that more children were walking independently at 30 months of age [65]. Due to the large hysterotomy scar that is formed as a result of the fetal surgery, it is recommended these patients have a cesarean delivery by 37 weeks of gestation (if they do not go into preterm labor) to decrease the risk of uterine rupture [66].

References

1 Lin CC and Santolaya-Forgas J. Current concepts of fetal growth restriction, Part I. Causes, classification and pathophysiology. *Obstetrics & Gynecology* 1998;**82**:1044–1055.

2 Boers KE, van Wyk L, van der Post JA *et al.* Neonatal morbidity after induction vs. expectant monitoring in intrauterine growth restriction at term: a subanalysis of the DIGITAT RCT. *American Journal of Obstetrics & Gynecology* 2012; **206**:e1–7.

3 American College of Obstetricians and Gynecology Practice Bulletin No.12: Intrauterine Growth Restriction. Washington, DC: ACOG, 2000.

4 Harman CR and Baschat AA. Arterial and venous Doppler in IUGR. *Clinical Obstetrics and Gynecology* 2003;**46**:931–946.
5 Ott WJ. Development of a fetal risk assessment score for the prediction of neonatal outcome in the growth-restricted fetus. *Journal of Maternal-Fetal and Neonatal Medicine* 2012; Epub. DOI: 10.3109/14767058.2012.679712.
6 Cosmi E, Ambrosini G, D'Antona D *et al.* Doppler, cardiotocography and biophysical profile changes in growth-restricted fetuses. *Obstetrics & Gynecology* 2005;**106**:1240–1245.
7 Walker DM *et al.* The Growth Restriction Intervention Trial: long-term outcomes in a randomized trial of timing of delivery in fetal growth restriction. *American Journal of Obstetrics & Gynecology* 2009;**204**:34 e1–e9.
8 Cyntrynbaum CS, Smith AC, Rubin T, and Weksberg R. Advances in overgrowth syndromes: clinical classification to molecular delineation in Sotos syndrome and Beckwith-Wiedemann syndrome. *Current Opinion in Pediatrics* 2005;**17**:740–746.
9 Faivre L, Rosseau T. Laurent N *et al.* Prenatal overgrowth and mosaic trisomy 15q25-qter including the IGF1 receptor gene. *Prenatal Diagnosis* 2004;**24**:393–395.
10 American College of Obstetricians and Gynecologists Practice Bulletin No. 30: Gestational Diabetes. Washington, DC: ACOG, 2001.
11 Ahmed S, Romejko-Wolniewicz E, Zareba-Szczudlik J, and Czajkowski K. Fetal macrosomia – an obstetrician's nightmare? *Neuroendocrinology letters* 2012;**33**:149–155.
12 Haram K, Pirhonen J, and Bergsjo P. Suspected big baby: a difficult clinical problem in obstetrics. *Acta Obstetricia et Gynecologica Scandinavica* 2002;**81**:185–194.
13 Hoffman MK, Bailit JL, Branch DW *et al.* A comparison of obstetric maneuvers for the acute management of shoulder dystocia. *Obstetrics & Gynecology* 2011;**117**:1272–1278.
14 Firshein DI, Hoyer LW, Lazarchick J *et al.* Prenatal diagnosis of classic hemophilias. *New England Journal of Medicine* 1979;**300**:937–941.
15 Shetty S and Ghosh K. Robustness of factor assays following cordocentesis in the prenatal diagnosis of hemophilia and other bleeding disorders. *Haemophilia* 2007;**13**:172.
16 Kulkarni R and Lusher JM. Intracranial and extracranial hemorrhages in newborns with hemophilia; a review of the literature. *Journal of Pediatric Hematology/Oncology.* 1999;**21**:289–295.
17 Creasy RK, Resnik R, Iams JD, Lockwood CJ, and Moore TR (eds). *Creasy & Resnick's Maternal-Fetal Medicine*, 6th edn. Philadelphia, PA: Saunders Elsevier, 2009
18 Peyvandi F, Jayandharan G, Chandy M *et al.* Genetic diagnosis of hemophilia and other inherited bleeding disorders. *Haemophilia* 2006;**12**:82.
19 Sage DJ. Epidurals, spinals, and bleeding disorders in pregnancy: a review. *Anaesthesia and Intensive Care* 1990;**18**:319.
20 Oberklaid F, Danks DM, Jensen F, Stace L, and Rosshandler S. Achondroplasia and hypochondroplasia. *Journal of Medical Genetics* 1979;**16**:140–146.
21 Shaing R, Thompson LM, Zhu Y-Z *et al.* Mutations in the transmembrane domain of FGFR3 cause the most common genetic form of dwarfism, achondroplasia. *Cell* 1994;**78**:335–342.
22 Kurtz AB, Filly RA, Wapner RJ *et al.* In utero analysis of heterozygous achondroplasia: variable time of onset as detected by femur length measurements. *Journal of Ultrasound in Medicine* 1986;**5**:137–140.
23 Lattanzi DR and Harger JH. Achondroplasia and pregnancy. *Journal of Reproductive Medicine* 1982;**27**:363–366.
24 Allanson JE and Hall JG. Obstetric and gynecologic problems in women with chondrodystropies. *Obstetrics & Gynecology* 1986;**67**:74–78.
25 Carstoniu J, Yee I, and Halpern S. Epidural anesthesia for caesarean section in an achondroplastic dwarf. *Canadian Journal of Anesthesia* 1992;**39**:708–711.
26 Roofthooft E, and Van de Velde M. Low-dose spinal anesthesia for caesarean section to prevent spinal-induced hypotension. *Current Opinion in Anaesthesiology* 2008; **21**:259–262.

27 Brons JT, Van Der Harten HJ, Wladimiroff JW *et al.* Prenatal ultrasonographic diagnosis of osteogenesis imperfecta. *American Journal of Obstetrics & Gynecology* 1988;**159**:176–181.
28 Constantine G, McCormack J, McHugo J, and Fowlie A. Prenatal diagnosis of severe osteogenesis imperfecta. *Prenatal Diagnosis* 1991;**11**:103–110.
29 Cubert R, Cheng EY, Mack S, Pepin MG, and Byers PH. Osteogenesis imperfecta: mode of delivery and neonatal outcome. *Obstetrics & Gynecology* 2001;**97**:66–69.
30 Carlson JW and Harlass FE. Management of osteogenesis imperfecta in pregnancy: a case report. *Journal of Reproductive Medicine* 1993;**38**:228–232.
31 Krishnamoorthy U, Vausse S, and Donnai P. 2002. Management of pregnancy complicated by maternal osteogenesis imperfecta. Report of a case with uterine rupture. *Journal of Obstetrics and Gynecology* 2002;**22**:316–322.
32 Young BK and Gorstein F. Maternal osteogenesis imperfecta. *Obstetrics & Gynecology* 1969;**31**:461–470.
33 Christodoulou S, Freemont AJ, McVey R, and Vause S. Prospective comparative case study of uterine collagen in a woman with osteogenesis imperfecta type 1 who had previously ruptured her uterus. *Journal of Obstetrics and Gynecology* 2007;**27**:738–739.
34 Parasuraman R, Taylor MJO, Liversedge H, and Gilg J. Pregnancy management in type III maternal osteogenesis imperfecta. *Journal of Obstetrics and Gynecology* 2007;**27**:619–621.
35 Canfield MA, Honein MA, Yuskiv N *et al.* National estimates and race/ethnic-specific variation of selected birth defects in the United States, 1999–2001. *Birth Defects Research: Clinical and Molecular Teratology* 2006;**76**:747–756.
36 Young ID, Cook JO, and Metha L. Changing demography of trisomy 18. *Archives of Disease in Childhood* 1986;**61**:1035–1036.
37 Goldstein H and Nielsen KG. Rates and survival of individuals with trisomy 13 and 18. *Clinical Genetics* 1988;**34**:366–372.
38 Wladimiroff JW, Stewart PA, Reuss A, and Sachs ES. Cardiac and extracardiac anomalies as indicators for trisomies 13 and 18: a prenatal ultrasound study. *Prenatal Diagnosis* 1989;**9**(7):515–520.
39 Carlson DE, Platt LD, and Medearis A. The ultrasound triad of fetal hydramnios, abnormal hand posturing, and any other anomaly predicts autosomal trisomy. *Obstetrics & Gynecology* 1992;**79**:731–734.
40 Benacerraf B, Miller WA, and Frigoletto FD. Sonographic detection of fetuses with trisomies 13 and 18: accuracy and limitations. *American Journal of Obstetrics & Gynecology* 1988;**158**:404–409.
41 Nicolaides KH, Snijders RJM, Godsen CM, Berru C, and Campbell S. Utrasonographically detectable markers of fetal chromosomal abnormalities. *Lancet* 1992;**340**:704–707.
42 Nyberg DA and Souter VL. Sonographic markers of fetal trisomies. *Journal of Ultrasound in Medicine* 2001;**20**:65–674.
43 Won RH, Currier RJ, Lorey F, and Towner DR. The timing of demise in fetuses with trisomy 21 and trisomy 18. *Prenatal Diagnosis* 2005;**25**:608–611.
44 Jacobs PA, Hassold TI, Henry A, Pettay D, and Takaesu N. Trisomy 13 ascertained in a survey of spontaneous abortions. *Journal of Medical Genetics* 1987;**24**:721–724.
45 Schnieder AS, Mennutu MT, and Zackai EH. High cesarean section rate in trisomy 18 births: a potential indication for late prenatal diagnosis. *American Journal of Obstetrics & Gynecology* 1981;**140**:367–370.
46 Stoll C, Alembik Y, Dott B, and Roth MP. Omphalocele and gastroschisis and associated malformations. *American Journal of Medical Genetics* 2008;**146**:1280–1285.
47 Copel JA, Pilu, and Kleinman CS. Congenital heart disease and extracardiac anomalies: associations and indications for fetal echocardiography. *American Journal of Obstetrics & Gynecology* 1986;**154**:1121–1132.

48 Lee SL, Beyer TD, Im SS *et al.* Initial nonoperative management and delayed closure for treatment of giant omphaloceles. *Journal of Pediatric Surgery* 2006;**41**:1403–1406.

49 How HY, Harris BJ, Pietrantoni M *et al.* Is vaginal delivery preferable to elective cesarean delivery in fetuses with a known ventral wall defect? *American Journal of Obstetrics & Gynecology* 2000;**182**:1527–1534.

50 Segel SY, Marder SJ, Parry S *et al.* Fetal abdominal wall defects and mode of delivery: a systematic review. *Obstetrics & Gynecology* 2001;**98**:867–873.

51 Lewis DF, Towers CV, Farite TJ *et al.* Fetal gastroschisis and omphalocele: is cesarean section the best mode of delivery. *American Journal of Obstetrics & Gynecology* 1990;**163**:773–775.

52 Hwang PJ and Kouseff BG. Omphalocele and gastroschisis: an 18-year review study. *Genetics in Medicine* 2004;**6**:232–236.

53 Roeper PJ, Harris J, and Lee G. Secular rates and correlates for gastroschisis in California (1986–1977). *Teratology* 1987;**35**:203–210.

54 Goldbaum G, Daling J, and Milham S. Risk factors for gastroschisis. *Teratology* 1990;**42**:397–403.

55 American College of Obstetricians and Gynecologists Practice Bulletin No. 77: Screening for Fetal Chromosomal Anomalies. Washington, DC: ACOG, 2007.

56 Paidas M, Crombleholme TM, and Roberston FM. Prenatal diagnosis and management of the fetus with an abdominal wall injury. *Seminars in Perinatology* 1994;**18**:182–195.

57 Ergun O, Barksdale E, Ergun FS *et al.* The timing of delivery of infants with gastroschisis influences outcome. *Journal of Pediatric Surgery* 2005;**40**:424–428.

58 Strauss RA, Balu R, Kuller JA *et al.* Gastroschisis: the effect of labor and rupture membranes on neonatal outcome. *American Journal of Obstetrics & Gynecology* 2003;**189**:1672–1678.

59 Shaer CM, Chescheir N, Schulkin J. Myelimeningocele: a review of the epidemiology, genetics, risk factors for conception, prenatal diagnosis and prognosis for affected individuals. *Obstetrical and Gynecological Survey* 2007;**62**:471–479.

60 Van den Hoff MC, Nicolaides KH, Campbell J, and Campbell S. Evaluation of the lemon and banana signs in one hundred thirty fetuses with open spina bifida. *American Journal of Obstetrics & Gynecology* 1990;**162**:322–327.

61 Kollias SS, Goldstein RB, Cogen PH, and Filly RA. Prenatally detected myelomeningoceles: sonographic accuracy in estimation of the spinal level. *Radiology* 1992;**185**:109–112.

62 Dinh DH, Wright RM, and Hanigan WC. The use of magnetic resonance imaging for the diagnosis of fetal intracranial anomalies. *Child's Nervous System* 1990;**6**:212–215.

63 Cuppen I *et al.* Influence of birth mode on early neurologic outcome in infants with myelomeningocele. *European Journal of Obstetrics & Gynecology and Reproductive Biology* 2001;**156**:18–22.

64 Shurtleff DB and Lemire RJ. Epidemiology, etiologic factors and prenatal diagnosis of open spinal dystrophies. *Neurosurgery Clinics of North America* 1995;**6**:183–193.

65 Adzick SN *et al.* A randomized trial of prenatal versus postnatal repair of myelomeningocele. *New England Journal of Medicine* 2011;**364**:993–1004.

66 Gupta N, Farrell JA, Rand L, Cauldwell CB, and Farmer D. Open fetal surgery for myelomeningocele. *Journal of Neurosurgery: Pediatrics* 2012;**9**:265–273.

CHAPTER 15

Labor and delivery management of the obese gravida

Jordan H. Perlow, Megan Jones, and John Ozimek

Division of Maternal-Fetal Medicine, Department of Obstetrics and Gynecology, Banner Good Samaritan Medical Center, Phoenix, AZ, USA

15.1 Intrapartum management

15.1.1 Introduction

Obesity complicating pregnancy has been uniformly shown to increase the risk for adverse maternal, fetal, and neonatal outcomes [1]. There is a direct correlation between the degree of obesity and the severity of associated complications, including diabetes, postpartum hemorrhage, fetal macrosomia, preterm delivery, intrauterine fetal death, and extended postpartum hospitalization neonatal intensive care unit (NICU) admissions [2]. The obese gravida is also at increased risk for developing preeclampsia, with one large study demonstrating that the risk of preeclampsia doubles with each 5–7 kg/m^2 increase in prepregnancy BMI [3]. Neonates born to mothers with BMI > 40 are at increased risk for peripheral nervous system, skeletal injury, respiratory distress syndrome, bacterial sepsis, seizures, and hypoglycemia, regardless of mode of delivery [4]. Preexisting conditions such as hypertension and diabetes mellitus are often exacerbated by pregnancy, and further increase the risk for additional complications, including hypertensive disorders of pregnancy, fetal macrosomia, and intrauterine growth restriction. Longstanding maternal hypertension and diabetes may also predispose to cardiomyopathy and renal disease, and consideration should be given to prepregnancy or early pregnancy cardiology consultation. These disorders should be recognized and medically optimized prenatally. This allows for appropriate counseling and optimization of maternal health, which will decrease the incidence of maternal or fetal complications. Optimal intrapartum management of the obese gravida requires that the obstetrician work closely with the labor and delivery nurse, obstetric

---

Management of Labor and Delivery, Second Edition. Edited by George A. Macones.

anesthesiologist, nurse anesthetist, and pediatric team to ensure that all are aware of, and prepared for, potential complications.

15.1.2 Labor position

Physiologic changes associated with obesity include: diminished lung volumes and capacities, decreased lung and chest wall compliance, decreased breathing efficiency and gas exchange, and relative hypoxia secondary to pulmonary shunt. For these reasons, careful consideration should be given to maternal position of the obese patient in labor. Optimal positioning can help to minimize maternal and fetal hypoxia, with the left lateral position being most preferable. This position optimizes maternal oxygenation and uteroplacental blood flow and prevents caval compression. A sitting position with the head and chest elevated may also improve maternal comfort, prevent airway closure, and improve oxygenation. Continuous pulse oximetry monitoring should be initiated to identify hypoxia and supplemental oxygen provided as needed. Epidural anesthesia should be considered, as the analgesia provided may decrease respiratory work by reducing pain [5].

15.1.3 Anesthesia

As anesthesia complications are higher in the setting of obesity and pregnancy [6,7], consultation with an anesthesiologist, either during the antepartum period or upon admission to labor and delivery, is advisable [8,9]. After general assessment of the patient's cardiovascular and pulmonary status, a thorough evaluation of the airway is essential. Anesthesia evaluation, ideally in the non-emergent situation, is advised, as it has been reported that 80% of all anesthesia-related maternal mortality occurred among obese patients, with inability to accomplish intubation noted as the principal cause [10]. In fact, nearly a third of these patients may experience difficult intubation [11]. Given the challenges of accurate blood pressure measurement in the obese patient population, and difficulty with intravenous access, consideration may be given for a central venous line and an arterial line if clinically indicated.

As one meta-analysis demonstrated that obesity more than doubled the risk of emergency cesarean section [12], it may be advisable to prophylactically place an epidural catheter early in labor. Early catheter placement may eliminate the need for general anesthesia (and its inherent increased risks) should an emergency cesarean section become necessary. Also, when compared to lean women, obese women experienced a significantly higher rate of initial epidural anesthesia failure requiring epidural catheter replacement [10]. Other technical difficulties during epidural catheter placement are more prominent among obese patients, including: more inadvertent dural puncture, a higher frequency of multiple attempts at placement, and higher rates of hypotension and fetal heart rate decelerations [13,14]. Ideally, epidural placement should occur in a non-emergent fashion, especially where obesity poses technical challenges with placement.

15.1.4 Aspiration prophylaxis

Anesthesiologists should be notified when a gravid obese patient is admitted to Labor and Delivery, or other areas of the hospital where the potential need for anesthesia intervention exists in a pregnant woman. Planning for potential complications is always preferable to responding to a crisis without being forewarned and thus, prepared. Anesthetic complications leading to maternal mortality have fortunately seen reductions in recent years; however, the risks remain substantial [15]. Aspiration of acidic gastric contents remains a life-threatening risk, particularly for the obese gravida. The risks are intensified among obese gravidae due to anatomic barriers to intubation, increased gastric contents with lower pH values, and a diminished barrier pressure due to the difference between lower esophageal sphincter tone and intragastric pressure [16]. As more attempts are needed to place regional anesthesia in obese women [6], the potential benefits of an early anesthesia evaluation to consider placement of an epidural catheter prophylactically, and to evaluate the patient for intubation risks, are apparent. This assessment, in addition to pharmacological therapies to reduce aspiration risk, is critical and is the most effective way to prepare for and minimize difficult intubation and its associated morbidity [17,5]. Although randomized trials are lacking, a practical approach that we individually consider includes an H2 antagonist (e.g. ranitidine hydrochloride 50 mg IV q 6–8 hrs in labor or 45 minutes prior to surgery). Sodium citrate with citric acid (Bicitra® [Willen Drug Company, Baltimore, MD]: 30 ml of 0.3 M) should be given to all patients prior to anesthesia, and one may also consider metoclopramide (10 mg IV over 1–2 min) 45 minutes prior to surgery to further reduce aspiration risks in this population [5].

15.1.5 Induction of labor

Induction of labor (IOL) is associated with higher risks of obstetrical complications when compared to spontaneous labor. While cesarean section carries greater risks for morbidity than successful induction of labor resulting in vaginal delivery, the greatest risk occurs in women who undergo cesarean delivery following prolonged labor, particularly among the obese population. Unfortunately, medical conditions associated with obesity such as hypertension and diabetes more frequently necessitate medically indicated preterm or early-term induction of labor. Obese women are also more likely to undergo induction of labor for post-dates. Overall, it has been reported that the rate of labor induction is approximately 1.6–2.1-fold higher among obese women when compared to their normal weight counterparts. Failure of induction is also more common among obese women.

A large population-based cohort study examined rates of induction failure stratified by BMI among 89,131 women who underwent IOL [18]. The authors found that the rate of IOL was associated with increasing BMI, with 28% of normal weight women and 34% of women with BMI > 40 kg/m^2 undergoing IOL.

They also reported that the rate of failed induction increased as BMI increased, with 13% of normal weight women, 20.2% with BMI 30–34.9, 24.2% with BMI 35–39.9, and 29% with BMI > 40 failing induction of labor. Rates of failed induction among the obese increased further with birth weight of > 4000 g and in those who had not had a previous vaginal delivery.

A second study, a secondary analysis that included 1273 patients, estimated the effect of BMI on the outcome of prostaglandin labor induction [19]. Patients were stratified by BMI and the duration and outcome of labor were analyzed. The authors found that increasing BMI correlated with an increased incidence of cesarean delivery from 21.3% in those with BMI < 30, to 29.8% in those with BMI 30–39.9, and 36.5% in those with BMI > 40. They also reported increased dose and duration of oxytocin, and increased median time to delivery as BMI increased.

15.1.6 Dysfunctional labor

Arrest of dilation, as historically defined by the Friedman labor curve, is often noted as the reason for cesarean delivery among obese patients in labor. Multiple studies have demonstrated, however, that the Friedman curve is not applicable to all women, particularly obese women. One recent retrospective cohort study of 5204 women with singleton, term pregnancies and vertex presentation compared the length of first stage of labor between women with BMI < 30 and BMI > 30 [20]. Findings indicated significantly longer duration (4–10 cm: 4.7 compared with 4.1 hrs) and slower progression of cervical dilation from 4 to 6 cm (1.9 compared with 2.2 hrs) among obese women. The authors concluded that obesity should be considered when defining normal labor. Another large retrospective, multicenter review of 118,978 gravidas with singleton, term cephalic gestations compared labor patterns by body mass index [21]. Findings were largely similar to the previous study. The authors concluded that the time difference to reach 10 cm dilation was 1.2 hours from the lowest to highest BMI category for nulliparas. Those with BMI > 40 took longer to reach active phase. Progression by centimeter from 4–10 cm was also shown to increase in duration as BMI increased. The authors suggest that labor management should be altered as appropriate for obese women. A third study analyzed the effect of obesity on labor progression in 612 nulliparous women with a term pregnancy [22]. The results support the findings of the previous two studies. The authors found that the median duration of labor from 4–10 cm was significantly longer for both overweight and obese women compared with normal weight women (7.5, 7.9, and 6.2 hrs, respectively) [22]. Thus, an awareness of the contemporary literature addressing length of labor is recommended so as to allow these patients to achieve vaginal delivery.

Interestingly, multiple studies indicate that increasing maternal BMI does not prolong the second stage of labor. In one large study, secondary analysis of 3739 nulliparous women who met inclusion criteria was performed to evaluate the length of the second stage of labor in relation to increasing maternal prepregnancy BMI [23]. The authors found that increasing maternal BMI was not associated with second stage duration: normal weight 1.1 hr, overweight 1.1 hr, and obese 1.0 hr. Second stage length was also examined according to increasing BMI in another study [21], where, again, second stage length was similar among BMI categories for nulliparous patients but actually decreased as BMI increased for multiparas.

Generally, the achievement of a successful vaginal delivery is preferred in the obese patient given that obese women who undergo cesarean delivery are at a higher risk of morbidities when compared to those women with a normal BMI [24–26]. Rates of wound infection, wound separation, dehiscence, anesthetic complications, and surgical injury are higher among obese women undergoing cesarean section [26–28]. Given a uniform body of evidence indicating higher rates of complications for the obese gravida undergoing cesarean delivery, it is important to reserve cesarean section for true obstetrical indications, where risk/benefit analysis has been undertaken and in the setting of careful patient counseling.

15.1.7 Trial of labor after cesarean

Following cesarean delivery, obese women are significantly less successful in achieving vaginal birth in subsequent pregnancies. Failed trial of labor after cesarean (TOLAC) rates among obese women are higher, and women with excessive weight gain also have lower TOLAC success rates [29]. Exact mechanisms of failure are unknown; however, contributing factors include induction of labor, nulliparity, macrosomia, and a recurrent indication prompting prior cesarean delivery [30]. Maternal and neonatal morbidity also increase with obesity in TOLAC. Maternal morbidity is increased sixfold, and uterine rupture rates double from 1 to 2% compared to those of patients of normal weight. Additionally, neonatal morbidity, including fractures, nerve injury, and lacerations, increases from 0.2 to 1%, though no difference in neonatal encephalopathy has been observed [31].

Obesity may reduce the likelihood of TOLAC success to no more than 15% [18], with significantly increased risks for infectious morbidity described. Therefore, in counseling the obese patient with respect to issues relating to TOLAC, realistic outcomes should be conveyed with significantly higher risks for cesarean delivery noted. If TOLAC is desired, the significantly higher failure rate, accompanied by the surgical, anesthetic, and perioperative morbidity risks that apply to a failed attempt, should be thoroughly discussed and documented [32]. Also worthy of discussion with patients is the anticipated longer delivery interval required from the initiation of surgery (skin incision). Thus, the ability to extract the fetus from the maternal abdomen in the emergent setting of uterine rupture would likely be impaired to some degree due to maternal obesity. Certainly, the degree of the patient's obesity as well as the individual body habitus of the patient should be taken into account.

15.1.8 Anticipated complications associated with macrosomia

Obese women are twofold more likely to give birth to infants weighing over 4500 g, and obesity has been shown to bc an independent risk factor for fetal macrosomia [33]. Thus, the obstetrical team should be well prepared for the complications associated with macrosomia, including shoulder dystocia, malpresentation, postpartum hemorrhage, and vaginal lacerations. Obtaining or confirming a recent estimated fetal weight by ultrasound on presentation to labor and delivery should be considered to facilitate and prepare for any anticipated complications, and to assist in guiding counseling regarding route of delivery. A large, 15-year, population-based cohort study comparing maternal outcomes in 142,404 obese and non-obese women demonstrated increased risk of shoulder dystocia and postpartum hemorrhage among obese patients [28]. The American College of Obstetricians and Gynecologists (ACOG) recommends consideration for delivery by cesarean section when the estimated fetal weight reaches 4500 g in pregnancy complicated by diabetes, and 5000 g otherwise (ACOG Practice Bulletin No. 22, November 2000; reaffirmed 2013). There are no evidence-based recommendations for modifying these recommendations based on maternal BMI.

15.2 Cesarean section

The obese gravida is at least twice as likely to be delivered by primary cesarean section, and furthermore, her risk for emergency cesarean section and perioperative morbidity is significantly higher. Over the last 20 years, the increasing prevalence of obesity has contributed significantly to the increasing cesarean rate in the United States. Even in a low-risk population receiving midwifery care, the incidence of obesity-related cesarean deliveries has tripled [34]. Obesity-specific risks associated with cesarean delivery include unsuccessful placement of the epidural catheter, prolonged operative and delivery times, increased blood loss, prolonged hospitalization, venous thrombosis, and nearly a 10-fold increase in endomyometritis and wound infection, as discussed below [2].

15.2.1 Factors contributing to cesarean delivery

The antepartum period allows time for the provider to counsel and prepare gravid patients for expectations during labor and delivery. Obesity is strongly associated with higher rates of diabetes and hypertensive disease, and the obese gravida should be aware of the higher indication for induction of labor due to these risk factors [33]. Even without maternal conditions prompting induction, rate of postterm induction is 50% greater among obese women, which indicates that abnormalities of spontaneous labor might exist in this population. During labor, obese women have slower cervical dilation rates and longer, protracted stages of labor. Rates of failed inductions in addition to abnormal labor courses are significantly higher [22]. Macrosomia is twofold greater, shoulder dystocia is threefold greater, and failed instrumental deliveries are twofold greater among obese women. Following delivery, neonatal morbidity is elevated, which is exemplified by lower Apgar scores and higher rates of NICU admissions, feeding difficulties, and neonatal trauma [35].

This information has prompted many studies to evaluate the incidence of cesarean delivery according to BMI, and the data are overwhelmingly consistent in demonstrating a strong correlation. Invariably, studies and meta-analyses suggest that cesarean delivery rates are directly and positively correlated to BMI, with average risks 1.5-, two-, and threefold higher in overweight (BMI > 25), obese (BMI > 30), and morbidly obese (BMI > 35) women, respectively, prior to conception [36]. Additionally, excessive weight gain in pregnancy can further increase the risks for cesarean delivery, even with an ideal BMI prior to conception. In a study involving 460,000 women with singleton gestations, cesarean delivery risk increased 80% if BMI increased > 10 throughout pregnancy [24].

15.2.2 Operative challenges and surgical approach

Even in experienced hands, cesarean delivery of obese women is physically and technically challenging. A skilled and mindful approach must be taken to accommodate the size of the patient, concurrent co-morbidities, and perioperative risks [1,37]. The approach should be one that assures the greatest likelihood for patient safety, with utilization of experienced obstetrical providers and staff in sufficient numbers, and appropriate equipment. Surgical equipment, tables, and instruments must be sized to accommodate the increased body mass and deeper operative field. Monitoring devices and equipment, such as blood pressure cuffs and sequential compression devices, must be fitted appropriately [11]. Peripheral IV access may be difficult, with ultrasound-guided placement having been shown in some studies to reduce the number of attempts, time to successful cannulation, and patient satisfaction [38].

Each patient should be individually assessed prior to surgical draping and skin preparation in order to best plan surgical incision placement. While vertical skin incisions are generally discouraged due to higher risks for wound complications [39], at times this may indeed provide the safest and best approach to accomplish cesarean delivery (e.g. history of multiple prior cesareans, other abdominal surgery, concern for the need for cesarean hysterectomy, history of pelvic adhesive disease, uterine myomata, etc.) for a given patient. Thus, many factors must be considered to determine the most appropriate type of incision during a cesarean delivery when pregnancy is complicated by obesity. Transverse incisions provide more tensile strength upon closure and less postoperative pain and respiratory compromise, but difficulty with visualization and retraction of the pannus can pose a problem [11]. Vertical skin incisions have been utilized with the idea to gain better exposure and minimize blood loss; however, longer operative times, greater blood loss, and higher infection rates up to 12-fold that of transverse incisions have been observed. Among transverse incisions, no difference in infection rates has been observed with supra- versus infraumbilical [40].

When the pannus can be retracted cephalad without causing significant respiratory compromise, and when such retraction allows for minimally unencumbered access to the lower abdomen, we proceed with pannus retraction utilizing Montgomery straps or simply using adhesive tape, utilizing the "ether screen" device on the surgical bed as a point of attachment, and create a transverse low abdominal skin incision (Pfannensteil)[11]. When cephalad retraction of the pannus does, however, compromise maternal respiratory function, or where such retraction results in a "vertical wall" of adipose tissue, precluding ready access to the lower abdomen, we prefer to leave the pannus *in situ*, and use a transverse periumbilical approach to skin incision placement.

Great care should be taken as one proceeds through subcutaneous tissue dissection, as large caliber veins are commonly found within the adipose tissue in this location, as well as just beneath the fascia. Particularly when the pannus is left *in situ*, great caution should be exercised in planning incision placement as care must be taken to direct the incision *into* the peritoneal cavity and not "through and through" the pannus. Clearly, a "hands-on" exam by an experienced practitioner will prove crucial in determining optimal incision placement. We also use a retractor such as the Alexis-O® (Applied Medical, Rancho Santa Margarita, CA) on an individualized basis to allow for retraction of the thick layer of subcutaneous fat circumferentially, which we have found helpful in allowing ideal exposure for uterine incision placement and delivery.

Operative time has been shown to be significantly greater, which contributes to a higher rate of neonatal and maternal morbidities. Data suggest operative times are 30% increased overall, and time from skin incision to delivery is increased 25% in obese women. Importantly, the risk for emergent cesarean delivery is markedly higher in this population, where operative time becomes critical with respect to maternal-fetal-neonatal outcomes. Awareness of these risks needs to be collectively addressed by members of the labor team to facilitate rapid preparation, delivery, and a safe operative course that minimizes complications [27].

Obstetrical hemorrhage, defined as blood loss > 1000 mL during cesarean delivery, is significantly more prevalent among obese women. Rates can rise to 35%, and studies worldwide involving thousands of obese gravid women report higher rates of estimated blood loss greater than 1500 cc. Obesity can increase the risk for substantial hemorrhage threefold, and this has been attributed to the technically difficult surgery, risks for emergent intervention, and higher rates of co-morbidities [33]. Thus, postpartum hemorrhage management protocols should be familiar to staff, and both mechanical and pharmacologic interventions designed to treat this life-threatening complication should be readily available.

A methodical approach to cesarean section is critical for a successful outcome for these high-risk patients, and consists of appropriate preparation, a focus on the task at hand, clear communication amongst the surgical team, and a deliberate approach devoid of distraction.

15.2.3 Avoiding postoperative complications

Postoperative wound complications rise significantly with increasing BMI, with type of incision, intraoperative management, and type of closure also contributing factors [41,42]. Controlling for other variables, women with a BMI > 30 showed a 15% incidence of postoperative wound infection while those with a BMI > 50 had an incidence of wound infections reaching 30% [43]. Additionally, obese women have higher rates of diabetes and other co-morbidities, which make tissue healing compromised. Other factors further increasing risk of wound infection include African American race, steroid use, endometritis, and incisions greater than 16 cm [42].

Prior to surgery, appropriate cleansing of the skin is important to decrease bacterial colonization, especially in the obese patient with many skin folds and a pannus. Either chlorhexidine or povidone-iodine are acceptable agents; however, the length of time for cleansing must be extended to 3–5 minutes of drying in an obese patient. Preoperative antibiotics effective against both gram positive and gram negative bacteria, such as a first-generation cephalosporin (e.g. cefazolin), is generally selected, and should be administered within 1 hour of skin incision. This approach has been demonstrated to decrease the rate of infection 60% in the general population. Maternal obesity, cesarean in labor, hematocrit < 30, and general anesthesia increase the risk for postoperative infection further, with rates reaching 30–60% depending on the number of combined risk factors. Among those with additional risk factors, antibiotics can decrease this risk to 15%. An additional dose of antibiotics is suggested in situations where EBL rises above 1500 cc or operative time persists greater than 4 hours [12]. As standard dosing of antibiotics is less likely to result in therapeutic tissue levels in obese patients, a 2 g dose of cefazolin is recommended rather than the usual 1 g dose [11].

To reduce the risk for significant wound complications, the subcutaneous tissue should be reapproximated in the obese gravida undergoing cesarean section. While subcutaneous drains have not been shown to be effective in minimizing wound disruption or infection [44], subcutaneous sutures have been shown to demonstrate this benefit. Meta-analyses comparing drain placement with none show no difference in seroma, hematoma, or infection, but several studies have actually shown a higher incidence of wound complications, fascial dehiscence, and hospital readmissions [45]. However, when subcutaneous tissue is greater than 2 cm in depth, reapproximation of this layer with suture material can decrease the incidence of wound disruption by 35% [46]. Placing a drain additionally, however, will increase the chance for failure of successful healing 5–10% [47].

Incision closure with staples allows shorter operative times but also two- to fourfold higher rates of wound disruption and patient dissatisfaction compared to subcuticular closure. No specific studies compare staple versus subcuticular closure solely in the obese population, but the baseline risks of an already prolonged operative time, increased postoperative infection rate, and co-morbidities affecting healing should be considered. If staple closure is used, then removal between 7 and 10 days in obese women shows superiority to the routine removal at 3 days postoperatively in order to minimize wound separation [40].

15.2.4 Venous thromboembolic prophylaxis

Venous thromboembolic disease is a life-threatening complication of pregnancy, and is often cited as one of the leading causes of obstetrically related maternal death in the developed world. Pregnancy, obesity, and surgery are all significant risk factors for venous thromboembolism (VTE). Opportunities for prevention exist through both mechanical and pharmacological interventions. Obesity places women at a 10-fold increased risk of VTE following cesarean delivery [48]. In retrospective reviews, more than half of all VTE occurred in women with BMI > 30.

Early postoperative ambulation, compression stockings, and pneumatic compression devices placed before the initiation of surgery and continued post-operatively have all been shown to decrease thromboembolic disease after many surgical procedures. There is only limited data on these interventions or on the efficacy of perioperative heparin prophylaxis for the prevention of thromboembolic disease after cesarean delivery [49], nor are there clinical trials evaluating compression stockings or pneumatic compression devices for the prevention of VTE following cesarean delivery, and there are only small, randomized clinical trials evaluating the efficacy of unfractionated heparin and low-molecular-weight heparin (LMWH) at the time of cesarean delivery for prevention of VTE [16]. Specific recommendations regarding VTE prophylaxis following cesarean delivery have been put forth by many professional organizations, including the Royal College of Obstetricians and Gynaecologists (RCOG), Society of Obstetricians and Gynaecologists of Canada (SOGC), and the American College of Chest Physicians (ACCP). Each of these recommendations is based on expert opinion.

The RCOG recommends that women who have an elective cesarean delivery with one or more risk factors, including obesity or an emergency cesarean delivery, be considered for thromboprophylaxis with LMWH for 7 days after delivery. These recommendations are based on case-control or cohort studies [50].

The SOGC recommends that thromboprophylaxis be considered in women undergoing cesarean delivery who have other risk factors (previous history of VTE, known thrombophilia, prolonged immobility, or obesity). Postoperative recommendations include either 5000 units of unfractionated heparin every 12 hours until fully mobile or 20 mg LMWH daily for 5 days [51].

The ACCP recommends that a thrombosis risk assessment be conducted on all women prior to cesarean delivery to assess their need for thromboprophylaxis. They recommend that women with 1 risk factor should receive either pharmacologic or mechanical prophylaxis, and women with > 1 risk factor receive both pharmacologic and mechanical prophylaxis [52]. Risk factors include: previous history of VTE, thrombophilia, concurrent autoimmune disease, age > 35, smoking, multifetal pregnancy, and obesity. Obesity carries the highest risk for VTE of the listed risk factors.

The Society for Maternal-Fetal Medicine published recommendations that obese patient receive mechanical thromboprophylaxis and that consideration be given to adding low-molecular-weight heparin or unfractionated heparin for additional risk factors (age > 35, parity > 3, gross varicose veins, current infection, preeclampsia, immobility for > 4 days preoperatively, major current illness and emergency cesarean section during labor, cesarean hysterectomy, thrombophilia, and previous deep vein thrombosis) or a BMI of ">40–50" [11,47].

In general, our approach. in addition to early ambulation, is to provide pneumatic compression devices preoperatively to all patients undergoing cesarean section and to add pharmacological prophylaxis with low-molecular-weight heparin for patients with additional risk factors and/or BMI > 40. We initiate low-molecular-weight heparin generally 12 hours postoperatively, given potential concerns of postoperative hemorrhage, including the risk of postepidural catheter hemorrhage in the setting of neuraxial anesthesia [49].

References

1 Gunatilake R and Perlow JH. Obesity and pregnancy: clinical management of the obese gravida. *American Journal of Obstetrics & Gynecology* 2011;**204**;106–119.

2 Scott-Pillai R, Spence D, Cardwell CR, Hunter A, and Holmes VA. The impact of body mass index on maternal and neonatal outcomes; a retrospective study in a UK obstetric population, 2004–2011. *BJOG* 2013;**120**(8):932.

3 O'Brien TE, Ray JG, and Chan WS. Maternal body mass index and the risk of preeclampsia: a systematic overview. *Epidemiology* 2003;**14**(3):368.

4 Blomberg M. Maternal obesity, mode of delivery, and neonatal outcome. *Obstetrics & Gynecology* 2013;**122**(1):50–55.

5 Perlow JH. Obesity in the obstetric intensive care patient. In: Foley MR, Strong Jr TH, and Garite TJ (eds). *Obstetric Intensive Care Manual*, 3rd edn. Chicago, IL: McGraw-Hill, 2011.

6 Perlow JH and Morgan MA. Massive maternal obesity and perioperative cesarean morbidity. *American Journal of Obstetrics & Gynecology* 1994;**170**(2):560.

7 Vricella LK, Louis JM, Mercer BM, and Bolden N. Anesthesia complications during scheduled cesarean delivery for morbidly obese women. *American Journal of Obstetrics & Gynecology* 2010;**203**:276 e1–5.

8 Soens MA, Birnbach DJ, Ranasinghe JS, and van Zundert A. Obstetric anesthesia for the obese and morbidly obese patient: an ounce of prevention is worth more than a pound of treatment. *Acta Obstetricia et Gynecologica Scandinavica* 2008;**52**(1):6–19.

9 Tan T and Sia AT. Anesthesia considerations in the obese gravida. *Seminars in Perinatology* 2011;**35**(6):350–355.

10 Hood DD and Dewan DM. Anesthetic and obstetric outcome in morbidly obese parturients. *Anesthesiology* 1993;**79**(6):1210.

11 Johnson D and Society for Maternal-Fetal Medicine (SMFM). Management of cesarean delivery in the morbidly obese woman. *Contemporary Obstetrics & Gynecology* Oct 1, 2012.

12 Poobalan AS, Aucott LS, Gurung T, Smith WC, and Bhattacharya S. Obesity as an independent risk factor for elective and emergency caesarean delivery in nulliparous women – systematic review and meta-analysis of cohort studies. *Obesity Reviews* 2009;**10**(1):28–35.

13 Ranta P, Jouppila P, Spalding M, and Jouppila R. The effect of maternal obesity on labour and labour pain. *Anaesthesia* 1995;**50**(4):322.

14 Vricella LK, Louis JM, Mercer BM, and Bolden N. Impact of morbid obesity on epidural anesthesia complications in labor. *American Journal of Obstetrics & Gynecology* 2011;**205**(4):370.e1.

15 Hawkins JL, Chang J, Palmer SK, Gibbs CP, and Callaghan WM. Anesthesia-related maternal mortality in the United States: 1979–2002. *Obstetrics & Gynecology* 2011;**117**:69–74.

16 Loubert C and Fernando R. Cesearean delivery in the obese parturient: anesthetic considerations. *Current Opinion in Anaesthesiology* 2007;**20**(3):175–180.

17 Roofhooft E. Anesthesia for the morbidly obese parturient. *Current Opinion in Anaesthesiology* 2009;**22**(3):341–346.

18 Wolfe KB, Rossi RA, and Warshak CR. The effect of maternal obesity on the rate of failed induction of labor. *American Journal of Obstetrics & Gynecology* 2011;**205**:128 e1–7.

19 Pevzner L, Powers BL, Rayburn WF, Rumney P, and Wing DA. Effects of maternal obesity on duration and outcomes of prostaglandin cervical ripening and labor induction. *Obstetrics & Gynecology* 2009;**114**(6):1315–1321.

20 Norman SM, Tuuli MG, Odibo AO, Caughery AB, Roehl KA, and Cahill AG. The effects of obesity on the first stage of labor. *Obstetrics & Gynecology* 2012;**120**(1):130–135.

21 Kominiarek MA, Zhang J, VanVeldhuisen P, Troendle J, Beaver J, and Hibbard JU. Contemporary labor patterns: the impact of maternal body mass index. *American Journal of Obstetrics & Gynecology* 2011;**205**:244 e1–8.

22 Vahratian A, Zhang J, Troendle JF, Savitz DA, and Siega-Riz AM. Maternal prepregnancy overweight and obesity and the pattern of labor progression in term nulliparous women. *Obstetrics & Gynecology* 2004;**104**(5 Pt 1):943.

23 Robinson BK, Mapp DC, Bloom SL, Rouse DJ, Spong CY, Varner MW *et al.* Increasing maternal body mass index and characteristics of the second stage of labor. *Obstetrics & Gynecology* 2011;**118**(6);1309–1313.

24 Dodd JM, Grivell RM, Nguyen AM, Chan A, and Robinson JS. Maternal and perinatal health outcomes by body mass index category. *Australian and New Zealand Journal of Obstetrics and Gynaecology* 2011;**51**:136–140.

25 Ovsen P, Rasmussen S, and Kesmodel U. Effect of prepregnancy maternal overweight and obesity on pregnancy outcome. *Obstetrics & Gynecology* 2011;**118**:305–312.

26 Usha Kiran TS, Hemmadi S, Bethel J, and Evans J. Outcome of pregnancy in a woman with an increased body mass index. *BJOG* 2005;**112**:768–772.

27 Alanis MC, Villers MS, Law TL, Steadman E, and Robinson CJ. Complications of cesarean delivery in the massively obese parturient. *American Journal of Obstetrics & Gynecology* 2010;**203**:271 e1–7.

28 Robinson HE, O'Connell CM, Joseph KS, and McLeod NL. Maternal outcomes in pregnancies complicated by obesity. *Obstetrics & Gynecology* 2005;**106**:1357–1364.

29 Juhasz G, Gyamfi C, Gyamfi P, Tocce K, and Stone JL. Effect of body mass index and excessive weight gain on success of vaginal birth after cesarean delivery. *Obstetrics & Gynecology* 2005;**106**(4):741–746.

30 Gunatilake RP, Smrtka MP, Harris B, Kraus DM, Small MJ, Grotegut CA *et al.* Predictors of failed trial of labor among women with an extremely obese body mass index. *American Journal of Obstetrics & Gynecology* 2013;**209**(6):562 e1–e5.

31 Goodall PT, Ahn JT, Chapa JB, and Hibbard JU. Obesity as a risk factor for failed trial of labor in patients with previous cesarean delivery. *American Journal of Obstetrics & Gynecology* 2005;**192**(5):1423–1426.

32 Wispelwey BP and Sheiner E. Cesarean delivery in obese women: a comprehensive review. *Journal of Maternal-Fetal and Neonatal Medicine* 2013;**26**(6):547–551.

33 Weiss JL, Malone FD, Emig D *et al.* Obesity, obstetric complications and cesarean delivery rate: A population-based screening study. *American Journal of Obstetrics & Gynecology* 2004;**190**:1091.

34 Suidan RS, Apuzzio JJ, and Williams SF. Obesity, comorbidities, and the cesarean delivery rate. *American Journal of Perinatology* 2012;**29**(8):623–628.

35 Crane JM, Murphy P, Burrage L, and Hutchens D. Maternal and perinatal outcomes of extreme obesity in pregnancy. *Journal of Obstetrics and Gynaecology Canada* 2013; **35**(7):606–611.

36 Davies GA, Maxwell C *et al.* Obesity in pregnancy. *Journal of Obstetrics and Gynaecology Canada* 2010;**32**(2):165–173.

37 James DC and Maher MA. Caring for the extremely obese woman during pregnancy and birth. *American Journal of Maternal Child Nursing* 2009;**34**(1):24–30.

38 Constantino TG, Parikh AK, Satz WA, and Fojtik JP. Ultrasonography-guided peripheral intravenous access versus traditional approaches in patients with difficult intravenous access. *Annals of Emergency Medicine* 2005;**46**(5):456–461.

39 Wall PD, Deucy EE, Glantz JC, and Pressman EK. Vertical skin incisions and wound complications in the obese parturient. *Obstetrics & Gynecology* 2003;**102**(5):952–956.

40 Sarsam SE, Elliott JP, and Lam GK. Management of wound complications from cesarean delivery. *Obstetrical and Gynecological Survey* 2005;**60**(7):462–473.

41 Conner SN, Verticchio JC, Tuuli MG, Odibo AO, Macones GA, and Cahill AG. Maternal obesity and risk of postcesarean wound complications. *American Journal of Perinatology* 2013;**31**(4)299–304.

42 McLean M, Hines R, Polinkovsky M, Stuebe A, Thorp J, and Strauss R. Type of skin incision and wound complications in the obese parturient. *American Journal of Perinatology* 2012;**29**(4):301–306.

43 Tipton AM, Cohen SA, and Chelmow D. Wound infection in the obese pregnant woman. *Seminars in Perinatology* 2011;**35**(6):345–349.

44 Gates S and Anderson ER. Wound drainage for cesarean section. *Cochrane Database of Systematic Reviews* 2005;(**1**):CD004549.

45 Hellums EK, Lin MG, and Ramsey PS. Prophylactic subcutaneous drainage for prevention of wound complications after cesarean delivery – a metaanalysis. *American Journal of Obstetrics & Gynecology* 2007;**197**(3):229–235.

46 Chelmow D, Rodriguez EJ, and Sabatini MM. Suture closure of subcutaneous fat and wound disruption after cesarean delivery: a meta-analysis. *Obstetrics & Gynecology* 2004;**103**(5 Pt 1):974–980.

47 Ramsey PS, White AM *et al.* Subcutaneous tissue reapproximation, alone or in combination with drain, in obese women undergoing cesarean delivery. *Obstetrics & Gynecology* 2005;**105**(5 Pt 1):967–973.

48 Marik PE. Venous thromboembolism in pregnancy. *Clinics in Chest Medicine* 2010; **31**(4):731–740.

49 Varner MW. Thromboprophylaxis for cesarean delivery. www.contemporaryobgyn.net June 2011: 30–33.

50 Royal College of Obestetricians and Gynaecologists. Green-top guideline No. 37a: Reducing the risk of thrombosis and embolism during pregnancy and the puerperium. Royal College of Obstetricians and Gynaecologists. London. November 2009;1–35.
51 Kent N, Leduc L, Crane J *et al.* Prevention and treatment of venous thromboembolism (VTE) in obstetrics. *Journal of the Society of Obstetricians and Gynaecologists of Canada* 2000;**22**(9):736–749.
52 Bates SM, Greer IA, Pabinger I, Sofaer S, and Hirsh J. Venous thromboembolism, thrombophilia, antithrombotic therapy and pregnancy: American College of Chest Physicians Evidence-Based Clinical Practice Guidelines (8th edn). *Chest* 2008;**133**(Suppl. 6):844s–886s.

CHAPTER 16

Intrapartum and postpartum infections

Scott A. Sullivan and Christopher Goodier
Department of Obstetrics and Gynecology, Medical University of South Carolina, Charleston, SC, USA

16.1 Introduction

Maternal and fetal infections may occur at any time during a pregnancy, ranging from the trivial to the potentially fatal. They may result from exposure to any number of bacteria, viruses, parasites, and fungi. Clinicians must maintain an index of suspicion and broad differential diagnosis when faced with signs or symptoms of infection. Timing of infection is also critical, as primary infection may occur in the antepartum, intrapartum, or postpartum periods. Even if remote from term, antepartum infections can have a significant impact on the management and outcome of labor, neonatal outcome, and the postpartum period.

16.2 Group B *Streptoccocus*

First identified as a significant pathogen in the 1970s, Group B *Streptoccocus* remains the leading cause of neonatal sepsis and meningitis in the United States [1]. Group B *Streptoccocus* (GBS) is an encapsulated gram positive bacterium also known as *S. Agalactiae*, which primarily infects infants and pregnant or postpartum women, although it can also affect the elderly or those with chronic diseases. Initial mortality rates from GBS sepsis were estimated as high as 50% in the 1970s and have decreased dramatically to 4–6% because of improved diagnosis, utilization of intrapartum antibiotics, and advances in neonatal care [2].

Over time, it became apparent that there were two distinct clinical entities associated with GBS infection in neonates: early onset (within the first 7 days of

Management of Labor and Delivery, Second Edition. Edited by George A. Macones.

life) and late onset (1 week to 3 months of life). Early-onset GBS sepsis carries a much higher morbidity and mortality and typically presents within the first 24–48 hours of life. It usually manifests as respiratory distress, cardiovascular instability, and periods of apnea suggesting pneumonia and sepsis. Late-onset GBS can present at any time after the first week of life; however, the median age is approximately day of life 36 [3]. The clinical course is usually milder than early-onset disease; however, like early-onset disease, sepsis is the most common presentation. GBS meningitis is more common in late-onset disease, occurring in approximately 25% of cases [1]. The incidence of early-onset disease has decreased from 1.7 cases/1000 live births to 0.4 cases/1000 live births since the 1990s with the advent of maternal screening and intrapartum antibiotics. Interestingly, the rate of late-onset disease has remained relatively constant at 0.4 cases/1000 live births [1].

16.2.1 Progress

After the identification of GBS sepsis as a major causation of neonatal mortality in the 1970s, there were many promising clinical trials performed showing a reduction in early-onset GBS sepsis in newborns if intrapartum antibiotics were administered to high-risk parturients during labor. Subsequent collaboration produced the first recommendations for intrapartum prophylaxis to prevent perinatal GBS sepsis, which were issued in 1996 by the American College of Obstetrics and Gynecology (ACOG) and the Centers for Disease Control (CDC). Recommendations were made to identify women who should receive intrapartum antibiotics using either a risk-based versus culture-based screening approach. The guidelines recommended intrapartum antibiotics for patients who had a positive GBS culture performed between 35 and 37 weeks of gestation or for women who had intrapartum risk factors including gestational age < 37 weeks, temperature > 100.4 °F, or ruptured membranes > 18 hours. Women who had significant GBS bacteria during pregnancy, or a previously affected neonate, were also recommended to get intrapartum prophylaxis. After the implementation of these guidelines, early-onset GBS sepsis declined by approximately 70% [1].

The guidelines were subsequently revised in 2002 with the most significant change recommending universal culture-based screening for all pregnant patients between 35 and 37 weeks of gestation. This recommendation was based upon a large population-based study by Schrag *et al.* in 2002, which demonstrated superiority of universal screening over the risk-based approach adopted in 1996 [4]. Risk-based use of intrapartum antibiotics should continue to be used for GBS unknown patients.

There is a controversy about patients with intact fetal membranes and planned cesarean section prior to the onset of labor. In general these patients do not need prophylactic antibiotics, regardless of gestational age. Therefore, the benefit of antenatal GBS culture is questionable. Some patients may experience

Table 16.1 GBS indications for treatment.

Intrapartum GBS prophylaxis indicated	Intrapartum GBS prophylaxis not indicated
• Previous infant with invasive GBS disease for GBS prophylaxis is present for current pregnancy) • GBS bacteriuria during any trimester of the current pregnancy* • Positive GBS vaginal-rectal screening culture in late gestation during current pregnancy* • Unknown GBS status at the onset of labor (culture not done, incomplete, or results unknown) and any of the following: – Delivery at <37 weeks' gestation – Amniotic membrane rupture > 18 hours – Intrapartum temperature > 100.4 F (> 38.0 C)¶ – Intrapartum NAAT** positive for GBS	• Colonization with GBS during a previous pregnancy (unless an indication • GBS bacteriuria during previous pregnancy (unless an indication for GBS prophylaxis is present for current pregnancy) • Negative vaginal and rectal GBS screening culture in late gestation† during the current pregnancy, regardless of intrapartum risk factors • Cesarean delivery performed before onset of labor on a woman with intact amniotic membranes, regardless of GBS colonization status or gestational age

Abbreviation: NAAT = Nucleic acid amplification tests.

*Intrapartum antibiotic prophylaxis is not indicated in this circumstance if a cesarean delivery is performed before onset of labor on a woman with intact amniotic membranes.

†Optimal timing for prenatal GBS screening is at 35–37 weeks' gestation.

¶If amnionitis is suspected, broad-spectrum antibiotic therapy that includes an agent known to be active against GBS should replace GBS prophylaxis.

**NAAT testing for GBS is optional and might not be available in all settings. If intrapartum NAAT is negative for GBS but any other intrapartum risk factor (delivery at <37 weeks' gestation, amniotic membrane rupture at ≥18 hours, or temperature ≥100.4°F [≥38.0°C]) is present, then intrapartum antibiotic prophylaxis is indicated.

Taken from MMWR at cdc.gov/mmwr. Prevention of Perinatal Group B Streptococcal Disease. Revised Guidelines from CDC, 2010

Source: CDC, 2010. Adapted from CDC, 2010 [2].

preterm premature rupture of membranes (PPROM) or preterm labor of course, or have an "unplanned" vaginal delivery. These scenarios are used to justify screening for patients with planned cesarean deliveries. At this point, either approach would appear to be reasonable.

Acceptance of the CDC guidelines improved screening for maternal GBS from 48% in the late 1990s to 85% in 2004 [1]. The most recent guidelines, published in 2010, were implemented in part to improve the suboptimal use of antibiotics in preterm pregnancies, as well as the utilization of second-line agents in penicillin allergic patients. Table 16.1 (CDC, 2010) lists the indications for intrapartum prophylaxis to help prevent early-onset GBS sepsis in newborns.

The guidelines also included language for the option of using a new GBS testing modality utilizing nucleic acid amplification tests (NAAT). The use of this testing is considered optional. If NAAT is available, the obstetrician can choose to perform intrapartum rectovaginal swab in patients with unknown GBS status and no risk factors necessitating treatment. Patients should receive intrapartum antibiotics if the test returns positive or if intrapartum risk factors develop, even if the NAAT returns negative.

Women in preterm labor or who present with PPROM should have a rectovaginal swab for routine GBS culture collected on admission and antibiotic prophylaxis should be started immediately. If the patient is not entering labor, GBS prophylaxis can be stopped. If the patient has PPROM and labor is not a concern, prophylactic antibiotics for latency should be continued until completion or for 48 hours if being used for GBS prophylaxis.

16.2.2 Risk factors

Approximately 10–30% of women are colonized with GBS in the vagina, with the gastrointestinal tract thought to be the primary reservoir. Maternal colonization is asymptomatic and can be transient or permanent. Black women have higher rates of positive cultures than other ethnicities [1].

The primary risk factor for early-onset GBS in infants seems to be maternal vaginal colonization. Boyer *et al.* performed a prospective study in the mid-1980s which showed that infants born to culture positive women were 25 times more likely to develop early-onset GBS sepsis than those of mothers whose screening cultures were negative. Parturients with GBS bacteriuria or a prior infant with GBS sepsis are thought to be more heavily colonized and at higher risk for infants born with early-onset disease. Other factors that increase the risk of early-onset disease include preterm delivery (<37 weeks of gestation), intrapartum chorioamnionitis, prolonged rupture of membranes (>12–18 hrs), and intrapartum fever [5,6]. There have been some observational studies that suggest the use of intrauterine monitors and five or more digital cervical exams after rupture of membranes may also increase the risk for early-onset GBS disease [2].

Unlike early-onset disease, the risk factors for late-onset GBS are not as well characterized. Risk factors include maternal colonization, race, and prematurity.

These risk factors account for about only 40–50% of GBS cases, thus the CDC recommends universal screening [7].

16.2.3 Pathogenesis

The highest risk factor for early-onset disease is maternal intrapartum colonization with GBS. These infections are vertically transmitted from mother to child as it ascends from the vagina into the amniotic fluid, although invasion can occur through intact membranes. While in the amniotic fluid, GBS bacterium replicates and colonizes infant mucous membranes. The infected amniotic fluid can also be aspirated by the neonate resulting in subsequent bacteremia and early-onset sepsis. Colonization acquired via passage through the birth canal is generally benign and many infants show no symptoms [2].

Late-onset GBS infectivity is not always acquired from vertical transmission. Maternal colonization does play an important role in up to 50% of cases; however, alternative modes of transmission also occur. Nosocomial infections help explain GBS disease in non-GBS infected mothers. Horizontal transmission has also been reported from mother to child, with breast milk being a primary source [1].

16.2.4 Diagnosis

GBS culture has been utilized as the primary test for the identification of women colonized with the bacteria. Screening cultures are recommended between 35 and 37 weeks due to the transient nature of GBS in pregnant women. The recommended timing for screening was based upon the work of Yancey and Boyer in the late 1980s and early 1990s [1]. GBS screening cultures include a single combined rectovaginal swab placed in a nonnutritive transport medium which is then incubated for 18–24 hours in an enrichment broth allowing for enhanced identification of the bacterium. Swabbing the rectum and vagina increases the yield 48% compared with screening the vagina alone [8]. An enrichment step allows for a decreased rate of false-negative tests by approximately 50% compared to direct plating [2].

Early testing is not predictive of colonization after 6 weeks, thus repeat testing should be performed if a patient had a negative test earlier in pregnancy [7].

The addition of the NAAT in some laboratories has recently been introduced as an option for intrapartum testing on patients with unknown GBS status. Between 7 and 11% of women deliver prior to screening at 35 weeks and this group (preterm infants) has a more severe course of early-onset disease, accounting for approximately 32–28% of early-onset cases [9]. The sensitivities of these tests range from 62.5 to 98.5% compared to culture, and vary by technique and length of time to get a result [2]. This test was designed to be more sensitive and rapid than the current enriched culture which has a 95–97% negative predictive value. Studies have shown that the sensitivity of NAAT to GBS improves to 93–100% with an enrichment step; however, this adds additional time and may not be practical. Without the enrichment step, the sensitivities of NAAT are not adequate when compared to the current gold standard, culture [2].

16.2.5 Antibiotic choices

Penicillin remains the primary agent for GBS positive individuals who are not allergic. Ampicillin is an acceptable alternative. Patients who are penicillin allergic should be queried regarding the type of reaction associated with the allergy. Those patients who do not have a history of anaphylaxis, respiratory distress, angioedema, or urticaria should receive cefazolin as a second-line agent. The 2010 CDC guidelines no longer recommend the use of erythromycin. For those patients who are penicillin allergic and are not candidates for cefazolin, antimicrobial sensitivities should be attempted on the GBS isolates.

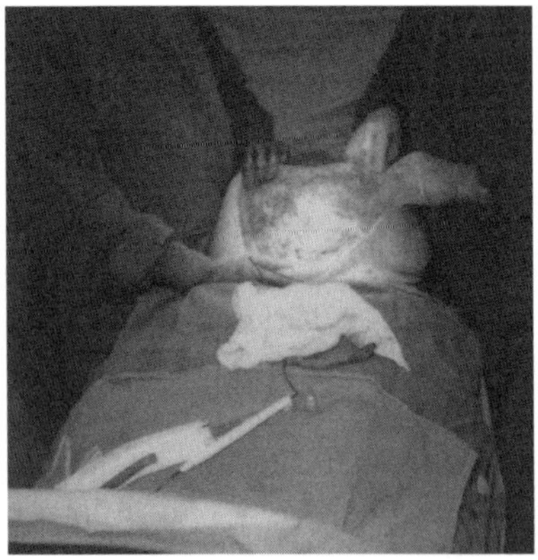

Figure 16.1 GBS treatment regimens. *Source*: CDC, 2010. Adapted from CDC, 2010 [2].

Laboratory sensitivity testing should include clindamycin and erythromycin. If the isolate is susceptible to both clindamycin and erythromycin, clindamycin should be utilized intrapartum. On the other hand, if the isolate is resistant to erythromycin, then follow-up testing for inducible clindamycin resistance should occur. If the result is negative, clindamycin can be safely used. If the isolate is resistant to clindamycin via susceptibility testing or demonstrates inducible resistance, vancomycin prophylaxis should be employed (Figure 16.1).

The CDC guidelines recommend at least 4 hours of intrapartum antibiotic treatment for protection of newborns against early-onset GBS sepsis, otherwise they are considered "high risk" and typically undergo invasive testing, such as complete blood count, white blood cell count, blood cultures, and possibly antibiotic treatment. There are no randomized control trials to validate this time interval; however, there have been some prospective studies that suggest a time frame of closer to 1–2 hours of intrapartum antibiotics is sufficient to reduce early-onset GBS disease [6]. The recommendations also state that no medically necessary obstetric procedures should be delayed in order to achieve 4 hours of intrapartum antibiotic prophylaxis in GBS positive mothers.

16.2.6 Future of Group B *Streptoccocus* prevention

While early-onset GBS sepsis has declined significantly since the 1980s, opportunities still remain, especially in the understanding of racial disparities. The development of rapid and accurate intrapartum testing for GBS colonization screening will help decrease the incidence of early-onset GBS sepsis. Unfortunately, universal screening and intrapartum prophylaxis have had no impact on the rate of late-onset GBS disease, which has remained flat over several decades, thus more research is needed. Vaccine trials are in development and an effective vaccination program would go a long way to the eradication of this life-threatening disease in newborns [10].

16.3 Varicella

16.3.1 Pathogenesis

Varicella zoster virus (VZV) is a member of the herpesvirus family and causes both varicella (chickenpox) and herpes zoster (shingles). VZV is found in worldwide geographic distributions but occurs more in tropical climates predominantly in the winter/spring [11]. Chickenpox is a common childhood illness with symptoms typically lasting 4–5 days, consisting of fever, malaise, and a vesicular rash. While the virus in children is relatively benign, exposure during pregnancy can have devastating maternal and fetal consequences. Transmission occurs by direct contact with fluid from skin lesions or respiratory droplets. Exposed persons are generally considered infectious 1–2 days prior to development of the rash, lasting until all lesions are healed (crusted over). Once the initial infectious period is complete, the virus goes dormant in dorsal root ganglia of sensory nerves and may be reactivated as herpes zoster at a later time, most commonly in the elderly or immunocompromised. Infection as a child is believed to confer lifelong immunity with virus-specific IgG antibodies, and approximately 90% of adults are immune [12,13]. Because of the high prevalence of natural immunity, the incidence of varicella infection is low, between 0.4–0.7/1000 pregnancies and 2–3/1000 pregnancies, depending on which study you read [12].

In adults, other complications include varicella pneumonia, hepatitis, and encephalitis. Varicella pneumonia is more common in pregnancy, especially the in third trimester, and should be regarded as a medical emergency requiring hospitalization, treatment, and supportive care as needed. Smokers tend to have the highest risk of varicella pneumonia, at 42–47% [12]. Mortality in the general population is 10–20% and has been reported as high as 40–45% in pregnancy. Modern intensive care likely has reduced this risk. Early identification and treatment are extremely important for this end. As mortality has decreased, perinatal complications such as preterm delivery have increased. Common symptoms include cough, dyspnea, malaise, hypoxia, and maternal fever [12].

16.3.2 Diagnosis

Varicella is a clinical diagnosis based on constellation of symptoms as well as the appearance of multiple vesicular lesions in different stages of healing. If a patient is exposed, she should initially be questioned about childhood varicella or prior vaccination. If this information is not known, serology can be obtained. If maternal exposure is suspected, fetal surveillance can be undertaken via ultrasound looking for limb abnormalities and intrauterine growth restriction (IUGR). In addition, amniotic fluid can be assessed via PCR or culture for varicella.

16.3.3 Risk to fetus

Neonatal infection occurs via three routes, including transplacental viremia, ascending infection during delivery, and via respiratory droplets [13]. Fetal complications depend on the timing of the initial infection and range from no effects to fetal death. Primary varicella infection in parturients can result in infection in up to 25% of pregnancies, although the rate of miscarriage is unchanged. Congenital varicella syndrome (CVS), first described in 1947 [13], occurs when there is maternal infection during the first half of pregnancy and is seen in up to 1–2% of infants, with second-trimester infections accounting for the majority of CVS [2–4]. Most reported cases of CVS occur prior to 20 weeks of gestation [14]. Common symptoms include low birth weight, limb hypoplasia, microcephaly, ocular abnormalities, skin lesions, and mental retardation. Ultrasound is the modality of choice to diagnose congenital varicella and should be performed on all pregnant women with primary varicella infection during the first or second trimester. Testing should be performed at least 5 weeks after infection or 16–22 weeks of gestational age to identify characteristic fetal anomalies; however, its sensitivity is unknown. Amniocentesis can also be utilized to identify the virus by culture or viral DNA by PCR in the amniotic fluid [15]. Varicella zoster immune globulin (VZIG) should be given to infants born to women who develop varicella between 5 days before and 48 hours after delivery, as well as premature infants < 28 weeks of gestation or < 1000 g at birth. Families should be counseled that treatment with VZIG does not assure prevention of congenital varicella, which carries a mortality rate of up to 30% [13].

Perinatal varicella, which was initially described in 1878 by Hubbard, occurs with late third-trimester maternal infection, specifically 5 days pre-delivery through 48 hours post-delivery. Between 17 and 30% of newborns of infected mothers have perinatal varicella, which typically manifests as fever and rash. Prior to the use of VZIG, mortality of these infants was as high as 30% but is now thought to be much lower [16]. Neonatal infection is thought to occur during the window of 5 days prior to delivery up until 2 days post-delivery because the neonate would not have protective maternal IgG antibodies via transplacental passage.

Current evidence suggests that maternal herpes zoster infection during pregnancy is not associated with birth defects as newborns possess maternal IgG antibodies preventing spread to infants [13].

16.3.4 Treatment

If non-immune or indeterminate status women are exposed during pregnancy, virus-specific IgG antibody testing should be conducted as soon as possible and within 10 days. IgG antibodies detected within 10 days of exposure are due to prior infection/vaccination and do not indicate current infection. Once diagnosis is confirmed, maternal isolation should be recommended so that she does not further spread the virus. If prior immunity cannot be confirmed, the treatment of the patient with VZIG as soon as possible and up to 72 hours (some authors describe 96 hrs) after exposure is recommended and can reduce severity of maternal disease, but does not eliminate the possibility of fetal infection [13,14]. Administration of antiviral medications within the first 24 hours of the development of maternal rash has been shown to decrease the duration of new lesion formation as well as the number of lesions. ACOG recommends the use of oral acyclovir, as it is the best studied and appears to be safe when used in pregnancy; however, no large controlled trials have been performed. The suggested dose is 800 mg 5x/day for 7–10 days. If the maternal varicella infection is complicated by pneumonia, intravenous acyclovir should be utilized (10–15 mg/kg every 8 hours for 5–10 days) as it may reduce maternal morbidity and mortality associated with varicella pneumonia [15].

16.3.5 Prevention

Preconception counseling should include documentation of childhood infection or prior vaccination. Serologic testing of all pregnant women with an indeterminate history of exposure or immunization to chickenpox has not been universally accepted. Active immunization with the varicella vaccine has been available since 1995 and should be completed in non-immune women at least 1 month (and preferably 3 months) prior to pregnancy, as it is a live-attenuated vaccine. While the vaccine is contraindicated in pregnancy due to the live virus, there are no case reports of adverse outcomes, thus termination is not recommended [14]. Close contacts of the neonate or susceptible pregnant woman should be considered for vaccination as well to prevent household transmission.

16.4 Urinary tract infections / pyelonephritis

Pregnancy physiological changes predispose women to a risk for urinary tract infections (UTI), which may manifest as asymptomatic bacteriuria (ASB), cystitis, or pyelonephritis. The enlarging uterus compresses the ureters and the bladder, resulting in a mechanical obstruction. Progesterone effect on smooth muscle slows ureteral contractions and urinary transit time. Increased glomerular filtration rate may increase the amount of glucose and protein substrate in the urine to enhance bacterial growth [17]. These changes create an environment favorable for ascending infection and bacterial growth (Figure 16.2). The incidence of UTI in pregnancy has been reported to be between 2 and 8% [18]. In addition, patients will not have signs or symptoms with ASB, and symptoms of UTI may be masked by common maternal symptoms of pregnancy and subsequently be under-reported.

Labor and the postpartum period carry additional risks for UTI. Patients may have in-dwelling catheters after a cesarean delivery, perineal trauma, or regional anesthesia. Laboring women also frequently are in/out catheterized as the second

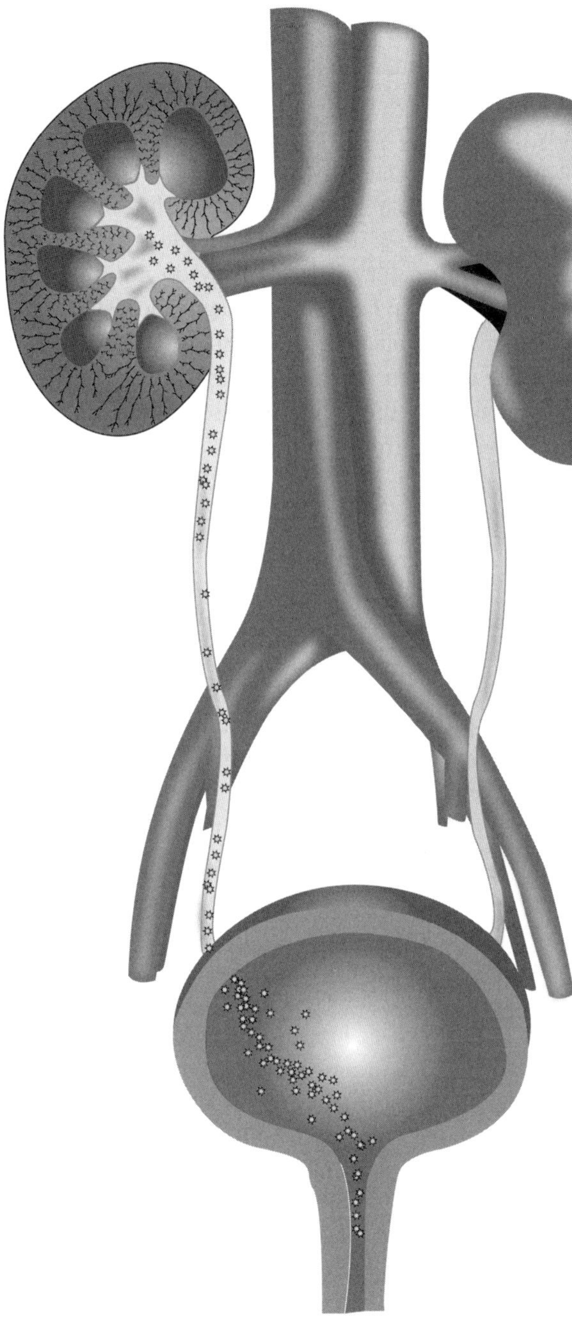

Figure 16.2 Ascending pyelonephritis.

stage approaches, or for operative vaginal delivery. Vaginal examinations and instrumentation likely increase these risks as well.

Given these increased risks, ACOG recommends screening every pregnant woman for ASB [19]. Undiagnosed ASB can lead to UTI and ultimately pyelonephritis. Screening is usually accomplished by a routine urine culture at the first prenatal visit, or in the first trimester. Greater than 10,000 colony-forming units/ml of a pathogenic bacteria is diagnostic. Treatment is guided by culture results and typical antibiotic coverage. In addition to a urine culture, patients are screened for evidence of ASB and UTI at every prenatal visit by way of a urine dipstick analysis. Leukocyte esterase and nitrites are indirect markers of infectious activity that may prompt the performance of a confirmatory culture. They do not have sufficient sensitivity and specificity on their own to be used as a diagnostic test [20]. Patients with hemoglobinopathies, neurogenic bladder, and frequent UTIs have increased incidence of ASB and should be screened via culture every trimester.

The usual causative organisms are the genital/GI flora, which may colonize the perineal area. *Escherichia coli* is a primary infectious agent, and represents a majority of UTI cases [21]. *Klebsiella, Staphylococcus, Enterobacter,* and *Proteus* species are also commonly encountered. Less commonly encountered organisms include *Enterococcus faecalis,* group B *Streptococcus* (GBS), *Pseudomonas,* and *Ureaplasma* species. If GBS is identified, there is a concern about higher risk for significant colonization and neonatal infection. They are treated in labor as if they have a genital positive culture.

ASB or UTI may be treated with simple oral regimens, guided by available sensitivities. First-generation cephalosporins or ampicillin are commonly used. Bacterial resistances vary by locale and organism, but may be over 40% against commonly used antibiotics like ampicillin. Nitrofurantoin, trimethaprim/sulfamethoxasole and fosfomycin are reasonable alternatives. Concerns have been raised about the use of trimethaprim/sulfamethoxasole in the first trimester, and nitrofurantoin in the third trimester. Theoretical concerns exist about use of quinolones in pregnancy, but they may be used if benefits outweigh the risks.

The ideal duration of treatment remains controversial, with differing regimens described in the available literature. Single-dose regimens have been described with reasonable rates of resolution [22]. However, longer courses of 3, 7, and 10 days are also described with higher rates of bacteriuria clearance. In general, short-course treatments are preferred to single-dose treatment in pregnancy [23].

Untreated or incompletely treated UTI may lead to pyelonephritis, or infection of the kidney. Classic symptoms include fever, flank or costovertebral angle tenderness, and systemic signs of malaise, chills, and sweats. Development of symptoms may be rapid and seemingly with little warning. The differential diagnosis may include chorioamnionitis, pneumonia, renal lithiasis, and appendicitis. A typical work-up consists of clinical examination, WBC, urinalysis, culture, and sensitivities. Renal imaging is not routinely required, but may be performed if there is significant concern for lithiasis, abscess, or obstruction.

Treatment of pyelonephritis may be either outpatient or inpatient, with some trials showing few outcome differences [24]. However, some experts favor inpatient, given the complexity and additional risks of pregnancy [21]. In any case, treatment revolves around targeted antibiotics and supportive care. Intravenous antibiotics are recommended for inpatient management, and may consistent of ceftriaxone, piperacillin/tazobactam, and cefoxitin. Gentamicin may also be added, or reserved for more complicated and resistant cases. Antibiotics are usually continued until the patient has been afebrile for 24 hours. Supportive care is also recommended, along with monitoring for preterm labor.

Pyelonephritis may lead to even more severe maternal infections, including urosepsis and acute respiratory distress syndrome. Patients may rapidly exhibit signs of shock and decompensation. Hypoxia, vital sign instability, mental status changes, acidosis, and non-reassuring fetal status (NRFS) may develop. Rapid recognition and treatment are essential to ensuring a good outcome. Patients should be treated in an ICU setting with multidisciplinary care. Generally, maternal resuscitation, reversal of acidosis, and hypovolemia will result in improved fetal status and heart rate tracings. Clinical judgment must be applied for when delivery is indicated. Prompt intensive care makes maternal death in this setting unusual, but there is a substantial risk for preterm labor, delivery for NRFS, and prolonged maternal hospitalization.

16.5 Parvovirus

Parvovirus B19 is the causative agent of erythema infectiosum, otherwise known as fifth disease. It has historically been called fifth disease because it was listed number five on a widely distributed classification of childhood infections. It is a relatively benign infection that predominantly affects children and produces a characteristic rash giving the appearance of "slapped cheeks." During the infectious period, myalgias and arthralgias are observed in children and even more commonly in adults [25]. Initially described by Cosart in the 1970s, it was later discovered that parvovirus is a potent inhibitor of erythropoiesis by infecting erythroid precursor cells and thus can precipitate aplastic crisis in susceptible patients. Transmission usually takes place via respiratory droplets; however, infection can also be disseminated via blood and blood products, as well as vertically from mother to fetus via transplacental passage [26].

Parvovirus B19 has its peak incidence each spring, but also shows an epidemiological cycle approximately every 4 years [25,26]. Infected individuals are thought to then have lifelong immunity with IgG antibodies. Approximately 60% of women of childbearing age possess these antibodies and vertical transmission in this group is thought to not occur [26]. The incidence of infection with parvovirus in pregnancy is 1–2%; however, it can increase to 10% during epidemics. While the risk of maternal transmission in confirmed cases of maternal infection ranges from 33 to 51%, associated fetal outcomes occur in only about 10% of newborns [26].

Approximately 50% of exposed mothers begin to show symptoms about 10 days to 2 weeks after exposure to infected individuals. The risk of vertical transmission is thought to be highest during the maternal peak viral load, which occurs about 7 days after exposure when IgM antibodies appear in serum [27].

16.5.1 Risk factors

In a study by Harger *et al.* in 1998 [28], the only statistically significant risk factor found for parvovirus infections in pregnant women was exposure by their own children. Other risk factors can include children's school teacher and day-care workers. There is no real prevention strategy, given that many infected people are asymptomatic, thus counseling of those pregnant patients with high risk of exposure should be performed.

16.5.2 Diagnosis

If maternal exposure to Parvovirus B19 is suspected during pregnancy, serologic examination with IgM and IgG antibodies should be performed. It is important to remember that B19V-specific IgM antibodies do not become detectable in serum until approximately 7–10 days after infection and decrease after 2–3 months [26].

The sensitivity of IgM enzyme immunoassay has been reported to be between 63 and 70% [26]. It is important to ensure that testing of maternal serum occurs at least 7–10 days after exposure, as levels of IgM may not be detected. In addition, B19 antibody testing may give false-negative results, as the antibodies can bind to viral particles, becoming undetectable in serum in low quantities [29]. Lastly, for fetuses with overt hydrops via ultrasound examination, IgM levels may be low or even undetectable, making the diagnosis harder. In these cases PCR analysis of maternal serum can be performed for confirmation of virus [25,26,30].

Testing the fetus is another option via amniocentesis with PCR of the amniotic fluid or percutaneous umbilical cord blood sampling (PUBS). This is usually warranted with ultrasound suspicion of fetal hydrops or anemia via middle cerebral artery (MCA) Doppler analysis. Neonatal serology is not very reliable due to the lack of production of IgG or IgM; however, B19 DNA via PCR would be appropriate [25].

The use of PCR to detect parvovirus DNA is extremely sensitive (almost 100%) and is very helpful in cases of immunocompromised or suppressed individuals, or where concerns remain even after maternal serology. It is important to note that B19 viral DNA levels may persist for years after acute infection and therefore low-positive PCR results do not 100% prove recent infection [31,32].

16.5.3 Pathogenesis

Fetal infection with parvovirus can be asymptomatic; however, it can also be associated with intrauterine fetal death, non-immune hydrops fetalis, and neurological manifestations [26]. The majority of fetal deaths will occur between 20 and 24 weeks; however, they can occur at any time throughout gestation. Fetal hydrops is estimated to occur in between 0 and 12.5% of infected mothers, depending upon the study, reaching its peak between 17 and 24 weeks [31]. This occurs because the half-life of red blood cells is shorter due to hepatic production at this gestation. Fetuses will initially show abdominal ascites and pericardial effusions, followed by a thickened placenta, skin edema, and pleural effusions as a result of severe anemia and high-output cardiac failure [25]. The interval from infection to manifestation of severe symptoms is 8–12 weeks and > 95% of fetal complications occur within 12 weeks following acute infection during pregnancy [30].

Encephalopathy and severe CNS abnormalities following intrauterine B19 infection are uncommon. Long term sequelae are unclear as data is limited to small studies which are inconclusive [25]. A large study by DeJong *et al.* fol lowed 28 children after intrauterine transfusion, and 11% were found to have neurodevelopmental impairment [33]. Mothers should be counseled that transfusion, while potentially life-saving, does not guarantee a favorable long-term outcome.

16.5.4 Fetal testing

In addition to serologic testing, ultrasound should be performed to serve as an adjunct if recent parvovirus infection is suspected, to look for signs of anemia and hydrops. Doppler ultrasonography of the MCA detects changes in blood flow due to increased cardiac output and decreased viscosity, while increases in peak systolic velocity (PSV) are a very sensitive test to identify fetal anemia [26]. MCA-PSV values higher than 1.5 multiples of the median are suggestive of severe fetal anemia, and indicative of the need for intervention. Several authors have found the sensitivity of MCA Dopplers to approach 100% when performed properly, and the specificity 85–95% [34]. This performance compares favorably to serial amniocentesis for OD450, and has the advantage of being non-invasive with little fetal risk.

Once fetal anemia is confirmed, PUBS is recommended for confirmatory diagnosis and possible intrauterine transfusion. Transfusion is the treatment of choice, as it can correct fetal anemia and may reduce the morbidity and mortality of B19V infection significantly. Unfortunately, performing PUBS carries a 3–5% rate of significant complications, including hemorrhage and the need for urgent delivery. In most cases, one transfusion is sufficient for fetal recovery, but there are exceptions. Following successful transfusion, it may take weeks for all fetal signs to disappear [26].

16.5.5 Management

Any pregnant woman who has either been exposed to parvovirus B19 or who develops compatible symptoms (e.g. rash, arthralgias, myalgias, low-grade temperature) should be assessed with IgM and IgG serology for parvovirus (see Figure 16.3). As noted earlier, if the patient is IgM−/IgG+, she has been exposed and has immunity, thus should be reassured that her exposure will not result in adverse consequences for her baby. If the IgG is negative and the IgM is negative after approximately 10 days post exposure, she is likely not infected with the virus. If the time frame of exposure is not able to be accurately confirmed, repeat serology in 2–4 weeks can be performed or elucidation of DNA via PCR can be requested; however, low levels of

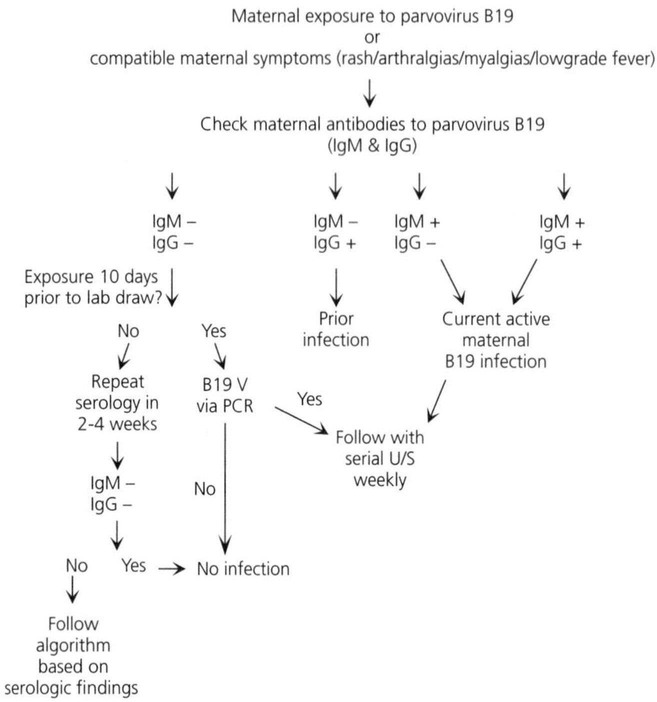

Figure 16.3 Parvo virus treatment flow diagram.

virus may be due to a remote infection. If the mother is IgM positive, the fetus should be monitored for the development of anemia and hydrops fetalis by ultrasound and MCA-PSV analysis weekly until 10–12 weeks post exposure.

If anemia is suspected, or overt hydrops is seen, an intrauterine transfusion should be entertained. Thrombocytopenia is another potential consequence of parvovirus infection; however, the utility of platelet transfusion is not recommended as the risks of volume overload and cardiac pathology outweigh the benefits [25]. If the fetus is near/at term, delivery should be considered, although transfusion of hydropic fetus in utero may be preferable as respiratory complications occurring in hydropic neonates can be prevented by allowing intrauterine recovery [26]. Pediatricians should be notified of the possibility of significant neonatal anemia even after in utero treatment. The majority of children who survive intrauterine or neonatal transfusion for parvovirus-induced fetal anemia and hydrops fetalis have a good neurodevelopmental prognosis [25].

16.6 Listeriosis

Listeria monocytogenes is a gram positive bacillus that is the cause of a rare but potentially serious infection. Pregnant patients and their neonates are particularly susceptible, accounting for 16% of all cases. Infection with listeriosis in pregnancy may result in preterm labor, preterm birth, perinatal death, and invasive neonatal disease [35].

Listeriosis is primarily felt to be a food-borne illness, with potential sources including unpasteurized cheeses, processed meats, incompletely washed fruits and vegetables, and possibly seafood. Infection is often asymptomatic in the mother or can be characterized by a viral syndrome that is usually mild and self-limited. Despite the mild maternal symptoms, neonatal consequences are severe. Perinatal death rates have been reported to be between 20 and 40% [36,37].

The neonatal infection is similar to GBS, in that a majority of cases are early onset or within 7 days of neonatal life. These cases are usually associated with sepsis and multi-organ system failure. Late-onset cases have also been reported and are often associated with meningitis and central nervous system involvement. Early onset is more likely to be associated with intrapartum transmission whereas late onset is more frequently by nosocomial transmission.

When diagnosed, treatment with penicillin or ampicillin is considered effective, and addition of gentamicin is sometimes also recommended. Most cases are not detected prior to the onset of neonatal disease or by placental pathology. Therefore avoidance of high-risk foods and patient education would seem to be the most effective prevention strategy. Clinicians should also maintain an index of suspicion for febrile illnesses, especially in the setting of preterm labor or unexplained perinatal death. Culturing listeria can be difficult, so consultation with microbiology or laboratory staff may be useful if you have a high clinical suspicion.

16.7 Human immunodeficiency virus / acquired immunodeficiency syndrome

The human immunodeficiency virus (HIV) is an RNA retrovirus that causes a chronic infection that is characterized by an immunocompromised state and opportunistic infections. Most infections in the United States are caused by the HIV-1 viral strain. Transmission of the virus is by contact with bodily fluids and may be from sexual activity, intravenous drug use, perinatal transmission, and, rarely, blood transfusion or organ donation.

Following acute infection there may be symptoms resembling a viral illness, including malaise, fevers, and sometimes lymphadenopathy. Some primary infections may be completely silent. Most patients will experience a long latent phase of infection where there may be no symptoms at all. This latent phase helps explain why a significant number of patients do not know they are infected, which increases the risk of further transmission. The latent phase may last upwards of 10 years but may now be increasing due to improved medical care.

Ultimately, patients will become symptomatic again as T-cells, specifically the CD4 subtype, are increasingly destroyed and the immune-compromise becomes more severe. They will develop a number of opportunistic infections that may include cytomegalovirus, pneumonias from various sources, fungal infections, and even lymphomas. These infections are the hallmarks of acquired immunodeficiency syndrome (AIDS). These infections may lead to disability and, ultimately, death.

Before the advent of perinatal therapy, the neonatal transmission of HIV was relatively common, over 25%. The landmark study, Pediatric AIDS Clinical Trials Group 076, demonstrated that the use of zidovudine prenatally, intrapartum, and for the neonate could decrease the rate of transmission by 70% [38]. Since that study, a number of other trials have demonstrated that aggressive perinatal and intrapartum care can further reduce transmission to 2% or less in most cases [39]. A multidrug regimen is often referred to as highly active antiretroviral therapy (HAART). It is estimated that currently there are fewer than 200 HIV-infected neonates born in United States [40]. The majority of these cases may be related to lack of prenatal care, non-compliance to recommended care, or failure to follow screening and treatment recommendations.

The choice of therapy may be made in conjunction with an infectious disease or maternal-fetal medicine specialist. The incidence of HIV drug resistance is increasing, sometimes even multidrug resistance. The use of virus-specific resistance studies may allow tailoring of treatment and improve maternal response. The general principles of HAART include a three-drug regimen with two nucleoside reverse transcriptase inhibitors (NRTI) and either one nonnucleoside reverse transcriptase inhibitor (NNRTI) or one protease inhibitor (PI). Use of the medications in pregnancy outweighs potential risks and a number of the agents have significant registry data now for fetal safety.

Zidovudine is usually included as one of the NRTI agents; lamivudine is acceptable as an alternative or as the second NRTI. Other options include stavudine, didanosine, and abacavir. Commonly used NNRTIs include nevirapine and efavirenz. Protease inhibitors may include lopinavir, ritonavir, and atazanavir. Combination products are also available to limit the number of pills that a patient must take every day, which may improve compliance.

The goal of treatment is to decrease the maternal viral load to as low as possible, even to the point of being undetectable. This decreases the risk of vertical transmission and increases the chances of a vaginal delivery if desired. Medications may have a number of side effects and must be managed carefully.

Given the availability of effective prophylactic treatments, the importance of screening for pregnant women is apparent. The CDC currently recommends universal screening with an opt-out approach. Patients must specifically decline the testing, otherwise it is performed with the remainder of the routine prenatal labs. The opt-out approach has been demonstrated to be a more effective screenings strategy then the opt-in approach, and does not require specific written consent [41]. Concerns about patient privacy and confidentiality remain, and test results must be handled with the utmost care.

Usual screening in the United States is performed by an zone immunoassay for both HIV-1 and HIV-2 strains. This assay is a screening test, and false positives are known to occur. Therefore, if a screen positive test is obtained, a confirmatory test must be performed. This is usually done before the notification to the patient. Various confirmatory tests exist, including immunofluorescent assays and the Western blot test. Once the confirmatory test is positive, then the patient may be notified and counseled about the diagnosis and the treatment options.

At the time of diagnosis or first prenatal care visit, patient should be evaluated with a viral load, a CD4 count, and comprehensive STI evaluation. They should also be evaluated for appropriate medical immunizations, including influenza, pneumococcus, hepatitis B, and meningococcus.

Patients should be counseled about the use of antiretroviral therapy, specifically highly active antiretroviral therapy. All pregnant women should be offered therapy regardless of their own health status or current viral load. If the patient has a diagnosis of AIDS, prophylaxis with sulfamethoxazole and trimethoprim for *Pneumocystis cariini* pneumonia is appropriate.

The use of cesarean section to reduce the incidence of vertical transmission has been shown to be efficacious in situations of high viral loads or limited prenatal care [42]. Patients should be offered this option in either situation of unknown viral load or in loads greater than 1000 copies per mL. This intervention has been demonstrated to reduce the incidence of vertical transmission from 28 to 8%. It is usually recommended that cesarean delivery be performed at 38 weeks, to minimize the risk of ruptured membranes or labor.

It is less clear whether cesarean delivery is also useful in settings of extremely low or non-detectable viral loads. The *a priori* risk of vertical transmission in these patients is 2% or less. Current available evidence does not demonstrate a clear decreased incidence from this very low level. However, it would take a very large prospect of trial to show a statistically significant decrease. At present it is considered reasonable to offer vaginal delivery at the patient's request, with good prenatal care and viral loads less than 1000 copies per mL. It is also reasonable to counsel patient about the theoretical benefit of cesarean section and the limitations of the current studies. Patients may make an informed decision about the route of delivery after counseling from their obstetric provider. If vaginal delivery is elected, expert opinion suggests avoidance of unnecessary amniotomy, internal monitoring, scalp pH testing, or other invasive maneuvers. The use of operative vaginal delivery is controversial, with primarily theoretical concerns about maternal and fetal trauma and admixing of bodily fluids. In general this is a relative contraindication, but if necessary due to the obstetric situation would still be reasonable.

Patients with HIV who have had insufficient prenatal care, or those with an unknown viral load who present in labor, are a management dilemma. Intrapartum treatment with zidovudine for the mother and neonatal treatment for 6 weeks may still significantly reduce the risk of vertical transmission. Studies outside of the United States have shown that treatment with niverapine intrapartum may similarly reduce the risk of transmission. If a patient comes into labor with no HIV screening then rapid HIV testing is reasonable. While the testing has improved significantly since introduction, the sensitivity and specificity is still not that of the screening and verification process. If the rapid screening test is positive then intrapartum therapy may be started until the confirmatory tests can be completed. If the test is a false negative and confirmatory tests are positive, neonatal treatment can still be undertaken.

The current recommendations in the United States are that patients with HIV infection should not breastfeed. The overall risk of transmission in breastfeeding is thought to be low but not zero. In countries where malnutrition is prevalent, breastfeeding may be reasonable.

16.8 Chorioamnionitis

Chorioamnionitis is an infection of the fetal environment including the amniotic fluid, amnion, chorion, placenta, and the umbilical cord. This infection, also called intra-amniotic infection, is primarily an ascending one, originating from the vagina and cervix (Figure 16.4). The incidence is estimated to be between 1 and 4% [43]. Pathogens consist of vaginal flora, opportunistic flora, and foreign pathogens. Hematogenous seeding has also been described, classically with listeria monocytogenese. Viruses and fungal organisms are rarely implicated in chorioamnionitis in an immunocompetent patient. The vast majority of infections are bacterial and polymicrobial. Commonly cultured organisms include: group B *Streptococcus*, *Escherichia coli*, ureaplasma, mycoplasma, and peptostreptococcus species [44].

A significant number of intra-amniotic infections follow rupture of the membranes, either spontaneous or artificial. This is due to the protective effect of the intact fetal membrane against infection. It provides a physical and immunologic barrier to ascending infection. A pregnancy has a number of other built-in defenses, including cervical mucus, which is thick and contains multiple elements of cellular immunity. Mucosal immunity in the vagina, cervix, and lower uterine segment consists of neutrophils, plasma cells, natural killer cells, and IgA antibodies. The vaginal flora in the absence of bacterial vaginosis consists of vast numbers of lactobacilli. These symbiotic organisms maintain an acidic vaginal PH and compete against potentially pathogenic or virulent organisms [21]. Lastly, the maternal and the fetal cellular and humeral immune systems are a last line of defense against opportunistic pathogens.

A number of situations may arise to limit or overcome these multiple lines of defense. Ruptured membranes, as previously mentioned, seem to allow a more direct ascending route of infection. PPROM especially seems to be a significant risk factor for intra-amniotic infection [45]. In addition, a shortened cervix seems to limit the effectiveness of the cervical mucosa barrier, perhaps through limiting the amount of cervical mucus, shortening the distance

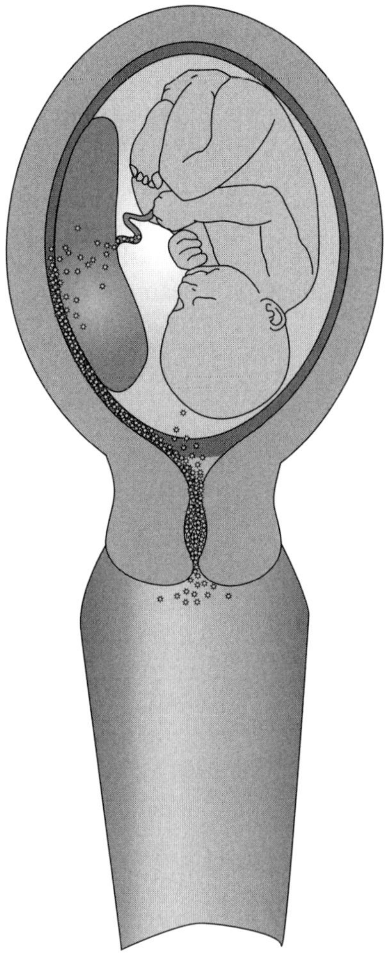

Figure 16.4 Chorioamnionitis.

between the vagina and fetal system, or through inflammatory or cytokine imbalances. There has been a significant amount of research to the basic science of how early chorioamnionitis develops and how cervical changes increase this risk. Alterations of the vaginal flora, including bacterial vaginosis and trichomoniasis, have been associated with the risks resulting in chorioamnionitis as well. The presence of significant numbers of *Gardnerella vaginalis* seems to allow the multiplication of facultative anaerobes and *mycoplasma* species that normally have a competitive disadvantage. Maternal medical compromise also raises the risk of chorioamnionitis. While HIV infection as well as serious chronic maternal medical conditions can compromise immunity, subtle impairments may arise from poor nutrition, concomitant sexually transmitted infections including chlamydia cervicitis, and possibly even human papilloma virus.

There are also a number of iatrogenic risk factors that are associated with chorioamnionitis. As previously mentioned, ruptured fetal membranes are a known risk factor. Usual indications are induction of labor or a prolonged labor. However, membranes that are ruptured longer than 18 hours have been strongly associated with the risk of infection. Vaginal examinations are also associated with chorioamnionitis. It is thought that the pushing of the examiner's fingers through the vaginal environment into the cervix and sometimes the lower uterine segment may inoculate areas that were previously sterile. There is no reliable evidence that sterile gloves as opposed to clean examining gloves are any less of a risk. Data exist that show a vaginal examination after PPROM is associated with shortened latency [46]. There are also data that link the number of vaginal examinations in labor to risk of clinical chorioamnionitis [47]. Since this data became available, institutions, especially ones associated in a teaching environment, have made a concerted effort to limit the number of vaginal examinations during labor.

The use of internal fetal monitors, which includes fetal scalp electrodes and intrauterine pressure monitors, is also associated with chorioamnionitis. Placement of these monitors involves the use of an examiner's hand in a very similar way to the previous cervical examinations. In addition, there is a foreign indwelling body that goes from the external environment, through the external genitalia, the vaginal environment, the cervical environment, and into the in utero environment; it is thought that this provides a conduit for ascending bacteria that may bypass maternal defense mechanisms. Given that there is very little evidence that internal monitors provide a benefit in terms of labor management or risk of cesarean section, their use should be generally limited, and for very specific indications.

The diagnosis of chorioamnionitis is usually made by clinical means via fever, maternal or fetal tachycardia, maternal abdominal pain, systemic symptoms including chills, sweats, or malaise, leukocytosis, purulent discharge, and sometimes dysfunctional uterine contraction patterns. Most patients will not have all of the symptoms listed but will have different combinations [48]. It requires a high index of clinical suspicion and should be entertained when any of the symptoms are present. However, there are a number of things that can cause false-positive symptoms, such as pain and maternal tachycardia, or fever after epidural placement. The definitive diagnosis usually requires amniotic fluid assessment and culture or pathological examination of the placenta and fetal membranes. In a laboring patient, it may not be practical or timely to obtain amniotic fluid testing given that cultures may take 24–48 hours. However, in situations such as PPROM or preterm labor there may be time to order this additional testing. Fluid is usually obtained through amniocentesis, which is somewhat invasive and expensive.

Treatment usually consists of antibiotics, maternal supportive care, and expedited delivery. Antibiotics are usually targeted to GBS, gram negative coverage, and anaerobic coverage, as most infections are polymicrobial.

Typical regimens may include a beta-lactam antibiotic, with or without gentamicin. In severe cases, anerobic coverage with clindamycin or metronidazole may be added. Attention should be paid to reduce maternal fever, with either antipyretics or cooling blankets. Hydration is also important, given the increased insensible losses with maternal fever and tachycardia. It is not clear what the optimal timing of delivery is with chorioamnionitis. The general principle of expedited delivery is to minimize the fetal exposure to an infectious environment. However, at present chorioamnionitis is not a stand-alone indication for cesarean delivery. Ensuring adequate contractions, regular labor progress, and induction of labor in settings of PPROM are recommended.

The risks associated with chorioamnionitis are dysfunctional labor, cesarean section, maternal sepsis, postpartum hemorrhage, endomyometritis, and neonatal sepsis. Long-term complications are also known to occur to fetuses exposed to the chorioamnionitis environment, including developmental delays and cerebral palsy. The risks are especially increased with premature fetuses.

There is an increasing research interest in the concept of the fetal inflammatory response syndrome (FIRS) [49]. Emerging evidence suggests that the fetal reaction to exposure to infectious agents includes an intense cascade of cytokines and cellular byproducts that may be useful in the immune response. However, as a byproduct, developing cells may be damaged or killed as collateral damage. Reactive free radicals, oxygen, and nitric species can be generated that can overwhelm the innate fetal protective cycle, for example glutathione. The cell death may continue for a significant period of time beyond the acute infection. Animal models seem to suggest that strong anti-inflammatory and anti-oxidant agents may be able to limit some of the cellular damage resulting from FIRS. N-acetylcysteine was able to significantly reduce white matter injury in an animal chorioamnionitis model [50].

In analyzing amniotic fluid for the diagnosis of chorioamnionitis, CBC, gram stain, and glucose are usually available rapidly whereas interleukin-6 and culture may take longer. CBC and gram stain can be diagnostic if very high numbers of organisms are seen. However, they generally lack sufficient sensitivity and specificity to be definitive. Low glucose levels, which may result from the metabolic activity of bacterial organisms, correlate well with culture results if the levels are extremely low, generally less than 15 mg/dL [51]. The expected glucose of amniotic fluid is usually two-thirds that of maternal levels, somewhere between 40 and 70 mg/dL. There are a number of factors that can affect the performance metrics of these tests: presence of maternal blood in the specimen, contaminants from maternal skin or the environment, insufficient amount of sample to run the tests, and machine and/or operator error. Culture, ultimately, is the best performing test for chorioamnionitis. However, limitations include the time it takes to obtain a result, in general 24–48 hours, which may be too late to allow timely intervention. In addition, some organisms are fastidious and difficult to culture out under ordinary circumstances, and this is especially true with anaerobic organisms and listeria monocytogenes. Interleukin-6, a well-known inflammatory cytokine, correlates well with the risk of clinical chorioamnionitis but is not available at every institution and may take a significant amount of time to return. If available, it may be used as an adjunct to the other mentioned tests for a marker for clinical infection.

Histologic chorioamnionitis is consistently reported to have a higher incidence than clinical chorioamnionitis [52]. It is usually defined by the presence of inflammatory cells in the fetal membranes, placenta, and the umbilical cord. These may consist of neutrophils, plasma cells, and, less commonly, areas of necrosis or even abscess. The discrepancy is likely due to a number of factors, including the subtlety of clinical symptoms, which may be missed, time lag between maternal and fetal response, systemic symptoms, and the likelihood that some inflammatory responses are not necessarily driven by frank bacterial infection. One confusing element in the study of chorioamnionitis is that differing authors use a clinical or histological basis for the diagnosis. While certainly overlapping and related, they are not always the same thing. On a practical level, the diagnosis of chorioamnionitis is a clinical one, due to both the timeliness of histological examination and the cost and availability of reliable placental pathology. When chorioamnionitis is suspected, a thorough placental examination is recommended to assess severity, the extent of tissue damage, and maternal response, if any. A culture of the placenta may also be considered for neonatal benefit.

16.9 Rubella

16.9.1 Epidemiology

Rubella, or German measles, a member of the togavirus family, is a viral exanthem that was initially identified in the late 1700s. It is a worldwide disease with major epidemics in the United States in 1935 and again in 1964. The virus is generally considered a mild, self-limiting disease only found in humans and is transmitted as an aerosol via the respiratory tract. The first rubella vaccine was developed in 1969 shortly after the last worldwide pandemic from 1963 to 1965 [53]. Prior to the introduction of the vaccine, rubella was most common in children less than 10 years of age, who then went on to have immunity as adults. It was not until the 1940s that an association between the virus and congenital defects was observed by an ophthalmologist named Gregg [54]. This was the first noted association between virus and neonatal sequelae [53]. Congenital rubella syndrome (CRS) can be devastating to neonates and classically presents as a triad of symptoms including cataracts, heart defects, and sensorineural deafness. There are many other transient and permanent sequelae, depending on gestational age at the time of infection, which can manifest many years later. Fortunately, CRS has become a rare disease in countries with effective vaccination programs; however, there are still sporadic cases. In the United States, via its dual vaccination program, seropositivity rates push 95% and the incidence of CRS is less than 2/100,000 live births [53].

16.9.2 Pathogenesis / clinical presentation

The rubella virus is transmitted via respiratory droplets and generally requires close contact. The incubation period is approximately 14 days and is followed by a prodromal period lasting up to 5 days consisting of low-grade temperatures, lymphadenopathy, arthralgias, and flu-like symptoms. This is followed by a maculopapular rash found on the face and chest lasting about 3 days. The rash spreads peripherally over time. In the non-pregnant population, recovery is spontaneous with subsequent immunity [55]. The significance of the rubella virus is derived from its effects on the fetus of infected pregnant mothers. Once the virus replicates, it spreads hematogenously and can infect the placenta, resulting in fetal exposure and the development of CRS [53]. The most influential factor in the development of CRS is gestational age at which neonatal infection occurs. While neonates can be infected at any gestational age, the most significant sequelae occur in the first trimester with more than 50% of fetuses developing abnormally. Spontaneous abortion may occur in up to 20% of cases when rubella occurs in the first 8 weeks of pregnancy [54].

This risk is greatly diminished in the second half of pregnancy, with no reported cases of CRS with maternal infection after the 20th week of gestation [55,56]. Infants, especially preterm, have an immature immune system which is unable to protect against vaccine-preventable infections [6]. Although the underlying mechanisms that cause fetal damage are not well understood, it is generally held that a fetus relies on the inefficient transport of maternal IgG in the first trimester to prevent infection. By the mid trimester the placental transport of maternal IgG improves considerably as well as the fetus's ability to mount its own response, significantly improving protection from the virus throughout the remainder of pregnancy. While the greatest risk for CRS occurs after a maternal primary infection, reinfection (despite protective IgG serum levels) can affect 5–8% of neonates if exposed in the first trimester [54].

At delivery, infants exposed to rubella infection can appear normal or have multiple, often severe, anomalies. Neonatal death within the first 2 years of life can occur in the most severely affected infants, who are usually exposed in the first trimester. As noted earlier, the classic triad of CRS incudes cataracts and hearing and heart defects. The most common anomaly is deafness. The most common heart defect is a patent ductus arteriosus and occurs in 30% of patients. Transient effects like low birth weight, thrombocytopenia, and hepatosplenomegaly typically resolve spontaneously in the first few weeks of life. There are several permanent, late-onset abnormalities, including developmental defects, hearing defects, diabetes mellitus, and eye defects [54].

Neonates with CRS can shed virus, thus must be cared for in isolation to help prevent spread of disease.

16.9.3 Diagnosis

Because it is a viral exanthem, manifesting with prodromal symptoms followed by a characteristic rash that spreads to the periphery, rubella can be difficult to distinguish clinically from other infective agents like parvovirus, measles, herpesvirus, and group A *Streptococcus*. In addition, about one-half of all rubella infections are subclinical, thus laboratory confirmation of rubella infection is required. Maternal serologic testing for IgM, IgG, and IgG avidity can be performed. IgM antibodies typically present about a week after onset of rash and persist for approximately 6 weeks, thus it is critical to perform testing in this window, given the potential to have a false negative if performed too early or too late [57].

According to the CDC, the laboratory diagnosis of rubella requires either (a) a positive serologic test for rubella IgM antibody, preferably via enzyme immunoassay, (b) a fourfold or greater rise in serum rubella IgG antibody level between samples collected within 7–10 days after onset of illness and repeated preferably 2–3 weeks later, or (c) isolation of rubella virus from nasal, blood, throat, urine, or cerebrospinal fluid specimens within 4 days after rash onset (although not all labs are equipped to perform this testing). Of note, rubella IgM test results in the serum can yield false positives, especially in patients with other viral infections like Epstein-Barr virus, cytomegalovirus, or parvovirus. In addition, the presence of rheumatoid factor can also cause false-positive results [58]. Women with a history of rubella vaccination should also be tested, since vaccination titers can wane over the years. If maternal serum taken within the first 12 days after contact is IgM negative and IgG positive, immunity can be assumed.

Once the maternal diagnosis of rubella is confirmed in pregnancy, there are several techniques that can be applied to determine if vertical transmission has occurred, including chorionic villus, fetal blood, and amniotic fluid testing via PCR for rubella antigen. Testing should be performed 6–8 weeks after maternal infection to ensure that virus or antibodies to it can be detected. Cordocentesis to obtain fetal blood is technically difficult before 20 weeks of gestation and data on chorionic villus sampling are limited. Amniocentesis seems to be the procedure of choice due to its decreased risk of complications [54]. It is important to note that maternal rubella infection during pregnancy does not always yield transmission of virus to the fetus, nor does fetal infection indicate the presence of abnormalities, including CRS [53,57]. This is especially the case if maternal infection occurs between 12 and 20 weeks of gestation. Fetal ultrasonography can be a useful adjunct to detect abnormalities consistent with CRS, such as growth restriction, microcephaly, cardiac malformations (septal defects), cataracts, and splenomegaly [59].

16.9.4 Treatment/prevention

There is no antiviral drug available to treat rubella or prevent transmission to the fetus. Rubella immunoglobulin is available; however, it has not proven to reduce the incidence of fetal infection, and is thus not recommended [55].

Because rubella is extremely teratogenic, primary prevention strategies have been employed to attain a goal of no cases of CRS. A universal vaccination program has virtually eradicated rubella in many populations; however, even in the United States there are still reported cases or persistent rubella infection and CRS in certain communities [53]. The primary purpose of rubella vaccination is to prevent congenital rubella infection and its early or late sequelae. Because of this, vaccination is targeted at children in order to help confer lifelong immunity beginning well before the reproductive years. However, it is important to note that vaccination strategies that target children alone should not be the sole strategy because of the potential for a shift to other susceptible groups. The United States and many other countries promote a dual vaccination strategy which includes children and susceptible adults. IgG antibodies persist in most vaccines for > 20 years after vaccination [54]. Obstetrics serves as a unique opportunity to test for and re-vaccinate patients whose titers are low so that perinatal transmission rates remain low. The current vaccine, the MMR, which was introduced in 1986 and contains live attenuated virus, is contraindicated in pregnancy.

Because it is a live virus, it is recommended that pregnancy be avoided for 1 month after vaccine administration to avoid congenital defects. Currently, pregnant women who have low rubella titers are offered the vaccine after delivery and prior to discharge from the hospital. There have been several studies that showed no statistical increase in adverse fetal effects or any cases of CRS, including a series of 94 cases showing no correlation between the rubella vaccination given 3 months pre- or postconception and major malformations [4]. Despite these data, a theoretical risk of 0.5–1.3% has been quoted if the vaccine is administered during the first trimester [60]. Parents should be given information related to the vaccine and its potential effects if inadvertent vaccination occurs while pregnant; however, there is no indication for termination of pregnancy [54].

16.10 Toxoplasmosis

16.10.1 Epidemiology

Toxoplasma gondii is an intracellular parasite and the causative agent of toxoplasmosis, which may give rise to congenital infection. It is estimated that 33% of world's population is infected with toxoplasmosis, with the highest prevalence found in Central America, Central Africa, and France [61,62]. In the United States, approximately 15% of women of childbearing age are seropositive. This results in approximately 400–4000 cases per year of congenital toxoplasmosis [62,63]. Overall, the risk of transmission to the fetus ranges from 0.6 to 1.7/1000 pregnant women [61].

The definitive host is a cat, both wild and domestic. Human infection occurs by eating undercooked meat containing viable cysts of the parasite, via food or water contaminated by the oocysts found in excrement of infected cats, or by the fecal–oral route. Intermediate hosts such as humans, birds, rodents, and other domestic animals can harbor infected cysts; however, they do not pass them in their feces like the definitive host. There is no evidence of direct human-to-human transmission except vertically from mother to fetus via transplacental passage from the circulation of mother with primary infection [62]. Congenital toxoplasmosis is the second most frequent intrauterine infection [61].

16.10.2 Risk factors

Risk factors increasing the risk of *T. gondii* include having a dog or a cat, cleaning litter trays, doing household work, ingesting unclean drinking water, having a lower educational level, having poor hygiene, eating raw meat/vegetables, and having contact with soil [61]. A review by Kravetz and Federman looked at multiple international studies and showed that undercooked meat and soil contact are most linked with seroconversion [64]. While the definitive host is a cat, owning a cat or changing cat litter was not found to be an independent risk factor for seroconversion with *T. gondii*. Indoor cats are typically fed pre-packaged foods and litter handlers use good hygiene when cleaning out litter boxes, thus these cats are not at risk for transmitting the oocysts. Outdoor cats that hunt or indoor cats that feed on raw meat are at risk for passing oocytes.

16.10.3 Diagnosis

Toxoplasmosis is primarily an asymptomatic infection. Approximately 10% of adults exhibit symptoms, with cervical lymphadenopathy being the most common clinical finding [62]. Fever, malaise, night sweats, and myalgias are also seen. In immunocompetent patients, immunity typically develops within 7–10 days of initial infection. While latent infections with toxoplasmosis are usually protective for both mother and neonate, reactivation may occur in immunocompromised hosts, thus patients with HIV [61,62] are at increased risk. The risk of congenital transmission of *T. gondii* depends upon the timing of maternal acquisition of the parasite. Approximately 90% of toxoplasmosis infections occur in the latter part of gestation. Vertical transmission rates increase from 10–15% in the first trimester to approximately 60% in the third trimester [65,66]. Serologic testing to detect antibodies to *T. gondii* via immunofluorescence antibody test, enzyme-linked immune filtration, and immunosorbant agglutination assay are available. All tests have a significant false-positive rate. IgM antibodies can be detected within a few days of infection and can remain elevated for several months. Interestingly, IgM titers can persist for years in up to 27% of healthy patients, yielding an approximately 1.3% false-positive rate [67]. Because of the difficulty in interpreting IgM testing, the FDA recommends confirmatory testing at a reference laboratory specializing in the diagnosis of toxoplasmosis. In the Unites States, the Palo Alto Medical Foundation offers a panel of tests including a dye test, determination of IgM, IgA, and IgE by ELISA, and IgG avidity testing, as well as a differential agglutination test to help determine if the infection is recent or has occurred in the past. IgG avidity increases over time; for example, a result greater than 20% suggests that the infection likely occurred > 20 weeks prior, although low avidity can be present for up to a year [62]. Gestational age at the time of infection helps guide which tests will be most helpful. If infection occurs at 16 weeks or less the IgG dye test, IgM ELISA, and IgG avidity are ordered and reflexed to other testing if needed. In pregnancies affected after 16 weeks, the agglutination test is substituted for the IgG avidity test in the initial panel, with reflex to the appropriate additional assay if confirmatory to help determine temporality of the infection. If the tests are consistent with a recent infection, treatment should be started.

If an acute maternal infection is confirmed, risk of congenital infection should be considered. The majority of neonatal *T. gondii* infections are asymptomatic. Congenital toxoplasmosis can result in chorioretinitis, which can be debilitating, as well as miscarriage, mental retardation, microcephaly, hydrocephalus, and seizures [63,64].

Fetal evaluation may consist of sonographic evaluation, amniocentesis, PUBS, or a combination of these. Common ultrasound findings include ventriculomegaly, ascites, intracranial calcifications, choroid plexus cysts, hepatosplenomegaly, and placentomegaly. The sensitivity of ultrasound for congenital infection is only about 20%; therefore, acute fetal infection is more accurately diagnosed with invasive testing via PUBS or amniocentesis. Serologic testing of fetal blood for *T. gondii* IgM or IgA is not possible before 22 weeks of gestational age, as the fetus does not produce these antibodies [62]. PCR on amniotic fluid has become the procedure of choice as it is rapid and accurate, with sensitivity of 83–97%, depending on the study [67].

16.10.4 Treatment

Once identified, an acute maternal infection warrants initiation of treatment with the antibiotic spiramycin until laboratory confirmation is confirmed. It concentrates in the placenta and thus reduces the risk of maternal–fetal transmission by > 50% [68]. It is only available in the United States through special permission through the CDC. If fetal infection is subsequently established, the addition of pyrimethamine (inhibitor of dihydrofolate reductase), sulfonamides, and folinic acid should be considered as this regimen has been shown to increase destruction of parasites in the placenta and in the fetus [69]. There are no randomized controlled trials to assess the effectiveness of antibiotic therapy. There are conflicting trials that showed anywhere from a fourfold reduction in congenital toxoplasmosis with treatment to no difference in the risk of congenital infection with or without antibiotic therapy. Gilbert *et al.* performed a prospective cohort trial of 1208 pregnant women in Europe who were treated for primary toxoplasmosis with spiramycin or pyrimethamine and found no difference in the risk of infection versus no treatment [70]. On the other hand, Ricci *et al.* published the results of a study of over 5200 susceptible pregnancies and were able to show a fourfold increase in the risk of congenital toxoplasmosis in neonates born to untreated mothers [71]. Because there are no randomized trials yet, ACOG recommends treatment. If an infant is diagnosed with congenital toxoplasmosis, the current recommendation is to treat with pyrimethamine, sulfadiazine, and leucovorin for up to 1 year [64].

16.10.5 Prevention

Prevention should include increased awareness and prenatal education, especially with regard to risk factors, such as handling of uncooked meats and vegetables, and methods to reduce exposure, such as hand washing, avoidance of raw/undercooked meat, use of appropriate food for cats (canned as opposed to raw), avoidance of cat litter, and wearing protective gloves if handling soil and cat litter [61].

Secondary prevention includes serologic monitoring of pregnant women who are at risk.

One report underscores that while obstetricians are generally knowledgeable about maternal infections, potential fetal outcomes, and preventative measures, the frequency with which these topics were discussed was low due to time constraints. ACOG recommends that pregnant women should be counseled regarding strategies to avoid infection with toxoplasmosis during pregnancy [63]. Given the low prevalence of toxoplasmosis in the United States, routine serologic screening during pregnancy is not recommended except in patients who are HIV positive.

16.11 Hepatitis B

Hepatitis B is a hepadnavirus that is a transmitted via bodily fluids and infects the liver. In approximately 10% of patients it develops into a chronic infection that is characterized by a lack of symptoms, normal liver function tests, and seropositivity to either HbsAg, HbcAg, HbeAg, or a combination [21]. A chronic infection may remain quiescent for many years. Reactivation or development of cirrhosis of the liver is possible in later years. In general, her pregnancy has no effect on the progression of hepatitis in the mother. In pregnancy, vertical transmission is known to occur and the risk increases with increasing viral load and with maternal positivity for HbeAg.

The current recommendations are to screen all pregnant women for the presence of HbsAg during routine prenatal screening [72]. Patients found to be positive require neonatal prophylaxis against transmission. Neonates are treated with hepatitis B immunoglobulin and hepatitis vaccinations at the time of birth. This significantly decreases their risk of vertical transmission.

Recent evidence has demonstrated that patients with a high viral load, for example those with greater than 100,000 copies per mL, may have lower rates of transmission from the additional treatment of lamivudine [73]. It is given daily during the last 4–8 weeks of pregnancy. The increasing evidence of the safety and efficacy of lamivudine for this indication argues for obtaining a hepatitis B viral load in the third trimester.

It is a larger goal to immunize as many patients as possible against hepatitis B. Most healthcare workers and children are now vaccinated as part of school or work vaccination programs. There remain, however, a significant number of patients who are still susceptible. Asking patients about their vaccination status is a key step toward identifying those who may be a candidate for vaccination [74]. Vaccination is considered safe in pregnancy and may be given on an accelerated-rate schedule to provide immunity before delivery [72]. The vaccination is accomplished in a three-injection series which may be accomplished within a 6-month span.

Intrapartum management consists primarily of avoiding invasive procedures as much as is practical. Planning for neonatal prophylaxis is the key step. There is no evidence that cesarean section is protective. Breastfeeding is considered safe in most cases.

16.12 Hepatitis C

Hepatitis C is an RNA flavivirus that is also transmitted via bodily fluids and infects the liver. This infection is particularly troublesome as there is no current vaccine available, no neonatal prophylaxis, and the majority of patients develop a chronic infection state. Vertical transmission is known to occur, seemingly related to the maternal viral load [75].

Patients who are infected are at high risk for co-infection with HIV, hepatitis B, and other STIs. Counseling and careful screening is needed. Avoidance of intrapartum invasive procedures is prudent. Breastfeeding is considered safe in most cases.

There has been interest in the use of cesarean section for the reduction of vertical transmission, similar to the HIV model. The preponderance of the available prospective studies do not support this concept [76]. The use of ribavirin and interferon has been reported in small, limited studies, but is not currently recommended.

16.13 Cytomegalovirus

Cytomegalovirus (CMV) is one of the most common causes of perinatal infection in the United States. It is estimated that nearly 40,000 pregnant women experience a primary infection during their pregnancy, with up to 8000 infants having permanent sequelae [77]. There are a number of factors that contribute to this high incidence, including the mild or absent symptoms associated with infection, and the incomplete upper protection provided by previous infection. Congenital infections may result from primary, recurrent, or reactivation infections. CMV is a member of the herpes virus family and may remain latent for years before reactivation.

Fetal CMV infection is frequently diagnosed by ultrasound findings, which may be growth restriction, polyhydramnios, echogenic bowel, intracranial or intra-abdominal calcifications, ventriculomegaly, or even fetal demise [78]. Maternal infection is usually silent or mildly symptomatic and, unless there is a known exposure, is rarely diagnosed at the time. If suspected from any sign or symptom, the usual first steps are to obtain maternal serum titers of CMV IgG and IgM. Negative titers would usually rule out an active infection. Hi IgM titers with negative IgG titers would be a diagnostic of an acute infection. Hi titers of both IgG and IgM can be confusing and then IgG of deep vein thrombosis testing may be of benefit. Older infections tend to have higher avidity, which may guide the clinician away from a recent infection diagnosis. Ultimately, to diagnose any fetal infection in the antenatal period requires amniocentesis and assay with a PCR for culture for CMV. If PCR confirms fetal infection, the patient should be counseled about her options, including observation, termination, in utero therapy, or postnatal therapy.

There is recent interest in the concept of in utero therapy for known or suspected fetal infections. Nigro and colleagues published a groundbreaking study in which the use of CMV IgG among pregnant women with confirmed CMV infections was able to decrease the incidence of congenital deafness, and in fact reverse some of the ultrasound findings, including calcifications [79]. It is not entirely clear how the mechanism of the CMV IgG is protective, and there were some limitations of the study. If confirmed in larger series, in utero treatment would seem to offer several advantages to traditional treatments such as neonatal ganciclovir.

If a readily available effective treatment became available then it would also seem to argue in favor of routine screening of a pregnant woman, given the high incidence of CMV, although this is controversial. There are also a number of potential vaccines undergoing evaluation at this time, which would add the possibility of primary prevention [80].

16.14 Herpes

Herpes simplex virus (HSV) is a common STI, compromised of both HSV-1 and HSV-2. Either subtype may be found in any anatomic location. The seroprevalence of pregnant women is reported to be approximately 7–28% [81]. Primary infections in pregnancy may be associated with spontaneous abortion, fetal death, IUGR, preterm, and structural birth defects. Congenital infection may be characterized by CNS and skin and ocular defects. Neonatal infections may also occur that can result in encephalitis, meningitis, and neonatal death. The estimated incidence of neonatal herpes is 1/3500 births [82].

Recurrent disease is much less likely to result in congenital HSV due to the presence of maternal IgG to the virus.

Active genital herpes lesions in the genital area are indications for cesarean delivery for the prevention of neonatal herpes infection. Cesarean section significantly reduces the risk of transmission. The use of third-trimester oral suppression for outbreak prophylaxis is also very effective at reducing both the risk of needing a cesarean for this indication and of neonatal complication [83]. Acyclovir or valacyclovir are the most commonly used agents for prophylaxis.

16.15 Wound infections

Wound infections can develop whenever a break in the epidermal barrier occurs. In the postpartum setting this most often is in the setting of a cesarean incision, but may also occasionally occur with perineal tears or episiotomy. The incidence of wound infections varies by patient and procedure, but most studies report a range of 2–10%. Obese patients have a consistently higher risk of wound disruption and infection, with as many as 1 in 3 patients experiencing a complication [84].

Prophylactic antibiotics have consistently been shown to decrease the incidence of postcesarean wound infection. Minimizing tissue destruction, limiting the time of surgery, and redosing antibiotics with significant blood loss have also been recommended. There is no current evidence that routine use of wound drains can decrease wound complications; in fact, some authors have found increased risks with their use [84,85].

Wound infections are typically polymicrobial and include opportunistic organisms, or those already existing on the skin or genital tract. Disruption of the skin, placement of foreign bodies, tissue destruction, decreased circulation, and oxygen tension may all contribute to an ideal growing environment for bacteria and other organisms. Causative organisms may include *Streptococcus, Staphylococcus,* mycoplasma, ureaplasma, facultative anaerobes, and other species. Wound cultures can be helpful to rule out methicillin-resistant *Staphylococcus aureus* (MRSA) and to guide therapy in cases that do not respond rapidly to wound care.

Treatment usually consists of wound opening, debridement, and draining of the infected exudate and tissue. Devitalized or dead tissue needs to be debrided to promote healing. The use of antibiotics is situational, based on the severity of the associated cellulitis. Coverage should be focused on *Staphylococcus* species and can be adjusted based on clinical factors or culture results. Opened wounds can either be left open to heal by secondary intention or closed secondarily once good granulation tissue is established.

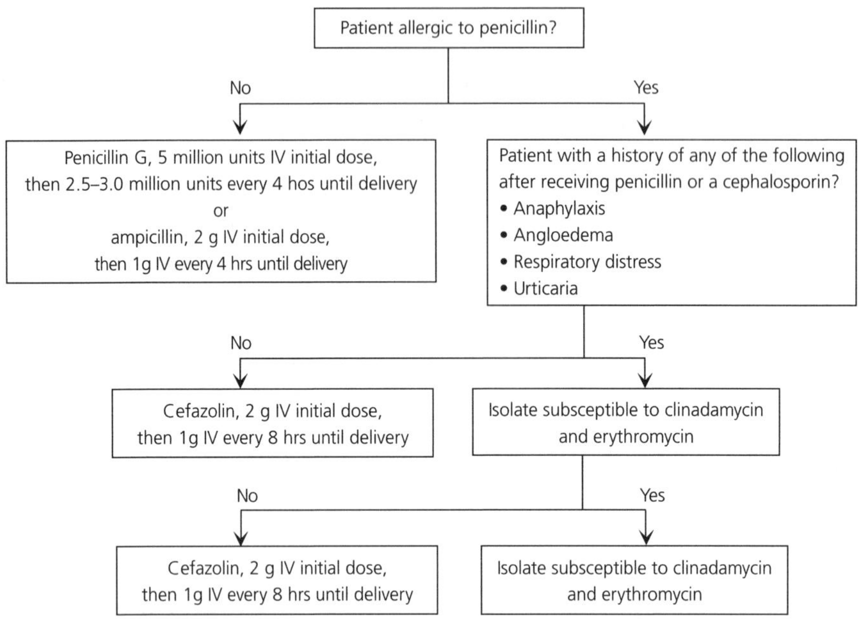

Figure 16.5 Necrotizing fasciitis.

Rarely, wound infections can lead to more severe infection, including necrotizing fasciitis. This occurs approximately in 1–2 cases per 1000 [86]. Necrotizing fasciitis is a rapidly spreading infection involving the superficial fascial and subcutaneous tissues. If not recognized and treated promptly it may result in severe morbidity or death. Skin changes may be the first sign of this dreaded complication, and can include discoloration, sloughing, bullous formation, and loss of integrity. Oddly, there may be no pain or patient complaint at first as the superficial nerves are destroyed. Late signs include acidosis, coagulopathy, and respiratory distress.

Rapid response and wide surgical debridement can reduce the risk of mortality with necrotizing fasciitis [86]. It is not uncommon to have to make multiple trips to the operating room for debridement (Figure 16.5). Broad-spectrum antibiotics are recommended as well as vigorous hydration and supportive care. The debridement is often so extensive that plastic and reconstructive surgery may be required for the surviving patient.

16.16 Endometritis

Endometritis is an infection of the endometrium and myometrium, characterized by abdominopelvic pain, fever, and occasionally leukocytosis, purulent discharge, and systemic symptoms [21]. This is a polymicrobial infection, usually consisting of genital, GI, or skin flora [87]. The diagnosis is a clinical one, with endometrial culture/biopsy rarely needed.

The incidence of endometritis following vaginal delivery is unusual, approximately 1/1000 deliveries. Following cesarean delivery, however, the incidence may range from 5 to 20%, depending on whether prophylactic antibiotics were given. Other risk factors include chorioamnionitis, prolonged labor or surgery, and use of internal monitors.

Clinicians must keep a wide differential diagnosis when considering endometritis, as there are several other conditions that can result in fevers and abdominal pain. A partial list includes UTI/pyelonephritis, pneumonia, atelectasis, wound infections, drug reactions, retained products of conception, and thromboembolic events. Serial examination, judicious use of laboratory testing, and cultures will help make a definitive diagnosis.

Treatment for endometritis is broad-spectrum antibiotics. Commonly used regimens include single agents such as piperacillin/tazobactam or ertapenem, or multi-agent regimens including gentamicin/clindamycin or metronidazole/gentamicin/ampicillin.

Patients who respond poorly to treatment or who continue to manifest symptoms and spiking temperatures for more than 72–96 hours post-diagnosis may have developed a pelvic abscess. These do not typically respond to IV antibiotic therapy alone. If there is suspicion for a pelvic abscess, diagnostic imaging is required. Ultrasound, computed tomography (CT), or magnetic resonance imaging may all be used for this purpose, but CT is most often used. Once confirmed, drainage is recommended to speed recovery. This could be accomplished by CT or ultrasound-guided drainage, colpotomy, laparoscopy, or, less commonly, laparotomy. The least invasive route that is effective would be preferred.

Prevention of endometritis is best accomplished with prophylactic antibiotics when appropriate. Patients undergoing cesarean section should receive antibiotics 15–60 minutes prior to the start of the surgery [88]. Following a vaginal delivery, patients who undergo manual extraction of the placenta or other instrumentation of the uterine cavity should be considered for antibiotic prophylaxis.

16.17 Septic pelvic thrombophlebitis

When a postpartum patient continues to have febrile morbidity despite treatment with antibiotics, serial examination, and time, other diagnoses must be considered. One of these is septic pelvic thrombophlebitis (SPT). This is a poorly characterized clinical scenario which usually involves a thrombosis of an ovarian vein [89]. Symptoms are extremely variable and can range from practically nothing to flank pain, abdominal pain, gastrointestinal symptoms, and pain with motion or tachycardia. Low-grade temperatures or slight temperatures are usually associated. Physical examination is often non-specific, with tenderness to palpation in the abdomen, flank, back, and pelvis all possible. There are two approaches to a patient who is suspected to have SPT. One is to perform imaging, usually with a CT of the abdomen and pelvis, although MRI is also reasonable. This modality looks for filling defects in the ovarian veins and other major pelvic vessels. This has the advantage of also being able to look for a pelvic abscess, which may often present in a similar fashion. The second approach would be to simply treat with anticoagulation: therapeutic doses of either unfractionated heparin or low-molecular-weight heparin for 7–14 days. A significant number of patients will experience resolution of their fevers and symptoms with this approach. Most clinicians with continue the broad-spectrum antibiotics, given that the treatment is somewhat empiric. Anticoagulation is also usually used with CT or MRI evidence of a thrombus.

It is unclear how frequent the occurrence of SPT is. Recent studies using magnetic resonance venography have demonstrated a 30% incidence of thrombosis in pelvic deep veins following spontaneous vaginal delivery [90]. These findings would suggest that SPT is sometimes overdiagnosed.

16.18 Mastitis

Mastitis is an inflammatory process of the breast usually caused by a bacterial infection (Figure 16.6). Symptoms may vary, but commonly include pain, erythema, swelling, fever, and systemic symptoms including chills and malaise. The incidence is also variable but was reported at 9.5% in one large series [91]. It may occur at any time in the postpartum period or during lactation, but the peak incidence is thought to be between 2 and 4 weeks postpartum. Mastitis may affect any postpartum patient, but risk factors such as nipple cracking or trauma, difficulties with breastfeeding, and previous history may increase the risk.

The diagnosis of mastitis is a clinical one, based largely on patient symptoms. The breast may or may not have erythema and edema associated as well. The affected breast will usually be tender on examination. A culture of breast milk is usually not indicated except in the usual circumstances, including treatment failures, immune-compromised patients, or suspected antibiotic resistance. Clinicians should attempt to differentiate mastitis from simple engorgement or breast abscess.

There are a few effective prevention strategies for mastitis. Maternal hand washing and attention to hygiene have been shown to decrease the incidence in the postpartum period [92]. Once diagnosed, attention should be toward symptomatic relief, antibiotic treatment, and the continuation of breastfeeding. This latter factor is important as it decreases milk stasis, which leads to a faster resolution of pain and a decreased incidence of breastfeeding discontinuation. If desired, the breast milk can be a pumped and discarded during the treatment phase.

Antibiotic treatment is targeted to the organisms commonly associated with mastitis. These include *Staphylococcus aureus, Staphylococcus epidermidis,* and, less

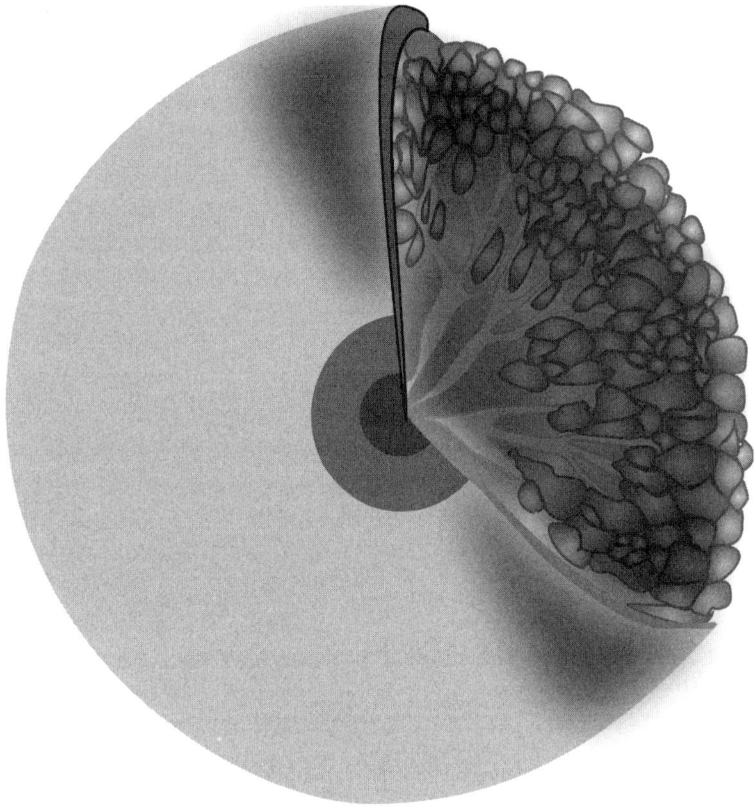

Figure 16.6 Mastitis.

commonly, MRSA, *Escherichia coli*, and various *Streptococcus* species. There is no evidence available to support a single-best treatment option [93]. Reasonable treatment options include trimethoprim/sulfamethoxazole, ciprofloxacin, cephalexin, and amoxicillin/clavulanate. Treatment is often recommended for 10–14 days.

References

1 Verani JR and Schrag SJ. Group B streptococcal disease in infants: progress in prevention and continued challenges. *Clinics in Perinatology* 2010;**37**:375–392.

2 Centers for Disease Control and Prevention. Prevention of perinatal group B streptococcal disease. Revised guidelines from CDC, 2010. *MMWR Recommendations and Reports* 2010;**59/RR-10**.

3 Jordan HT, Farley MM, Craig A *et al.* Revisiting the need for vaccine prevention of late-onset neonatal group B streptococcal disease: a multistate, population based analysis. *Pediatric Infectious Disease Journal* 2008;**27**(12):1057–1064.

4 Schrag SJ, Zell ER, Lynfield R *et al.* A population-based comparison of strategies to prevent early-onset GBS disease in neonates. *New England Journal of Medicine* 2002;**347**(4):233–239.

5 Boyer KM and Gotoff SP. Strategies for chemoprophylaxis of GBS early-onset infections. *Antibiotics and Chemotherapy* 1985;**35**:267–280.
6 Illuzi JL and Bracken MB. Duration of intrapartum prophylaxis for neonatal group B streptococcal disease. A systematic review. *Obstetrics & Gynecology* 2006;**108**(5):1254–1265.
7 Valkenberg-van den Berg AW, Houtman-Roelofsen RL, Oostvogel PM *et al.* Timing of group B *Streptococcus* screening in pregnancy: a systematic review. *Gynecologic and Obstetric Investigation* 2010;**69**:174–183.
8 El Helali N, Nguyen JC, Ly A, Giovangrandi Y, and Trinquart L. Diagnostic accuracy of a rapid real-time polymerase chain reaction assay for universal intrapartum group B *Streptococcus* screening. *Clinical Infectious Diseases* 2009;**49**:417–423.
9 Platt MW, McLaughlin JC, Gilson GJ *et al.* Increased recovery of group B *Streptococcus* by the inclusion of rectal culturing and enrichment. *Diagnostic Microbiology and Infectious Disease* 1995;**21**:65–68.
10 Edwards MS. Group B streptococcal conjugate vaccine: a timely concept for which the time has come. *Human Vaccines* 2008;**4**:444–448.
11 Arvin AM. Varicella-zoster virus. *Clinical Microbiology Reviews* 1996;**9**(3):361–381.
12 Sauerbrei A and Wutzler P. Herpes simplex and varicella-zoster virus infections during pregnancy: current concepts of prevention, diagnosis and therapy. Part 2: Varocella-zoster virus infections. *Medical Microbiology and Immunology* 2007;**196**:95–102.
13 Enders G. Serodiagnosis of Varicella-Zoster virus infection in pregnancy and standardization of the ELISA IgG and IgM antibody tests. *Developments in Biological Standardization* 1982;**52**:221–236.
14 Tan MP and Koren G. Chickenpox in pregnancy: revisited. *Reproductive Toxicology* 2006;**21**:410–420.
15 American College of Obstetrics and Gynecology Practice Bulletin No. 20: Perinatal Viral and Parasitic Infections. Washington, DC: ACOG, 2000.
16 Gardella C and Brown ZA. Managing varicella zoster infection in pregnancy. *Cleveland Clinic Journal of Medicine* 2007;**74**(4):290–296.
17 Lucas MJ and Cunningham FG. Urinary infection in pregnancy. *Clinical Obstetrics and Gynecology* 1993;**36**:855–868.
18 Patterson TF and Andriole VT. Bacteriuria in pregnancy. *Infectious Disease Clinics of North America* 1987;**1**:807–822.
19 American College of Obstetrics and Gynecology Educational Bulletin No. 245. Antimicrobial Therapy for Obstetric Patients. Washington, DC: ACOG, 1998.
20 Doern GV, Saubolle MA, and Sewell DL. Screening for bacteruria with the LB urine strip test. *Diagnostic Microbiology and Infectious Disease* 1986;**4**:355.
21 Faro S and Soper D. *Infectious Diseases in Women.* Philadelphia, PA: WB Saunders Co, 2001: 354–368.
22 Harris RE, Gilstrap LC, III, and Pretty A. Single-dose antimicrobial therapy for asymptomatic bacteriuria during pregnancy. *Obstetrics & Gynecology* 1982;**59**:546–549.
23 Patterson TF and Andriole VT: Detection, significance and therapy of bacteriuria in pregnancy. *Infectious Disease Clinics of North America* 1997;**11**:593.
24 Millar LK, Wing DA, Paul RH, and Grimes DA. Outpatient treatment of pyelonephritis in pregnancy: a randomized controlled trial. *Obstetrics & Gynecology* 1995;**864**:1560–1564.
25 Dijkmans AC, de Jong EP, Dijkmans BAC, Lopriore E, Vossen A, Walther FJ *et al.* Parvovirus B19 infection in pregnancy. *Current Opinion in Obstetrics and Gynecology* 2012;**24**:95–101.
26 de Jong EP, de Haan TR, Kroes ACM, Beersma MFC, Oepkes D, and Walther FJ. Parvovirus B19 infection in pregnancy. A Review. *Journal of Clinical Virology* 2006;**36**:1–7.
27 De Haan TR, Oepkes D, Beersma MFC, and Walther FJ. Aetiology, diagnosis and treatment of hydrops foetalis. *Current Pediatric Reviews* 2005;**1**:63–72.

28 Harger JH, Adler SP, Koch WC, and Harger GF. Prospective evaluation of 618 pregnant women exposed to parvovirus B19: risks and symptoms. *Obstetrics & Gynecology* 1998;**91**:413–420.
29 Bredla S, Plentz A, Wenzel JJ, Pfisterc H, Möst J, and Modrow S. False-negative serology in patients with acute parvovirus B19 infection. *Journal of Clinical Virology* 2011;**51**:115–120.
30 Enders M, Schalasta G, Baisch C, Weidner A, Pukkila L, Kaikkonen L *et al.* Human parvovirus B19 infection during pregnancy – value of modern molecular and serological diagnostics. *Journal of Clinical Virology* 2006;**35**:400–406.
31 Landolsi H, Yacoubi MT, Bouslama L, Lahmar A, Trabelsi A, Hmissa S *et al.* Detection of the human Parvovirus B19 in nonimmune hydrops fetalis using immunohistochemistry and nested-PCR in formalin-fixed and paraffin-embedded placenta and fetal tissues. *Pathologie Biologie* 2009;**57**:e1–e7
32 Lindblom A, Isa A, Norbeck O, Wolf S, Johansson B, Broliden K *et al.* Slow clearance of human parvovirus B19 viremia following acute infection. *Clinical Infectious Diseases* 2005;**41**:1201–1203.
33 de Jong EP, Lindenburg IT, van Klink JM *et al.* Intrauterine transfusion for parvovirus B19 infection: long-term neurodevelopmental outcome. *American Journal of Obstetrics & Gynecology* 2012;**206**:204 e1–e5.
34 Mari, G. Doppler ultrasonography in obstetrics from the diagnosis of fetal anemia to the treatment of intrauterine growth-restricted fetuses. *American Journal of Obstetrics & Gynecology* 2009;**200**(6):613 e1–9. Epub 2009/2/6.
35 Jackson KA, Iwamoto M, and Swerdlow D. Pregnancy-associated listeriosis. *Epidemiology & Infection* 2010;**138**:1503–1509.
36 Gellin BG and Broome CV. Listeriosis. *Journal of the American Medical Association* 1989;**261**:1313.
37 Lorber B. Listeriosis. *Clinical Infectious Diseases* 1997;**24**:1–11.
38 Connor EM, Sperling RS, Gelber R *et al.* Reduction of maternal-infant transmission of human immunodeficiency virus type 1 with zidovudine treatment. Pediatric AIDS Clinical Trials Group Protocol 076 Study Group. *New England Journal of Medicine* 1994;**331**(18):1173–1180.
39 Centers for Disease Control and Prevention (CDC). Achievements in public health. Reduction in perinatal transmission of HIV infection – United States, 1985–2005. *Morbidity and Mortality Weekly Report* 2006;**55**(21):592–597.
40 McKenna MT and Hu X. Recent trends in the incidence and morbidity that are associated with perinatal human immunodeficiency virus infection in the United States. *American Journal of Obstetrics & Gynecology* 2007;**197**(3Suppl. 3):S10–16.
41 Committee on Pediatric AIDS. HIV testing and prophylaxis to prevent mother-to-child transmission in the United States. *Pediatrics* 2008;**122**(5):1127–1134.
42 European Mode of Delivery Collaboration. Elective caesarean-section versus vaginal delivery in prevention of vertical HIV-1 transmission: a randomised clinical trial. The European Mode of Delivery Collaboration. *Lancet* 1999;**353**(9158):1035–1039.
43 Gibbs RS and Duff P. Progress in pathogenesis and management of clinical intraamniotic infection. *American Journal of Obstetrics & Gynecology* 1991;**164**:1317.
44 Tita ATN and Andrews WW. Diagnosis and management of clinical chorioamnionitis. *Clinics in Perinatology* 2010;**37**(2):339–354.
45 Berghella V. *Obstetric Evidence-Based Guidelines*. Taylor and Francis. 2007: **139**.
46 Lewis DF, Major CA, Towers CV *et al.* Effects of digital vaginal examinations on latency period in PPROM. *Obstetrics & Gynecology* 1992;**80**(4):630–634.
47 Soper DE, Mayhall CG, and Dalton HP. Risk factors for intra-amniotic infection: a prospective epidemiologic study. *American Journal of Obstetrics & Gynecology* 1989;**161**(3):562–566.
48 Newton ER. Chorioamnionitis and intraamniotic infection. *Clinical Obstetrics and Gynecology* 1993;**36**:795.
49 Gotsch F, Romero R, Kusanovic JP *et al.* The fetal inflammatory response syndrome *Clinical Obstetrics and Gynecology* 2007;**50**(3):652–683.

50 Chang EY, Zhang J, Sullivan S *et al.* NAC attenuates the maternal and fetal pro-inflammatory response to intrauterine LPS injection in an animal model of preterm birth and brain injury. *Journal of Maternal-Fetal and Neonatal Medicine* 2011;**24**(5):732–740. Epub 2011/1/10.

51 Kirshon B, Rosenfeld B, Mari G *et al.* Amniotic fluid glucose concentration: a rapid and simple method for the detection of intra-amniotic infection in preterm labor. *American Journal of Obstetrics & Gynecology* 1991;**164**:818.

52 Dong Y, St Clair PJ, Ramzy I *et al.* A microbiologic and clinical study of placental inflammation at term. *Obstetrics & Gynecology* 1987;**70**:175.

53 Duszac RS. Congenital Rubella Syndrome – major review. *Optometry* 2009;**80**:36–43.

54 Best JM. Rubella. *Seminars in Fetal & Neonatal Medicine* 2007;**12**:182 e192.

55 Signore C. Rubella. *Primary Care Update for OB/GYNS*. 2001;**4**(4);133–137.

56 Santis MD, Cavaliere AF, Straface G, and Caruso A. Rubella infection in pregnancy. A review. *Reproductive Toxicology* 2006;(**21**):390–398.

57 MMWR. Control and prevention of rubella: evaluation and management of suspected outbreaks, rubella in pregnant women, and surveillance for congenital rubella syndrome. *MMWR Recommendations and Reports* 2001;**50**(RR12):1–23.

58 Van den Berg JP, Westerbeek EAM, Berbers GAM, and van Elburg RM. Transplacental transport of IgG antibodies to preterm infants: a review of the literature. *Early Human Development* 2011;**87**:67–72.

59 Degani S. Sonographic findings in fetal viral infections: a systematic review. *Obstetrical and Gynecological Survey* 2006;**61**(5):329–336.

60 Morice A, Ullao-Gutierrez, and Avila-Aguero ML. Congenital rubella syndrome: progress and future challenges. *Expert Review of Vaccines* 2009;**8**(3):323–331.

61 Bojar I and Szymanska J. Environmental exposure of pregnant women to infection with *Toxoplasma gondii* – state of the art. *Annals of Agricultural and Environmental Medicine* 2010;**17**:209–214.

62 Beazley DM and Egerman RS. Toxoplasmosis. *Seminars in Perinatology* 1998;**122**(4):332–338.

63 Elmore SA, Jones JL, Conrad PA, Patton S, Lindsay DS, and Dubey JP. *Toxoplasma gondii*: epidemiology, feline clinical aspects, and prevention. *Trends in Parasitology* 2010;**26**(4):190–196.

64 Kravetz JD and Federman DG. Toxoplasmosis in pregnancy. A review. *American Journal of Medicine* 2005;**118**:212–216.

65 Hohlfeld P, Daffos F, Costa JM, Thulliez P, Forestier F, and Vidaud M. Prenatal diagnosis of congenital toxoplasmosis with a polymerase-chain-reaction test on amniotic fluid. *New England Journal of Medicine* 1994;**331**:695–699.

66 Foulon W, Villena I, Stray-Pedersen B, Decoster A, Lappalainen M, Pinon JM *et al.* Treatment of toxoplasmosis during pregnancy: a multicenter study of impact on fetal transmission and children's sequelae at age 1 year. *American Journal of Obstetrics & Gynecology* 1999;**180**:410–415.

67 Abdul-Ghani R. Polymerase chain reaction in the diagnosis of congenital toxoplasmosis: more than two decades of development and evaluation. *Parasitology Research* 2011;**108**:505–512.

68 Mombro M, Perathoner C, Leone A, Nicocia M, Moiraghi Ruggenini A *et al.* Congenital toxoplasmosis: 10-year follow up. *European Journal of Pediatrics* 1995;**154**:635–639.

69 Stray-Pedersen B. Treatment of toxoplasmosis in the pregnant mother and newborn child. *Scandinavian Journal of Infectious Diseases* 1992;**84**:23–31.

70 Gilbert R and Gras L. European multicentre study on congenital toxoplasmosis. Effect of timing and type of treatment on the risk of mother to child transmission of *Toxoplasma gondii*. *BJOG* 2003;**110**:112–120.

71 Ricci M, Pentimalli H, Thaller R *et al.* Screening and prevention of congenital toxoplasmosis: an effectiveness study in a population with a high infection rate. *Journal of Maternal-Fetal and Neonatal Medicine* 2003;**14**:398–403.

72 American College of Obstetricians and Gynecologists. Practice Bulletin No. 86: Viral Hepatitis in Pregnancy. *Obstetrics & Gynecology* 2007;**110**(4):941–956. PMID: 17906043.

73 van Zonneveld M, van Nunen AB, Niesters HG, de Man RA, Schalm SW, and Janssen HL. Lamivudine treatment during pregnancy to prevent perinatal transmission of hepatitis B virus infection. *Journal of Viral Hepatitis* 2003;**10**(4):294–297. PMID: 12823596.

74 Centers for Disease Control and Prevention, Workowski KA, and Berman SM. Sexually transmitted diseases treatment guidelines, 2006. *MMWR Recommendations and Reports* 2006;**55**(RR-11):1–94.

75 Ohto H, Terazawa S *et al.* Transmission of hepatitis C virus from mothers to infants. The Vertical Transmission of Hepatitis C Virus Collaborative Study Group. *New England Journal of Medicine* 1994;**330**:744–750.

76 Tajiri H, Miyoshi Y, Funada S, Etani Y, Abe J, Onodera T *et al.* Prospective study of mother-to-infant transmission of hepatitis C virus. *Pediatric Infectious Disease Journal* 2001;**20**:10–14.

77 Colugnati F, Staras S, Dollard S, and Cannon M. Incidence of cytomegalovirus infection in the general population in pregnant women in the United States. *BMC Infectious Diseases* 2007;**7**:71.

78 Watt-Morse ML, Laife SA, and Hill SA. The natural history of fetal CMV infection as assessed by serial ultrasound and fetal blood sampling. *Prenatal Diagnosis* 1995;**15**:567.

79 Nigro G, Adler S, La Torre R *et al.* Passive immunization during pregnancy for CMV infection. *New England Journal of Medicine* 2005;**353**:1350–1362.

80 Schleiss M. CMV vaccine development. *Current Topics in Microbiology and Immunology* 2008;**325**:361–382.

81 Patrick DM, Dawar M, Cook DA, Krajden M, Ng HC, and Rekart ML. Antenatal seroprevalence of herpes simplex virus type 2 (HSV-2) in Canadian women: HSV-2 prevalence increases throughout the reproductive years. *Sexually Transmitted Diseases* 2001;**28**:424–428.

82 Brown ZA, Wald A, Morrow RA, Selke S, Zeh J, and Corey L. Effect of serologic status and cesarean delivery on transmission rates of herpes simplex virus from mother to infant. *Journal of the American Medical Association* 2003;**289**:203–209.

83 Sheffield JS, Hollier LM, Hill JB, Stuart GS, and Wendel GD. Acyclovir prophylaxis to prevent herpes simplex virus recurrence at delivery: a systematic review. *Obstetrics & Gynecology* 2003;**102**:1396–1403.

84 Alanis M, Villers M, Law T *et al.* Complications of cesarean delivery in the massively obese parturient. *American Journal of Obstetrics & Gynecology* 2010;**203**(3):271–277.

85 Gates S and Anderson E. Wound drainage for cesarean section. *Cochrane Database of Systematic Reviews* 2005;(**1**):CD004549.

86 Goepfert AR, Guinn DA, and Andrews WW. Necrotizing fasciitis after cesarean delivery. *Obstetrics & Gynecology* 1997;**89**:409.

87 Phillips LE, Faro S Martens MG *et al.* Postcesarean microbiology of the high risk patient treated for endometritis. *Current Therapeutic Research* 1987;**42**:1157.

88 American College of Obstetrics and Gynecology Committee Opinion No. 465. *Antimicrobial Prophylaxis for Cesarean Section – Timing of Administration.* Washington, DC: ACOG, 2010.

89 Duff P and Gibbs RS. Pelvic vein thrombophlebitis: diagnostic dilemma and therapeutic challenge. *Obstetrical and Gynecological Survey* 1983;**38**:365.

90 Khalil H, Avruch L, Olivier A *et al.* The natural history of ovarian vein thrombosis on magnetic resonance venography after vaginal delivery. *American Journal of Obstetrics & Gynecology* 2012;**206**(4):356 e1–4. Epub 2012/1/13.

91 Foxman B, D'Arcy H, Gillespie B, Bobo JK, and Schwartz K. Lactation mastitis: occurrence and medical management among 946 breastfeeding women in the United States. *American Journal of Epidemiology* 2002;**155**(2):103–114.

92 Peters F and Flick-Filliés D. Hand disinfection to prevent puerperal mastitis. *Lancet* 1991;**338**(8770):831.

93 Jahanfar S, Ng CJ, and Teng CL. Antibiotics for mastitis in breastfeeding women. *Cochrane Database of Systematic Reviews* 2009;(1):CD005458.

CHAPTER 17

Obstetric anesthesia

Emily J. Baird, Richard C. Month, and Valerie A. Arkoosh

Department of Anesthesiology and Critical Care, Perelman School of Medicine, University of Pennsylvania, Philadelphia, PA, USA

17.1 A brief history of obstetric anesthesia

17.1.1 The first obstetric anesthetics

The first written account of obstetric anesthesia occurred on January 19, 1847; on this date, James Young Simpson, a 36-year-old Professor of Midwifery at the University of Edinburgh, became the first to administer an anesthetic for delivery [1]. Only a short three months and three days after its first public use as an anesthetic, Dr Simpson administered inhaled diethyl ether to a young woman with a deformed pelvis. Later that year, he first demonstrated the utility of chloroform as a general anesthetic and rapidly incorporated it into his obstetric practice.

Reaction to the use of anesthesia for delivery was swift. Many, including Simpson himself, questioned the effect of ether on the delivery process. Shortly after his first administration of labor anesthesia, he wrote, "It will be necessary to ascertain anesthesia's precise effect, both upon the action of the uterus and on the assistant abdominal muscles; its influence, if any, upon the child; whether it has a tendency to hemorrhage or other complications"[2]. This concern for the effect of anesthesia on the delivery process continues to this day.

In addition to these medical concerns there was a philosophical difference as to the nature and function of labor pain. Some, including Simpson, felt that pain was without physiologic value and, therefore, should be counteracted; others felt that all pain served some purpose, and, as such, should not be disrupted. Explanations for the utility of labor pain ranged from normal physiology to biblical fiat [3]:

> Unto the woman he said, "I will greatly multiply thy sorrow and thy conception; in sorrow thou shalt bring forth children..." Genesis 3:16

Management of Labor and Delivery, Second Edition. Edited by George A. Macones.

Ultimately, the demands of patients for painless childbirth led to the widespread adoption of labor analgesia. The first American woman to receive anesthesia for delivery was Fanny Longfellow, the wife of Henry Wadsworth Longfellow; she described ether for childbirth as "... certainly the greatest blessing of this age"[4]. But it was the administration of ether to Queen Victoria by John Snow for the birth of her last two children (Prince Leopold in 1853 and Princess Beatrice in 1857) that brought the administration of ether for delivery into the mainstream [5]. The process remained more or less unchanged for approximately 50 years.

17.1.2 New anesthetics for labor

The concept of *Dämmerschlaff*, or "twilight sleep," was introduced to obstetrics in the early 1900s. As popularized by Gauss, it involved intravenous opioids and scopolamine to provide amnesia and relative comfort during labor [6]. Analogous to the introduction of ether half a century earlier, physicians were initially resistant to intravenous analgesia for labor. In response to the incessant demands of uncomfortable patients, twilight sleep was used with increasing frequency over the first half of the 20th century. Unfortunately, this new form of obstetric anesthesia was not without risk. While Gauss and his contemporaries recommended relatively conservative doses of narcotics (no more than 10 mg subcutaneous morphine for the entire labor), others changed the technique. Use of increased amounts of opioids (as high as 50 mg) and the administration of additional agents (such as barbiturates or inhaled agents) preceded reports suggestive of adverse neonatal outcomes [7]. These reports influenced the work of Virginia Apgar. Dr Apgar, as Director of Anesthesia at Columbia University, published her simple, reliable system for evaluating neonates in 1953 [8]. For the first time, subjective and non-standardized descriptions of neonatal outcomes were replaced with a sensitive, reproducible, numerical score. The Apgar score played a large part in making the condition of the child the new standard for evaluating obstetric management.

In parallel with the advent of twilight sleep was the growth of regional anesthesia. The first papers describing the obstetric use of spinal, lumbar epidural, and caudal anesthesia for labor appeared between 1900 and 1930; however, due to a relative lack of drugs and methods of administration, its popularity remained relatively low [9]. With the introduction of a small malleable needle that remained in the sacral canal throughout labor, the use of regional anesthesia grew in the 1940s [10]. Small, flexible plastic catheters eventually replaced needles, making epidurals even more popular, and obstetricians began using them more frequently and earlier in labor. The modern era of labor analgesia heralds a clear understanding of the difference between anesthesia and labor analgesia, with a corresponding reduction in dose of local anesthetic and addition of adjunct medications like opioids that provide analgesia without maternal motor blockade. The spinal route of administration is increasingly popular. Research continues to seek the ideal balance between pain relief, maternal and neonatal safety, and obstetric outcome.

17.2 Anesthetic implications of the physiology of labor and delivery

Pregnancy, labor, and delivery have profound effects on maternal physiology, a number of which effects have direct implications on the anesthetic care of these patients.

17.2.1 Endotracheal intubation considerations

Difficult intubation in the general operative population has ranged between 1:2230 and 1:22,000, while in the obstetric population, the rate of difficult intubation is reported at 1:180 [11–13]. Vascular engorgement and decreases in intravascular colloid oncotic pressure lead to oropharyngeal and tracheal edema. The decrease in airway diameter, coupled with friable mucous membranes, impede laryngeal visualization and endotracheal intubation [14].

Changes in oxygen consumption and pulmonary mechanics also contribute to the challenge in managing a parturient's airway. Oxygen consumption increases 33% over baseline at term, and functional residual capacity decreases by 20% [15]. The combination of these changes leads to an increase in the rate of arterial oxygen desaturation during periods of apnea. The time to 90% desaturation decreases from nine minutes in a non-pregnant, healthy female to two minutes at term gestation. Controlled ventilation of the term parturient must consider the 25% reduction in $PaCO_2$ noted in the term parturient. Progesterone-induced stimulation in respiration leads to a respiratory acidosis with metabolic compensation. Ventilation with standard endpoints (end-tidal CO_2 of 35–40 mmHg) may lead to respiratory acidosis.

Aspiration of gastric contents is a concern at term. The gravid uterus creates a functional hiatal hernia by displacing the lower esophageal sphincter, while progesterone leads to relaxation of the lower esophageal sphincter. Gastric volume is increased at term, especially during labor, due to decreased peristalsis. For these reasons, the American Society of Anesthesiologists recommends all patients at risk for endotracheal intubation receive a nonparticulate antacid, prokinetic agent (metoclopramide), and/or H2 blocker [16].

17.2.2 Hemodynamic considerations

Maternal hemodynamic parameters change profoundly during pregnancy, labor, and delivery. Cardiac output increases by 50% at term and then continues to increase to a maximum 100% over baseline through labor and delivery. The immediate postpartum period is characterized by an increase of 150% over non-pregnant values. Normalization of cardiac output occurs by two weeks postpartum. While generally well tolerated in parturients, this increase in cardiac output can be problematic in patients with preexisting cardiac disease.

Several cardiovascular adaptations prepare the parturient for the inevitable blood loss occurring with delivery. Total blood volume increases by approximately 45–50% at term, with a 55% increase in plasma volume and a 30% increase in red cell mass [17]. This functional hemodilution leads to less red cell loss per unit volume during periods of bleeding. Vascular capacitance is decreased at delivery by the volume of the intervillous space (500 mL or more); this blood does not need to be replaced to maintain postpartum intravascular volume [18]. Contraction of the gravid uterus, necessary for hemostasis, results in autotransfusion of approximately 750 mL immediately after delivery. Finally, hemoconcentration begins shortly after delivery, with maternal blood volume decreasing from ~95 mL/kg at term to ~75 mL/kg in the postpartum period [19]. These factors cause blood loss to be well tolerated at term and should be taken into account when evaluating for the need for transfusion.

17.2.3 Musculoskeletal considerations

Musculoskeletal changes during pregnancy can enhance the difficulty of placement of neuraxial anesthesia. With enlargement of the gravid uterus and the resultant anterior displacement of the parturient's center of mass, the lumbar lordosis is enhanced leading to decreased width of the intervertebral spaces [17].

17.3 Pain sensation in pregnancy, labor, and delivery

17.3.1 Physiologic changes leading to elevated pain threshold

Labor is painful. Melzack found that > 50% of women described labor pain as severe (using descriptors such as "excruciating" and "unbearable"), with only traumatic amputation of a finger and complex regional pain syndrome found to be more painful than childbirth! [20]. Notwithstanding, there are a number of maternal adaptations that decrease the pain of labor. Women experience an elevation in pain threshold at term and during labor; the mechanism of this is unclear, but may be related to progesterone (which has analgesic and sedative properties) and endogenous opioids (endorphins and enkephalins) [21,22]. Also, changes related to nerve tissue sensitivity beginning early in pregnancy decrease neural pain transmission and increase nerve sensitivity to local anesthetics [23].

These physiologic changes lead to an overall decrease in the anesthetic requirements for the term parturient. Volatile anesthetic requirements fall by 40% at term, as does the dose of most induction agents (with the notable exception of propofol, for which the induction dose does not change) [24–26]. Neuraxial local anesthetic requirements are reduced and duration is longer in the term parturient compared to non-pregnant controls. Specifically, intrathecal local anesthetic requirements fall by approximately 25%, while epidural blockade spread increases by nearly 20% at term [27,28].

17.3.2 Pain pathways in labor

Pain transmission in labor falls into two distinct categories: early and late labor pain. The character, path, and location of pain vary starkly during these two periods.

Early labor pain (primarily during the early first stage of labor) results almost entirely from cervical dilation, as there are few sensory nerves in the uterine fundus at term. Sensory nerves pass from the cervix and lower uterine segment through the paracervical plexus and hypogastric nerve. From there they travel with the lumbar sympathetic chain and synapse in the dorsal horn of spinal levels T10–L1 [29]. These C-fibers are comparatively narrow, unmyelinated, and conduct slowly; the resultant pain is *visceral, poorly localized* pain, *referred* from the cervix to the lower abdomen and pelvis.

Late labor pain (late first stage, second stage, and third stage of labor) results from movement of the fetus through the pelvis and vagina. This activates perineal, cervical, and vaginal sensory nerves, which travel in the pudendal nerve and synapse at the S2–S4 spinal levels. These Aδ fibers are comparatively thick, myelinated, and conduct quickly; the resultant pain is *somatic* and *highly localized to the perineum*. Note that early labor pain continues through the late stages of labor; late labor pain *adds* to the pain of early labor, it does not replace it. This implies that ideal labor analgesia would cover pain between T10 and S4.

17.3.3 Pain pathways in cesarean delivery

Cesarean delivery involves a much wider spread of sensory innervation than labor and vaginal delivery. While somatic sensation of the skin, pelvic organs, and pelvic floor synapses at the same lumbosacral levels as does labor pain, visceral innervation of the abdominal and pelvic organs can travel with the sympathetic chain and synapse as high as the T5 level. Therefore, the anesthetic goal for cesarean delivery should be a sensory block extending from the T4 level (the nipple line) through the sacrum.

As the diaphragm has both sensory and motor innervation via the vagus nerve (C3–C5), surgical manipulation of the underside of the diaphragm may result in maternal discomfort, nausea, vomiting, or hiccups, despite a T4 sensory level [30]. Opioids, either systemic or neuraxial, help alleviate these symptoms.

17.4 Management of pain in labor and delivery

The management of labor pain can be divided into non-pharmacologic and pharmacologic methods.

17.4.1 Non-pharmacologic methods

Non-pharmacologic methods, which may reduce but not completely relieve labor pain, include continuous labor support by a trained layperson, massage, bathing during active labor, hypnosis, intradermal water injection, transcutaneous electrical nerve stimulation (TENS), and acupuncture. Most of these methods have not been tested in rigorous scientific trials; thus, it is hard to comment on the efficacy of various approaches. Small trials of acupuncture and hypnosis have shown some benefit [31]. There is insufficient evidence to determine whether or not biofeedback, sterile water injection, aromatherapy, or TENS are more effective than placebo or other forms of labor analgesia [32]. Nonetheless, these methods have few if any adverse side effects and the individual patient may find any of these methods beneficial. These methods may be especially useful for patients with a contraindication to pharmacologic methods of pain relief.

17.4.2 Pharmacologic methods

A variety of pharmacologic methods are used to provide labor analgesia. These methods can be categorized by route of delivery: either systemic or neuraxial.

17.4.2.1 Systemic labor analgesia

Options for systemic analgesia during the first stage of labor include intravenous opioid agonist-antagonists (e.g. butorphanol or nalbuphine), or pure opioid agonists (e.g. meperidine, fentanyl, remifentanil, hydromorhpine, or morphine). Parenteral opioids can be given intermittently or by patient-controlled devices. Additionally, though rarely available in the United States, inhalation analgesia can be produced by a combination of nitrous oxide and oxygen (Entonox®, BOC Healthcare, United Kingdom).

A recent Cochrane review analyzed 57 randomized controlled trials involving more than 7000 women that compared intramuscular or intravenous opioids, including patient-controlled analgesia. The authors included in their analysis studies that compared one opioid with another opioid or placebo, or a non-pharmacological intervention (TENS), or inhaled analgesia. Overall, the evidence was of poor quality with small sample sizes and low statistical power. Parenteral opioids provided some pain relief and moderate satisfaction with analgesia in labor, although up to two-thirds of women who received opioids reported moderate or severe pain and/or poor or moderate pain relief one or two hours after administration. Opioid medications were associated with maternal nausea, vomiting, and drowsiness. There was no clear evidence of adverse effects on the newborn. There was insufficient evidence to assess which opioid drug provides the best pain relief with the least adverse effects or the highest maternal satisfaction [33]. There is some evidence, however, that compared with other opioids women receiving meperidine experienced more drowsiness and nausea [32].

Table 17.1 Systemic opioids commonly used for labor pain relief.

Opioid	Common intermittent dose	Suggested PCA dose
Meperidine	IV: 25–50 mg/1–2 h	50 mg loading dose, 5 mg bolus, 10 min lockout interval Total dose limit 200 mg
Fentanyl	IV: 50–100 mcg/h	50 mcg loading dose, 20 mcg bolus, 5 min lockout interval Dose limit 240 mcg/h
Remifentanil	N/A	40 mcg loading dose, 40 mcg bolus, 2 min lockout interval Dose limit 1200 mcg/h
Nalbuphine	IV: 10 mg/3 h	N/A
Butorphanol	IV: 1–2 mg/2–4 h	N/A

Source: Anderson D. A review of systemic opioids commonly used for labor pain relief. *Journal of Midwifery & Women's Health* 2011;56:222–239. Reproduced with permission of Elsevier.

Despite lack of efficacy and the side-effect profile, patient preference or the presence of a contraindication to a neuraxial technique may necessitate the use of parenteral opioids. Doses for several commonly used opioids are listed in Table 17.1. Patient-controlled analgesia (PCA) is an increasingly popular method for delivering systemic opioids during labor. A recent randomized trial compared the analgesic efficacy of remifentanil with meperidine and fentanyl (n = 54) using PCA. Pain scores decreased in all groups but remained above 4.5 cm (10-cm scale). Remifentanil was associated with the greatest decrease in pain score but this was significant only at 1 hour. Three hours after the initiation of treatment pain scores no longer differed significantly from baseline values in any group. Significantly more parturients receiving meperidine crossed over to epidural analgesia. Overall satisfaction scores were highest with remifentanil but women receiving remifentanil had significantly more sedation and pruritus. Women receiving remifentanil or fentanyl had more observed periods of desaturation ($SaO2 < 95\%$). There were no significant differences in fetal outcome among the groups [34].

17.4.2.2 Inhaled analgesia

Inhaled labor analgesia involves the self-administration of sub-anesthetic concentrations of inhaled anesthetics. The pharmacologic endpoint is moderate pain relief without compromising wakefulness or protective laryngeal reflexes. In comparative studies, halogenated anesthetics (generally not available for labor analgesia in the United States) provide better pain relief than nitrous oxide in the first stage of labor. Nitrous oxide provides more effective relief than placebo. Halogenated agents result in more drowsiness compared with nitrous oxide; however, the side effects of nitrous oxide include nausea, vomiting, dizziness, and drowsiness [35].

Where available, these medications are an acceptable choice for women who do not want, or have a contraindication to, other systemic or neuraxial medications.

17.4.2.3 Neuraxial labor analgesia

Modern neuraxial labor analgesia is typically administered using an epidural, combined spinal epidural (CSE), or continuous spinal technique. In the absence of a contraindication, neuraxial labor analgesia is initiated at maternal request. In 2008, the American College of Obstetricians and Gynecologists and the American Society of Anesthesiologists reaffirmed their 2004 joint opinion, saying:

> Labor causes severe pain for many women. There is no other circumstance where it is considered acceptable for an individual to experience untreated severe pain, amenable to safe intervention, while under a physician's care. In the absence of a medical contraindication, maternal request is a sufficient medical indication for pain relief during labor. [36]

Supporting this recommendation, a number of recent meta-analyses and randomized controlled trials have concluded that there is no difference in the cesarean delivery rate between women who received epidural analgesia compared with intravenous analgesia [37–42]. Additionally, a large randomized trial comparing early epidural placement (median cervical dilatation 2 cm) versus placement later in labor found no difference in the rate of cesarean delivery[41]. Finally, the use of intrathecal analgesia and the concentration of local anesthetic used in an epidural also do not impact the cesarean delivery rate [39,41,43,44]. Although the concentration of local anesthetic in an epidural does not impact cesarean delivery rate, it can influence the rate of spontaneous vaginal delivery. The Comparative Obstetric Mobile Epidural Trial found significantly lower instrumental vaginal delivery rates in patients who received either low-dose CSE or low-dose epidural techniques compared with the traditional epidural group [43].

17.4.3 Maternal side effects

Neuraxial techniques more effectively manage the pain of labor compared with other techniques but may produce maternal side effects. A recent comprehensive Cochrane review of pain management for women during labor concluded that neuraxial techniques effectively manage labor pain and that women receiving epidural analgesia were more likely to experience hypotension, motor blockade, fever, or urinary retention [32]. A recent meta-analysis found no risk of long-term back pain [45]. Unintentional dural puncture with the 16- or 18-gauge epidural needle results in postdural puncture headache in approximately 65% of women, of which approximately 50% will require epidural blood patch to resolve the headache [46]. Although very rare, serious adverse side effects have been reported following neuraxial analgesia or anesthesia such as respiratory depression from intrathecal opioids, infection (both meningitis and epidural abscess), nerve root damage, and inadvertent intravenous or intrathecal injection of medication intended for the epidural space.

17.4.4 Neonatal outcome

A 2002 systematic review of randomized controlled or high-quality prospective-cohort studies comparing epidural analgesia to systemic opioids during labor found the incidence of a 1-minute Apgar score < 7 and need for neonatal naloxone was significantly higher in the parenteral opioid group. The incidence of fetal heart rate abnormalities, intrapartum meconium, 5-minute Apgar score < 7, low umbilical artery pH, and initiation or maintenance of breastfeeding did not differ between the groups [37].

17.4.5 Fetal heart rate abnormalities

Although epidural analgesia is not associated with an increased incidence of fetal heart rate abnormalities compared with systemic opioids, fetal bradycardia following *intrathecal* opioid injection, typically as part of a CSE technique, has been observed. A 2002 meta-analysis of randomized comparisons of any intrathecal opioid (+/− local anesthetic) with any regimen that did not employ intrathecal opioids found a significant increase in the risk of transient fetal bradycardia. The risk of cesarean delivery due to fetal heart rate abnormalities was no different between the two groups [47]. Proposed theories related to the cause of fetal bradycardia including the following: (1) the rapid onset of analgesia achieved with intrathecal opioids and the corresponding rapid reduction in epinephrine allows the unopposed action of oxytocin and norepinephrine to produce uterine hypertonus and vasoconstriction; (2) reduced maternal blood pressure and cardiac output leads to uteroplacental hypoperfusion; (3) omission of local anesthetic which blocks sympathetic fibers and causes uterine vasodilation; and (4) omission of fluid preload [48]. A case-control study found that lack of fetal head engagement and the presence of variable fetal heart rate decelerations were associated with prolonged fetal heart rate deceleration after intrathecal bupivacaine with fentanyl [49]. Of note, each of the above studies utilized higher doses of intrathecal opioids than are typically used in current practice. Whether or not this dose reduction has changed the incidence of fetal bradycardia is unreported. Nonetheless, there is no evidence of adverse neonatal impact of transient fetal heart rate changes associated with the initiation of labor analgesia.

17.4.6 Maternal fever

Maternal temperature increases in some women who receive epidural labor analgesia without evidence for an infectious cause; this has led to concern that there could be a negative impact on the neonate from fetal exposure to hyperthermia and inflammation. Although an association between epidural analgesia and fever is apparent, causation remains controversial. A recent Cochrane meta-analysis of studies comparing epidural analgesia with parenteral or no analgesia found that epidural analgesia was associated with an increase in maternal fever during labor [45]. A prospective study of 81 women undergoing induction of labor found a significant linear trend of temperature over time that correlated with significantly longer time from rupture of membranes to delivery and a higher body mass index. Epidural analgesia had no effect on the temperature trend [50]. Although causation is not proven, the potentially serious consequences of fever during labor are prompting a number of investigations into possible etiologies as well as preventive therapies. The mechanism(s) by which epidural analgesia may produce maternal hyperthermia during labor remains unclear but many studies find evidence of maternal inflammation mediated through increased levels of pro-inflammatory cytokines. The interested reader is referred to two excellent reviews of the topic [51,52].

17.4.7 Breastfeeding

Following concern that epidural fentanyl during labor may negatively impact breastfeeding, Wilson *et al.* compared breastfeeding initiation and duration in approximately 1400 nulliparous women randomized to either epidural with only local anesthesia, CSE initiated with intrathecal fentanyl, epidural with low-dose fentanyl infusion, or no neuraxial analgesia. Women were interviewed in the hospital and sent a postal survey at 12 months. At 24–48 hours after delivery there was no difference in initiation of breastfeeding among women in the three epidural groups and the non-epidural group. Closer evaluation of the non-epidural subgroup revealed that women who received intravenous meperidine reported significantly less initiation of breastfeeding compared to all epidural groups ($p = 0.002$). There were no significant differences among the groups at 12 months in the mean duration of breastfeeding. These authors conclude that epidural fentanyl does not impact breastfeeding initiation or mean duration [53].

17.5 Neuraxial techniques

17.5.1 Epidural

Lumbar epidural analgesia is a safe and versatile technique that can be used to provide labor analgesia or surgical anesthesia. Low-concentration local anesthetics, usually with an opioid, are injected into the epidural space with the goal of achieving a T10–L1 sensory block during the first stage of labor. After the initial bolus, subsequent medication is given by continuous infusion or by a patient-controlled epidural pump. An additional volume of medication may be required to achieve adequate sacral analgesia for the second stage of labor.

17.5.2 Combined-spinal epidural

The combined-spinal epidural technique involves injecting the first dose of medication, typically an opioid with or without a small dose of local anesthetic, into the cerebrospinal fluid, followed by insertion of a catheter into the epidural space. This technique offers the advantage of rapid onset of analgesia, within 1 to 2 minutes of injection of the intrathecal dose, coupled with the ability to extend the duration of the block using the epidural catheter. Because of the rapid onset and low dose of local anesthetic needed to achieve pain relief, CSE can be particularly helpful for the woman in advanced labor requesting analgesia. A recent meta-analysis of CSE versus low-dose epidural analgesia found CSE produced significantly faster onset of effective analgesia and more pruritus. There was no difference in maternal satisfaction, need for rescue analgesia, mobilization in labor, incidence of postdural puncture headache, urinary retention, nausea/vomiting, hypotension, need for labor augmentation, mode of delivery, umbilical pH, Apgar score, or admission to the neonatal intensive care unit [54]. At least two studies suggest that CSE may be associated with more rapid cervical dilation in nulliparous patients compared with traditional epidural analgesia [41,55].

17.5.3 Continuous spinal

The continuous spinal technique involves placement of a catheter into the intrathecal space, allowing for continuous use of spinal opioids and local anesthetics. This significantly decreases maternal systemic exposure to these medications and enables the use of a mostly opioid technique to provide labor analgesia, thus minimizing the use of local anesthetics. A continuous intrathecal catheter also enables a rapid conversion to anesthesia for cesarean delivery. This technique is useful for any woman in labor but can be of particular benefit for those with previous spinal surgery, morbid obesity, and certain cardiac co-morbidities (where the ability to very carefully titrate medication increases the likelihood of hemodynamic stability). This technique is currently limited by the lack of small-bore "microcatheters," which were removed from the US market by the Food and Drug Administration (FDA) in the early 1990s after several reports of cauda equina syndrome associated with their use in nonobstetric patients. A subsequent FDA-sanctioned randomized trial found the microcatheter technique to be safe and effective in obstetric patients [56]. Although there are currently no microcatheters available in the United States, the continuous spinal technique can be performed using a standard epidural catheter, and is frequently employed following an unintended dural puncture with an epidural needle. Currently, ongoing clinical trials are testing a new intrathecal catheter design and, if found to be safe and effective, may lead to more frequent use of this technique.

17.5.4 Contraindications to neuraxial techniques

Absolute contraindications to neuraxial techniques include patient refusal, intracranial mass, coagulopathy, infection at the site of needle insertion, and herpes simplex viremia. Use of neuraxial techniques must also be given careful consideration when maternal hemodynamic instability or systemic bacteremia is present. The potential maternal and fetal risks and benefits must be considered in deciding the appropriate timing and mode of analgesia or anesthesia. Initial and ongoing communication among all members of the labor floor team will result in the best outcomes for both mother and neonate.

17.6 Surgical anesthesia for the parturient

17.6.1 Cesarean delivery

The choice of anesthesia for cesarean delivery depends on several factors, including the urgency of the situation, maternal co-morbidities, and maternal preference. In almost all circumstances a neuraxial technique is preferred to general anesthesia. A neuraxial technique has several advantages, including a decreased risk of failed intubation and aspiration of gastric contents, decreased fetal exposure to anesthetic medications, and the ability of the mother to witness the birth of her child.

17.6.2 Neuraxial techniques

Any of the neuraxial techniques described for labor analgesia can be used for cesarean delivery anesthesia. Regardless of which technique is chosen, a long-acting lipid-insoluble opioid such as preservative-free morphine can be administered for postoperative analgesia. Given that a T4 dermatome level is required for adequate maternal comfort, hypotension is an expected side effect of any neuraxial technique. Currently, many centers employ low-dose phenylephrine infusions or intermittent phenylephrine boluses to maintain maternal blood pressure within 20 mmHg of baseline. A systematic review of seven randomized controlled trials comparing the efficacy and safety of ephedrine with phenylephrine for the prevention and treatment of hypotension during spinal anesthesia for cesarean delivery found that although there was no difference between the two medications for the prevention or treatment of hypotension, women given phenylephrine had neonates with higher umbilical arterial pH values and less negative arterial base excess. The risk of fetal acidosis, defined as $pH < 7.20$, was similar between the two groups [57].

Spinal anesthesia has some advantages for cesarean delivery, including rapid onset, a dense block, and a low failure rate. Unfortunately, this technique is limited by a finite duration of action, thus, it is not an optimal choice if a prolonged surgical time is anticipated. In contrast, epidural anesthesia can provide a nearly unlimited duration of anesthesia. In the parturient with a functioning *labor* epidural *in situ*, administration of a higher concentration of local anesthesia can lead to the achievement of surgical anesthesia within 5 minutes. However, producing surgical levels of anesthesia with a newly placed epidural can take as long as 25 to 30 minutes. In a meta-analysis of 10 trials comparing spinal versus epidural anesthesia for cesarean section, no difference was found between the techniques in failure rate, need for additional intraoperative analgesia, need for conversion to general anesthesia, maternal satisfaction, need for postoperative pain relief, or neonatal intervention. Women with spinal anesthesia had a quicker time from the start of the anesthetic to the start of the surgery and an increased need for treatment of hypotension [58].

Despite a strong preference for neuraxial techniques for cesarean delivery, certain clinical situations require general anesthesia. As discussed previously, a number of physiologic changes of pregnancy enhance the risk of general anesthesia, including risk of difficult intubation, risk of gastric aspiration, increased oxygen demand, and decreased oxygen reserve. The case fatality risk ratio for general compared with neuraxial anesthesia between 1985 and 1990 was 16.7. The majority of the deaths attributed to general anesthesia were related to airway management issues and respiratory events [59]. Although the incidence of failed intubation in parturients, about 1 in 275 women, has remained fairly constant, awareness of these risks has prompted development of failed intubation algorithms, new airway devices, and practice of airway rescue techniques on labor units. Implementation of these collective processes has reduced maternal risk at induction of general anesthesia [60]. Between 1997 and 2002 the case fatality risk ratio decreased to 1.7 and there was no statistical difference between general anesthesia and neuraxial techniques ($p = 0.2$) [61]. Of note, recent data suggest that maternal deaths related to anesthesia are now occurring at emergence of anesthesia and in the early postpartum period related to hypoventilation and airway obstruction [62,63]. Thus, in addition to ongoing efforts to improve the quality of care in obstetric post-anesthesia care units, frequent communication between obstetric and anesthesia providers with the goal of avoiding general anesthesia whenever possible continues to be recommended.

17.6.3 Infiltration block

On rare occasions, such as inability to intubate, contraindication to neuraxial anesthesia, and/or extreme maternal instability, local anesthetic infiltration may provide the safest anesthetic for emergent cesarean delivery. Originally described in 1975 [64], a more recent case report describes the technique for cesarean delivery in a 150-kg patient with fetal demise [65]. The technique involves sequential injection of tissue layers using large volumes of low-concentration lidocaine (0.5% or 1%) with epinephrine. The total dose administered must remain below 5–7 mg/kg of lidocaine, or toxicity may manifest.

17.7 Non-delivery surgical anesthesia for the parturient

17.7.1 Maternal considerations

Maternal implications of antepartum and immediate postpartum surgery are similar to those for cesarean delivery with some minor exceptions. Surgery during early pregnancy (<20 weeks of gestation) may be associated with a smaller likelihood of airway edema and thus less chance of difficult airway. Likewise, early pregnancy may be associated with less abdominal displacement and therefore less chance of gastric aspiration; however, this decrease is negated (and possibly reversed) by intra-abdominal inflammation (such as caused by appendicitis or cholecystitis). Otherwise, the physiologic alterations of pregnancy discussed above should be taken into account. All patients undergoing anesthesia (general or neuraxial) require application of standard monitors (blood pressure, pulse oximeter, electrocardiogram, and temperature probe). Left uterine displacement should be maintained after 20 weeks of gestation.

17.7.2 Fetal considerations

The major fetal concerns regarding anesthesia typically involve teratogenicity and direct fetal effects. Risk versus benefit should always be taken into account when considering any anesthetic during pregnancy.

17.7.2.1 Teratogenicity

17.7.2.1.1 Systemic anesthetic agents

Early studies implicated many commonly used neurologically active agents, including opioids, in teratogenesis [66]. Further testing in animals and humans has not been able to replicate these results and, in fact, strongly suggests that opioids, in clinically relevant doses, are not teratogenic [67,68]. Sedative/anxiolytic drugs, specifically barbiturates and benzodiazepines, have been implicated in teratogenicity in animal models [69,70]; however, this has not been replicated in humans at clinically relevant doses [71]. Finally, common induction agents, including propofol, thiopental, and ketamine, have been deemed pro-neuroapoptotic in the developing brain in rodent models [72]. The degree to which this translates to human development is still unclear.

17.7.2.1.2 Inhalation anesthetic agents

The role of volatile anesthetics in neurodegeneration of the developing brain has been debated extensively [73]. In addition to direct neurodegeneration and neuroapoptosis in animal models, recent data in humans show a correlation between in utero or early childhood exposure to general anesthesia and various neurodevelopmental and behavioral problems [74,75]. The extent to which these changes are directly attributable to general anesthesia is controversial.

17.7.2.1.3 Local and regional anesthetic agents

Many local anesthetics have been shown to be directly neurotoxic in doses several-fold higher than the therapeutic window [76]. However, subsequent study has not duplicated these results at clinically relevant concentrations [77]. In addition, local anesthetic administered in the epidural or subarachnoid space equilibrates so minimally with the intravascular space that maternal blood levels remain only a small fraction of the safe level during treatment. As such, local anesthetic agents are generally considered not to be teratogenic.

17.7.3 Direct fetal effects of anesthetic agents

The fetus is separated from the maternal circulation by a lipid bilayer, in much the same way as the brain is separated from the peripheral circulation (i.e. the blood-brain barrier). As such, most anesthetic agents cross the placenta and have direct fetal effects. Typically, this is noted during continuous fetal monitoring; during opioid-induced fetal sleep, the fetal heart tracing will show a decrease in baseline (not typically below 110) and a reduction in variability and accelerations. These changes should be considered iatrogenic, as they will resolve after discontinuation of the anesthetic.

Of note, drugs that are highly charged (such as succinylcholine, nondepolarizing muscle relaxants, glycopyrrolate, and neostigmine) and drugs with molecular weight over 1000 Daltons (heparins, including low-molecular-weight heparins) do not typically cross the placenta in appreciable amounts. Exceptions to this include vancomycin (molecular weight 1449 Daltons) and ampicillin (positively charged), both of which cross the placenta readily. Also, highly lipophilic drugs, such as fentanyl and sufentanil, may bind to lipids in the placental membrane itself, decreasing total transfer to the fetus.

17.7.4 Cervical cerclage

Adequate sensory anesthesia for transvaginal cervical cerclage requires blockade of sensory nerves from both the cervix (T10–L1) and vagina and perineum (S2–S4). Typically this can be achieved with neuraxial anesthesia; both spinal and epidural anesthesia have been used for cerclage placement, with spinal anesthesia providing the most reliable and rapid onset of anesthesia. Few studies have compared outcomes for patients receiving general versus neuraxial anesthesia for cervical cerclage. One retrospective analysis of 489 procedures found no difference in fetal outcomes between the two techniques [78].

Maternal or fetal indications may dictate the use of general anesthesia for cerclage placement. In the setting of bulging uterine membranes, volatile anesthetics can provide uterine relaxation to allow for their reduction. With general anesthesia, airway management depends on maternal co-morbidities and gestational age. Parturients beyond 20 weeks of gestation are typically considered to have a full stomach and require rapid sequence induction and endotracheal intubation, while parturients prior to this gestational age may be safely managed with a laryngeal mask airway.

Transvaginal cerclage removal can usually be done without anesthesia. However, anesthesia similar to that required for placement is sometimes required depending on the patient and the initial procedure (i.e. Shirodkar cerclage).

17.7.5 Dilation and evacuation

Anesthetic management for dilation and curettage (D&C) or dilation and evacuation (D&E) varies widely, depending on patient co-morbidities, procedure timing, and patient expectations. Intravenous conscious sedation is usually sufficient for a first trimester D&C. This can be achieved with intravenous opioids (morphine, meperidine), benzodiazepines (midazolam, lorazepam), or other agents (propofol, ketamine) titrated to patient comfort. Prior to 20 weeks of gestation, full stomach is usually not a concern and strict maintenance of airway reflexes is not imperative.

Sedation is usually insufficient for second trimester D&E; as such, regional or general anesthesia is often utilized. For general anesthesia, method of induction and airway control depends on gestational age and aspiration risk. Most patients beyond 20 weeks of gestational age will require rapid sequence induction and endotracheal intubation for D&E. Those at earlier gestational ages may be safely and successfully managed with a laryngeal mask airway. Uterine relaxation, if required, can be provided with increased doses of volatile anesthetic [79].

Regional anesthesia, administered via the epidural or spinal routes, should reach a dermatome level of T10 or higher for adequate patient comfort. Concomitant administration of intravenous opioid analgesics or anxiolytics may contribute to patient comfort and satisfaction. Care must be exercised in the case of intrauterine fetal demise, as this may be associated with disseminated intravascular coagulation (DIC) and increased risk of epidural hematoma.

17.7.6 Retained placenta

Retained placenta complicates as many as 3.3% of deliveries, often resulting in postpartum hemorrhage [80]. Manual extraction of the retained placenta or formal D&E is often required in these cases. Anesthetic management of these procedures depends highly on maternal hemodynamic status, degree of hemorrhage, and surgical requirements.

Intravenous conscious sedation, with ketamine, fentanyl, propofol, and/or midazolam, may be sufficient to provide anesthesia for a minor procedure, such as vaginal examination and rapid placental extraction. In this case, care must be taken to ensure maintenance of protective airway reflexes to avoid pulmonary aspiration.

Regional anesthesia should be strongly considered for patients who are hemodynamically stable. This may be administered through an *in situ* epidural catheter, or spinal anesthesia may be administered de novo. The goal of either technique is a sensory level to at least T10. Uterine relaxation to facilitate placental extraction can be achieved with small doses of nitroglycerine. Nitroglycerine, with a half-life of 1 to 3 minutes, provides rapid and reliable uterine relaxation through release of nitric oxide [81]. Intravenous bolus doses of 50–200 mcg and sublingual doses of 1 mg of nitroglycerine have successfully been used for placental extraction [82,83]. Since neuraxial anesthesia causes near maximal dilation of the capacitance veins of the lower extremities, nitroglycerine does not have clinically significant hemodynamic effects [83].

General anesthesia may be considered for patients who are hemodynamically unstable or who need more profound uterine relaxation for extraction of the retained placenta. Uterine relaxation may be assisted with high-dose volatile anesthetic; all volatile anesthetics in current clinical use cause a dose-dependent decrease in uterine tone. In these cases, large volume fluid resuscitation, including blood resuscitation, may be needed as well as uterotonics following removal of the placenta.

17.7.7 Postpartum tubal ligation

More than 350,000 women undergo postpartum tubal ligations (PPTL) annually in the United States, accounting for half of US tubal ligations each year [84]. Anesthesia for PPTL can be achieved in several different ways. The majority of tubal ligations worldwide are performed under local anesthesia with sedation [85]. The technique, described by Cruikshank, involves intravenous sedation followed by subcutaneous lidocaine for skin incision and large-volume (80 mL of 0.5% solution) intraperitoneal lidocaine for anesthesia [86]. All patients in this study reported complete anesthesia and all stated they would have the same procedure again.

In the United States, the majority of PPTL procedures occur under regional anesthesia, either via reactivation of a labor epidural or spinal anesthesia. Regional anesthesia provides more definitive anesthesia than does the local anesthesia technique described above. A sensory T6 level is usually needed to provide sufficient patient comfort for PPTL by minilaparotomy. If the procedure is within 24 hours of delivery, use of an *in situ* labor epidural has an 87% success rate at providing adequate anesthesia; however, after 24 hours, the risk of epidural failure begins to climb [87]. If no labor epidural is present or concern for epidural failure is high, spinal anesthesia is an attractive option, providing a dense, rapid block of short duration.

General anesthesia for PPTL is an option for those women who either refuse or are not candidates for neuraxial anesthesia. Guidelines for induction and maintenance of general anesthesia in the immediate postpartum period are similar to those outlined above for cesarean delivery. Although airway edema and uterine gastric displacement dramatically improve following delivery, the risk of difficult intubation and/or aspiration is still present. As such, rapid sequence induction and endotracheal intubation are still recommended. Anesthetic requirements return to baseline between 12 and 36 hours postpartum; titration to effect is prudent [88,89].

17.7.8 Nonobstetric procedures

Approximately 1 in 500 pregnant women will require nonobstetric surgery during their pregnancy [90,91]. The most common indications for antepartum nonobstetric surgery include trauma, appendicitis (~1 in 1500 pregnancies), bowel obstruction (~1 in 2000 pregnancies), and cholecystitis (~1 in 2000 pregnancies) [90]. If possible, elective surgery should be delayed until after pregnancy and non-elective surgery should be postponed until the second trimester; this is beyond the period of organogenesis and teratogenicity and before the period of highest risk of preterm labor.

Local or regional anesthesia, with minimal fetal drug exposure, is preferred. For intra-abdominal and some emergency procedures, general anesthesia may be the only feasible option. Mechanical ventilation should be adjusted to normocarbia for pregnancy (end-tidal CO_2 between 30 and 34 mmHg). Normotension should be maintained to ensure adequate uteroplacental perfusion. Nitrous oxide use may be considered, as short-term clinical doses of nitrous oxide have not been shown to have a negative effect on the fetus. Systemic anxiolysis and opioids are likely of minimal consequence if delivery of the fetus is not imminent.

17.8 Hypertensive diseases of pregnancy

As hypertension is the most common medical disorder during pregnancy in the United States, it is among the most common problems faced in obstetric anesthesia management. While *gestational hypertension* is usually associated with similar outcomes to normotensive pregnancies and, therefore, does not require specialized intervention, *preeclampsia* and *eclampsia* can be associated with severe alterations in maternal physiology that can affect the administration of anesthesia.

17.8.1 Management of labor anesthesia

It is recommended that all parturients with preeclampsia receive early epidural analgesia. Epidural analgesia provides high-quality analgesia, decreasing circulating catecholamines, and thus the hypertensive response to pain [92]. In addition, neuraxial anesthesia-induced sympathectomy increases intervillous blood flow, especially in patients with severe preeclampsia [93]. Finally, an *in situ* epidural catheter can be extended for urgent cesarean delivery should the need arise, avoiding the administration of general anesthesia.

While the administration of epidural anesthesia does not vary greatly compared to healthy patients, patients with preeclampsia are at risk of thrombocytopenia or coagulopathy due to hepatic involvement, both of which increase the risk of epidural hematoma. Safe platelet ranges for neuraxial anesthesia in pregnancy remain controversial. Although prior consensus opinion suggested a platelet count of greater than 100,000/mm^3 was required for epidural placement, recent reports support the safety of epidural anesthesia in patients with platelet counts as low as 70,000/mm^3 [94,95]. Growing consensus among obstetric anesthesiologists is that the risk of a neuraxial procedure in the parturient increases in the setting of platelet counts $< 50{,}000$/mm^3. Neuraxial anesthesia considered in the setting of a platelet count between 50,000 and 70,000/mm^3 should strongly weigh the risk versus benefit to the patient. It is also important to document, if possible, the *trend* in platelet count. A rapidly falling platelet count makes it difficult to predict the true platelet number at the time of placement of a neuraxial anesthetic. While patients with mild preeclampsia rarely require serial platelet counts, in patients with severe preeclampsia, a platelet count within 6 hours of epidural placement should be obtained. In the event of a falling platelet count, measurements could be as frequent as every 1–3 hours. All patients at risk of coagulopathy (e.g. HELLP syndrome, severe preeclampsia, DIC, fetal demise) should have coagulation studies, including partial thromboplastin time (PTT), prothrombin time (PT), and international normalized ratio (INR), prior to administration of neuraxial anesthesia; a normal or near-normal INR is required for administration of epidural anesthesia [96].

17.8.2 Management of anesthesia for cesarean delivery

Epidural anesthesia has long been considered the optimal technique for cesarean delivery in patients with preeclampsia. It allows for slow titration of anesthesia to avoid major fluctuations in maternal hemodynamics, thus improving uteroplacental blood flow.

Spinal anesthesia in patients with preeclampsia has a history of controversy. Historically, spinal anesthesia was avoided in preeclamptic patients due to the concern for severe hypotension. However, recent investigations dispel this concern; multiple studies have demonstrated no difference in nadir blood pressure between patients receiving epidural versus spinal anesthesia [97,98]. In fact, there is evidence that patients with preeclampsia may actually require less vasopressor and have less reduction in blood pressure after spinal anesthesia than do healthy parturients, though this data remains controversial [99].

General anesthesia raises many concerns for the preeclamptic patient. Airway management, already a concern during pregnancy, is more difficult in preeclampsia due to nondependent edema of the oropharynx and trachea. Small caliber endotracheal tubes and alternative airway devices (such as the laryngeal mask airway) should always be immediately available.

All patients have a hypertensive response to laryngoscopy. However, the response in patients with preeclampsia can be exaggerated, leading to potentially catastrophic increases in blood pressure. A number of short-acting antihypertensives have been shown to successfully attenuate this response, including labetalol, esmolol, sodium nitroprusside, nitroglycerine, and hydralazine [100–102]. The ultra-short-acting opioid remifentanil has had similar success in attenuating hemodynamic response to intubation [103]. No matter the method, the goal is to maintain blood pressure within +/- 20 mmHg of baseline maternal blood pressure in order to reduce maternal risk of intracerebral hemorrhage and to maintain adequate perfusion of the placenta. Invasive arterial blood pressure measurement should be considered, especially for women with severe preeclampsia.

Treatment of hypotension is also complicated by preeclampsia. While mildly preeclamptic women respond normally to vasopressors, there is conflicting data that severely preeclamptic women may have an exaggerated response to phenylephrine, ephedrine, and epinephrine. Judicious use of vasopressors, and avoidance of epinephrine-containing local anesthetic solutions (including epidural test doses), is therefore recommended. As in healthy women, population-level benefit of intravenous fluid preloading in preeclamptic women has not been reliably demonstrated. Because of this, and because of an increased risk of pulmonary edema in preeclampsia, routine prehydration prior to neuraxial blockade is not recommended.

Magnesium therapy presents multiple challenges during general anesthesia. Magnesium inhibits the release of acetylcholine at the neuromuscular junction, decreases sensitivity to acetylcholine, and depresses the excitability of the muscle fiber membrane. As such, patients receiving magnesium therapy may have a prolonged response to nondepolarizing muscle relaxants, sometimes resulting in extended periods of endotracheal intubation [104]. This differs from the depolarizing muscle relaxant succinylcholine, which works by mimicking acetylcholine at the motor end plate. While there is a theoretical decrease in potency and increase in block latency, neither of these effects is clinically significant [105]. Care should be taken when using nondepolarizing muscle relaxants in patients receiving magnesium therapy, with small doses titrated using a peripheral nerve stimulator.

Magnesium causes calcium channel-mediated smooth muscle relaxation of the uterus, leading to the theoretical risk of uterine atony; in fact, Bateman *et al.* found that hypertensive diseases of pregnancy were an independent predictor of uterine atony and postpartum hemorrhage with an odds ratio of 2.5 [106]. As such, patients receiving magnesium who subsequently require a cesarean delivery should have immediate access to uterotonic drugs and an active blood type and antibody screen.

Similarly, since magnesium acts by antagonizing calcium at the calcium channel, synergy has been described between magnesium and calcium channel-blocking drugs. Profound, refractory hypotension has been seen with co-administration of magnesium and both dihydropyridine and nondihydropyridine calcium channel blockers. While safe concomitant use has been described, it is prudent to avoid calcium channel blockade in patients receiving magnesium if alternatives are available [107].

17.8.3 Anesthetic management of the eclamptic patient

Overall, anesthetic management of the eclamptic patient varies little from the management of the preeclamptic patient. Seizure management is primarily symptomatic, and only rarely does an eclamptic seizure necessitate endotracheal intubation. Conscious patients without concern for increase in intracranial pressure may be managed with neuraxial anesthesia. Patients with persistent seizures are at risk for increased intracranial pressure, and anesthetic management should be tailored accordingly.

17.9 Management of obstetric hemorrhage

17.9.1 Introduction

Obstetric hemorrhage remains the leading cause of maternal death and severe morbidity worldwide [108–110]. Although obstetric hemorrhage may occur during the antepartum period, more than 80% of cases develop postpartum [111]. Failure of the uterus to contract following separation and expulsion of the placenta can lead to considerable bleeding as blood flow to the uterine spiral arteries is between 600 and 800 mL/min at term. Successful management of obstetric hemorrhage requires an appreciation of potential risk factors for bleeding, early recognition of bleeding, and aggressive treatment.

17.9.2 Causes of obstetric hemorrhage

Uterine atony is the most common cause of postpartum bleeding, accounting for 79% of obstetric hemorrhage [106]. It is more likely to occur in the presence of one or more of the following: grand multiparity; uterine distention from multiple gestations, polyhydramnios, or fetal macrosomia; abnormal placentation including placenta previa, placenta accreta, or placental abruption; chorioamnionitis; induced or prolonged labor; and/or retained placenta.

While pregnancy is normally characterized as a hypercoagulable state, with an increase in activity of many coagulation factors (VII, VIII, IX, X, XII, von Willebrand factor, and fibrinogen) and a decrease in activity of anticoagulant protein S, inherited or acquired coagulation disorders can disrupt these protective pro-hemostatic changes. Parturients with hereditary hematologic disorders, most frequently including von Willebrand disease, hemophilia, and platelet disorders, are at an increased risk of significant obstetric bleeding. In addition, pregnancy-related conditions, including preeclampsia, placental abruption, intrauterine fetal demise, and amniotic fluid embolism, have been implicated in the development of a coagulopathy.

Finally, operative or instrumented delivery, which occurs more commonly in the setting of obesity, preeclampsia, cardiac disease, abnormal placentation, and chorioamnionitis, is also associated with increased blood loss. Although there are several risk factors for hemorrhage, the majority of women with excessive obstetric bleeding do not have identifiable predictors [106]. Therefore, all parturients should be considered at risk of obstetric hemorrhage, and extreme vigilance must be exercised in the assessment of blood loss during and after delivery.

17.9.3 Diagnosis of obstetric hemorrhage

The timely diagnosis of an obstetric hemorrhage can be challenging. Visual assessment of blood loss is complicated by the presence of amniotic fluid contributing to the volume of fluid measured at delivery. In addition, blood loss concealed in surgical drapes and sponges is often unaccounted [112]. Hemodynamic parameters prove similarly unhelpful as most pregnant women tolerate excessive blood loss with limited perturbations in blood pressure and heart rate. Peripheral and splanchnic vasoconstriction facilitates the relocation of blood from venous capacitance vessels to the central circulation, allowing the blood pressure to remain near normal until blood loss exceeds 1500 mL in most parturients. Laboratory evaluation is generally too slow to meaningfully reflect the dynamic changes in hemoglobin and coagulation status occurring during an obstetric hemorrhage. Given the challenges in the accurate assessment of blood loss during delivery, extreme vigilance is necessary to ensure the early recognition and treatment of obstetric hemorrhage.

17.9.4 Treatment of obstetric hemorrhage

17.9.4.1 Crystalloid

There is no consensus on the optimal resuscitation of obstetric bleeding. Maintenance of circulating blood volume is necessary to prevent tissue and organ hypoperfusion. Rapid restoration of intravascular volume is generally initiated with the use of warmed, non-dextrose-containing crystalloid, administered in a ratio of 3:1 in relation to estimated blood loss. Given that infusion of large volumes of fluid can lead to dilutional acidosis, interstitial edema, and impairment of microcirculation, synthetic colloid solutions (e.g. hydroxyethyl starch) should be considered early in resuscitation efforts. Although synthetic colloids are effective in timely restoration of circulating volume, there have been some reports that large infusions can lead to impaired clot formation and increased blood loss [113,114]. To avoid undesirable side effects of excessive synthetic colloid infusions, administration of hydroxyethyl starch solutions should be limited to 30 mL/kg.

17.9.4.2 Red blood cells

Prolonged resuscitation with crystalloid or other volume expanders is not recommended and transfusion of red blood cells (RBCs) should be considered early in resuscitation efforts. Although crystalloid can restore intravascular volume, RBCs are needed to insure adequate oxygen-carrying capacity of blood and avoid acidosis. The transfusion of one unit of RBCs is expected to increase hemoglobin (Hb) by 1 g/dL, or hematocrit (Hct) by 3–5%. Data from clinical trials to guide management of RBC transfusion in obstetric hemorrhage is lacking and suggested guidelines for other surgical situations are often broad and of questionable transference. The 2006 American Society of Anesthesiologist Practice Guidelines for Perioperative Blood Transfusion states transfusion is usually unnecessary in patients with Hb > 10 g/dL but generally indicated when Hb < 6 g/dL [115]. The specific Hb value at which blood is given should be tailored to the individual patient and based on the coexistence of co-morbidities, cardiovascular parameters, and anticipated additional blood loss. Traditionally, transfusion with RBC in the obstetric setting was centered on maintaining an Hb around 7 g/dL. Many experts now recommend setting the Hb target higher, around 10 g/dL during active bleeding, to improve overall coagulation [116,117].

Coagulation involves the interplay between RBCs, plasma coagulation factors, platelets, and endothelium. Adequate RBC mass is essential in optimizing the interactions between platelets and the vessel wall. As RBC mass decreases, both blood viscosity and resistance to blood flow markedly decreases. As a result, anemia leads to the fast transit of platelets through central luminal flow, reducing the crucial interactions between platelets and endothelial cells mandatory for primary hemostasis. Therefore, transfusion of RBCs can improve not only oxygen-carrying capacity but coagulation, as well.

17.9.4.3 Coagulation factors

An acquired coagulopathy, resulting from dilutional and consumptive effects on clotting factors, frequently complicates obstetric hemorrhage. Rapid volume replacement with crystalloid and RBCs can lead to dilution of plasma coagulation factors and platelets. Critical levels of prothrombin, factor V, factor VII, and platelets are reached after a loss of > 200% calculated blood volume, whereas life-threatening levels of fibrinogen are reached after a loss of only 140% [118]. Rapid bleeding characteristic of obstetric hemorrhage can also lead to the *consumption* of clotting factors, platelets, and fibrinogen. Disseminated intravascular coagulation, characterized by widespread intravascular activation of the coagulation system with loss of localization and control of hemostatic and fibrinolytic processes, often manifests as an early feature in obstetric hemorrhage. Obstetric complications such as amniotic fluid embolism, placental abruption, uterine infection, and intrauterine fetal demise are associated with early-onset and severe DIC [119]. Activation of fibrinolysis in DIC leads to the production of D-dimers and fibrin-degradation products, which interfere with platelet function and can impair myometrial contractility, further contributing to blood loss [111]. Confirmatory laboratory tests, including PT, activated partial thromboplastin time (aPTT), fibrinogen concentration, and platelet counts, are useful in guiding the diagnosis and treatment of coagulopathy in the obstetric setting.

The prompt implementation of pro-hemostatic interventions is crucial in preventing complications from uncontrolled coagulopathy. Normal coagulation is generally maintained if the concentration of coagulation factors remains above 30%. Fresh frozen plasma (FFP) is frequently indicated in the setting of obstetric hemorrhage, with each unit increasing coagulation factor levels by approximately 8% [120]. Although traditional guidelines suggest FFP should be used only in the setting of an elevated PT or aPTT, recent data emerging from the trauma literature endorse more aggressive repletion of coagulation factors. Specifically, resuscitation using an FFP:RBC transfusion ratio of approximately 1:1 was associated with a decrease in blood loss and improved survival in combat-related trauma [121,122]. Although data from the trauma literature are persuasive, caution should be exercised in the wholesale adoption of a high FFP:RBC ratio until efficacy and safety are demonstrated in the obstetric population. Resuscitation should also include prevention and treatment of hypothermia, acidosis, and hypocalcemia, which can impede optimal function of transfused coagulation factors.

Fibrinogen may play a unique role in the diagnosis and management of obstetric hemorrhage. In a recent multivariate analysis, fibrinogen was the only marker associated with the occurrence of severe postpartum hemorrhage, with a 100% positive predictive value when below 200 mg/dL [123]. Hypofibrinogenemia, secondary to dilutional and consumptive coagulopathy, can be difficult to correct with FFP. To increase fibrinogen plasma level by 100 mg/dL, 30 mL/kg of FFP is necessary, increasing the risk of pulmonary edema and other hypervolemic complications [124]. In contrast, 10 pooled units of crypoprecipitate (~100 mL), which contains a concentrated source of fibrinogen, factor VIII, fibrinogen, fibronectin, von Willebrand factor, and factor XIII, will increase fibrinogen levels by approximately 70 mg/dL. Fibrinogen, which is critical not only for clot strength but also in speed of clot initiation and propagation, should be considered early in the course of obstetric hemorrhage. Although standard teaching recommends fibrinogen replacement with levels < 100 mg/dL, a recent in vitro study showed that a fibrinogen level of 200 mg/dL was required to improve clot formation, with optimal clot formation at levels of 250 mg/dL [118].

17.9.4.4 Platelets

In the setting of obstetric hemorrhage, platelet transfusion is indicated when the platelet count is less than $50{,}000/mm^3$. One unit of donor platelets increases the platelet count from 5000 to $10{,}000/mm^3$. Although not required, ABO compatibility increases the lifespan of transfused platelets. In addition, Rh sensitivity can occur in an Rh-negative recipient due to the presence of a few red cells in an Rh-positive unit.

17.9.4.5 Procoagulants

The prevalence and severity of coagulopathy accompanying obstetric hemorrhage has led to interest in additional procoagulant agents including recombinant activated factor VII (rFVIIa) and tranexamic acid (TxA). rFVIIa is a synthetic vitamin K–dependent glycoprotein which aids in hemostasis via activation of the extrinsic pathway of the coagulation cascade. Although currently only approved for use in hemophilia, factor VII deficiency, and Glanzmann's thrombasthenia, several groups have explored use of rFVIIa in treatment of obstetric hemorrhage [125–127]. Although all of these studies report significant reduction in bleeding following administration of rFVIIa, caution must be exercised in interpreting these results, which were derived from retrospective, uncontrolled studies. In addition, there is some concern that use of rFVIIa may contribute to subsequent thrombotic complications [128].

With the absence of sufficient efficacy and safety data, rFVIIa should only be considered after failure of conventional therapies, including invasive treatment (such as embolization or conservative surgery), but prior to obstetric hysterectomy. rFVIIa should not be used to compensate for an inadequate blood transfusion therapy, and administration of RBCs, FFP, cryoprecipitate, and platelets is essential in the treatment of severe obstetric hemorrhage. The effectiveness of rFVIIa depends on an optimal hemostatic environment including Hct > 30%, platelet count > 50,000/mm^3, fibrinogen > 100 mg/dL, arterial pH > 7.20, normocalcemia, and temperature > 34°C. The suggested bolus dose of rFVIIa is 60–90 ug/kg and, when effective, an improvement in bleeding is seen within 15 minutes. The half-life of rFVIIA is 2 hours in non-bleeding patients; the dose may be repeated within 30–60 minutes if hemostasis is not achieved [126].

The evidence for use of TxA is even more limited than for use of rFVIIa; however, since fibrinolysis is extremely common in obstetric hemorrhage, TxA could theoretically be very effective. TxA is an antifibrinolytic agent that inhibits the activation of plasminogen into plasmin. A recent prospective randomized trial involving vaginal deliveries complicated by greater than 800 mL blood loss reported a significant decrease in blood loss, bleeding duration, and transfusion requirement in patients receiving TxA [129]. The only adverse effects associated with TxA include transient blurred vision and nausea [129–131]. Despite the lack of clinical evidence, the WHO supports use of TxA in obstetric hemorrhage given the ease of administration, low cost, and absence of major adverse events. Previous studies support a 1–4 g bolus followed by an infusion of 1 g/hr for 6 hours [129].

17.9.5 Intraoperative blood salvage

Given the expense and potential complications associated with transfusion of heterologous blood products, the use of intraoperative blood salvage has recently gained popularity in cardiovascular, trauma, and general surgery. Intraoperative blood salvage involves recycling the patient's scavenged blood, thus reducing transfusion requirements. The technique involves centrifuging, washing, filtering, and returning blood salvaged from the surgical field [132]. Of note, platelets, activated clotting factors, and complement are removed in the processing of the scavenged blood. The resulting autologous blood has a relatively high hematocrit (60–80%) and is similar to regular blood in pH, morphology, osmotic stability, and 2,3-DPG content [133]. Transfusion of autologous blood avoids the risk of alloimmunization, viral transmission, and hemolytic transfusion reactions. In addition, blood obtained from intraoperative salvage likely has higher survival and oxygen-carrying abilities than stored blood.

The use of intraoperative blood salvage has yet to gain widespread acceptance in obstetric hemorrhage because of the theoretical concern of inducing an amniotic fluid embolism (AFE). Studies of blood scavenged and processed during cesarean delivery demonstrate the concentration of alpha-fetoprotein, phospholipids, tissue factor, fetal squamous cells, and other cellular debris is similar to that found in maternal circulation at delivery [134,135]. Given that recent evidence suggests AFE is an anaphylactic reaction, rather than an embolic event, it is unlikely that the use of intraoperative blood salvage increases the risk of AFE [136]. Rebarber *et al.* performed a retrospective, multicenter study of 139 patients in whom autologous blood transfusion was performed during cesarean delivery [137]. The range of autotransfused volumes was between 200 and 11,250 mL and there were no cases of AFE or acute respiratory distress syndrome. Of note, blood salvage techniques do not separate fetal from maternal RBCs. Salvaged blood containing rhesus (Rh)-positive fetal blood could immunize an Rh-negative mother. Therefore, if salvaged blood is given to an Rh-negative mother, an appropriate dose of anti-D immunoglobulin must be administered.

17.10 Anesthetic implications of specific maternal co-morbidities

17.10.1 Cardiovascular disease in pregnancy

The occurrence of cardiac disease in the parturient has steadily increased over the past few decades, with a current estimated prevalence of 0.2–3.0% [138]. Recent advancements in surgical techniques and medical management have allowed children born with congenital heart diseases (CHD) to survive to childbearing age. In addition, developments in reproductive technology have facilitated a cohort of older women, with increased prevalence of *acquired* cardiac valvular and ischemic disorders, to become pregnant. Given the heterogeneity of cardiac lesions encountered in this population, it is difficult to quantify the risk of pregnancy with coexisting cardiovascular disease. In general, maternal outcomes correlate with the functional classification of the parturient as outlined by the New York Heart Association (NYHA) (Table 17.2). Specifically, NYHA class I or II is associated with < 1% maternal mortality; whereas a mortality rate of 6.8% has been reported for parturients with an NYHA class III or IV [139,140]. Successful obstetric and anesthetic management of the parturient with cardiac disease depends on a thorough understanding of the hemodynamic compromise accompanying *specific* cardiac lesions and the interplay with the physiologic changes of pregnancy.

Table 17.2 New York Heart Association functional capacity.

Class I	No limitation of physical activity
Class II	Slight limitation of physical activity
Class III	Marked limitation of physical activity
Class IV	Inability to carry on any physical activity without discomfort

Source: AHA medical/scientific statement. 1994 revisions to classification of functional capacity and objective assessment of patients with diseases of the heart. *Circulation* 1994;90(1): 644. Reproduced with permission of Lippincott Williams & Wilkins.

Table 17.3 Central hemodynamic assessment of normal term pregnancy.

Hemodynamic parameter	Non-pregnant	Pregnant
Cardiac output (L/min)	4.3 +/– 1.0	6.2 +/– 1.0
Heart rate (bpm)	70 +/– 10	83 +/– 10
SVR (dyne.sec.cm)	1530 +/– 520	1210 +/– 226
PVR (dyne.sec.cm)	119 +/– 47	78 +/– 22
MAP (mmHg)	86 +/– 8	90 +/– 6
PCWP (mmHg)	6.3 +/– 2.1	7.5 +/– 1.8
CVP (mmHg)	3.7 +/– 2.6	3.6 +/– 2.5

Source: Clark SL *et al.* Central hemodynamic assessment of normal term pregnancy. *American Journal of Obstetrics & Gynecology* 1989;161: 1449–1444. Adapted with permission of Elsevier.

The principal danger for a pregnant woman with a heart lesion is cardiac decompensation from the additional physiologic demands of pregnancy. Pregnancy is characterized by a progressive cardiopulmonary stress that peaks in the third trimester and dramatic hemodynamic changes occurring with labor and delivery, many of which are discussed earlier in this chapter (see Section 17.2) and are outlined in Table 17.3. These dynamic fluid shifts cause further stress on an already compromised cardiac lesion and may promote dysrhythmias or cardiac failure.

Although discussion of *specific* heart lesions is beyond the scope of this chapter, it is accurate to assume that pregnancies complicated with cardiac disease are at a significantly higher risk of adverse maternal and neonatal outcomes. In a prospective study of over 1000 parturients, maternal complications, defined as pulmonary edema, arrhythmia, stroke, and/or death, occurred in 13% of the pregnancies [141]. Likewise, there was a 20% risk of fetal complications including prematurity, small-for-gestational-age, and death [141]. The risk of cardiac event during parturition is increased in the setting of left heart obstruction and/or dysfunction and/or a history of previous cardiac-related events, including arrhythmia, heart failure, or stroke.

Although care must be individualized to the cardiac lesion and patient condition, certain basic hemodynamic goals are applicable to the anesthetic management of most cases. Maintenance of normal sinus rhythm and avoidance of sudden alterations in heart rate are crucial in the preservation of cardiac output. Although it is important to maintain adequate preload, sudden increases in central blood volume can lead to pulmonary edema in pregnant patients with cardiovascular compromise. In addition, sudden decreases in afterload and systemic vascular resistance can compromise cardiac perfusion, further worsening cardiac function.

Both general and regional anesthesia can have significant cardiovascular effect on a parturient with cardiac disease. General anesthesia is associated with

Table 17.4 Regional anesthesia in the patient receiving antithrombotic or thrombolytic therapy.

Medication	Dose	Minimum time between last anticoagulation dose and neuraxial procedure
Heparin	5000 units SQ q8 hr	No time restriction
	7500 units SQ q8 hr	8 hr
	Continuous IV infusion	aPTT < 40 sec
Enoxaparin	40 mg SQ qday	12 hrs (longer in renal impairment)
(Lovenox®)	40 mg SQ q12 hr	12 hrs (longer in renal impairment)
	1.5 mg/kg SQ qday	24 hrs (longer in renal impairment)
	1.0 mg/kg q12 hr	24 hrs (longer in renal impairment)
Dalteparin	5000 units SQ qday	12 hrs (longer in renal impairment)
(Fragmin®)	100 units/kg SQ q12 hr	24 hrs (longer in renal impairment)
	200 units/kg SQ qday	24 hrs (longer in renal impairment)
Fondaparinux	2.5 mg SQ qday	48 hrs (longer in renal impairment)
(Arixtra®)	5 mg SQ qday	72 hrs (longer in renal impairment)
Aspirin/NSAIDs		No time restriction

Source: Horlocher TT *et al*. Regional anesthesia in the patient receiving antithrombotic or thrombolytic therapy. American Society of Regional Anesthesia and Pain Medicine evidence-based guidelines, 3rd edn. *Regional Anesthesia and Pain Medicine* 2010;35:64–101. Adapted with permission of Elsevier.

sympathetic stimulation caused by laryngoscopy; increased pulmonary vascular resistance and decreased preload resulting from positive pressure ventilation; and decreased cardiac contractility due to inhalation agents. The sympathectomy accompanying regional anesthesia can lead to dramatic decreases in preload and afterload. If a neuraxial technique is deemed the preferred mode of anesthesia, the anticoagulation status of the parturient must be considered. Many women with cardiac disease are treated with anticoagulants to avoid thromboembolism, and the American Society of Regional Anesthesiology guidelines should be considered prior to performing any neuraxial procedure (Table 17.4).

Regardless of the mode of delivery, the American Congress of Obstetricians and Gynecologists and the American Heart Association vehemently discourage the routine use of antibiotics for infective endocarditis prophylaxis during delivery [142,143]. The risk of bacteremia following a normal delivery is exceedingly low (0.5%), with infective endocarditis being much more likely to result from frequent exposure to random bacteremias associated with daily activities than from genitourinary tract procedures. The haphazard use of antibiotics is not without significant risk. Antibiotics may cause maternal allergic reactions and fetal toxicity. In addition, the indiscriminate administration of antibiotics may promote the emergence of bacterial strains that are virulent and resistant to currently available antibiotics. The use of antibiotic prophylaxis for infective endocarditis should be reserved for parturients with a cardiac condition associated with the highest risk

Table 17.5 Prevention of bacterial endocarditis.

High risk: Endocardial prophylaxis *recommended*	Prosthetic cardiac valve History of endocarditis Complex cyanotic CHD Surgically constructed systemic pulmonary shunt
Moderate risk: Endocardial prophylaxis *not* recommended	Acquired valve dysfunction Hypertropic obstructive cardiomyopathy Mitral valve prolapse
Low risk: Endocardial prophylaxis *not* recommended	Atrial septal defect Ventricular septal defect Patent ductus arteriosus History of coronary artery bypass graft History of pacemaker or defibrillator

Source: Dajani AS *et al.* Prevention of bacterial endocarditis. Recommendations by the AHA. *Circulation* 1997;96:358–366. Reproduced with permission of Lippincott Williams & Wilkins.

Table 17.6 Prevention of bacterial endocarditis.

Endocarditis prophylaxis	Ampicillin 2 g IV + Gentamicin 1.5 mg/kg IV
Endocarditis prophylaxis (penicillin allergy)	Vancomycin 1 g IV + Gentamicin 1.5 mg/kg IV

Source: Dajani AS *et al.* Prevention of bacterial endocarditis. Recommendations by the AHA. Circulation 1997;96:358–366. Reproduced with permission of Lippincott Williams & Wilkins.

of adverse outcome (Table 17.5) *and* an established infection that could cause bacteremia, such as chorioamnionitis or pyelonephritis. If these two conditions are met, the underlying infection should be treated in the usual fashion and treatment should include a regimen effective for infective endocarditis prophylaxis (Table 17.6).

17.10.2 Obesity

Obesity is emerging as an international health epidemic with approximately 1.6 billion adults currently classified as overweight or obese [144]. Although the physiologic changes of pregnancy are typically associated with a 10–15-kg weight gain, a parturient is generally considered obese when her BMI is greater than 30 kg/m^2 and morbidly obese if her BMI exceeds 40 kg/m^2 [144]. The prevalence of obesity in pregnancy has doubled in the past 20 years, with incidence now ranging from an alarming 18.5 to 38.3% [145]. Superimposing pregnancy on organ systems already stressed due to the physiologic demands of obesity leads to a substantial increase in both obstetric and anesthetic risk.

Similar to pregnancy, obesity impacts virtually every organ system. Effective management of the obese parturient depends on a thorough understanding of the interplay between the pathophysiologic changes accompanying both conditions. The combination of obesity and pregnancy can lead to significant compromise of the pulmonary system. Increased thoracoabdominal fat deposition, in conjunction with cephalad movement of the diaphragm by the gravid uterus, leads to a substantial reduction in lung volumes. Ventilation-perfusion (V/Q) mismatch follows as reduced functional residual capacity (FRC) leads to airway closure in dependent portions of the lung. Arterial oxygen partial pressure (P_aO_2) is further compromised by the increased oxygen consumption characteristic of both obesity and pregnancy. The increased incidence of obstructive sleep apnea in obese parturients contributes to additional risk of clinically significant desaturations. Hypoxemia resulting from V/Q mismatch, increased oxygen consumption, and obstructive sleep apnea can have significant implications, including systemic hypertension, pulmonary hypertension, arrhythmias, and intrauterine fetal growth restriction.

The cardiovascular system is similarly influenced by the cumulative stresses of obesity and pregnancy. Supine hypotensive syndrome is compounded by abdominal adiposity. Pregnancy and obesity independently increase blood volume, stroke volume, and cardiac output; obesity has been estimated to enhance cardiac output by ~40 mL/min for every 100 g of adipose tissue [146]. High plasma levels of leptin, insulin, and inflammatory mediators, characteristic of obesity, lead to endothelial dysfunction with increased peripheral vascular resistance [147]. Obesity-induced endothelial dysfunction mitigates the afterload reduction typically occurring in pregnancy, resulting in a threefold higher incidence of hypertension in parturients with a BMI exceeding 30 kg/m^2 [148]. Myocardial adaptation to hypertension leads to left ventricle hypertrophy and, in severe cases, dilation and systolic dysfunction. The additive contribution of myocardial hypertrophy, fat deposition in conducting systems, elevated catecholamines, and obstructive sleep apnea have been implicated in the more common occurrence of fatal arrhythmias in obese parturients [149].

Obesity is associated with higher rates of gestational diabetes mellitus, with a rate of 24.5% in obese parturients compared with 2.2% in non-obese controls [150]. Both pregnancy and obesity are insulin-resistant conditions. In addition, obese pregnant women have a higher incidence of preexisting type II diabetes mellitus [149]. Insulin insufficiency during pregnancy can have serious repercussions, including fetal congenital malformations and macrosomia, as well as maternal cardiovascular and renal complications.

The gastrointestinal changes accompanying pregnancy and obesity contribute to an increased risk of gastric regurgitation and pulmonary aspiration. Both conditions are independently associated with elevated intra-abdominal pressure, relaxation of the lower esophageal sphincter, and reduced gastrointestinal motility. The combination of obesity and pregnancy leads to an additional risk of gastric regurgitation, with gastric volume greater than 25 mL and pH less than 2.5 being present in 86% and 88% of obese parturients, respectively [151]. Gastric emptying may be further compromised by autonomic dysfunction accompanying preexisting diabetes mellitus.

Labor is adversely impacted by obesity. Obese women are more likely to progress past term gestation and frequently require induction of labor. Despite increased use of oxytocin and early amniotomy, labor augmentation is associated with a higher failure rate in obese parturients (14.6%) compared with non-obese women (7.9%) [152]. The increased occurrence of fetal macrosomia, cephalopelvic disproportion, and maternal soft tissue dystocia contributes to higher rates of shoulder dystocia (OR 3.6; 95% CI 2.1–6.3) [152]. Unfortunately, maternal body habitus may hinder maneuvers to manage shoulder dystocia, increasing both maternal and fetal complications. Obese parturients are more likely to require both instrumental delivery and cesarean section. The incidence of operative delivery correlates with increases in BMI. Weiss *et al.* reported the rate of cesarean delivery in nulliparous women to be 20.7% for normal weight parturients (BMI 18.5–24.9 kg/m^2), 33.8% for class I obese parturients (BMI 30–34.9 kg/m^2), and 47.4% for class II obese parturients (BMI 35–39.9 kg/m^2) [148]. Obese pregnant women are also at increased risk of complications associated with operative delivery, including postpartum hemorrhage, maternal infection, and wound dehiscence [153].

Because the obese parturient is more likely to require an instrumental or emergent cesarean delivery, adequate labor analgesia should be established early in the course of labor. Neuraxial placement is frequently complicated by inability to palpate anatomic landmarks and limited back flexion. Difficulty in identifying the epidural space leads to an increased occurrence of accidental dural puncture in the obese parturient. Fortunately, higher intra-abdominal pressures are believed to decrease the egress of cerebrospinal fluid, and postdural puncture headaches occur less commonly in obese patients. Additional care are should be exercised in initiating and maintaining a neuraxial block in the obese parturient. Increased epidural fat and engorgement of the epidural veins may decrease the capacity of the epidural and subarachnoid space. If local anesthesia is not cautiously titrated, an unanticipated high block can occur, resulting in both hemodynamic and respiratory compromise.

General anesthesia is typically avoided in the obese parturient. Dramatic reductions in the FRC, in conjunction with increased oxygen consumption, lead to clinically significant oxygen desaturation following even brief periods of apnea. Reduced chest wall compliance and increased intra-abdominal pressure can hinder attempts at mask ventilation. In addition, pregnancy is associated with a greater occurrence of difficult intubation, and obesity compounds this risk. Increased blood volume and elevated estrogen levels lead to capillary engorgement, mucosal edema, and a distorted, friable airway. The anatomy is further compromised by oropharyngeal soft tissue adiposity accompanying obesity. The elevated intra-abdominal pressure, higher gastric volumes, and elevated gastroesophageal junction comprise characteristics of obese parturients that predispose these women to pulmonary aspiration. Given the risk associated with general anesthesia, neuraxial techniques are overwhelmingly preferred for operative deliveries.

17.10.3 Systemic lupus erythematosus

Systemic lupus erythematosus (SLE), with a prevalence of approximately five cases per 10,000 population [154], is the most common collagen vascular disease seen in pregnancy. SLE is a multisystem autoimmune disease with diverse clinical and immunologic manifestations. With a female to male preponderance of 10–15:1 and a mean age of onset of 25 years [155], this chronic inflammatory disease occurs most frequently in women during their childbearing years. The clinical course is highly variable and characterized by relapses and remissions. Exacerbations are precipitated not only by pregnancy but also by circumstances often encountered during parturition, including infection and new medication exposure. Maternal and fetal prognosis is related to severity of disease, with increased morbidity associated with high disease activity, diffuse organ involvement, and lower socioeconomic class.

Although the precise etiology of SLE is unknown, the complex interactions between genetic (HLA B8, DR2, DR3 haplotypes), hormonal (estrogen), immunological, and environmental (viruses, ultraviolet light) factors have been implicated in the initiation and progression of the disease. Clinical manifestations are mediated by antibody formation and/or the deposition of immune complexes. The leading theory on the development of SLE involves impaired clearance of apoptotic cells causing the release of intracellular autoantigens and aberrant sensitization. Genetic defects in immune regulation and/or environmental triggers may further contribute by facilitating proliferation of autoantibody-producing B cells and defective helper and suppressor T cells. Formation and deposition of antibody-antigen immune complexes within specific organs may subsequently activate inflammatory responses causing direct tissue damage. Clinical manifestations are also a result of autoantibodies binding cell surface molecules or serum components, leading to their removal from the circulation [156].

The pervasiveness of autoantibodies and immune complexes in SLE can result in perturbations in virtually every organ system. Clinical manifestations are generally categorized as articular and systemic, with the most common disease pattern consisting of a mixture of constitutional complaints (fatigue, weight loss, fever) combined with musculoskeletal, dermatologic, hematologic, and serologic involvement. SLE is associated with a symmetrical, nonerosive, oligoarticular arthritis involving primarily peripheral joints, most commonly the hands, wrists, elbows, knees, and ankles. The episodic and migratory arthritis manifests as joint tenderness, swelling, and/or effusion. Dermatologic characteristics include a malar rash (erythema over malar eminences), discoid rash (erythematosus raised patches with keratotic scaling), and photosensitivity (skin reaction to sunlight). Common hematological sequelae of SLE consist of hemolytic anemia, thrombocytopenia, and leucopenia. Although mild thrombocytopenia (100,000 – 150,000/μL) can occur in up to 50% of parturients with SLE, platelet counts less than 50,000/μL are noted in less than 10% of patients. Antibodies against specific clotting factors, including factors VIII, IX, XII, and XIII, may further disrupt coagulation. Leucopenia, antibody granulocyte dysfunction, decreased complement levels, and functional asplenia contribute to the increased risk of infections in parturients with SLE.

The potential for serious SLE complications increases with involvement of the cardiac, pulmonary, renal, and/or central nervous systems. Cardiac abnormalities, including valvular disorders, conduction anomalies, pericarditis, and pericardial effusions, occur in 50% of patients with SLE, and 25% will have significant cardiovascular complications [157,158]. Furthermore, SLE-mediated coronary artery vasculitis and accelerated atherosclerosis contribute to an increased risk of myocardial ischemia and infarction. Pulmonary manifestations commonly include pleuritis, interstitial pneumonitis, and pulmonary hypertension. Pulmonary function tests frequently demonstrate a restrictive pattern with decreased diffusion capacity. The most worrisome pulmonary complication, pulmonary angiitis with lung hemorrhage, complicates only 2% of SLE cases [159]. SLE glomerulonephritis, characterized by proteinuria, hypertension, and decreased creatinine clearance, progresses to end-stage renal disease in 10–20% of cases. Neurologic and psychiatric impairment occurs in 50% of patients with SLE, with the most serious complications including stroke, seizures, and peripheral neuropathies.

SLE is associated with considerable risk of maternal complications. Preeclampsia, with associated proteinuria, hypertension, and renal insufficiency, occurs in 5–38% of SLE parturients [160]. Even in the absence of preeclampsia, 12% of pregnant women with SLE experience irreversible progression of renal dysfunction [161]. Finally, the presence of antiphospholipid and anticardiolipin antibodies is associated with an increased risk of maternal thrombotic complications. Although vaginal delivery is preferred, cesarean section occurs in approximately 40% of parturients with SLE [162]. The delivery mode is frequently influenced by maternal and fetal status, with worsening renal function, refractory hypertension, and/or fetal distress necessitating cesarean delivery.

Fetal well-being is significantly impacted by the presence and severity of maternal SLE, with complications including intrauterine growth restriction, prematurity, neonatal lupus, and fetal demise. The severity of maternal disease impacts fetal loss, which occurs in 20–30% of SLE pregnancies [163].

Anesthetic management of the parturient with SLE requires careful preoperative assessment, given the diverse systemic effects of the disease. Although there are no contraindications to a specific type of anesthesia, the involvement of different organ systems may favor a particular technique. Since 15% of individuals have a peripheral neuropathy, with sensory more common than motor nerve involvement, it is imperative to evaluate for preexisting neurologic deficits. Although SLE arthritis rarely involves the spine, the presence of severe thrombocytopenia or coagulation defects may make regional anesthesia less desirable. In contrast, a neuraxial technique may be preferred in the presence of SLE-mediated laryngeal disease. Cricoarytenoid arthritis and recurrent laryngeal nerve palsy may affect as many as 30% of patients with SLE [164]. Associated airway obstruction may compromise airway management and/or predispose the patient to postextubation stridor. Therefore, successful management of the parturient with SLE requires a thorough appreciation for the diverse manifestations and clinical implications of this potentially devastating disease.

17.10.4 Rheumatoid arthritis

Rheumatoid arthritis, with a prevalence of 1% in the United States, is a chronic systemic disorder characterized by a symmetric polyarthritis [154]. Activation of the cellular immune response, via an unknown inciting event, results in synovial proliferation with progressive joint destruction and deformity. In addition, the diffuse deposition of immune complexes in extra-articular small vessel walls contributes to the varied systemic manifestations of rheumatoid arthritis. The course of this debilitating disease is marked by exacerbations and remissions and the prognosis is highly variable. Effective management of the parturient with rheumatoid arthritis is dependent on a thorough understanding of the involvement of multiple organ systems and the associated obstetric and anesthetic implications.

The hallmark of rheumatoid arthritis is symmetrical synovitis involving the wrists, knees, shoulders, and metacarpal-phalangeal joints. Although joint destruction and deformity is the most prevalent manifestation of rheumatoid arthritis, it is important to appreciate that this devastating disease can impact virtually every organ system. Cardiac involvement, including pericardial thickening and effusion, cardiac valve fibrosis, and/or intracardiac rheumatoid nodules, can lead to decreases in cardiac reserve, endocarditis, and/or conduction disturbances, respectively. Although pleural effusions are the most common pulmonary manifestations, rheumatoid arthritis may also cause pulmonary fibrosis, costochondritis, and pulmonary nodules. Pulmonary fibrosis and/or costochondral involvement may lead to restrictive changes resulting in ventilation-to-perfusion mismatch and decreased arterial oxygenation. Nerve compression and/or deposition of immune complexes in the walls of blood vessels supplying nerves may lead to peripheral neuropathies. It is important to determine and document the extent of neurologic impairment prior to any obstetric or anesthetic procedure in a parturient with rheumatoid arthritis. Hematologic compromise, including anemia, neutropenia, and thrombocytopenia, may also complicate the pregnancy course of rheumatoid patients. Specifically, anemia due to poor utilization of iron stores or chronic blood loss can contribute to reduced oxygen transport and intrauterine fetal growth restriction. Neutropenia increases the risk of infectious complications. Finally, thrombocytopenia, although rarely clinically significant, may increase their risk of spinal hematoma and/or postpartum hemorrhage.

It is imperative that providers caring for the rheumatoid parturient are aware of the specific anesthetic implications of various disease manifestations. Although larger, axial joints are frequently spared, 5% of patients with rheumatoid arthritis have osteophytes and ligament calcification in the lumbosacral spine, which can impact the success of regional anesthesia. Determination of affected joints' permissible range of activity is crucial prior to initiating any anesthetic technique. The associated destruction of supporting ligaments and cartilage results in instability of rheumatoid joints. Forcing motion beyond the disease-imposed limits may lead to further damage. In addition, care should be taken in the padding of affected joints during labor and delivery to provide further protection against unanticipated harm.

If general anesthesia is indicated, rheumatoid-mediated airway manifestations may make endotracheal intubation particularly challenging and dangerous. Airway compromise can occur at the temporomandibular joint, cricoarytenoid joint, and/or cervical spine. Temporomandibular joint involvement may impede oral opening, hindering mask ventilation and endotracheal intubation. Diminished or absent movement of the cricoarytenoid joint, suggested by the presence of hoarseness or stridor, results in narrowing of the glottic opening and subsequent interference with translaryngeal passage of the endotracheal tube. Patients with cricoarytenoid joint dysfunction are also at increased risk of joint dislocation and postextubation laryngeal obstruction. Cervical spine involvement has been reported in 25–50% of patients with longstanding rheumatoid arthritis [165]. Visualization of trachea during direct laryngoscopy may be difficult or impossible if cervical neck extension is limited. In addition, these patients are at increased risk of atlantoaxial instability and subluxation in which disruption of the transverse ligament allows anterior movement of C1 on C2 during neck flexion. The displaced odontoid process can compress the cervical spinal cord and/or impair blood flow through the vertebral arteries resulting in neurologic injury, quadriparesis, or sudden death. Radiographs can help elucidate the severity of cervical spine disease and have been recommended by some groups prior to any elective procedure in a patient with rheumatoid arthritis [166].

17.10.5 Multiple sclerosis

Multiple sclerosis is a chronic inflammatory neurologic condition occurring most frequently in women of childbearing age. Although a genetic susceptibility and an environmental exposure are known prerequisites, the precise pathogenesis of multiple sclerosis is still incompletely understood. Presumably, it involves a maladaptive immune reaction with a virus or other environmental antigen initiating a T-cell mediated response to myelin. Inflammation and demyelination at multiple sites within the brain and spinal cord interfere with neural transmission and expose affected axons to potentially injurious elements within the central nervous system. Demyelinated plaques eventually form over the exposed axonal segments but recovery is incomplete.

Multiple sclerosis is widely variable in its presentation, with periods of exacerbations and remissions punctuating its overall progressive course. Manifestations of multiple sclerosis reflect sites of demyelination within the central nervous site. Inflammation of the optic nerves is heralded by visual disturbances; whereas gait disturbances indicate cerebellar involvement. Demyelination within the spinal cord commonly manifests as lower extremity weakness, urinary incontinence, and/or sexual impotence. In addition, brain stem involvement can produce diplopia, trigeminal neuralgia, cardiac dysrhythmias, and/or autonomic dysfunction.

The interplay of pregnancy and multiple sclerosis may have significant implications for the parturient. Spinal cord lesions above T6 can affect the perception of uterine contractions, although this degree of disease is unusual for most parturients with multiple sclerosis. In general, multiple sclerosis does not appear to affect the course of labor or the obstetric management of delivery. Pregnancy, however, may influence the course and progression of multiple sclerosis [167–170]. Estrogen and progesterone are powerful immunomodulatory molecules associated with immunotolerance in pregnancy. Increased levels of these hormones during pregnancy appear to temporarily antagonize the subset of pro-inflammatory T cells implicated in multiple sclerosis. There is a 70% reduction in relapse risk during the third trimester of pregnancy, with a corresponding rebound increase in relapse risk during the first 3 months postpartum [167]. Overall, pregnancy does not appear to adversely affect long-term multiple sclerosis outcomes and some evidence suggests it might be beneficial. Previous studies have demonstrated an increased time between diagnosis of disease and being wheelchair-bound for patients who had previously been pregnant compared to nulliparous women (18.6 years compared with 12.5 years) [168]. In contrast, a recent multivariate regression analysis reported a median disease duration of 17 years with no independent association between pregnancy and time to secondary progression in 277 women with multiple sclerosis [169]. Therefore, it is still unclear whether pregnancy is protective in multiple sclerosis disease progression or merely a marker of less severe disease.

Anesthesia, in the form of labor analgesia or surgical anesthesia, is often indicated in parturients with multiple sclerosis. Neuraxial anesthesia is especially effective in preventing the development of autonomic dysreflexia in patients with spinal cord dysfunction above the T6 level. In patients with less severe disease, neuraxial analgesia may still prove beneficial in reducing maternal stress, preventing the use of intravenous opioids, and avoiding general anesthesia. Despite the benefits of neuraxial anesthesia in the parturient, some providers are reluctant to administer an epidural and/or spinal because of the concern of exposing demyelinated areas of the spinal cord to the potential neurotoxic effects of local anesthetic agents. Many reports suggest labor epidural analgesia is safe and effective in patients with multiple sclerosis [167,171], with no difference in relapse rate or disease progression compared to non-epidural controls [167,170].

However, other studies have implied epidural anesthesia for cesarean delivery is associated with an increased risk of relapse. The increased incidence of relapse rate with epidural anesthesia used for cesarean versus vaginal delivery suggests the concentration of local anesthesia may influence disease progression [171].

The significance of local anesthetic effect site concentration on relapse rate is further emphasized by the observation that spinal anesthesia is associated with greater exacerbations of multiple sclerosis than epidural anesthesia. Two series reported a small number of relapses in patients with multiple sclerosis receiving spinal anesthesia [172,173]. The mechanism by which spinal anesthesia may exacerbate multiple sclerosis is unknown but potentially reflects local anesthetic neurotoxicity. Demyelination and the lack of a protective nerve sheath may render the spinal cord more susceptible to potential neurotoxic effects of local anesthetics. Epidural anesthesia is potentially less neurotoxic than spinal anesthesia because the concentration of local anesthetics in the white matter of the spinal cord is four times less after epidural anesthesia. Although it is still unclear whether the relapses are a result of spinal anesthesia or other postoperative conditions known to exacerbate multiple sclerosis (emotional stress, infection, hyperpyrexia), it is prudent for anesthesia providers to use the minimal effective concentration of local anesthesia during labor and delivery.

17.10.6 Myasthenia gravis

Myasthenia gravis is an autoimmune disease, with a prevalence of approximately 1:20,000, most commonly afflicting women of childbearing age [174]. It is characterized by a maladaptive immune response against the nicotinic acetylcholine receptors or other muscle membrane proteins present on the neuromuscular end plate of skeletal muscles. Although the precise pathogenesis of myasthenia gravis is unclear, it is generally agreed that antibodies directed against postsynaptic components lead to an increased degradation and/or decreased formation of functional acetylcholine receptors. The end result is a 70–80% reduction in functional acetylcholine receptors present on the neuromuscular end plate. With this dramatic decrease in acetylcholine receptors, the margin of safety for neuromuscular transmission is profoundly reduced and the number of activated postsynaptic receptors may be insufficient to trigger a muscle action potential.

Myasthenia gravis is a chronic disorder, characterized by a slow and insidious onset followed by periods of relapses and remission. The reduction in activated acetylcholine receptors translates clinically into weakness and fatigability of skeletal muscles, with improvement in symptoms following a period of rest. A disease classification based on severity of skeletal muscle groups affected has been described (Table 17.7, Table 17.8, and Table 17.9) [175]. The disease demonstrates a predilection for muscles innervated by the cranial nerves. Ptosis and diplopia, from extraocular muscle involvement, are the most common initial complaints. Involvement of the bulbar (pharyngeal and laryngeal) muscles is heralded by dysphagia, dysarthria, and difficulty eliminating oral secretions.

Table 17.7 Anesthetic implications of systemic lupus erythematosus.

Organ system	Disease manifestation	Anesthetic implication
Cardiovascular	Pericarditis	Limited cardiac reserve
	Pericardial effusions	
	Valvular disorder	
	Conduction anomalies	Conduction disturbances
	Atherosclerosis	
Respiratory	Pleuritis	Limited pulmonary reserve
	Interstitial pneumonitis	
	Pulmonary hypertension	
Gastrointestinal	Dysphagia	Aspiration risk
Renal	Glomerulonephritis	Renal dysfunction
Neurological	Cognitive dysfunction	Consent issues
	Peripheral neuropathy	Preexisting neurologic deficits
	Stroke	
	Seizure	
Hematological	Anemia	Reduced oxygen transport
	Thrombocytopenia	Increase risk of bleeding
	Leukopenia	Increased risk of infection

Table 17.8 Anesthetic implications of rheumatoid arthritis.

Organ system	Disease manifestation	Anesthetic implication
Airway	TMJ dysfunction	Difficult intubation
	Laryngeal deviation	
		Subluxation with laryngoscopy
Skeletal	Cervical spine instability	Subluxation with laryngoscopy
	Calcification of lumbar ligaments	Difficult neuraxial anesthesia
	Lumbar spine osteophytes	
Cardiovascular	Pericarditis	Limited cardiac reserve
	Pericardial effusion	Conduction disturbances
	Myocarditis	
	Myocardial nodules	
Respiratory	Pulmonary effusion	Limited respiratory reserve
	Pulmonary fibrosis	
	Pulmonary nodules	
	Costochondritis	
Neurological	Nerve root compression	Preexisting neurologic deficits
	Neurovascular disease	
Hematological	Anemia	Reduced oxygen transport

Extremity and truncal weakness can occur in any combination and are generally asymmetric in distribution. Although smooth muscle is not affected, cardiac manifestations may include focal myocarditis, atrial fibrillation, atrioventricular conduction delay, and left ventricular diastolic dysfunction. The thymus may

Table 17.9 Clinical classification of myasthenia gravis.

Type 1	Involvement of only extraocular muscles
Type 2a	Mild, generalized myasthenia No respiratory crisis
Type 2b	Moderate, generalized myasthenia No respiratory crisis
Type 3	Severe Acute onset with rapid deterioration (<6 months) Respiratory crisis
Type 4	Severe Slow onset (>2 years) Respiratory crisis

play a role in pathogenesis as 90% have histologic abnormalities such as thymoma, thymic hyperplasia, or thymic atrophy.

Anesthetic management of the myasthenic parturient requires a thorough evaluation of the distribution and extent of skeletal muscle involvement as well as an understanding of the potential interaction of the disease with medications commonly used in labor. Drugs potentiating muscle weakness should be avoided as much as possible, including magnesium sulfate, calcium channel blockers, terbutaline, furosemide, and aminoglycoside antibiotics [176]. Neuraxial anesthesia can be safely and effectively used for labor and delivery. Epidural anesthesia not only increases maternal satisfaction, but early initiation reduces the stress, pain, and fatigability associated with disease exacerbations. Furthermore, adequate neuraxial analgesia mitigates the need for systemic medications, including opioids and benzodiazepines, which may contribute to central respiratory depression. Neuraxially induced muscle relaxation may compound the weakness caused by myasthenia gravis and a level greater than T4 can compromise the integrity of respiratory function and airway patency in patients with significant disease.

General anesthesia may be indicated for cesarean delivery in patients with significant bulbar or respiratory compromise. Endotracheal intubation not only facilitates control over oxygenation and ventilation, but also decreases the risk of pulmonary aspiration of gastric contents. Extreme caution must be exercised in administering muscle relaxants to patients with myasthenia gravis. Patients with poorly controlled disease are exquisitely sensitive to nondepolarizing muscle relaxants (vecuronium, rocuronium, cisatracurium) and small doses can produce significant muscle weakness and respiratory distress. In contrast, myasthenic patients are relatively resistant to the effects of depolarizing muscle relaxants (succinylcholine), although this is rarely clinically relevant in the doses typically administered for tracheal intubation. In addition, high end-tidal concentrations of volatile inhalation agents can induce neuromuscular blockade of ~ 40%. Therefore, adequate respiratory and bulbar strength must be confirmed prior to extubating a parturient with myasthenia gravis.

17.10.7 Spinal dysraphism

Spinal dysraphism is a global term describing a group of congenital spine and spinal cord abnormalities resulting from the maldevelopment of the ectodermal, mesodermal, and neuroectodermal tissue. Although there is certainly overlap in the pathophysiology and clinical manifestations of neural tube disorders, there are important differences in the associated central nervous system anatomy with each specific disorder [177]. Unfortunately, there is limited information about the anesthetic implications of *specific* neural tube defects, with most recommendations extrapolated from case reports or small, retrospective studies. A thorough understanding of the unique characteristics and clinical implications of specific neural tube disorders is imperative in providing a safe, effective anesthetic in the parturient.

Spina bifida occulta, with an incidence of 17–30%, results from failed fusion of the posterior neural arch *without* herniation of meninges or neural elements [178]. The defect is generally limited to a single lumbosacral vertebra, with 60% of spina bifida occulta occurring between L4 and S2 levels [179]. The clinical significance of an isolated bony arch abnormality has yet to be determined, with many considering spina bifida occulta a normal variant. Although spina bifida occulta is associated with a higher incidence of posterior disc herniation and chronic back pain, it is rarely complicated by more significant neurologic issues. The isolated finding of a defective laminar arch rarely complicates the administration of neuraxial anesthesia. Given that spina bifida occulta can be associated with abnormal posterior supporting ligaments (interspinous ligament and ligamentum flavum), it is prudent to perform regional anesthesia at a site remote from the level of anomaly to avoid inadvertent dural puncture. In addition, parturients should be informed of the possibility of inadequate or failed analgesia since the epidural space may be discontinuous at the defect level. Therefore, although analgesia may be less effective, regional anesthesia can be safely administered in parturients with spina bifida occulta and well-preserved neurologic function.

Occult spinal dysraphism describes a group of abnormalities characterized by a bony spine defect with one or more associated spinal cord anomalies, including tethered spinal cord, intraspinal lipomas, dermal sinus tracts, dermoid cysts, fibrous bands, syringocele, diplomyelia (duplication of spinal cord), and diastematomyelia (split cord). Tethered spinal cord (TSC), a commonly encountered anomaly with occult spinal dysraphism, generally occurs in the low thoracic or lumbosacral region and is frequently associated with a low-lying spinal cord. Neurologic deterioration, including urinary incontinence, scoliosis, lower extremity weakness, and sensory changes, results from traction on the conus medularis. Although only

30% of parturients with occult spinal dysraphism manifest obvious neurologic impairment, many have a history of minor neurologic and/or orthopedic issues [179]. Cutaneous stigmata, including hemangiomas, skin dimples, cutaneous lipomas, hyperpigmented areas, tufts of hair, and hypertrophic or atrophic skin, heralds the presence of underlying cord abnormalities in 50–70% of parturients with occult spinal dysraphism [180].

The presence of cutaneous manifestations warrants further neurologic evaluation. Several case reports have highlighted the risk of undiagnosed tethered spinal cord and neurologic injury following regional anesthesia in individuals with occult spinal dysraphism. TSC is associated with not only a low-lying, but also a more posteriorly located spinal cord, increasing the likelihood of direct needle trauma during administration of regional anesthesia. Magnetic resonance imaging (MRI) is imperative in determining the degree and character of associated neurologic anomalies. Consideration should be given to avoiding neuraxial anesthesia in the absence of imaging with suspected occult spinal dysraphism. In addition, care must be given to obstetric positioning. Prolonged squatting and/or lithotomy position exacerbates traction on a tethered spinal cord and should be avoided. Therefore, occult spinal dysraphism is a congenital spinal anomaly with obstetric and anesthetic implications that may lead to significant neurologic impairment if not appropriately appreciated.

Spinal bifida cystica, with an incidence of approximately ~1 in 2000 births, is the most debilitating of the neural tube disorders [181]. Failure of neural arch closure facilitates herniation of meninges (meningocele) or meninges and neural elements (myelomeningocele) through the defect. Although previously associated with > 50% mortality, improvements in surgical treatment have enhanced survival to 70%, allowing more affected females to reach childbearing age.

There are obvious challenges and unpredictability of regional anesthesia for this subset of parturients: one study of five women with spina bifida cystica receiving epidural anesthesia showed three women had "normal" blocks; one had a "high" block (T3 level after 10 mL of 0.25% bupivicaine); and one patient had inadequate analgesia with sacral sparing [182]. Given the inconsistent involvement of neural elements with spina bifida cystica, neuraxial anesthesia should not be attempted in the absence of a thorough evaluation. Operative reports should be obtained to define the manner and extent of previous surgeries. MRI can provide further insight into the location and character of residual spinal defects and the presence of scar tissue that may influence subsequent neuraxial anesthesia attempts. A regional technique should be avoided if elevated intracranial pressure and obstruction to cerebrospinal fluid flow is suspected. In this circumstance, a dural puncture, accidental or otherwise, can lead to herniation and associated sequelae. As such, the functionality of existing ventriculoperitoneal (VP) shunts should be evaluated and alternative forms of anesthesia, including general, local nerve blocks, and/or parenteral opioids, should be pursued in the presence of a dysfunctional VP shunt. Regardless of the mode of anesthesia, a thorough neurologic exam, and record of any deficits, should be documented before, during, and after any procedure. In addition, other organ systems, especially cardiac, renal, musculoskeletal, and genitourinary, should be assessed due to the increased incidence of associated anomalies with spinal bifida cystica. Discussion with the patient should include a thorough explanation of risk-to-benefit ratio of various anesthetic techniques and the increased potential for technical difficulty and incomplete blockade with neuraxial anesthesia.

17.10.8 Von Willebrand's disease

Von Willebrand's disease (VWD), with a prevalence of 1% in the general population, is the most common hereditary bleeding disorder. VWD is characterized by a deficiency in the quality and/or quantity of von Willebrand's factor (VWF), a protein that influences the hemostatic potential of both platelets and factor VIII. VWF mediates the adhesion of platelets to exposed endothelium at the site of vascular injury. In addition, VWF substantially increases the half-life and effectiveness of factor VIII by forming a nonconvalent complex which both resists clearance from the circulation and localizes factor VIII to the site of endothelium compromise [183]. VWD encompasses a spectrum of VWF deficits that vary in pathophysiology, manifestations, and treatment.

Although VWD universally involves an abnormality in VWF, variation in the specific quantitative or qualitative defect of VWF has led to further subclassification [184]. Type 1 VWD, which accounts for approximately 80% of cases, is characterized by a deficiency of structurally and functionally normal VWF. Whereas type 1 VWD confers a mild to moderate risk of bleeding, type 2 VWD imparts a more severe phenotype. Type 2 VWD, referring to a *functional* abnormality in VWF, is further divided into four subtypes based on the nature of the qualitative defect in the VWF protein. Type 2A VWD is characterized by a reduction in the larger, more active VWF multimers, resulting in decreased pro-hemostatic interactions with *both* factor VIII and platelets. The mutation in type 2B VWD stimulates *increased* platelet binding via the GPIb binding site. Enhanced binding subsequently leads to thrombocytopenia as platelet-VWF aggregates are sequestered from circulation and degraded. In contrast, type 2M VWD is characterized by a defect in the GPIb binding site leading to *decreased* platelet interaction and inefficient platelet adhesion at the site of vascular injury. The mutation in type 2N VWD causes impaired formation of the stabilizing factor VIII:VWF complex, resulting in increased factor VIII proteolysis and decreased circulating levels. The most severe bleeding manifestations occur with type 3 VWD, in which there is complete absence of VWF.

Pregnancy, generally characterized as a prothrombotic state, significantly impacts the parturient with VWD. As pregnancy progresses, escalating estradiol concentration leads to an increase in many coagulation factors, including a threefold increase in VWF and a twofold increase in factor VIII [185–187]. The influence of pregnancy-induced elevated VWF and factor VIII levels depends on the specific VWD defect. In type 1 VWD, characterized by a deficiency in functionally normal VWF, parturients generally experience an improvement in bleeding symptoms as coagulation levels increase into the hemostatic range. Parturients with type 2 VWD do not experience improvement in their hemostatic potential and, in some cases, demonstrate worsening of symptoms, as the upregulated VWF is functionally defective. The elevated levels of abnormal VWF in type 2B VWD result in increased pro-degradation platelet interactions and progressive thrombocytopenia. Type 3 VWD, with absent production of VWF, is not improved with pregnancy.

The hemostatic management of parturients with VWD depends on the specific VWF defect. Desmopressin (1-deamino-8-D-arginine vasopressin; DDAVP) is the preferred treatment for women with type 1 VWD who do not achieve normalization of VWF and factor VIII levels during parturition. Desmopressin, a synthetic analogue of antidiuretic hormone, acts via type 2 vasopressin receptors to release VWF and factor VIII into the systemic circulation [184]. Administration can occur either intravascularly (0.3 mcg/kg) or intranasally (150 mcg per metered-dose inhalation), with a maximum dose of 300 mcg via either route. After intravascular or intranasal administration, peak coagulation effects occur at approximately 45 minutes or 100 minutes, respectively. Although individual responses may vary, desmopressin generally results in a two- to fivefold increase in circulating levels of VWF and factor VIII lasting for 8–10 hours [188]. The dose can be repeated every 12 hours, although frequent readministration is discouraged because of the risk of serious side effects. Desmopressin is not effective, and can be potentially detrimental, in type 2 and type 3 VWD.

In type 1 VWD patients who fail to achieve an adequate response to desmopressin, as well as patients with type 3 VWD and most forms of type 2 VWD, plasma-derived factor VIII-VWF concentrate is the preferred pro-hemostatic agent. Infusions of heterologous factor VIII-VWF concentrate lead to an increase in functionally normal levels of VWF and factor VIII, independent of autologous production and stores. Although the different preparations of factor VIII-VWF concentrate (Alphanate SD/HT® [Grifols Biologicals, Inc., Los Angeles, California], Humate-P® [CSL Behring, King of Prussia, Pennsylvania], and Wilate ® [Octapharma, Lachen, Switzerland]) vary in the ratio of factor VIII to VWF and the method used to inactivate viruses, all forms are effective. The dose depends on baseline levels of factor VIII and VWF, with doses of 40–60 IU/kg recommended for women with factor VIII:C and/or VWF: Ristocetin Cofactor (RCo) levels less than 10 IU/dL. Proportionally lower doses can be administered to women with VWF:RCo levels higher than 10 IU/dL [184]. Infusions of factor VIII-VWF concentrate are generally maintained after delivery, at doses of 20–40 IU/kg every 8 to 24 hours, for 3 to 5 days postpartum [184].

FFP or cryoprecipitate can be considered in emergency situations in which desmopressin or factor VIII-VWF concentrates are not available or the specific type of VWD is unknown. Because of the higher risk of viral transmission, FFP and cryoprecipitate are generally considered second-line treatment. Regardless of the pro-hemostatic agent used, laboratory monitoring should guide treatment. Hemostatic agents should be considered postpartum when factor VIII:C levels are less than 50 IU/dL. Care should to taken to avoid supranormal factor VIII:C levels, which are associated with an increased risk of venous thromboembolism [184].

Anesthetic management of the parturient with VWD requires a thorough understanding of the specific VWF defect and awareness of appropriate pro-hemostatic options. Preanesthetic evaluation should include formulation of a plan (in conjunction with a hematologist) for optimizing coagulation status, and a review of the bleeding risks associated with labor and delivery. Regional anesthesia is safe in women whose coagulation factor levels have either normalized spontaneously or have been supplemented with hemostatic agents. Levels of VWF:RCo and FVIII:C greater than 50 IU/dL are associated with minimum risk when performing a neuraxial procedure [184]. Most parturients with type 1 VWD achieve spontaneous normalization of coagulation factors at term; whereas all women with type 3 VWD require prophylactic treatment. In contrast, presentation of type 2 VWD is variable, with many women not requiring prophylactic treatment unless for surgical delivery or perineal trauma [184]. A recent systematic review of neuraxial techniques in patients with bleeding disorders identified 74 procedures performed on 72 patients with VWD, type 1 (n = 71), type 2 (n = 2), and type 3 (n = 1) disease [189]. The majority (n = 64) had normalization of VWF levels without hemostatic treatment, whereas those remaining received hemostatic augmentation. Neuraxial procedures were performed in all 72 patients without any bleeding complications. In contrast, use of nonsteroidal anti-inflammatory agents is generally discouraged in the setting of VWD, as the antiplatelet effects may exacerbate bleeding risk. Therefore, management of the parturient with VWD requires an appreciation of the specific VWF defect and its interaction with hemostasis, parturition, and anesthetic options.

References

1 Ball C. James Young Simpson, 1811–1870. *Anaesthesia and Intensive Care* 1996;**24**(6):639.

2 Simpson WG (ed.) *The Works of Sir James Y. Simpson*. Adam and Charles Black: Edinburgh. 1871: 199–200. Available at: http://archive.org/details/worksofsirjamesy01simp (accessed May 20, 2015).

3 Levinson A. The three Meigs and their contribution to pediatrics. *Annals of Medical History* 1928;**10**:138–148.

4 Wagenknecht E. Mrs. *Longfellow: Selected Letters and Journals of Fanny Appleton Longfellow*. New York: Longmans, Green and Co., 1956. Available at: archive.org/details/mrslongfellowsel013699mbp (accessed May 20, 2015).

5 Caton D. John Snow's practice of obstetric anesthesia. *Anesthesiology* 2000;**92**(1):247–252.

6 Macht DI, Herman NB, and Levy CS. A quantitative study of cutaneous analgesia produced by various opium alkaloids. *Proceedings of the National Academy of Sciences of the United States of America* 1915;**1**(12):582–585.

7 Knipe WHW. The Freiburg method of Dämmerschlaf or twilight sleep. *American Journal of Obstetrics and Diseases of Women and Children* 1914; **70**:884–909.
8 Apgar V. A proposal for a new method of evaluation of the newborn infant. *Current Researches in Anesthesia & Analgesia* 1953;**32**(4):260–267.
9 Bonar BE and Meeker WR: The value of sacral nerve block anesthesia in obstetrics. *Journal of the American Medical Association* 1923; **81**(13):1079–1083.
10 Southworth JL and Hingson RA. Continuous caudal analgesia in surgery. *Annals of Surgery* 1943;**118**(6):945–970.
11 Samsoon GL and Young JR. Difficult tracheal intubation: a retrospective study. *Anaesthesia* 1987;**42**(5):487–490.
12 Cook TM, Woodall N and Frerk C. Major complications of airway management in the UK: results of the Fourth National Audit Project of the Royal College of Anaesthetists and the Difficult Airway Society. Part 1: anaesthesia. *British Journal of Anaesthesia* 2011;**106**(5):617–631.
13 Tao W, Edwards JT, Tu F, Xie Y, and Sharma SK. Incidence of unanticipated difficult airway in obstetric patients in a teaching institution. *Journal of Anesthesia* Jan **31**, 2012.
14 Dobb G. Laryngeal oedema complicating obstetric anaesthesia. *Anaesthesia* 1978;**33**(9): 839–840.
15 Pernoll ML, Metcalfe J, Schlenker TL, Welch JE, and Matsumoto JA. Oxygen consumption at rest and during exercise in pregnancy. *Respiration Physiology* 1975;**25**(3):285–293.
16 Practice guidelines for obstetric anesthesia: an updated report by the American Society of Anesthesiologists Task Force on Obstetric Anesthesia. *Anesthesiology* 2007;**106**(4):843–863.
17 Conklin KA. Maternal physiological adaptations during gestation, labor, and the puerperium. *Seminars in Anesthesia* 1991;**10**:221–234.
18 Adams JQ and Alexander AM Jr. Alterations in cardiovascular physiology during labor. *Obstetrics & Gynecology* 1958;**12**(5):542–549.
19 Lund CJ and Donovan JC. Blood volume during pregnancy. Significance of plasma and red cell volumes. *American Journal of Obstetrics & Gynecology* 1967;**98**(3):394–403.
20 Melzack R. The myth of painless childbirth (the John J. Bonica lecture). *Pain* 1984;**19**(4):321–337.
21 Cogan R and Spinnato JA. Pain and discomfort thresholds in late pregnancy. *Pain* 1986;**27**(1):63–68.
22 Abboud TK, Sarkis F, Hung TT *et al.* Effects of epidural anesthesia during labor on maternal plasma beta-endorphin levels. *Anesthesiology* 1983;**59**(1):1–5.
23 Fagraeus L, Urban BJ, and Bromage PR. Spread of epidural analgesia in early pregnancy. *Anesthesiology* 1983;**58**(2):184–187.
24 Palahniuk RJ, Shnider SM, and Eger EI, II. Pregnancy decreases the requirement for inhaled anesthetic agents. *Anesthesiology* 1974;**41**(1):82–83.
25 Morgan DJ, Blackman GL, Paull JD, and Wolf LJ. Pharmacokinetics and plasma binding of thiopental. II: Studies at cesarean section. *Anesthesiology* 1981;**54**(6):474–480.
26 Higuchi H, Adachi Y, Arimura S, Kanno M, and Satoh T. Early pregnancy does not reduce the C(50) of propofol for loss of consciousness. *Anesthesia & Analgesia* 2001; **93**(6):1565–1569, table of contents.
27 Abouleish EI. Postpartum tubal ligation requires more bupivacaine for spinal anesthesia than does cesarean section. *Anesthesia & Analgesia* 1986;**65**(8):897–900.
28 Kalas DB, Senfield RM, and Hehre FW. Continuous lumbar peridural anesthesia in obstetrics. IV. Comparison of the number of segments blocked in pregnant and nonpregnant subjects. *Anesthesia & Analgesia* 1966;**45**(6):848–851.
29 Cleland JP. Paravertebral anaesthesia in obstetrics. *Surgery, Gynecology, and Obstetrics* 1933; **57**:51–62.

30 Burns SM and Barclay PM. Regional anaesthesia for caesarean section. *Current Anaesthesia & Critical Care* 2000;**11**(2):73–79.
31 Smith CA, Collins CT, Cyna AM, and Crowther CA. Complementary and alternative therapies for pain management in labour. *Cochrane Database of Systematic Reviews* 2006;(**4**):CD003521.
32 Jones L, Othman M, Dowswell T *et al.* Pain management for women in labour: an overview of systematic reviews. *Cochrane Database of Systematic Reviews* 2012;(**3**):CD009234.
33 Ullman R, Smith LA, Burns E, Mori R, and Dowswell T. Parenteral opioids for maternal pain relief in labour. *Cochrane Database of Systematic Reviews* 2010;(**9**):CD007396.
34 Douma MR, Verwey RA, Kam-Endtz CE, van der Linden PD, and Stienstra R. Obstetric analgesia: a comparison of patient-controlled meperidine, remifentanil, and fentanyl in labour. *British Journal of Anaesthesia* 2010;**104**(2):209–215.
35 Klomp T, van Poppel M, Jones L, Lazet J, Di Nisio M, and Lagro-Janssen AL. Inhaled analgesia for pain management in labour. *Cochrane Database of Systematic Reviews* 2012;(**9**):CD009351.
36 American College of Obstetricians and Gynecologists Committee Opinion No. 295. Pain relief during labor. *Obstetrics & Gynecology* 2004;**104**(1):213.
37 Leighton BL and Halpern SH. The effects of epidural analgesia on labor, maternal, and neonatal outcomes: a systematic review. *American Journal of Obstetrics & Gynecology* 2002;**186** (5 Suppl. Nature):S69–77.
38 Liu EH and Sia AT. Rates of caesarean section and instrumental vaginal delivery in nulliparous women after low concentration epidural infusions or opioid analgesia: systematic review. *BMJ* 2004;**328**(7453):1410.
39 Sharma SK, McIntire DD, Wiley J, and Leveno KJ. Labor analgesia and cesarean delivery: an individual patient meta-analysis of nulliparous women. *Anesthesiology* 2004;**100**(1):142–148; discussion 146A.
40 Halpern SH, Muir H, Breen TW *et al.* A multicenter randomized controlled trial comparing patient-controlled epidural with intravenous analgesia for pain relief in labor. *Anesthesia & Analgesia* 2004;**99**(5):1532–1538, table of contents.
41 Wong CA, Scavone BM, Peaceman AM *et al.* The risk of cesarean delivery with neuraxial analgesia given early versus late in labor. *New England Journal of Medicine* 2005;**352**(7):655–665.
42 Sharma SK, Alexander JM, Messick G *et al.* Cesarean delivery: a randomized trial of epidural analgesia versus intravenous meperidine analgesia during labor in nulliparous women. *Anesthesiology* 2002;**96**(3):546–551.
43 Effect of low-dose mobile versus traditional epidural techniques on mode of delivery: a randomised controlled trial. *Lancet* 2001;**358**(9275):19–23.
44 Chestnut DH, McGrath JM, Vincent RD Jr *et al.* Does early administration of epidural analgesia affect obstetric outcome in nulliparous women who are in spontaneous labor? *Anesthesiology* 1994;**80**(6):1201–1208.
45 Anim-Somuah M, Smyth RM, and Jones L. Epidural versus non-epidural or no analgesia in labour. *Cochrane Database of Systematic Reviews* 2011;(**12**):CD000331.
46 Russell IF. A prospective controlled study of continuous spinal analgesia versus repeat epidural analgesia after accidental dural puncture in labour. *International Journal of Gynecology & Obstetrics* 2012;**21**(1):7–16.
47 Mardirosoff C, Dumont L, Boulvain M, and Tramer MR. Fetal bradycardia due to intrathecal opioids for labour analgesia: a systematic review. *BJOG* 2002;**109**(3):274–281.
48 Reynolds F. The effects of maternal labour analgesia on the fetus. *Best Practice & Research Clinical Obstetrics & Gynaecology* 2010;**24**(3):289–302.
49 Gaiser RR, McHugh M, Cheek TG, and Gutsche BB. Predicting prolonged fetal heart rate deceleration following intrathecal fentanyl/bupivacaine. *International Journal of Gynecology & Obstetrics* 2005;**14**(3):208–211.

50 Frolich MA, Esame A, Zhang K, Wu J, and Owen J. What factors affect intrapartum maternal temperature? A prospective cohort study: maternal intrapartum temperature. *Anesthesiology* 2012;**117**(2):302–308.
51 Goetzl L. Epidural analgesia and maternal fever: a clinical and research update. *Current Opinion in Anaesthesiology* 2012;**25**(3):292–299.
52 Segal S. Labor epidural analgesia and maternal fever. *Anesthesia & Analgesia* 2010; **111**(6):1467–1475.
53 Wilson MJ, MacArthur C, Cooper GM, Bick D, Moore PA, and Shennan A. Epidural analgesia and breastfeeding: a randomised controlled trial of epidural techniques with and without fentanyl and a non-epidural comparison group. *Anaesthesia* 2010;**65**(2):145–153.
54 Simmons SW, Taghizadeh N, Dennis AT, Hughes D, and Cyna AM. Combined spinal-epidural versus epidural analgesia in labour. *Cochrane Database of Systematic Reviews* 2012;(10):CD003401.
55 Tsen LC, Thue B, Datta S, and Segal S. Is combined spinal-epidural analgesia associated with more rapid cervical dilation in nulliparous patients when compared with conventional epidural analgesia? *Anesthesiology* 1999;**91**(4):920–925.
56 Arkoosh VA, Palmer CM, Yun EM *et al.* A randomized, double-masked, multicenter comparison of the safety of continuous intrathecal labor analgesia using a 28-gauge catheter versus continuous epidural labor analgesia. *Anesthesiology* 2008;**108**(2):286–298.
57 Lee A, Ngan Kee WD, and Gin T. A quantitative, systematic review of randomized controlled trials of ephedrine versus phenylephrine for the management of hypotension during spinal anesthesia for cesarean delivery. *Anesthesia & Analgesia* 2002;**94**(4):920–926, table of contents.
58 Ng K, Parsons J, Cyna AM, and Middleton P. Spinal versus epidural anaesthesia for caesarean section. *Cochrane Database of Systematic Reviews* 2004;(**2**):CD003765.
59 Hawkins JL, Koonin LM, Palmer SK, and Gibbs CP. Anesthesia-related deaths during obstetric delivery in the United States, 1979–1990. *Anesthesiology* 1997;**86**(2):277–284.
60 McDonnell NJ, Paech MJ, Clavisi OM, and Scott KL. Difficult and failed intubation in obstetric anaesthesia: an observational study of airway management and complications associated with general anaesthesia for caesarean section. *International Journal of Gynecology & Obstetrics* 2008;**17**(4):292–297.
61 Hawkins JL, Chang J, Palmer SK, Gibbs CP, and Callaghan WM. Anesthesia-related maternal mortality in the United States: 1979–2002. *Obstetrics & Gynecology* 2011;**117**(1):69–74.
62 Mhyre JM, Riesner MN, Polley LS, and Naughton NN. A series of anesthesia-related maternal deaths in Michigan, 1985–2003. *Anesthesiology* 2007;**106**(6):1096–1104.
63 Wong CA. Saving mothers' lives: the 2006–8 anaesthesia perspective. *British Journal of Anaesthesia* 2011;**107**(2):119–122.
64 Ranney B and Stanage WF. Advantages of local anesthesia for cesarean section. *Obstetrics & Gynecology* 1975;**45**(2):163–167.
65 Gautam PL, Kathuria S, and Kaul TK. Infiltration block for caesarean section in a morbidly obese parturient. *Acta Obstetricia et Gynecologica Scandinavica* 1999;**43**(5):580–581.
66 Geber WF and Schramm LC. Congenital malformations of the central nervous system produced by narcotic analgesics in the hamster. *American Journal of Obstetrics & Gynecology* 1975;**123**(7):705–713.
67 Fujinaga M, Stevenson JB, and Mazze RI. Reproductive and teratogenic effects of fentanyl in Sprague-Dawley rats. *Teratology* 1986;**34**(1):51–57.
68 Fujinaga M, Mazze RI, Jackson EC, and Baden JM. Reproductive and teratogenic effects of sufentanil and alfentanil in Sprague-Dawley rats. *Anesthesia & Analgesia* 1988;**67**(2):166–169.
69 Finnell RH, Shields HE, Taylor SM, and Chernoff GF. Strain differences in phenobarbital-induced teratogenesis in mice. *Teratology* 1987;**35**(2):177–185.

70 Safra MJ and Oakley GP Jr. Association between cleft lip with or without cleft palate and prenatal exposure to diazepam. *Lancet* 1975;**2**(7933):478–480.

71 Rosenberg L, Mitchell AA, Parsells JL, Pashayan H, Louik C, and Shapiro S. Lack of relation of oral clefts to diazepam use during pregnancy. *New England Journal of Medicine* 1983;**309**(21):1282–1285.

72 Pesic V, Milanovic D, Tanic N *et al.* Potential mechanism of cell death in the developing rat brain induced by propofol anesthesia. *International Journal of Developmental Neuroscience* 2009;**27**(3):279–287.

73 Yon JH, Daniel-Johnson J, Carter LB, and Jevtovic-Todorovic V. Anesthesia induces neuronal cell death in the developing rat brain via the intrinsic and extrinsic apoptotic pathways. *Neuroscience* 2005;**135**(3):815–827.

74 Sprung J, Flick RP, Katusic SK *et al.* Attention-deficit/hyperactivity disorder after early exposure to procedures requiring general anesthesia. *Mayo Clinic Proceedings* 2012;**87**(2):120–129.

75 Wilder RT, Flick RP, Sprung J *et al.* Early exposure to anesthesia and learning disabilities in a population-based birth cohort. *Anesthesiology* 2009;**110**(4):796–804.

76 Sturrock JE and Nunn JF. Cytotoxic effects of procaine, lignocaine and bupivacaine. *British Journal of Anaesthesia* 1979;**51**(4):273–281.

77 Teiling AK, Mohammed AK, Minor BG, Jarbe TU, Hiltunen AJ, and Archer T. Lack of effects of prenatal exposure to lidocaine on development of behavior in rats. *Anesthesia & Analgesia* 1987;**66**(6):533–541.

78 Crawford JS and Lewis M. Nitrous oxide in early human pregnancy. *Anaesthesia* 1986;**41**(9):900–905.

79 Turner RJ, Lambros M, Kenway L, and Gatt SP. The in-vitro effects of sevoflurane and desflurane on the contractility of pregnant human uterine muscle. *International Journal of Gynecology & Obstetrics* 2002;**11**(4):246–251.

80 Combs CA and Laros RK Jr. Prolonged third stage of labor: morbidity and risk factors. *Obstetrics & Gynecology* 1991;**77**(6):863–867.

81 Vinatier D, Dufour P, and Berard J. Utilization of intravenous nitroglycerin for obstetrical emergencies. *International Journal of Gynecology & Obstetrics* 1996;**55**(2):129–134.

82 DeSimone CA, Norris MC, and Leighton BL. Intravenous nitroglycerin aids manual extraction of a retained placenta. *Anesthesiology* 1990;**73**(4):787.

83 Bullarbo M, Tjugum J, and Ekerhovd E. Sublingual nitroglycerin for management of retained placenta. *International Journal of Gynecology & Obstetrics* 2005;**91**(3):228–232.

84 Westhoff C and Davis A. Tubal sterilization: focus on the U.S. experience. *Fertility and Sterility* 2000;**73**(5):913–922.

85 Pati S andCullins V. Female sterilization. Evidence. *Obstetrics and Gynecology Clinics of North America* 2000;**27**(4):859–899.

86 Cruikshank DP, Laube DW, and De Backer LJ. Intraperitoneal lidocaine anesthesia for postpartum tubal ligation. *Obstetrics & Gynecology* 1973;**42**(1):127–130.

87 Goodman EJ and Dumas SD. The rate of successful reactivation of labor epidural catheters for postpartum tubal ligation surgery. *Regional Anesthesia and Pain Medicine* 1998;**23**(3):258–261.

88 Chan MT and Gin T. Postpartum changes in the minimum alveolar concentration of isoflurane. *Anesthesiology* 1995;**82**(6):1360–1363.

89 Zhou HH, Norman P, DeLima LG, Mehta M, and Bass D. The minimum alveolar concentration of isoflurane in patients undergoing bilateral tubal ligation in the postpartum period. *Anesthesiology* 1995;**82**(6):1364–1368.

90 Coleman MT, Trianfo VA, and Rund DA. Nonobstetric emergencies in pregnancy: trauma and surgical conditions. *American Journal of Obstetrics & Gynecology* 1997;**177**(3):497–502.

91 Kort B, Katz VL, and Watson WJ. The effect of nonobstetric operation during pregnancy. *Surgery, Gynecology, and Obstetrics* 1993;**177**(4):371–376.

92 Howell CJ and Chalmers I. A review of prospectively controlled comparisons of epidural with non-epidural forms of pain relief during labour. *International Journal of Gynecology & Obstetrics* 1992;**1**(2):93–110.

93 Jouppila P, Jouppila R, Hollmen A, and Koivula A. Lumbar epidural analgesia to improve intervillous blood flow during labor in severe preeclampsia. *Obstetrics & Gynecology* 1982;**59**(2):158–161.

94 Rasmus KT, Rottman RL, Kotelko DM, Wright WC, Stone JJ, and Rosenblatt RM. Unrecognized thrombocytopenia and regional anesthesia in parturients: a retrospective review. *Obstetrics & Gynecology* 1989;**73**(6):943–946.

95 Beilin Y, Zahn J, and Comerford M. Safe epidural analgesia in thirty parturients with platelet counts between 69,000 and 98,000 mm(-3). *Anesthesia & Analgesia* 1997;**85**(2):385–388.

96 Horlocker TT, Wedel DJ, Benzon H *et al.* Regional anesthesia in the anticoagulated patient: defining the risks (the second ASRA Consensus Conference on Neuraxial Anesthesia and Anticoagulation). *Regional Anesthesia and Pain Medicine* 2003;**28**(3):172–197.

97 Wallace DH, Leveno KJ, Cunningham FG, Giesecke AH, Shearer VE, and Sidawi JE. Randomized comparison of general and regional anesthesia for cesarean delivery in pregnancies complicated by severe preeclampsia. *Obstetrics & Gynecology* 1995;**86**(2):193–199.

98 Hood DD and Curry R. Spinal versus epidural anesthesia for cesarean section in severely preeclamptic patients: a retrospective survey. *Anesthesiology* 1999;**90**(5):1276–1282.

99 Aya AG, Mangin R, Vialles N *et al.* Patients with severe preeclampsia experience less hypotension during spinal anesthesia for elective cesarean delivery than healthy parturients: a prospective cohort comparison. *Anesthesia & Analgesia* 2003;**97**(3):867–872.

100 Report of the National High Blood Pressure Education Program Working Group on High Blood Pressure in Pregnancy. *American Journal of Obstetrics & Gynecology* 2000;**183**(1):S1–S22.

101 Hood DD, Dewan DM, James FM, III, Floyd HM, and Bogard TD. The use of nitroglycerin in preventing the hypertensive response to tracheal intubation in severe preeclampsia. *Anesthesiology* 1985;**63**(3):329–332.

102 Bansal S and Pawar M. Haemodynamic responses to laryngoscopy and intubation in patients with pregnancy-induced hypertension: effect of intravenous esmolol with or without lidocaine. *International Journal of Gynecology & Obstetrics* 2002;**11**(1):4–8.

103 Ngan Kee WD, Khaw KS, Ma KC, Wong AS, Lee BB, and Ng FF. Maternal and neonatal effects of remifentanil at induction of general anesthesia for cesarean delivery: a randomized, double-blind, controlled trial. *Anesthesiology* 2006;**104**(1):14–20.

104 Yoshida A, Itoh Y, Nagaya K *et al.* Prolonged relaxant effects of vecuronium in patients with deliberate hypermagnesemia: time for caution in cesarean section. *Journal of Anesthesia* 2006;**20**(1):33–35.

105 James MF, Cork RC, and Dennett JE. Succinylcholine pretreatment with magnesium sulfate. *Anesthesia & Analgesia* 1986;**65**(4):373–376.

106 Bateman BT, Berman MF, Riley LE, and Leffert LR. The epidemiology of postpartum hemorrhage in a large, nationwide sample of deliveries. *Anesthesia & Analgesia* 2010;**110**(5):1368–1373.

107 Aali BS and Nejad SS. Nifedipine or hydralazine as a first-line agent to control hypertension in severe preeclampsia. *Acta Obstetricia et Gynecologica Scandinavica* 2002;**81**(1):25–30.

108 Mercier FJ and Bonnet MP. Use of clotting factors and other prohemostatic drugs for obstetric hemorrhage. *Current Opinion in Anaesthesiology* 2010;**23**(3):310–316.

109 Hogan MC, Foreman KJ, Naghavi M *et al.* Maternal mortality for 181 countries, 1980–2008: a systematic analysis of progress towards Millennium Development Goal 5. *Lancet* 2010;**375**(9726):1609–1623.

110 Knight M, Callaghan WM, Berg C *et al.* Trends in postpartum hemorrhage in high resource countries: a review and recommendations from the International Postpartum Hemorrhage Collaborative Group. *BMC Pregnancy and Childbirth* 2009;**9**:55.

111 McLintock C and James AH. Obstetric hemorrhage. *Journal of Thrombosis and Haemostasis* 2011;**9**(8):1441–1451.

112 Stafford I, Dildy GA, Clark SL, and Belfort MA. Visually estimated and calculated blood loss in vaginal and cesarean delivery. *American Journal of Obstetrics & Gynecology* 2008;**199**(5):519 e511–517.

113 Kozek-Langenecker SA. Effects of hydroxyethyl starch solutions on hemostasis. *Anesthesiology* 2005;**103**(3):654–660.

114 Westphal M, James MF, Kozek-Langenecker S, Stocker R, Guidet B, and Van Aken H. Hydroxyethyl starches: different products – different effects. *Anesthesiology* 2009; **111**(1):187–202.

115 Practice guidelines for perioperative blood transfusion and adjuvant therapies: an updated report by the American Society of Anesthesiologists Task Force on Perioperative Blood Transfusion and Adjuvant Therapies. *Anesthesiology* 2006;**105**(1):198–208.

116 Mercier FJ and Van de Velde M. Major obstetric hemorrhage. *Anesthesiology Clinics* 2008;**26**(1):53–66, vi.

117 Eugster M and Reinhart WH. The influence of the haematocrit on primary haemostasis in vitro. *Thrombosis and Haemostasis* 2005;**94**(6):1213–1218.

118 Bolliger D, Szlam F, Molinaro RJ, Rahe-Meyer N, Levy JH, and Tanaka KA. Finding the optimal concentration range for fibrinogen replacement after severe haemodilution: an in vitro model. *British Journal of Anaesthesia* 2009;**102**(6):793–799.

119 Letsky EA. Disseminated intravascular coagulation. *Best Practice & Research Clinical Obstetrics & Gynaecology* 2001;**15**(4):623–644.

120 Santoso JT, Saunders BA, and Grosshart K. Massive blood loss and transfusion in obstetrics and gynecology. *Obstetrical and Gynecological Survey* 2005;**60**(12):827–837.

121 Holcomb JB, Jenkins D, Rhee P *et al.* Damage control resuscitation: directly addressing the early coagulopathy of trauma. *Journal of Trauma* 2007;**62**(2):307–310.

122 Borgman MA, Spinella PC, Perkins JG *et al.* The ratio of blood products transfused affects mortality in patients receiving massive transfusions at a combat support hospital. *Journal of Trauma* 2007;**63**(4):805–813.

123 Charbit B, Mandelbrot L, Samain E *et al.* The decrease of fibrinogen is an early predictor of the severity of postpartum hemorrhage. *Journal of Thrombosis and Haemostasis* 2007;**5**(2):266–273.

124 Johansson PI and Stensballe J. Effect of Haemostatic Control Resuscitation on mortality in massively bleeding patients: a before and after study. *Vox Sanguinis* 2009;**96**(2):111–118.

125 Franchini M, Lippi G, and Franchi M. The use of recombinant activated factor VII in obstetric and gynaecological haemorrhage. *BJOG* 2007;**114**(1):8–15.

126 Franchini M, Franchi M, Bergamini V, Salvagno GL, Montagnana M, and Lippi G. A critical review on the use of recombinant factor VIIa in life-threatening obstetric postpartum hemorrhage. *Seminars in Thrombosis and Hemostasis* 2008;**34**(1):104–112.

127 Phillips LE, McLintock C, Pollock W *et al.* Recombinant activated factor VII in obstetric hemorrhage: experiences from the Australian and New Zealand Haemostasis Registry. *Anesthesia & Analgesia* 2009;**109**(6):1908–1915.

128 Yank V, Tuohy CV, Logan AC *et al.* Systematic review: benefits and harms of in-hospital use of recombinant factor VIIa for off-label indications. *Annals of Internal Medicine* 2011;**154**(8):529–540.

129 Ducloy-Bouthors AS, Jude B, Duhamel A *et al.* High-dose tranexamic acid reduces blood loss in postpartum haemorrhage. *Critical Care* 2011;**15**(2):R117.

130 Henry DA, Carless PA, Moxey AJ *et al.* Anti-fibrinolytic use for minimising perioperative allogeneic blood transfusion. *Cochrane Database of Systematic Reviews* 2007;(**4**):CD001886.

131 Ferrer P, Roberts I, Sydenham E, Blackhall K, and Shakur H. Anti-fibrinolytic agents in post partum haemorrhage: a systematic review. *BMC Pregnancy and Childbirth* 2009;**9**:29.

132 Williamson KR and Taswell HF. Intraoperative blood salvage: a review. *Transfusion* 1991;**31**(7):662–675.
133 Tevet A, Grisaru-Granovsky S, Samueloff A, and Ioscovich A. Peripartum use of cell salvage: a university practice audit and literature review. *Archives of Gynecology and Obstetrics* 2012;**285**(2):281–284.
134 Catling SJ, Williams S, and Fielding AM. Cell salvage in obstetrics: an evaluation of the ability of cell salvage combined with leucocyte depletion filtration to remove amniotic fluid from operative blood loss at caesarean section. *International Journal of Gynecology & Obstetrics* 1999;**8**(2):79–84.
135 Waters JH, Biscotti C, Potter PS, and Phillipson E. Amniotic fluid removal during cell salvage in the cesarean section patient. *Anesthesiology* 2000;**92**(6):1531–1536.
136 Benson MD, Kobayashi H, Silver RK, Oi H, Greenberger PA, and Terao T. Immunologic studies in presumed amniotic fluid embolism. *Obstetrics & Gynecology* 2001;**97**(4):510–514.
137 Rebarber A, Lonser R, Jackson S, Copel JA, and Sipes S. The safety of intraoperative autologous blood collection and autotransfusion during cesarean section. *American Journal of Obstetrics & Gynecology* 1998;**179**(3 Pt 1):715–720.
138 Kuczkowski KM. Labor analgesia for the parturient with cardiac disease: what does an obstetrician need to know? *Acta Obstetricia et Gynecologica Scandinavica* 2004;**83**(3):223–233.
139 Chang J, Elam-Evans LD, Berg CJ *et al.* Pregnancy-related mortality surveillance – United States, 1991–1999. *MMWR Surveillance Summaries* 2003;**52**(2):1–8.
140 Cox PB, Gogarten W, and Marcus MA. Maternal cardiac disease. *Current Opinion in Anaesthesiology* 2005;**18**(3):257–262.
141 Siu SC, Sermer M, Colman JM *et al.* Prospective multicenter study of pregnancy outcomes in women with heart disease. *Circulation* 2001;**104**(5):515–521.
142 Wilson W, Taubert KA, Gewitz M *et al.* Prevention of infective endocarditis: guidelines from the American Heart Association: a guideline from the American Heart Association Rheumatic Fever, Endocarditis, and Kawasaki Disease Committee, Council on Cardiovascular Disease in the Young, and the Council on Clinical Cardiology, Council on Cardiovascular Surgery and Anesthesia, and the Quality of Care and Outcomes Research Interdisciplinary Working Group. *Circulation* 2007;**116**(15):1736–1754.
143 Pocock SB and Chen KT. Inappropriate use of antibiotic prophylaxis to prevent infective endocarditis in obstetric patients. *Obstetrics & Gynecology* 2006;**108**(2):280–285.
144 Obesity: preventing and managing the global epidemic. Report of a WHO consultation. *World Health Organization Technical Report Series* 2000;**894**:i–xii, 1–253.
145 Yogev Y and Catalano PM. Pregnancy and obesity. *Obstetrics and Gynecology Clinics of North America* 2009;**36**(2):285–300, viii.
146 Veille JC and Hanson R. Obesity, pregnancy, and left ventricular functioning during the third trimester. *American Journal of Obstetrics & Gynecology* 1994;**171**(4):980–983.
147 Saravanakumar K, Rao SG, and Cooper GM. Obesity and obstetric anaesthesia. *Anaesthesia* 2006;**61**(1):36–48.
148 Weiss JL, Malone FD, Emig D *et al.* Obesity, obstetric complications and cesarean delivery rate – a population-based screening study. *American Journal of Obstetrics & Gynecology* 2004;**190**(4):1091–1097.
149 Mace HS, Paech MJ, and McDonnell NJ. Obesity and obstetric anaesthesia. *Anaesthesia and Intensive Care* 2011;**39**(4):559–570.
150 Kumari AS. Pregnancy outcome in women with morbid obesity. *International Journal of Gynecology & Obstetrics* 2001;**73**(2):101–107.
151 Vaughan RW, Bauer S, and Wise L. Volume and pH of gastric juice in obese patients. *Anesthesiology* 1975;**43**(6):686–689.
152 Dixit A and Girling JC. Obesity and pregnancy. *Journal of Obstetrics and Gynaecology* 2008;**28**(1):14–23.

153 Norman JE and Reynolds RM. The consequences of obesity and excess weight gain in pregnancy. *Proceedings of the Nutrition Society* 2011;**70**(4):450–456.

154 Lawrence RC, Helmick CG, Arnett FC *et al.* Estimates of the prevalence of arthritis and selected musculoskeletal disorders in the United States. *Arthritis & Rheumatology* 1998;**41**(5):778–799.

155 Lahita RG. The role of sex hormones in systemic lupus erythematosus. *Current Opinion in Rheumatology* 1999;**11**(5):352–356.

156 D'Cruz DP, Khamashta MA, and Hughes GR. Systemic lupus erythematosus. *Lancet* 2007;**369**(9561):587–596.

157 Mandell BF. Cardiovascular involvement in systemic lupus erythematosus. *Seminars in Arthritis and Rheumatism* 1987;**17**(2):126–141.

158 Roldan CA, Shively BK, and Crawford MH. An echocardiographic study of valvular heart disease associated with systemic lupus erythematosus. *New England Journal of Medicine* 1996;**335**(19):1424–1430.

159 Raj R, Murin S, Matthay RA, and Wiedemann HP. Systemic lupus erythematosus in the intensive care unit. *Critical Care Clinics* 2002;**18**(4):781–803.

160 Mok CC and Wong RW. Pregnancy in systemic lupus erythematosus. *Postgraduate Medical Journal* 2001;**77**(905):157–165.

161 Petri M. Systemic lupus erythematosus and pregnancy. *Rheumatic Disease Clinics of North America* 1994;**20**(1):87–118.

162 Chakravarty EF, Nelson L, and Krishnan E. Obstetric hospitalizations in the United States for women with systemic lupus erythematosus and rheumatoid arthritis. *Arthritis & Rheumatology* 2006;**54**(3):899–907.

163 Molad Y, Borkowski T, Monselise A *et al.* Maternal and fetal outcome of lupus pregnancy: a prospective study of 29 pregnancies. *Lupus* 2005;**14**(2):145–151.

164 Espana A, Gutierrez JM, Soria C, Gila L, and Ledo A. Recurrent laryngeal palsy in systemic lupus erythematosus. *Neurology* 1990;**40**(7):1143–1144.

165 Conlon PW, Isdale IC, and Rose BS. Rheumatoid arthritis of the cervical spine. An analysis of 333 cases. *Annals of the Rheumatic Diseases* 1966;**25**(2):120–126.

166 Macarthur A and Kleiman S. Rheumatoid cervical joint disease – a challenge to the anaesthetist. *Canadian Journal of Anesthesia* 1993;**40**(2):154–159.

167 Vukusic S, Hutchinson M, Hours M *et al.* Pregnancy and multiple sclerosis (the PRIMS study): clinical predictors of post-partum relapse. *Brain* 2004;**127**(Pt 6):1353–1360.

168 Runmarker B and Andersen O. Pregnancy is associated with a lower risk of onset and a better prognosis in multiple sclerosis. *Brain* 1995;**118** (Pt 1):253–261.

169 Koch M, Uyttenboogaart M, Heersema D, Steen C, and De Keyser J. Parity and secondary progression in multiple sclerosis. *Journal of Neurology, Neurosurgery & Psychiatry* 2009;**80**(6):676–678.

170 Confavreux C, Hutchinson M, Hours MM, Cortinovis-Tourniaire P, and Moreau T. Rate of pregnancy-related relapse in multiple sclerosis. Pregnancy in Multiple Sclerosis Group. *New England Journal of Medicine* 1998;**339**(5):285–291.

171 Bader AM, Hunt CO, Datta S, Naulty JS, and Ostheimer GW. Anesthesia for the obstetric patient with multiple sclerosis. *Journal of Clinical Anesthesia* 1988;**1**(1):21–24.

172 Bamford C, Sibley W, and Laguna J. Anesthesia in multiple sclerosis. *Canadian Journal of Neurological Sciences* 1978;**5**(1):41–44.

173 Stenuit J and Marchand P. [Sequelae of spinal anesthesia]. *Acta Neurologica et Psychiatrica Belgica* 1968;**68**(8):626–635.

174 Kurtzke JF. Epidemiology of myasthenia gravis. *Advances in Neurology* 1978;**19**:545–566.

175 Osserman KE. Studies in myasthenia gravis. I. *New York State Journal of Medicine*1956; **56**(16):2512–2522.

176 Barrons RW. Drug-induced neuromuscular blockade and myasthenia gravis. *Pharmacotherapy* 1997;**17**(6):1220–1232.

177 Kreeger RN and Hilvano A. Anesthetic options for the parturient with a neural tube defect. *International Anesthesiology Clinics* 2005;**43**(4):65–80.

178 Kaufman BA. Neural tube defects. *Pediatric Clinics of North America* 2004;**51**(2):389–419.

179 Avrahami E, Frishman E, Fridman Z, and Azor M. Spina bifida occulta of S1 is not an innocent finding. *Spine (Phila Pa 1976)* 1994;**19**(1):12–15.

180 Yamane T, Shinoto A, Kamegaya M, and Shinada Y. Spinal dysraphism. A study of patients over the age of 10 years. *Spine (Phila Pa 1976)* 1991;**16**(11):1295–1297.

181 Arca MJ and Teich S. Current controversies in perinatal care: fetal versus neonatal surgery. *Clinics in Perinatology* 2004;**31**(3):629–648.

182 Tidmarsh MD and May AE. Epidural anaesthesia and neural tube defects. *International Journal of Gynecology & Obstetrics* 1998;**7**(2):111–114.

183 De Meyer SF, Deckmyn H, and Vanhoorelbeke K. Von Willebrand factor to the rescue. *Blood* 2009;**113**(21):5049–5057.

184 Lipe BC, Dumas MA, and Ornstein DL. Von Willebrand disease in pregnancy. *Hematology/Oncology Clinics of North America* 2011;**25**(2):335–358, viii.

185 Kujovich JL. Von Willebrand disease and pregnancy. *Journal of Thrombosis and Haemostasis* 2005;**3**(2):246–253.

186 Sanchez-Luceros A, Meschengieser SS, Marchese C *et al.* Factor VIII and von Willebrand factor changes during normal pregnancy and puerperium. *Blood Coagulation & Fibrinolysis* 2003;**14**(7):647–651.

187 Kjellberg U, Andersson NE, Rosen S, Tengborn L, and Hellgren M. APC resistance and other haemostatic variables during pregnancy and puerperium. *Thrombosis and Haemostasis* 1999;**81**(4):527–531.

188 Mannucci PM. Treatment of von Willebrand's disease. *New England Journal of Medicine* 2004;**351**(7):683–694.

189 Choi S and Brull R. Neuraxial techniques in obstetric and non-obstetric patients with common bleeding diatheses. *Anesthesia & Analgesia* 2009;**109**(2):648–660.

CHAPTER 18
Postpartum care

Audrey Lyndon[1], Kirsten Wisner[2], and Kristina J. Hung[3]
[1] *School of Nursing, University of California, San Francisco, CA, USA*
[2] *Salinas Valley Memorial Hospital, Seaside, CA, USA*
[3] *San Francisco General Hospital and Trauma Center, San Francisco, CA, USA*

18.1 Goals of care

Dramatic physiologic, psychological, and emotional changes occur for women and their families after birth. The overarching goal of postpartum care is to provide a safe, family-centered environment where women and providers engage in shared decision making to select treatment plans that promote physiologic and emotional adaption and family bonding [1]. The birth process and the fourth stage of labor are dynamic and present potential risk to mother and baby. Most births proceed without incident and most women require minimal assistance with successful adaptation in the postpartum period, but providers must be prepared to respond to complications and emergencies. Providers should prioritize supporting natural physiologic processes with minimal intervention while remaining attuned to early recognition of complications.

18.2 Postpartum physiologic changes

The reproductive system undergoes a process of organ involution lasting 6–8 weeks involving the gradual return of the uterus, cervix, and vagina to their prepregnant states.

18.2.1 Uterus

Following delivery of the placenta, the uterus weighs an estimated 1000 g and rests midline within the pelvis, halfway between the symphysis pubis and umbilicus. By 12 hours, the uterine fundus is within 1–2 cm of the umbilicus. Over the

Management of Labor and Delivery, Second Edition. Edited by George A. Macones.

first postpartum week, fundal height descends approximately 1 cm/day; is palpable at 4–5 cm below the umbilicus by day 7, and shrinks within the true pelvis by day 16 [2]. Uterine weight decreases to 500, 300, and ≤ 100 g at 1, 2, and 4 weeks, respectively. Complete involution occurred by 8 weeks in all studied subjects. Serial ultrasound demonstrated uterine rotation of 100–180 degrees from retroversion on days 1–3; to midline on day 7; to a progressively anteverted position on days 28 and 56 [3].

Uterine involution includes repair of the site of placental detachment, as well as regeneration and remodeling of the entire endomyometrium. Hemostasis is achieved at the placental detachment site via arterial smooth muscle contraction, endarteritis in uterine vasculature, and compression of deeper myometrial vessels from forceful uterine contractions [4]. As early as 5 hours postpartum, doubling of the internal elastic lamina and thickening of the uterine vessel intima occurs [5]. Repetitive contractions immediately reduce the placental detachment site dimension from 18 to 9 cm. The initial endometrial slough that occurs with delivery of the placenta eliminates a portion of the decidua basalis at the level of the stratum spongiosum and penetrates the myometrial layer within several days. By the end of week 1, a superficial necrotic layer is clearly demarcated from the viable deeper layers of the endomyometrium. This is eliminated in lochia via exfoliation, leaving the remaining glandular endomyometrium to regenerate over the next 6 weeks [4].

Uterine tissue remote from the placental site is restored to its prepregnant state more quickly. Reversal of the estrogen-mediated hypertrophy and hyperplasia of myometrial cells begin immediately as proteolytic enzymes and macrophages eliminate excess intracellular proteins and cytoplasm, reducing cell volume and size. The decidual layer remaining after placental delivery differentiates into a superficial and basal layer by 2–3 days. Superficial granulation tissue, formed partly by leukocyte infiltration, necroses and is eliminated in lochia. New endometrium is formed from the remaining gland-rich basal layer. A proliferative mucosa is first recognizable by day 8–9. The endometrium is structurally restored to its non-pregnant state by day 16 [6].

18.2.2 Cervix and vagina

Immediately following vaginal birth, the cervix is edematous with interstitial hemorrhages, retaining much of the vascular hypertrophy and hyperplasia present at term. Restoration of the endocervical lining, glands, and stroma begins by day 4; however, pregnancy-induced vascular changes persist beyond the first week [7]. For the first several days, the cervix has minimal tone, and is dilated 2–3 cm. By the end of week 1, it has grossly returned to its prepregnant state, with cellular alterations persisting for 2–4 months [8,9]. Increased vascularity and edema within the vaginal walls obliterate vaginal rugae, causing a smooth and edematous appearance following birth. By 3 weeks, rugae return, and restoration of vaginal epithelium is achieved at 6–10 weeks.

18.2.3 Lochia

Lochia is generated from uterine involution and endometrial repair. Three forms are observed which typically progress from rubra (red or reddish brown), to serosa (pinkish-brown), to alba (whitish-yellow). Lochial transitions may be influenced by breastfeeding duration and parity [10].

Lochia rubra has a fleshy odor and is usually seen up to day 3–4. It contains blood, decidual cells, vernix, meconium and lanugo, and chorioamniotic remnants. From day 4 to 4 weeks, the progressively lightened discharge lochia serosa is present, and may contain blood, decidual tissue, exudates, mucous, microorganisms, erythrocytes, and leukocytes. Alba may present from 3–6 weeks, and contains decidual cells and leukocytes. Median total duration of lochia has been reported as 27 days in two large studies [11,12], with median ranges in subsamples in the largest study varying in length from 22 to 34 days [12].

18.2.4 Return of menses and ovulation

The return of menses and ovulation is variable, and may be influenced by breastfeeding patterns. Lactation disrupts secretion of gonadotropin-releasing hormone (GnRH), causing suppression of leutenizing hormone (LH) and follicle stimulating hormone (FSH). As lactation frequency decreases, GnRH secretion normalizes, causing LH release and resumption of a normal follicular cycle [13,14]. Most non-lactating women will resume menstruating by 6–8 weeks postpartum [15,16]. Wide variation exists in the percentage of first menses that are anovulatory (29–80%). Even when preceded by ovulation, many (30–100%) first postpartum menses may be subfertile due to inadequate corpus luteum function [15,17]. Given the erratic return of ovulation and variable effects of lactation on fertility, contraceptive planning prior to discharge to home is critically important.

18.2.5 Cardiovascular and hematologic

Cardiac output (CO) increases by as much as 80% immediately postpartum. Venous return and stroke volume increase through autotransfusion of blood from the uteroplacental unit, mobilization of extravascular fluid, and relief of venacaval obstruction by the gravid uterus. Cardiac output returns to pre-labor values by 24–48 hours [18,19].

Left atrial dimensions increase up to 3 days after delivery. In addition to increased preload from increased venous return, elevated atrial natriuretic levels originating from atrial myocytes may facilitate dieresis and natriuresis early in the postpartum period [20]. The most dramatic reductions in heart rate, stroke volume, cardiac output, systemic vascular resistance, and hemoglobin and hematocrit occur by 2 weeks [21]. However, remnants of pregnancy-related elevations in CO, mean arterial pressure, left ventricular end-diastolic and stroke volume have been observed as late as 6–12 months following delivery [18,22].

While the left atrium is restored to normal size by day 10, enlarged left ventricular wall dimensions and dilation of the semilunar valves may persist beyond 6 months [21].

18.2.6 Renal, hepatic, and gastrointestinal

Marked renal hyperfiltration occurs immediately postpartum, but glomerular filtration rate, serum creatinine clearance, and renal plasma flow return to normal limits by 2–6 weeks [23,24]. Regression of pregnancy-induced anatomic changes (increased kidney length, and ureteral and pelvocaliceal dilation) may take up to 3 months [25]. While of no apparent physiologic consequence, some degree of pelvocaliceal dilation may persist for years. Diuresis and naturesis begin by day 4, with restoration of fluid and sodium balance completed by day 21 [24].

Serial evaluations of hepatic enzymes indicated that aspartate transaminase (AST), alanine transaminase (ALT), and total bilirubin all peak by postpartum day 5 and normalize within 10 days. Gamma glutamyl transferase elevates later (day 5–10), and alkaline phosphatase – already elevated by as much as 300% during pregnancy – rises intrapartum and may take up to 13 days to normalize [26]. Mode of birth may affect postnatal values of AST and ALT, with cesarean birth causing steeper elevations [26]. Serum triglycerides, high-density lipoproteins (HDLs), and very low-density lipoproteins (VLDLs) return to non-pregnant levels by 6 weeks postpartum. Elevations in low-density lipoproteins (LDLs), as well as alterations in LDL composition, may persist beyond 20 weeks [27].

Lower esophageal sphincter pressure normalizes as early as 2 days [28] and as late as 1–4 weeks postpartum [29]. During pregnancy, gallbladder motility decreases creating a predisposition to sludge formation. While gallbladder volume may return to normal by 2 weeks, existing stones or sludge may delay the return to normal volumes [28,30]. Gastrointestinal motility decreases intrapartum, which may cause bloating and distension in the first few days postpartum. Most women will have a bowel movement by day 2–3, and resume regular bowel function within 1–2 weeks.

18.2.7 Endocrine

Similar patterns of decline in levels of FSH, LH, human chorionic gonadatropin (HCG), progesterone, and estrogen are seen for several weeks in breastfeeding and non-breastfeeding women. In both groups, levels of FSH, HCG, and LH all decline for about 3 weeks, at which time LH stabilizes, HCG is virtually undetectable, and FSH gradually increases until reaching normal follicular phase levels. Progesterone drops rapidly within the first week and remains low in both groups for up to 7 weeks [31]. Prolactin levels are significantly lower in non-breastfeeding women by 72 hours postpartum and fall rapidly thereafter reaching prepregnant levels by 1–3 weeks [31,32]. In breastfeeding women, prolactin levels decline gradually, remaining higher than non-pregnant values for at least 6 weeks. Breastfeeding causes surges of prolactin release within 30 minutes of initiation of suckling, with the most dramatic surges observed 10–40 days postpartum. After 80 days, suckling has little effect on prolactin release [32]. Estrogen follows a similar pattern of decline in both groups for about 3 weeks; thereafter non-lactating women demonstrate a steady increase, while levels in breastfeeding women remain suppressed.

18.2.8 Respiratory

Most pregnancy-induced respiratory changes resolve within several weeks. Resting minute ventilation, which is increased by 20–50% at term, declines 10–25% by 72 hours postpartum, and reaches prepregnant values by a few weeks. Static lung volumes rapidly normalize after birth as the diaphragm and lungs are relieved of uterine compression. Functional residual capacity and residual volume, reduced by up to 30 and 25% respectively in pregnancy, are restored to baseline within 48 hours. Chest wall expansion can take 24 weeks to return to normal. The subcostal angle remains approximately 20% wider compared to a non-pregnant baseline [33].

18.2.9 Integumentary

Most women (≥90%) experience some skin hyperpigmentation during pregnancy in the genital region or nearby skin folds, areola, or demarcation lines (linea nigra). Hyperpigmentation usually regresses postpartum, although complete elimination may not occur. Melasma of the face may take up to a year to disappear, lingering longer in approximately 30% of women. Vascular changes such as spider angiomas, arterial spiders, spider nevi, and nevi aranei should fade or disappear within 3 months. Erythema of the palmar surfaces or finger pads, and mottling, cyanosis, or pallor of the palm usually disappears within a week [34]. Rare pruritic rashes of pregnancy usually clear within a few weeks.

Gingivitis begins to regress at term and may take several months to disappear. Edema from venous congestion and increased vessel permeability resolves quickly as hemodynamic and vascular stability is achieved early in the postpartum period. Hemorrhoids and varicosities should improve, but often are not completely eliminated. Striae resulting from tears in dermal connective tissue will fade considerably [34].

Telogen gravidarum refers to postpartum hair loss at 1–5 months. Hair follicles cycle through a several-year cycle of anagen (growth), telogen (resting), and catagen (involution). During pregnancy, telogen is delayed, causing a lengthened anagen phase, netting increased hair volume. Postpartum, conversion from anagen to telogen accelerates, resulting in a release of hair follicles and noticeable shedding of hair [35]. Shedding is complete by 3–6 months, with regrowth occurring by 9 months [36].

18.2.10 Metabolic

Approximately 11 kg of maternal weight gain during pregnancy is attributed to maternal and fetal components. Maternal tissues including blood components and extracellular fluid, uterine, breast, and adipose tissue contribute about 6 kg. The remaining 5 kg is attributed to the fetus, placenta, and amniotic fluid [37]. An average of 4.5–5.8 kg is shed during birth from loss of fetal weight, associated tissues, and blood. Additional losses of 2–5 kg result from diuresis, perspiration, and uterine involution after birth. The most significant weight loss is usually seen in the first 3 months, with gradual declines up to 6 months. Most women retain about 1 kg for each pregnancy. Lower parity, age, and prepregnant weight are associated with faster and greater weight loss [38]. Similarly, breastfeeding is associated with more weight loss postpartum, with an additional loss of 1.5 lb for each week of breastfeeding. Conversely, exceeding recommended guidelines for weight gain is associated with increased retention of weight at 1 year postpartum [39].

18.3 The fourth stage of labor

Rapid changes in the uterine vasculature at the site of placental detachment and dramatic shifts in maternal hemodynamic status make the immediate recovery period a particularly vulnerable time for the mother. The profound physiologic changes associated with pregnancy and the immediate postpartum period can mask signs of decompensation and reveal previously unappreciated problems such as cardiac compromise. Heightened surveillance of hemodynamic status and uterine involution can assist the clinical team in recognizing and responding to complications.

Physiologic monitoring in the immediate postpartum period should be guided by type and severity of any co-morbidities and risk factors, complications during labor and birth, and type of anesthesia or analgesia used. Sensitivity and responsiveness to the psychosocial, emotional, and cultural needs of the mother and infant should be prioritized along with the provision of timely clinical interventions aimed at maintaining or achieving stability. Assessment of maternal heart rate, blood pressure, respiratory rate, pain level, fundal height and tone, and amount and characteristics of lochia should be assessed every 15 minutes for the first 2 hours following vaginal birth; for cesarean birth, monitoring should also include oxygen saturation, and regression of surgical block or parameters for recovery from general anesthesia [40]. Most maternal and infant assessments can be accomplished with the infant skin-to-skin on the maternal chest following both types of birth, thus facilitating early and uninterrupted interaction between the mother and infant. The trajectory of normal postpartum adaptation during inpatient recovery is outlined in Table 18.1.

Table 18.1 Trajectory of normal recovery in the inpatient period.

	Immediate recovery	PPD 1	PPD 2	PPD 3	PPD 4
Fundal height	Midline, between umbilicus and pubis	• First 12h may ↑ or ↓ 1–2 cm • ≥12h, ↓ 1cm/day, midline • Usually retroverted [3]	↓ 1 cm/day, midline, usually retroverted [3]		
Lochia	• Rubra • Small clots normal if accompanied by light-moderate bleeding	• Rubra • Gradual ↓ for first several days • Excess bleeding, clots, cramping or slow fundal descent may indicate subinvolution of placental site or retained placental fragments • Retained placental fragments can secrete progesterone and cause delayed lactogenesis II [41]			• Rubra • Serosabegin
Breastfeeding	• Initiate skin-to-skin immediately • Maintain skin-to-skin during recovery period or through first feeding [42,43]	• Assess: latch, mother's response to infant cues • Teaching: demand-supply, infant cues, positioning, and latch • 8–12 feeds/day [44] • Assess for stress/fatigue, may delay lactogenesis II [45]		Lactogenesis II : • Dramatic ↑ milk volume • Usually begins around 60h PP • Delayed if > 72h PP • Delayed lactogenesis II may affect ability to sustain and/or exclusively breastfeed [43]	
Cardiac function [18]	• Cardiac output ↑ up to 80% • Stroke volume and heart rate ↑	• Cardiac output to pre-labor values by 24–48h • Stroke volume remains ↑ • Dramatic ↓ in HR after 24h		• Gradual ↓ in cardiac output throughout PP period • Dramatic ↓ in stroke volume after 48h	
Fluid balance		Edema may ↑ due to mobilization of extravascular fluids			Diuresis usually begins PPD 4 [24]
Perineum	• Cleanse with plain water • Observe for unresponsive pain; signs/symptoms of infection • Increased risk of wound breakdown with severe lacerations				
CS special considerations	• ↑ VTE risk, especially in presence of other risk factors (see Table 18.8) [46] • Five- to 20-fold increased risk of infectious morbidity [47]				

(continued)

Table 18.1 (*continued*)

	Immediate recovery	PPD 1	PPD 2	PPD 3	PPD 4
CS wound assessment	• Scant bleeding or serosa normal, monitor drainage for ↑ bleeding • Dressing dry, intact	S/S of wound infection: • Purulent drainage, fever, pain, erythema, induration, spontaneous wound dehiscence, and/or abscess [48] • Most wound infections occur after discharge; educate patient re: signs and symptoms requiring follow-up [49,50]			
Infection surveillance		↑ temperature during first 24h may be normal	Monitor for signs and symptoms of infection: • Temperature > 38°C, 2x, 4–6h apart ≥ 24h after birth, or > 38.5°C at any time [51,52] • Uterine/parametrial tenderness, abnormal discharge or odor, leukocytosis, tachycardia, slow fundal descent [51–53]		

18.3.1 Skin-to-skin contact

Healthy infants should be placed skin-to-skin on their mother's chest immediately after birth, and remain so at least until after the first breastfeeding, unless medically contraindicated [54,42]. Early skin-to-skin contact benefits both mother and infant, and facilitates breastfeeding. In contrast, early separation of the mother and neonate may be harmful and have long-term behavioral consequences for both mother and infant [55,56].

Early skin-to-skin contact is associated with less breast engorgement pain, lower maternal anxiety, and increased maternal satisfaction and confidence [57]. Infant benefits include thermal regulation and stability, decreased crying, higher blood glucose, and cardio-respiratory stability [57]. Skin-to-skin contact promotes neurobehavioral organization, which correlates with improved breastfeeding behaviors [58,59], resulting in higher rates of successful breastfeeding initiation and increased breastfeeding duration [57].

Skin-to-skin contact should be provided as soon as possible after birth, regardless of the mode of birth, and supported and encouraged through the recovery and early postpartum period, since the mother provides the ideal environment for successful newborn transition to the extrauterine environment. The naked infant should lie prone on a mother's bare chest, with the infant's back covered by warm blankets and a cap on the infant's head. After cesarean births, skin-to-skin contact is initiated within a half hour after the infant is able to respond, which is typically immediately with regional anesthesia [60]. Routine medications and assessments can be done during skin-to-skin, and newborn weighing and bathing delayed to promote uninterrupted contact in the critical first hours of life [54].

18.3.2 Breastfeeding

Keys to successful breastfeeding include initiation within the first hour after birth and early skin-to-skin contact [61]. Early breastfeeding benefits the infant, decreases postpartum bleeding, and promotes uterine involution [44]. The mother's breasts should remain unwashed, without scented products applied, since olfaction plays a role in attracting the infant to the mother's breast [62].

A healthy newborn can spontaneously latch on to the mother's breast unassisted and suckle within the first hour of life [54]. Early and undisturbed skin-to-skin contact promotes early self-regulation leading to self-attachment onto the breast [62,63]. Infants go through inborn sequential behaviors including: a birth cry, relaxation (no activity), awakening (small head and limb movements), active head and limb movements, crawling (pushing or shifting the body), resting (may include mouth activity or sucking on the hand), familiarization (brushing or licking of the areola and nipple), and finally suckling of the nipple and sleeping [62].

Breastmilk feeding benefits mothers, infants, and society. Mothers who breastfeed lower their risk of ovarian cancer, breast cancer, and type 2 diabetes [64]. Infants who are breastfed have a lower risk of acute otitis media, asthma, lower respiratory infections, sudden infant death syndrome (SIDS), non-specific gastroenteritis, obesity, types 1 and 2 diabetes, atopic dermatitis, and childhood leukemia [64]. Infant formula lacks the growth factors and protective qualities of human milk. Early ingestion of even small amounts of artificial milk changes the gut flora [65]. If 90% of infants in the United States were exclusively breastfed until 6 months of age, the United States would save an estimated $13 billion and over 900 deaths would be prevented annually [66].

Human breastmilk has a complex array of over 200 components that change significantly throughout the postpartum period; it is comprised of bioactive substances that target the developing human brain and immune system [65]. Colostrum is a thick, yellowish fluid with anti-infective properties appearing in the first few days after birth in volumes of 2–20 mL per feeding [65]. Colostrum is high in protein, potassium, sodium, chloride, fat-soluble vitamins, carotenoids, and pancreatic secretory trypsin inhibitor, which plays a crucial role in protecting and preparing the intestines for future food. Colostrum is highly concentrated with antioxidants, antibodies, and immunoglobulins, and is especially beneficial to preterm infants. Transitional milk appears 6–13 days postpartum, evolving into mature milk within 2 weeks [65]. Breastmilk contains water, lipids, proteins, carbohydrates, microminerals and vitamins, including thiamin (vitamin B1), folate, riboflavin (vitamin B12), pyridoxine (vitamin B6), niacin, pantothenate, biotin, ascorbic acid (vitamin C), and vitamins A, D, E, and K [65].

The breast is supported by Cooper's ligaments, supplied with blood through the internal mammary and lateral thoracic arteries, and enervated by the second to fifth intercostal nerves. The breast is composed of glandular and adipose tissue. Each breast contains 15–20 connected lobes with 10–100 alveoli per lobule [67]. Alveoli, the basic units of the breast's glandular tissue, are composed of acinar units [68], and are surrounded by myoepithelial cells which contract and eject milk into the ductules. Each breast contains nine main ducts on average, which open to the surface at the nipple [68,69]. The areola surrounds the nipple; both contain erectile smooth muscles. Montgomery tubercles on the areola are made up of sebaceous and mammary milk glands, which secrete a fluid that is associated with earlier onset of lactogenesis II and increased weight gain in breastfeeding infants [70]. Milk is secreted into the alveoli and stored there until oxytocin causes the letdown reflex triggering contraction of myoepithelial cells and milk ejection [68].

Breast size is not associated with milk production; however, mothers with hypoplastic breasts, or who have had breast augmentation or reduction, require increased follow-up, monitoring of infant weight gain, and lactation support [65]. These mothers need to stimulate their breasts frequently through breastfeeding, hand expression, or pumping to maximize their milk supply. Flat, retracted, or inverted nipples are common, but most will protrude with stimulation and areolar softening [65].

Lactogenesis I refers to the mammary gland development during pregnancy [71]. In the postpartum period, lactogenesis II is marked by dramatic increases in milk volume 3–4 days after birth, triggered by the drop in progesterone following placental delivery. Establishment of lactation involves increased levels of prolactin, cortisol, insulin, thyroid-stimulating hormone, prolactin-inhibiting factor, and oxytocin [68,71]. Lactation is maintained as milk is removed and produced to match the infant's intake [68].

The American Academy of Pediatrics recommends exclusive breastfeeding for the first 6 months of life, and continued breastfeeding with the introduction of complementary foods for a year or more [44]. Contraindications to breastfeeding are listed in Table 18.2. Breastfeeding on demand is important until the milk supply is well established. Infants should breastfeed 8–12 times in a 24-hour period [44]. Feedings should not be scheduled; parents should be encouraged to feed on demand by watching for infant feeding cues, such as mouthing, rooting, physical activity, or increased alertness [44,63,71]. Infants may feed frequently several times and then have a longer break, or alternate feedings from one or both breasts [71]. Crying is a late hunger sign, and it may be more difficult to obtain an appropriate latch once the infant reaches this point. Mother and infant should remain together (rooming-in) throughout their hospital stay to facilitate frequent breastfeeding [60].

Appropriate positioning for breastfeeding involves close, comfortable, and supportive positioning for both mother and infant, with the infant's head and

Table 18.2 Contraindications to breastfeeding.

Condition	Comments
HTLV-1, HTLV-2	
Maternal HIV	Contraindicated in developed nations
Active untreated tuberculosis	Expressed milk can be given by different care provider
Active herpes simplex lesion on breast	
Newborn galactosemia	
Medication	
Chemotherapeutic agents	Express and discard milk to maintain supply if contraindication is temporary
Amphetamines	
Statins	
Ergotamines	

Adapted from American Academy of Pediatrics, Breastfeeding and the use of human milk [50] and American Academy of Pediatrics, Sample hospital breastfeeding policy for newborns [54].

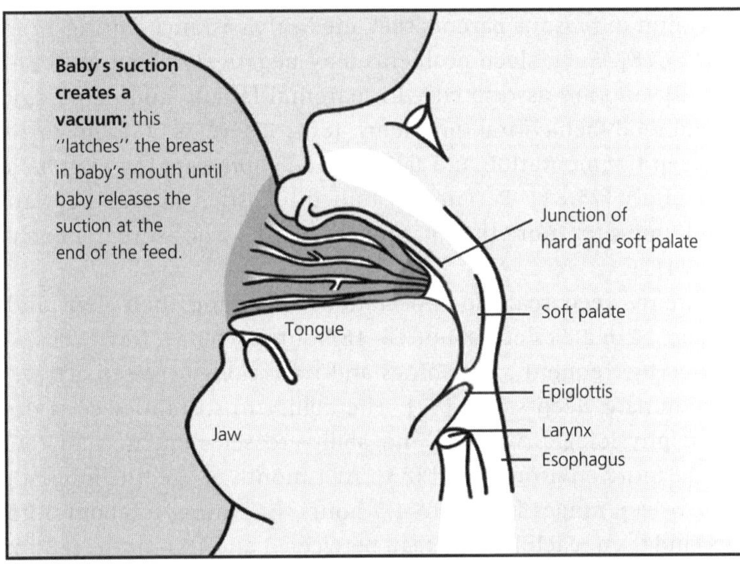

Figure 18.1 Anatomy of a proper latch. *Source*: Rebecca Glover. Reproduced with permission of Rebecca Glover.

body aligned over his or her hips and head free to tilt back [63]. The latch is asymmetric, where the infant's head tilts back and the jaw drops into the breast, and more areola is seen at the infant's top lip (Figure 18.1). Latching onto the breast with a wide-open mouth protects the mother's nipple and maximizes milk transfer [63]. Semi-reclined maternal positioning known as "biological nurturing" may elicit primitive neonatal reflexes aiding successful breastfeeding [72]. Mothers should be encouraged to completely empty one breast before offering the other to maximize transfer of the higher fat hind milk [65].

Fatigue and stress can lower prolactin and increase cortisol levels, delaying lactogenesis [45]. Mothers with depression need early support as they report more breastfeeding difficulties and lower breastfeeding self-efficacy [73]. Depressed mothers should be encouraged to continue breastfeeding since breastfeeding is associated with lower levels of depressive symptoms [45,73] and breastfeeding mothers get more sleep [74].

18.3.3 Maternal-infant sleep

New mothers experience shortened, highly fragmented sleep and often spend hours awake each night [75]. Tiredness is the most common complaint in the postpartum period. Two-thirds of mothers report tiredness as a problem during the first 2 months, and over half of mothers report it as a major problem through the first year [76]. Mothers experience a decline in sleep efficiency postpartum, with increased nighttime awakenings and increased daytime sleepiness [77].

Sleep disturbance related to infant waking, crying, and feeding is among the most common reasons parents seek medical assistance during an infant's first year [75,78]. Such sleep problems may negatively affect mother-infant bonding [79], and are associated with parental fatigue and depression, and future childhood behavioral problems [80]. There is a high correlation between sleep fragmentation and fatigue, and short napping may have little restorative effect [75,81]. Parents of studied breastfed infants slept an average of 40–45 minutes more than parents of infants who were not exclusively breastfed [74].

New parents need realistic expectations regarding their own and their infant's sleep. Neonates sleep about 16–18 hours each day. Newborns' sleep is characterized by frequent awakenings and transitions between active, quiet, and indeterminate sleep states [82]. The ability to sustain sleep is developmental and physiologic, whereas the ability to self-regulate and return to sleep may be more environmental [83]. At 1 month of age, the longest period of sustained sleep ranges from 3 to 4.5 hours, increasing to about 6 hours at 2 months, and then reaching a plateau between 3 and 12 months [83]. Infants are increasingly able to self-regulate and return to sleep without assistance during this time. The duration of self-regulated sleep usually exceeds 7 hours by 3 months [83].

Mother-infant bed sharing is associated with increased duration of breastfeeding; increased number, but shorter duration, of nocturnal awakenings [84]; and increased total sleep time for breastfeeding mothers [75]. Conversely, evidence suggests bed sharing is associated with sudden infant death syndrome (SIDS) among smokers. This association is less clear among nonsmokers [84]. Safe infant sleep guidelines include recommendations for supine positioning. Prone positioning is associated with higher risk of SIDS, more difficult arousability, and lower levels of cerebral oxygenation [85].

18.3.4 Psychological/psychosocial adaptation

New mothers experience disruptions in daily life, relationships, self-identity, work, and commitments [86]. In the 1960s, Rubin described the "transition to motherhood" as phases that include: taking-in, taking-hold, and letting-go [87,88]. The taking-in phase encompasses the first few days as the mother recovers from birth by sleeping, eating, exhibiting a "passively dependent" behavior, and discussing details of her birth to move into the present [87]. During taking-hold, she focuses on the tasks of mothering, and may become anxious about her new responsibilities [87]. She becomes acutely interested in the care of her infant and any difficulty may be experienced as failure [89]. During letting-go, roles or identities that are no longer compatible with her new role as a mother are relinquished, and she expands her focus outside of herself and her newborn [88,90].

In the 1980s, Mercer defined maternal role attainment as a process of achieving role competence and integrating social norms regarding mothering behaviors into her role and maternal identity [91]. The landscape of parenting has changed dramatically since these theories were developed. Even by the mid-1980s, research suggests that few mothers were as dependent as Rubin described in the 1960s [92]. A more modern-day understanding values the diverse, complex, and changing experience of each individual woman, including evolving gender roles and family structure [93,94]. The early theories do not account for the large variation in women's inner experience before, during, and after birth. It can be disempowering to a woman when "appropriate mothering" is homogenized and the reality of her lived experience is ignored or overlooked [93]. Postpartum care should be individualized, with high value placed on engaging with each woman rather than completing a set of routine examinations and documentation [95]. In addition to the normal physical and emotional changes of birth, a woman may have a variety of psychosocial issues that impact her health, including domestic violence, a history of physical or sexual abuse, substance abuse, depression, social isolation, mental illness, or a lack of financial, interpersonal, or social support [95].

Maternal behavior observed by clinicians may not be consistent with a woman's perception of her maternal competence [96]. Furthermore, health professionals should consider differences in cultural beliefs and traditional postpartum practices since conflict between cultural practices and advice given by health professionals can reduce women's confidence [97]. A woman-centered approach involves actively listening to each woman's story and factors she feels impact her changing experience, acknowledging the woman as a powerful expert on her own life processes [95]. Promoting continuity of care throughout and after pregnancy can aid in this communication and support [95].

18.3.5 Contraception

Planning for postpartum contraception should begin during pregnancy. Choice of contraception should be guided by venous thromboembolism (VTE) risk, breastfeeding practices, timing, and patient preference. Other considerations

Table 18.3 CDC categories for classifying hormonal contraceptives and intrauterine devices.

1. A condition for which there is no restriction for the use of the contraceptive method
2. A condition for which the advantages of using the method generally outweigh the theoretical or proven risks
3. A condition where the theoretical or proven risks usually outweigh the advantages of using the method
4. A condition that represents an unacceptable health risk if the contraceptive method is used

include cost, access to health care, and potential exposure to sexually transmitted infections.

The World Health Organization [98] and the Centers for Disease Control [99] have published guidelines regarding postpartum initiation of contraception and specific contraceptive use in the presence of certain co-morbidities, risk factors, and breastfeeding (Table 18.3). While most recommendations contained in these two guidelines are the same, some differences exist and are summarized in Table 18.4.

18.3.5.1 Centers for disease control medical eligibility criteria

For breastfeeding and non-breastfeeding women, condoms, spermicides, and the copper intrauterine device (Cu-IUD) inserted immediately postpartum (<10 min following placental delivery) are assigned a category 1. If not placed immediately, the Cu-IUD is assigned a category 2 in both groups (≥10 min to ≤ 4 weeks), as is the levonorgestrel-releasing IUD (LNG-IUD) if placed ≤ 4 weeks. Both IUDs are category 1 if placed ≥ 4 weeks postpartum [99,100]. Expulsion rates are higher for IUDs placed in the immediate postpartum period overall when compared to insertion ≥ 6 weeks postpartum [101,102]. However, expulsion rates are lower if placed within the first 10 minutes following placental delivery compared to placement up to 72 hours [103], and are lower for immediate placement after cesarean when compared to vaginal birth [102].

The risks of combined hormonal contraceptives (CHCs; combined oral contraceptive pill, hormonal patch, and vaginal ring) within the first 21 days postpartum are considered unacceptably high for all women, largely due to the heightened risk of venous thromboembolism [104], and concerns over the effect of CHCs on milk production and infant growth in lactating women. From 21 to 42 days, the risks associated with CHCs generally outweigh the benefits in women who have other risk factors for VTE, but benefits outweigh theoretical or proven risks for non-lactating women without VTE risk factors.

For breastfeeding women without risk factors for VTE, CHCs are not advised for 21–30 days postpartum, but benefits outweigh risks thereafter. There are no restrictions on the use of progestin-only contraceptives (POCs; progestin-only pills, depot medroxyprogesterone acetate injections) and implants in non-lactating women throughout the postpartum period, and for breastfeeding women after day 30.

Table 18.4 Recommendations for postpartum hormonal, intrauterine, and barrier contraceptive use.

Method	WHO (1–4)		CDC (1–4)	
Breastfeeding status:	BF	NBF	BF	NBF
BF = breastfeeding				
NBF = non-breastfeeding				
Cu-IUD:				
Immediate[a]	1	1	1	1
Delayed PP[b]	3	3	2	2
≥4 weeks	1	1	1	1
Puerperal sepsis	4	4	4	4
LNG-IUD:				
Immediate	3	1	2	2
Delayed PP	3	3	2	2
≥4 weeks	1	1	1	1
Puerperal sepsis	4	4	4	4
CHCs:				
With other VTE risk factors:				
<21 days	4	3/4[c]	4	4
21 to < 30 days[d]	4	2/3	3	3
30–42 days[e]	4	2/3	3	3
Without other VTE risk factors:				
<21 days	4	3	4	4
21 to < 30 days	4	2	3	2
30–42 days	4	2	2	2
≥42 days to < 6 months[f]	3	1	2 (>42d)	1(>42d)
≥6 months[g]	2			
POCs:				
<21 days	3	1	2	1
21 to < 30 days	3	1	2	1
30–42 days	3	1	1	1
≥42 days to < 6 months	1	1		
≥6 months	1			
Condoms	1	1	1	1
Diaphragm and cervical cap	Contraindicated in first 6 weeks postpartum			

Abbreviations: CHC-combined hormonal contraception; Cu-IUD-copper IUD; LNG-IUD-levonorgestrel-releasing IUD; POC-progestin-only contraception, PP-postpartum VTE-venous thromboembolism.

[a] Immediate postpartum placement is defined by CDC as < 10 min from placental expulsion, and by WHO as < 48 hrs postpartum.

[b] Delayed postpartum placement is defined by CDC as 10 min to < 4 weeks, and by WHO as ≥ 48 hrs to < 4 weeks postpartum.

[c] WHO assigns range values to certain categories (i.e. 2/3 or 3/4) signifying that each woman's risk profile is unique. Providers then assign the category based on the number, severity and combination of risk factors, allowing for the application of clinical judgment.

[d–g] WHO guidelines do not use the interval of 21–30 days. Other time intervals differ between the CDC and WHO guidelines. See specific sections within each guideline [98–100].

Before 30 days, the benefits of POCs generally outweigh the risks in breastfeeding women. This is based on data from animal studies and anecdotal clinical evidence regarding progesterone's effect on infant growth and development and on early milk production. Data from high-quality clinical trials are lacking.

Fitting for a diaphragm or cervical cap should be delayed until 6 weeks postpartum when involution of the cervix is complete [9]. Likewise, if this method was used before pregnancy, refitting should occur at 6 weeks since the cervix's shape and dimensions can change following birth. A risk category is not assigned to female surgical sterilization since no medical conditions absolutely contradict its use, but if not done within a few days postpartum, sterilization is generally delayed until after uterine involution is complete [105].

The lactational amenorrhea method (LAM) relies on breastfeeding as a contraceptive method. Exclusive, regular breastfeeding in the presence of amenorrhea during the first 6 months postpartum is associated with a 98% contraceptive efficacy rate [106]. Regular feeding means no between-feeding intervals of greater than 4 or 6 hours for daytime or nighttime feedings, respectively. Exclusive breastfeeding is defined as supplemental food comprising no more than 5–10% of feedings. At 6 months postpartum in exclusively breastfeeding women, LAM has an efficacy rate of 94%. Women should be counseled to initiate other forms of birth control should they begin menstruating, when supplemental feeds are introduced, or at 6 months if high-efficacy contraception is desired [106].

18.4 Complications

18.4.1 Hemorrhage

Postpartum hemorrhage remains a leading cause of maternal mortality throughout the world [107]. Although US hemorrhage-related deaths have declined steadily since the late 1980s, postpartum hemorrhage still accounts for about 10% of US pregnancy-related deaths and approximately one-third of maternal deaths globally [107,108]. While the US mortality profile for pregnancy-related hemorrhage has improved, the rate of postpartum hemorrhage increased from 2.3 to 2.9% between 1994 and 2006 in a nationally representative sample [109]. Critical issues for successful prevention and management of postpartum hemorrhage include risk assessment, early recognition of excessive bleeding, and timely interventions to support maternal fluid volume and oxygenation while simultaneously identifying and addressing the underlying etiology [110,111].

The leading etiology of postpartum hemorrhage is uterine atony [107,109,112]. This is primarily a function of the remodeling of the uterine artery vasculature in pregnancy: uterine arteries are incapable of autoregulation after placental separation, and depend on firm and sustained myometrial contraction for constriction of blood flow. The atonic uterus allows rapid, large-volume blood loss through maximally dilated uterine arteries. Hemorrhage may also be caused by decidual factors such as abnormal placentation, systemic factors such as coagulation disorders or coagulopathy, and local injuries such as lacerations, uterine rupture, and uterine inversion [110].

Risk factors for postpartum hemorrhage are listed in Table 18.5 by etiology. While the majority of postpartum hemorrhage occurs in women without risk factors, preparation can be enhanced through implementation of a systematic approach to risk assessment for all women, including assessment of prenatal risk factors such as anemia, abnormal placentation, and inherited coagulopathies. Intrapartum risk factors should be assessed upon admission and throughout labor and birth for both static (e.g. known coagulation disorder) and dynamic risks (e.g. prolonged labor, chorioamnionitis) [110,111].

Prenatal risk factor identification facilitates amelioration of risk through treatment and/or coordination of necessary resources [110,111]. For example, severe prenatal anemia that is insufficiently responsive to oral iron can be treated with IV iron sucrose, and arrangements for birth at a tertiary center and special equipment or personnel (e.g. for intraoperative cell salvage) made for women diagnosed with placenta accreta. Specific plans, including optimization of antenatal hemoglobin levels and consideration of cell salvage, acute normovolemic hemodilution, and acceptability of various products, should be made in advance for women who may refuse some or all types of blood component replacement [111,113].

Table 18.5 Etiology and risk factors for postpartum hemorrhage.

Cause	Risk factor(s)
Uterine atony	Polyhydramnios, multifetal gestation, grand multiparity, macrosomia, rapid or prolonged labor, chorioamnionitis, uterine relaxants
Obstetric trauma	Operative delivery, macrosomia, precipitous delivery, episiotomy
Retained placenta	Placenta accreta/increta/percreta, placental succenturiate lobe, previous cesarean delivery, placenta previa
Acquired coagulopathy	Anticoagulant use, placental abruption, amniotic fluid embolism, preeclampsia, retained intrauterine fetal demise
Inherited coagulopathy	von Willebrand disease, hemophilia, idiopathic thrombocytopenic purpura
Uterine rupture	Previous uterine surgery, internal podalic version, prolonged labor, midforceps delivery, uterotonic use, high parity
Uterine inversion	Uterine atony, excessive cord traction, macrosomia, fundal placentation, oxytocin use, primiparity, placenta accreta, uterine anomalies
Cesarean delivery	General anesthesia, obesity, preeclampsia, chorioamnionitis
General	History of hemorrhage, inadequate prenatal care

Source: Haeri & Dildy [110]. Reproduced with permission of Elsevier.

Timely recognition and early identification of the etiology of hemorrhage aid successful management [110,114]. Issues in recognition include clinician capacity for accurate estimation of blood loss, and understanding of signs and symptoms of hemorrhage. Postpartum hemorrhage is typically defined by estimated blood loss or by percent change in hematocrit. Historically, blood loss greater than 500 or 1000 mL after a vaginal or cesarean birth, respectively, or a 10% reduction in hematocrit, constitute postpartum hemorrhage [115]. Both approaches have limitations. Use of changes in hematocrit is problematic, as significant and potentially life-threatening delays in care can occur if treatment is deferred until laboratory results are obtained [111]. Visual estimation of blood loss is problematic because clinicians underestimate and overestimate blood volumes in the postpartum setting, tending to overestimate small blood volumes and significantly underestimate large blood volumes [116–119]. Education regarding blood volumes [118–121] and the use of graduated drapes and gravimetric methods of assessment of blood loss can improve accuracy [121–123]. A standardized approach to routine quantification of blood loss using graduated drapes and cylinders, monitoring of irrigation fluid volume, and weighing of blood-soaked materials for all births is recommended [111].

A second issue in recognition of hemorrhage is appropriate vigilance regarding the norms for vital signs and clinical symptoms after birth. The physiologic changes of pregnancy create the opportunity for rapid and massive blood loss. Signs clinicians associate with blood loss, such as low blood pressure, are late signs: hypovolemic shock is typically already present by the time hypotension is apparent. Earlier signs include tachycardia, widening pulse pressure, and increased respiratory rate. "Early warning" systems or vital sign trigger tools, such as the Modified Early Obstetric Warning System [124], can help clinicians proactively recognize hemorrhage. Reviews of mortality cases indicate the importance of identifying a working diagnosis addressing etiology of hemorrhage and quickly moving through escalating levels of therapy rather than repeating procedures or doses of uterotonic medications that have been ineffective [110,111,114]. The principle issues to be addressed in responding to obstetric hemorrhage are summarized in Table 18.6, and the most common uterotonic agents are listed in Table 18.7. Recent changes in hemorrhage management include less aggressive use of crystalloid, more aggressive blood product replacement, and the use of 1:1:1 ratios of fresh frozen plasma, red blood cell products, and platelets [125–127]. These changes are based on advances in management of massive trauma outside of the obstetric setting. No randomized controlled trials support the effectiveness of these practices. Some centers recommend the use of recombinant factor VIIa (rfVIIa) prior to proceeding to hysterectomy in cases of uncontrolled bleeding [125], but this strategy remains controversial due to the potentially significant side effects of rfVIIa and difficulty obtaining prospective data regarding effectiveness. Optimization of transfusion therapy is necessary prior to rfVIIa administration [128].

Table 18.6 Key issues in hemorrhage management, by stage of hemorrhage.

Stage 0	Stage 1	Stage 2	Stage 3
All births	Cumulative blood loss > 500 mL vaginal birth or > 1000 mL cesarean birth OR >15% change in vital signs; increased bleeding; or any of the following: HR ≥ 110; BP ≤ 85/45; SaO_2 < 95%	Continued bleeding or vital sign instability and < 1500 mL cumulative blood loss	Cumulative blood loss > 1500 mL; > 2 units packed red blood cells administered, vital signs unstable, or suspicion of DIC
• Risk assessment • Active management of third stage of labor • Vigorous fundal massage • Quantification of blood loss	• Call for help • Large bore IV access, oxygen, keep warm, empty bladder • Oxytocin, additional uterotonic agent • Quantify and communicate blood loss • Type and cross match • Inspect for uncontrolled bleeding at all levels • Identify underlying etiology	• Consider additional uterotonic agent • Bimanual uterine massage • Second large bore IV • Obtain blood; administer on clinical signs – do not wait for laboratory results • Maintain fluid volume • Maintain oxygenation warmth, empty bladder • Obtain serial blood counts and clotting factors • Mobilize additional resources (e.g. blood bank) to prepare for massive transfusion • Sequentially work though procedures to treat etiology and apply definitive therapy	• Activate massive transfusion protocol with high ratio of FFP:RBC:platelets (1:1:1) • Obtain additional personnel • Maintain fluid volume • Maintain oxygenation, warmth, empty bladder • Prevent hypothermia and acidemia • Obtain serial blood counts and clotting factors • Conservative or definitive surgery: selective embolization, uterine artery ligation, hysterectomy

Abbreviations: DIC, disseminated intravascular coagulation; FFP, fresh frozen plasma; RBC, red blood cells.

Adapted from the California Maternal Quality Care Collaborative *OB Hemorrhage Care Guidelines: Checklist* 2010: http://www.cmqcc.org/ob_hemorrhage, and Pacheco LD, Saade GR, Gei AF *et al.* Cutting-edge advances in the medical management of obstetrical hemorrhage [125].

Techniques that may be necessary to control bleeding depending on etiology include balloon tamponade, compression sutures, selective arterial embolization (in centers with available expertise and resources), uterine artery ligation, and hysterectomy. It is important that personnel have the skills and training to use

Table 18.7 Uterotonics.

Agent	Side effect
Oxytocin (Pitocin®)	Premature ventricular contractions, hypotension
Prostaglandin E1 (misoprostol, Cytotec®)	Nausea, vomiting, abdominal pain, diarrhea, headache
Methylergonovine (Methergine®)	Hypertension exacerbation, coronary vasospasms, increased systemic vascular resistance/mean arterial pressure/central venous pressure, pulmonary edema, intracranial hemorrhage and seizures, retinal detachment
Prostaglandin 15-methyl F2α (Hemabate®)	Bronchoconstrictions (avoid in asthmatics), increased cardiac output and peripheral vascular resistance, decreased systemic vascular resistance and coronary artery perfusion, diarrhea
Prostaglandin E2 (Dinoprostone®)	Decreased systemic vascular resistance and mean arterial pressure, increased cardiac output, nausea, vomiting, diarrhea, tachypnea
Recombinant factor VIIa (NovoSeven®)	Increased thromboembolism risk

Source: Haeri & Dildy [110]. Reproduced with permission of Elsevier.

these techniques when necessary, keeping in mind that embolization is not appropriate for the acutely unstable or massive hemorrhage where hysterectomy may be lifesaving and the coordination of resources for embolization may waste precious time [114].

In the case of uterine inversion, uterotonics should be discontinued and management of hemorrhage attended to simultaneously with attempted manual replacement (Figure 18.2 and Figure 18.3). Uterine relaxation with nitroglycerine or terbutaline may be needed to facilitate replacement, and surgical intervention needed if manual replacement is unsuccessful [129].

To reduce morbidity and prevent maternal mortality, it is essential that all obstetric units have a well-organized approach to hemorrhage management supported by clear algorithms, specified vital sign and clinical condition trigger parameters, protocols for responding to changes in condition, a massive transfusion protocol, strong interdepartmental collaboration, regular interdisciplinary drills, and systematic assessment of opportunities for improvement [111,114,130].

18.4.2 Thromboembolism

Thromboembolism is a leading cause of death in developed countries including the United States and the United Kingdom [107,131]. Manifesting as cardiac arrest or stroke, arterial thromboembolism accounts for approximately 20% of pregnancy-associated cases of thromboembolism. Venous thromboembolism (VTE) accounts for the remaining 80%. Of pregnancy-associated VTEs, 80% are deep vein thromboses (DVTs), and the remaining 20% are pulmonary emboli (PEs) [132].

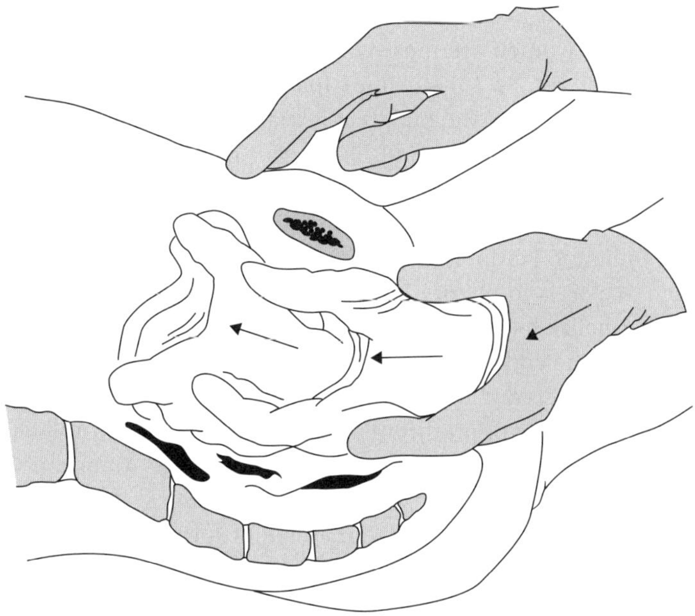

Figure 18.2 The uterine fundus can be replaced by steady upward pressure from the provider's upturned hand.

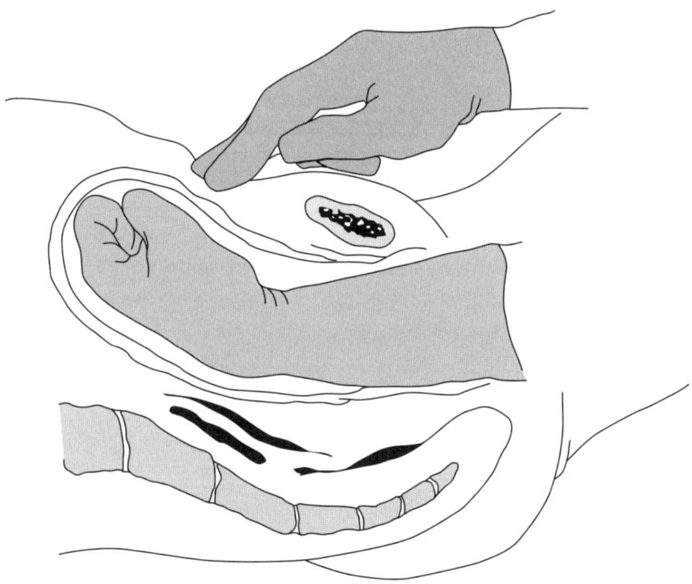

Figure 18.3 After replacement, the provider's hand should remain in place while contractions are stimulated.

While pregnancy is associated with a four- to sixfold increase in the risk of developing a VTE, women are most vulnerable to VTE during the postpartum period, where the risk is 15–60 times that for non-pregnant women [104, 133–135]. Changes shifting the maternal hematologic system towards hypercoagulability include elevated levels of fibrinogen, factors V, VII, VIII, IX, X, XII, and von Willenbrand factor, and decreased levels of the natural anticoagulant free protein S, acquired resistance to anticoagulant protein C, and increased tissue factor inhibitor. Fibrinolytic capacity is diminished from elevated levels of plasminogen activator inhibitors-1 (PAI-1) and -2 (PAI-2). Most hematologic parameters normalize by 4–8 weeks postpartum, and VTE risk returns to near-baseline levels by the end of week 6 [136–139].

Previous thrombosis and the presence of inherited thrombophilias (homozygosity for factor V Leiden or prothrombin G20210A) are the most significant risk factors for pregnancy-associated VTE [134,136,140]. The American College of Chest Physicians [46] classification of medical and clinical VTE risk is summarized in Table 18.8. Extremes of maternal age (15–19 and ≥ 35) and African American race may also increase risk [132,133]. Advanced maternal age (≥35) is a significant risk factor for the development of PE postpartum [135].

The threshold for recommending anticoagulation is lower in the postpartum period as VTE risk is higher. Furthermore, aside from breastfeeding, fetal effects are no longer a concern. Postpartum treatment recommendations are summarized and contrasted with antepartum management in Table 18.9. Postpartum treatment often includes bridging from low-molecular-weight heparin (LMWH) to a vitamin K antagonist (VKA), usually warfarin. This involves initiating the

Table 18.8 Baseline risk of postpartum VTE of > 3%.

Major risk factor: presence of ≥ 1 factor	Minor risk factor: presence of ≥ 2 factors
Immobility (strict bed rest for ≥ 1 week antepartum)	BMI ≥ 30
Postpartum hemorrhage ≥ 1,000 mL w/surgery	Multiple pregnancy
Previous VTE	Postpartum hemorrhage ≥ 1000 mL
Preeclampsia with fetal growth restriction	Smoking ≥ 10 cigarettes/d
Thrombophilia	Fetal growth restriction
Antithrombin deficiency	Thrombophilia
Factor V Leiden (homozygous or heterozygous)	Protein C deficiency
Prothrombin G20210A (homozygous or heterozygous)	Protein S deficiency
Medical conditions	Preeclampsia
Systemic lupus erythematosus	
Heart disease	
Sickle cell disease	
Blood transfusion	
Postpartum infection	

Source: Bates *et al.*, 2012 [46]. Adapted with permission of American College of Chest Physicians.

Table 18.9 VTE recommendations for antepartum and postpartum management: comparison.

Clinical scenario	Antepartum management	Postpartum management
Prior VTE receiving long-term anticoagulation	Full- or 75%-dose LMWH	Resume long-term anticoagulation
Prior VTE, not receiving long-term anticoagulation • Unprovoked VTE • Estrogen-related VTE (i.e. OCP, pregnancy)	Prophylactic or intermediate-dose low-molecular-weight heparin (LMWH) or vitamin K antagonist** (VKA) x 6 weeks	Prophylactic or intermediate-dose LMWH or VKA x 6 weeks
Prior VTE, not receiving long-term anticoagulation • VTE associated with a transient major provoking risk factor	Clinical vigilance	Prophylactic or intermediate-dose LMWH or VKA x 6 weeks
No prior VTE; homozygous factor V Leiden or prothrombin gene mutation (regardless of family hx)	Prophylactic or intermediate-dose LMWH or VKA x 6 weeks	Prophylactic or intermediate-dose LMWH or VKA x 6 weeks
No prior VTE; other thrombophilia, + family hx	Clinical vigilance	Prophylactic or intermediate-dose LMWH or VKA x 6 weeks
No prior VTE; other thrombophilia, no family hx	Clinical vigilance	Clinical vigilance

[a] VKA assumes target INR of 2.0–3.0.

Source: Bates, 2011 [136]. Adapted with permission of Elsevier.

VKA during treatment with LMWH, and discontinuing the latter when an INR of at least 2.0 is achieved. When anticoagulation therapy has been suspended ahead of birth, it should be resumed when acute bleeding risk has subsided, generally by 12 and 24 hours after vaginal and cesarean birth, respectively. Following epidural anesthesia, treatment may be reinitiated 2 hours after catheter removal for prophylactic doses and after 24 hours for full-dose therapy [136].

Most women (>80%) with a pregnancy-related DVT will present with pain and swelling in an extremity [140,141], usually left sided [134,142]. Compression ultrasonography of the proximal veins is the recommended initial diagnostic test. If results are unclear, or iliac involvement is suspected, magnetic resonance venography may be indicated. Diagnosis of PE is via ventilation/perfusion scanning. Indeterminate studies in women without DVT should be confirmed by angiography or spiral computed tomography to prevent unnecessary treatment in current and future pregnancies [140].

18.4.3 Postpartum hypertension

Postpartum hypertension (PPHTN) is a serious and potentially underappreciated problem that may persist from pregnancy (preexisting chronic or gestational hypertension or preeclampsia) or arise for the first time in the postpartum period. The overall prevalence of PPHTN in unknown. The prevalence of new-onset PPHTN (including preeclampsia) is between 0.3 and 27.5% [143]. In 89 patients with eclampsia presenting over a 5-year period, 33% of cases occurred postpartum. One-third of postpartum cases occurred within the first 48 hours after birth [144]. While the index of suspicion for preeclampsia should be high, the list of differential diagnoses for PPHTN is extensive (Table 18.10), and includes volume overload and medication-induced hypertension. An evaluation and management algorithm developed by Sibai [143] is displayed in Figure 18.4.

Management of preeclampsia with magnesium sulfate for seizure prophylaxis does not differ in the postpartum period: therapy should be instituted promptly and maintained for at least 24 hours [143]. Postpartum hypertensive crisis is the acute onset of severe systolic (≥160 mmHg) or diastolic (≥110 mmHg) hypertension lasting ≥ 15 minutes. The severity of the systolic hypertension may be the strongest predictor of risk for cerebral injury [145]. The goal for antihypertensive treatment in this situation is to maintain blood pressures in the range

Table 18.10 Differential diagnosis of postpartum hypertension.

Etiology	Key findings to consider
New-onset hypertension-preeclampsia	Onset 3–6 days postpartum without headaches
Volume overload	Large volume of fluids, regional analgesia, delayed mobilization
Medications/drugs	Nonsteroidal analgesics, ergot derivatives
Ibuprofen, indomethacin	Peripheral and cerebral vasoconstriction, headaches
Phenylpropanolamine, ephedrine	Peripheral and cerebral vasoconstriction, headaches
Ergotamine, ergonovine	Vasoconstriction, headaches, nausea, vomiting, seizures
Persistence of GH-preeclampsia	Preexisting condition antepartum/in labor
Late-onset eclampsia	Headaches, visual changes, seizures, absent neurologic deficits
HELLP syndrome	Nausea/vomiting, epigastric pain, low platelets, increased liver enzymes
Preexisting/undiagnosed hypertension	Hypertension prior to pregnancy, or < 20 weeks
Preexisting renal disease	Proteinuria or hematuria < 20 weeks
Hyperthyroidism	Palpitations tachycardia, sweating, dry skin, heart failure
Primary hyperaldosteronism	Refractory hypertension, hypokalemia, metabolic alkalosis
Pheochromocytoma	Paroxysmal hypertension, headaches, chest pain, hyperglycemia
Renal artery stenosis	Hypertension that is refractory to treatment
Cerebral vasoconstriction syndrome	Sudden thunderclap headaches, visual changes, neurologic deficits
Cerebral venous thrombosis/stroke	Onset 3–7 days, gradual or acute headaches, seizures, neurologic deficits
TTP/hemolytic uremic syndrome	Hemolysis, severe thrombocytopenia, neurologic symptoms, normal liver enzymes

Source: Sibai, 2012 [143]. Reproduced with permission of Elsevier.

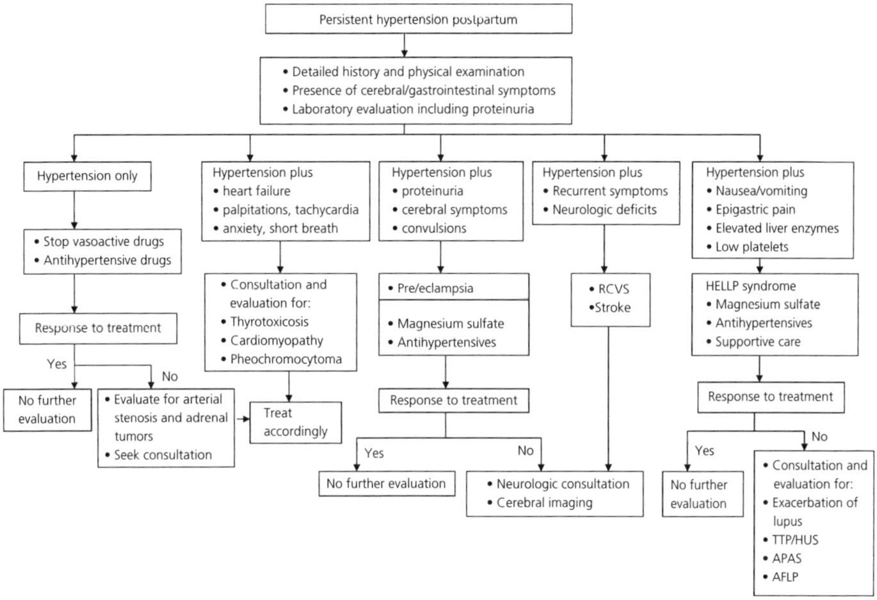

Figure 18.4 Management algorithm for persistent postpartum hypertension. *Source*: Sibai, 2012 [144]. Reproduced with permission of Elsevier.

of 140–160/90–100. Intravenous labetalol and intravenous hydralazine are the first-line choices for initial management [145]. Subsequent oral medication such as nifedipine or labetalol may be needed to maintain blood pressure control. Oral nifedipine may be preferred for blood pressure control in women with volume overload, as it increases renal blood flow and diuresis. It may also be appropriate for acute treatment of severe hypertension in women without IV access [146].

Postpartum headache may also signify preeclampsia. Of 95 women with a new-onset severe headache at greater than 24 hours after birth, 23 (24%) had preeclampsia/eclampsia with blood pressures ranging from 145 to 188 mmHg systolic and 92 to 130 mmHg diastolic [147]. Tension-type headache was more common (39%), but migraine and spinal headache were less common (11% and 16%, respectively). As with hypertension, the differential diagnosis for postpartum headache is extensive, and several etiologies are life threatening (Table 18.11). Thus the work-up of postpartum headache unresponsive to mild analgesia should include evaluation of hypertension and neurologic deficit, and may include cerebral imaging [147] (Figure 18.5).

18.4.4 Cardiac disease

Dramatic shifts in cardiac indices occur immediately after birth. Ventricular pressures, stroke volume, and cardiac output rise substantially and may cause clinical deterioration in women with severe cardiac disease [148].

Table 18.11 Differential diagnosis of postpartum headache.

Primary headache
Migraine headache
Tension-type headache (includes benign ordinary headache)
Orgasmic headache
Secondary headache
Postdural puncture headache
Preeclampsia/eclampsia
Cerebral venous sinus thrombosis*
Stroke (ischemic or hemorrhagic)*
Ruptured aneurysm or malformation
Hypertensive encephalopathy or bleeding
Cerebral arterial thrombosis or embolism
Posterior reversible encephalopathy syndrome
Postpartum cerebral angiopathy*/Call-Fleming syndrome
Pituitary apoplexy
Pseudotumor cerebri
Subarachnoid hemorrhage*
Meningitis*

* Life threatening.
Source: Stella *et al.*, 2007 [147]. Reproduced with permission of Elsevier.

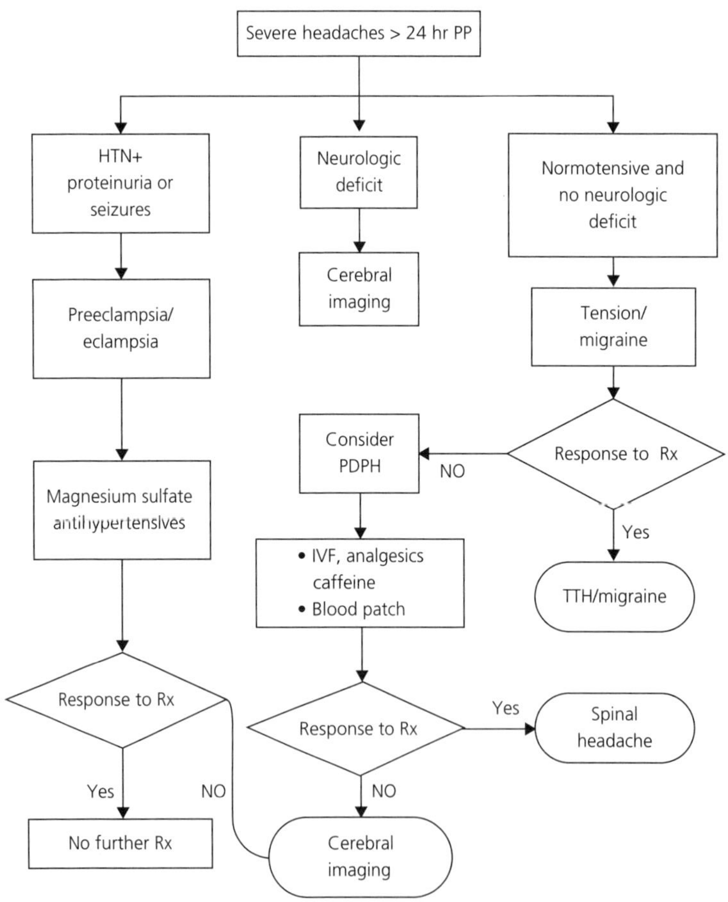

Figure 18.5 Evaluation of severe postpartum headache. *Source*: Stella *et al.*, 2007 [148]. Reproduced with permission of Elsevier.

Providers should be alert to signs of cardiac decompensation, especially in women with known cardiac disease or risk factors (≥35 years old, obesity, smoking, parity > 3, family history, diabetes, or hypertension), and include cardiac dysfunction in the differential diagnosis when signs and symptoms of cardiac or respiratory compromise are present [114].

Cardiac disease is now the leading cause of pregnancy-related death in the United States, the United Kingdom, and Canada [107,149,150]. An estimated 77% of pregnancy-related cardiac deaths between 1998 and 2005 occurred postpartum. Seventeen percent of deaths related to cardiovascular conditions, and 48% caused by cardiomyopathy, occurred after 42 days postpartum [107]. Deaths related to congenital heart disease and pulmonary hypertension have decreased, perhaps reflecting advances in the care, counseling, and management of patients with these disorders. Conversely, deaths from ischemic heart disease, myocardial infarction, and cardiomyopathy have risen [107,131].

Women aged ≥ 40 have a fivefold increased risk of pregnancy-related mortality compared to women aged 25–29 [151]. Obesity and smoking may predispose women to adverse outcomes. In the United Kingdom, over 60% of women who died from cardiac disease were overweight or obese, and all of the women who died from myocardial infarction or ischemic heart disease had identifiable risk factors [131].

A common problem is failure to recognize and respond to symptoms associated with acute coronary syndromes and to accurately interpret electrocardiogram findings in pregnant or postpartum women [131]. Cardiac syndromes should be included in the differential diagnosis for all women presenting with severe pain in the chest or subscapular region requiring opioid pain management. Symptoms associated with coronary syndromes are severe chest pain radiating to the neck, jaw, or back, agitation, vomiting, breathlessness, tachycardia, tachypnea, and orthopnea. Pulmonary edema may present as dyspnea and wheezing. Aortic dissection, a growing contributor to pregnancy-related death, can present as sternal or subscapular pain with systolic hypertension, agitation, dizziness, and vomiting. Peripartum cardiomyopathy may manifest as late as 5 months postpartum. Providers should investigate reports of breathlessness, persistent peripheral edema, orthopnea, tachypnea, or tachycardia on any follow-up visit during this time period. Appropriate screening includes chest X ray and electrocardiogram [114,131,152].

Unless severe, regurgitant valvular lesions are usually well tolerated in pregnancy. Stenotic lesions, such as mitral stenosis, may present for the first time during the peripartum period. Signs of cardiac decompensation related to mitral stenosis often progress from dyspnea, orthopnea, to paroxysmal nocturnal dyspnea. Clinical findings may include tachycardia, tachyarrythmias (usually atrial fibrillation), worsening pulmonary edema, and left atrial enlargement. Without treatment, the woman may suffer cardiac failure [152,153].

18.4.5 Perineal trauma

The perineum may be swollen, bruised, or have surgical or spontaneous tears after vaginal birth. Use of synthetic suture material for laceration or episiotomy repair may decrease perineal pain and subsequent dyspareunia [154]. In most cases, perineal pain is treated adequately with the same medications provided for cramping or afterpains. Although topical local anesthetics and cool ice or gel packs are commonly used to reduce swelling and pain, evidence regarding the safety and efficacy of these approaches is limited [155,156]. Significant perineal pain unresponsive to nonsteroidal anti-inflammatory medication should alert the provider to potential additional problems such as hematoma or infection. Perineal cleanliness can be maintained with lukewarm water sprayed gently over the area.

Lacerations that include anal sphincter damage (third- and fourth-degree lacerations) occur in 2–19% of vaginal births [157], although rates seem to be decreasing with decreased episiotomy and forceps use [158]. Severe lacerations can cause pain, sexual dysfunction, urinary and fecal incontinence, and increased risk of perineal wound infection [144,157]. While some experts recommend prophylactic antibiotics for severe lacerations, a 2010 Cochrane review found insufficient evidence to recommend antibiotic prophylaxis [159]. In a case-control study of 59 cases of perineal wound breakdown, risk factors for wound breakdown were similar to risk factors for anal sphincter injury [157,158,160–162] (Table 18.12). Operative birth and perineal trauma can result in dyspareunia and difficulties with postpartum sexual function that can persist for 6 months or more, although it is difficult to determine the independent effects of episiotomy, perineal trauma, and operative birth versus other factors potentially associated with these events [154]. While postpartum sexual dysfunction is common (41–83% at 2–3 months), few women discuss these issues with their obstetrician or midwife [154].

Table 18.12 Risk factors for anal sphincter injury and perineal wound breakdown.

Anal sphincter injury	Perineal wound breakdown
Nulliparity	Episiotomy
Occiput posterior presentation	Third-/fourth-degree laceration
Episiotomy	Operative delivery
Forceps	Meconium
Prolonged second stage	Prolonged second stage
Combination of episiotomy and forceps	Operative delivery and mediolateral episiotomy
Shoulder dystocia	
Increased birthweight (>3500–4000 g)	

Source: Data from Fitzgerald *et al.*, 2007 [160], Hamilton *et al.*, 2011 [161], and Williams & Chames, 2006 [162].

18.4.6 Postpartum mood disorders

Giving birth is life changing and stressful, and depression is a normal human response to a stressful event [45]. Mild depressive symptoms (tearfulness, mood lability, and feeling overwhelmed) known as "the baby blues," may last a few hours to a few weeks, affect up to 80% of women [163], and do not impair a mother's ability to function [164]. Postpartum depression, however, impairs the mother's functional ability and is more common than other medical complications [164]. The rate of postpartum depression is 10–15% in the United States [165]. It affects mothers of every ethnicity, nationality, and socioeconomic status worldwide [45].

Co-morbidities associated with postpartum depression include postpartum anxiety disorders, eating disorders, and substance abuse. Postpartum psychosis is the most severe form of postpartum mental illness, affecting 0.1–0.2% of women. It typically has an abrupt onset at 3–14 days postpartum and occurs most often among women with bipolar disorder [45,163].

A common misconception is that hormonal changes cause depression in new mothers; however, evidence supporting this explanation is limited. Research suggests that increased levels of pro-inflammatory cytokines from physical and psychological stressors in the third trimester and postpartum create an inflammatory response that places women at risk for depression [166]. Additional risk factors include infant characteristics such as difficult temperament, prematurity, or illness, and maternal factors such as unrealistic expectations of motherhood, low self-esteem and self-efficacy, previous depression, and a history of trauma, abuse, or perinatal loss. Social risk factors include stressful life events, poverty, limited maternity leave, partner-associated stress and interpersonal violence, and insufficient social support [45]. The risk of interpersonal violence increases by 19% prenatally and by 25% in the postpartum period, and can negatively affect the progress of postpartum depression for months or years after the birth [167]. Conversely, social support is protective [45].

Sleep deprivation and fatigue are both a symptom and a catalyst for postpartum depression and psychosis. Mothers who are extremely tired or report sleep disturbances unrelated to baby care should be closely monitored [45]. Hypothyroidism presents with depression-like symptoms, including fatigue, and can be screened for by testing TSH levels and free or total T4 [45].

Postpartum mood disorders harm both mothers and infants. Depressed mothers may disengage and ignore their infant's cues, or interact angrily and intrusively. The infant may withdraw or shut down, or react to the mother with anger or frustration [45]. Children of depressed mothers may have impaired cognitive skills, language and emotional development, and long-term behavioral issues [163]. Long-term maternal effects include increased risk of cardiovascular disease, poor eating habits, substance abuse, and relationship dysfunction [45].

Severe consequences of postpartum mood disorders include suicide and infanticide. Obsessive thoughts of infant harm are common among depressed mothers, although an infant may not be at increased risk unless the mother also portrays psychotic symptoms or behaviors [168]. All women with such negative thought patterns need professional care. Most mothers are ashamed to disclose thoughts of harming their infant, and are more likely to seek help by disclosing suicidal ideation [168]. Healthcare practitioners should validate the difficulty of the mother's experience without expressing great alarm, which can intensify the mother's negative thought patterns [45].

Routine screening for depression should continue throughout the first year postpartum in both maternal and infant care settings [164]. Screening tools include the Edinburgh Postnatal Depression Scale and the Postpartum Depression Screening Scale. If symptoms of depression are identified, further work-up for a diagnosis of depression, and screening for substance abuse, risk of suicide or infanticide, symptom severity, and need for psychiatric hospitalization are indicated [45].

Antidepressant medications increase the amount of monamine neurotransmitters in the brain and have anti-inflammatory effects [45]. Tricyclic antidepressants (TCAs) are the least expensive, but have significant side effects and are a potential suicide risk since they are lethal at high doses. Selective serotonin reuptake inhibitors (SSRIs) have fewer side effects and simpler dosing, but have the potential for drug-drug interactions. Monoamine oxidase inhibitors are highly effective, but are contraindicated in breastfeeding and have the potential for hypertensive crisis or death if taken with tyramine (in red wine and cheeses) [45]. With few exceptions, TCAs and SSRIs are generally compatible with breastfeeding [169], and the risks associated with *not* breastfeeding outweigh the risk of breastfeeding on the medication. The infant should be monitored for adverse effects and infant exposure minimized by taking the medication immediately after breastfeeding [163].

Complementary and alternative therapies, including omega-3 polyunsaturated fatty acids, exercise, cognitive behavioral therapy, and interpersonal therapy, may be used as primary or adjunctive therapy [45]. The omega-3 polyunsaturated fatty acids eicosapentaenoic acid (EPA) and docosahexaenoic acid (DHA) have anti-inflammatory effects and can lower perinatal depression scores [170]. Exercise helps to oppose pro-inflammatory cytokines and safely lower postpartum depression [45,171]. St John's wort is an effective, safe treatment, even if breastfeeding, for mild to moderate postnatal depression, with efficacy similar to or greater than synthetic antidepressants [45,169,172]. However, it should not be combined with other antidepressants [45,169].

18.4.7 Perinatal loss

Some 17% of recognized pregnancies end in spontaneous fetal loss, with the majority occurring in the first trimester [173]. The terms *miscarriage* refers to losses prior to 20 weeks, and *stillbirth* to losses ≥ 20 weeks. Stillbirth occurs in about 6 of 1000 (live births + fetal deaths) in the United States. About half occur between 20 and 27 completed weeks, and the other half at ≥ 28 weeks of gestation. Significant racial disparities exist, with non-Hispanic black women having the highest risk of stillbirth [174].

Causes of fetal loss vary by gestational age. Using a systematic protocol to evaluate the cause of stillbirth, VanderWielen *et al.* [175] identified a single cause in 70% of cases. Of these, 40% were placental, 21.5% fetal, and 12.7% maternal. Standardized protocols aimed at evaluating stillbirth causes can assist in identifying the etiology (which is often multifactorial), and guide the care and management of future pregnancies [175–179]. Recommendations may include referral to a geneticist; fetal autopsy and laboratory studies; examination of the placenta, umbilical cord, and membranes; and maternal evaluation derived from a detailed medical history, laboratory studies, or physical examination.

Grief associated with fetal loss can have lasting effects. While the gestational age of the baby has little bearing on the intensity and duration of a couple's grief, the number of prior losses has been positively correlated to severity and duration of anxiety, depression, and post-traumatic stress (PTS) [180,181]. While depression and anxiety may decrease over time, PTS can take longer to resolve. PTS in fathers has been associated with greater distancing from their children [182]. Fathers may also face special challenges while grieving if expected to be a source of primary comfort to the mother as well as manage their own distress [182].

Parental role development occurs over time [183]. Fetal loss abruptly interrupts this process, leaving parents in limbo, somewhere between "parent" and "not parent." Hence the grief process is related to threats to the newly emerging sense of self in addition to the loss of the baby. Mothers have reported the profound significance of mementos to validating their sense of themselves as a mother – a role that continues despite the loss, but is complicated and threatened by the absence of a living baby [184]. Helping families create memories (photos, memory boxes, footprints), and honoring the rituals and traditions that are meaningful to them, can facilitate parental role development, and validate the depth and complexity of their loss (Figure 18.6).

Many providers identified inadequacies in preparation for dealing with bereaved parents, and reported feeling uncomfortable supporting patients dealing with loss. These feelings are associated with heightened clinician distress [185]. Clinicians should monitor their own assumptions and experiences with loss, and provide support that is patient-centered, authentic, attentive, and seeks to understand the significance of the event for the parents [186]. Open-ended responses convey support and availability, and allow parents to assign their own meaning to the experience [187,188]. Suggestions for active listening support and other constructive responses are listed in Table 18.13.

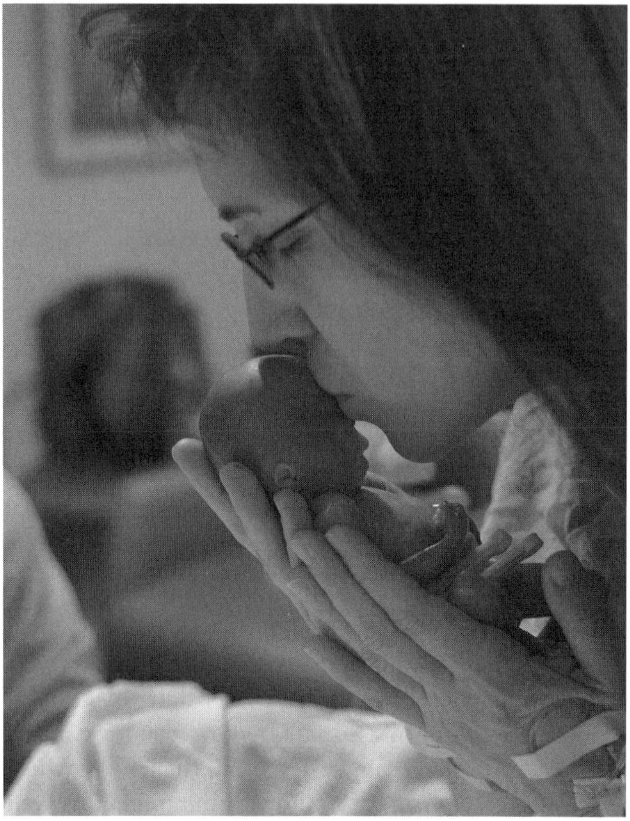

Figure 18.6 Sensitive photography assists families with creating mementos after perinatal loss. *Source*: Todd Hochberg. Reproduced with permission.

Table 18.13 Helpful and unhelpful responses for grieving parents.

Constructive, facilitating	Unconstructive, limiting
Behaviors and actions: • Listening • Being quiet • Gentleness • Kindness • Bathing, holding, nurturing the infant • Encouraging/supporting taking maternity or paternity leave • Provide foot/hand molds, footprints, pictures Statements: • I'm sorry • I'm here, and I want to listen • How are you handling this? • What can I do for you? • Tell me about … • Using validating language – "mother," "father," and the baby's name	Behaviors and actions: • Rushing • Not acknowledging infant • Unnecessary clinical interruptions • Maintaining clinical demeanor • Treating baby like an object Statements: • At least you didn't know the baby • You can have another • He/she is in a better place now • You should/can get pregnant right away and put this behind you

Source: Data from Lathrop *et al.*, 2011 [184] and Capitulo, 2005 [188].

Acknowledgments

Dr Lyndon is supported in part by the National Center for Research Resources, the National Center for Advancing Translational Sciences, and the Office of the Director, National Institutes of Health (NIH), through UCSF-CTSI Grant Number KL2 TR000143. The contents of this chapter are solely the responsibility of the authors and do not necessarily represent the official views of the NIH.

References

1 Quality patient care in labor and delivery: a call to action. *Journal of Obstetric, Gynecologic, & Neonatal Nursing* 2012;**41**:151–153.
2 Cluett ER, Alexander J, and Pickering RM. What is the normal pattern of uterine involution? An investigation of postpartum uterine involution measured by the distance between the symphysis pubis and the uterine fundus using a paper tape measure. *Midwifery* 1997;**13**:9–16.
3 Mulic-Lutvica A, Bekuretsion M, Bakos O *et al.* Ultrasonic evaluation of the uterus and uterine cavity after normal, vaginal delivery. *Ultrasound in Obstetrics & Gynecology* 2001;**18**: 491–498.
4 Anderson WR and Davis J. Placental site involution. *American Journal of Obstetrics & Gynecology* 1968;**102**:23–33.
5 Wakasa T, Wakasa K, Nakayama M *et al.* Change in morphology and oxytocin receptor expression in the uterine blood vessels during the involution process. *Gynecologic and Obstetric Investigation* 2009;**67**:137–144.
6 Sharman A. Post-partum regeneration of the human endometrium. *Journal of Anatomy* 1953;**87**:1–10.
7 Glass M and Rosenthal AH. Cervical changes in pregnancy, labor, and the puerperium. *American Journal of Obstetrics & Gynecology* 1950;**60**:353–362.
8 Kaufman RH, Topek NH, and Abbott JP. Postpartum cervical cytology. *Obstetrics & Gynecology* 1958;**12**:189–194.
9 McLaren H. The involution of the cervix. *BMJ* 1952;**1**:347–352.
10 Sherman D, Lurie S, Frenkel E *et al.* Characteristics of normal lochia. *American Journal of Perinatology* 1999;**16**:399–402.
11 Visness CM, Kennedy KI, and Ramos R. The duration and character of postpartum bleeding among breast-feeding women. *Obstetrics & Gynecology* 1997;**89**:159–163.
12 The World Health Organization multinational study of breast-feeding and lactational amenorrhea. IV. Postpartum bleeding and lochia in breast-feeding women. *Fertility and Sterility* 1999;**72**:441–447.
13 McNeilly AS, Tay CC, and Glasier A. Physiological mechanisms underlying lactational amenorrhea. *Annals of the New York Academy of Sciences* 1994;**709**:145–155.
14 Rogers IS. Lactation and fertility. *Early Human Development* 1997;**49**(Suppl.)S185–190.
15 Jackson E and Glasier A. Return of ovulation and menses in postpartum nonlactating women: a systematic review. *Obstetrics & Gynecology* 2011;**117**:657–662.
16 Wang IY and Fraser IS. Reproductive function and contraception in the postpartum period. *Obstetrical and Gynecological Survey* 1994;**49**:56–63.
17 McNeilly AS. Neuroendocrine changes and fertility in breast-feeding women. *Progress in Brain Research* 2001;**133**:207–214.

18 Hunter S and Robson SC. Adaptation of the maternal heart in pregnancy. *British Heart Journal* 1992;**68**:540–543.

19 Robson SC, Dunlop W, and Hunter S. Haemodynamic changes during the early puerperium. *BMJ* 1987;**294**:1065.

20 Pouta AM, Rasanen JP, Airaksinen KE *et al.* Changes in maternal heart dimensions and plasma atrial natriuretic peptide levels in the early puerperium of normal and pre-eclamptic pregnancies. *British Journal of Obstetrics and Gynaecology* 1996;**103**:988–992.

21 Robson SC, Hunter S, Moore M *et al.* Haemodynamic changes during the puerperium: a Doppler and M-mode echocardiographic study. *British Journal of Obstetrics and Gynaecology* 1987;**94**:1028–1039.

22 Clapp JF, III and Capeless E. Cardiovascular function before, during, and after the first and subsequent pregnancies. *American Journal of Cardiology* 1997;**80**:1469–1473.

23 Hladunewich MA, Lafayette RA, Derby GC *et al.* The dynamics of glomerular filtration in the puerperium. *American Journal of Physiology – Renal physiology* 2004;**286**:F496–503.

24 Jaffe DJ. Postpartum evaluation of renal function. *Clinical Obstetrics and Gynecology* 1985;**28**:298–309.

25 Bailey RR and Rolleston GL. Kidney length and ureteric dilatation in the puerperium. *Journal of Obstetrics and Gynaecology of the British Commonwealth* 1971;**78**:55–61.

26 David AL, Kotecha M, and Girling JC. Factors influencing postnatal liver function tests. *BJOG* 2000;**107**:1421–1426.

27 Montes A, Walden CE, Knopp RH *et al.* Physiologic and supraphysiologic increases in lipoprotein lipids and apoproteins in late pregnancy and postpartum. Possible markers for the diagnosis of "prelipemia." *Arteriosclerosis* 1984;**4**:407–417.

28 Everson GT. Gastrointestinal motility in pregnancy. *Gastroenterology Clinics of North America* 1992;**21**:751–776.

29 Richter JE. Review article: the management of heartburn in pregnancy. *Alimentary Pharmacology & Therapeutics* 2005;**22**:749–757.

30 Van Bodegraven AA, Bohmer CJ, Manoliu RA *et al.* Gallbladder contents and fasting gallbladder volumes during and after pregnancy. *Scandinavian Journal of Gastroenterology* 1998;**33**:993–997.

31 Bonnar J, Franklin M, Nott PN *et al.* Effect of breast-feeding on pituitary-ovarian function after childbirth. *BMJ* 1975;**4**:82–84.

32 Tyson JE, Hwang P, Guyda H *et al.* Studies of prolactin secretion in human pregnancy. *American Journal of Obstetrics & Gynecology* 1972;**113**:14–20.

33 Hegewald MJ and Crapo RO. Respiratory physiology in pregnancy. *Clinics in Chest Medicine* 2011;**32**:1–13, vii.

34 Wong RC and Ellis CN. Physiologic skin changes in pregnancy. *Seminars in Dermatology* 1989;**8**:7–11.

35 Lynfield YL. Effect of pregnancy on the human hair cycle. *Journal of Investigative Dermatology* 1960;**35**:323–327.

36 Harrison S and Sinclair R. Telogen effluvium. *Clinical and Experimental Dermatology* 2002;**27**:389–395.

37 Pitkin RM. Nutritional support in obstetrics and gynecology. *Clinical Obstetrics and Gynecology* 1976;**19**:489–513.

38 Crowell DT. Weight change in the postpartum period. A review of the literature. *Journal of Nurse-Midwifery* 1995;**40**:418–423.

39 Gould Rothberg BE, Magriples U, Kershaw TS *et al.* Gestational weight gain and subsequent postpartum weight loss among young, low-income, ethnic minority women. *American Journal of Obstetrics & Gynecology* 2011;**204**:52 e1–11.

40 American Academy of Pediatrics & American College of Obstetricians & Gynecologists. *Guidelines for Perinatal Care*. Elk Grove Village, IL: AAP & ACOG, 2007.

41 Neville MC and Morton J. Physiology and endocrine changes underlying human lactogenesis II. *Journal of Nutrition* 2001;**131**:3005S–3008S.
42 Forster DA and McLachlan HL. Breastfeeding initiation and birth setting practices: a review of the literature. *Journal of Midwifery & Womens Health* 2007;**52**:273–280.
43 Brownell E, Howard CR, Lawrence RA *et al.* Delayed onset lactogenesis II predicts the cessation of any or exclusive breastfeeding. *Journal of Pediatrics* 2012 May 9.
44 American Academy of Pediatrics. Breastfeeding and the use of human milk. *Pediatrics* 2012;**129**:e827–841.
45 Kendall-Tackett K. *Depression in New Mothers: Causes, Consequences and Treatment Alternatives.* New York: Routledge, 2010.
46 Bates SM, Greer IA, Middeldorp S *et al.* VTE, thrombophilia, antithrombotic therapy, and pregnancy: Antithrombotic Therapy and Prevention of Thrombosis, 9th edn: American College of Chest Physicians evidence-based clinical practice guidelines. *Chest* 2012;**141**(Suppl. 2):e691S–736S.
47 Smaill FM and Gyte GM. Antibiotic prophylaxis versus no prophylaxis for preventing infection after cesarean section. *Cochrane Database of Systematic Reviews* 2010;(**1**):CD007482.
48 Tharpe N. Postpregnancy genital tract and wound infections. *Journal of Midwifery & Womens Health* 2008;**53**:236–246.
49 Leth RA, Moller JK, Thomsen RW *et al.* Risk of selected postpartum infections after cesarean section compared with vaginal birth: a five-year cohort study of 32,468 women. *Acta Obstetricia et Gynecologica Scandinavica* 2009;**88**:976–983.
50 Yokoe DS, Christiansen CL, Johnson R *et al.* Epidemiology of and surveillance for postpartum infections. *Emerging Infectious Diseases* 2001;**7**:837–841.
51 Brumfield CG, Hauth JC, and Andrews WW. Puerperal infection after cesarean delivery: evaluation of a standardized protocol. *American Journal of Obstetrics & Gynecology* 2000;**182**:1147–1151.
52 Larsen JW, Hager WD, Livengood CH *et al.* Guidelines for the diagnosis, treatment and prevention of postoperative infections. *Infectious Diseases in Obstetrics and Gynecology* 2003;**11**:65–70.
53 Maharaj D. Puerperal pyrexia: a review. Part I. *Obstetrical and Gynecological Survey* 2007;**62**:393–399.
54 American Academy of Pediatrics. Sample hospital breastfeeding policy for newborns. *Safe and Heathy Beginnings: A Resource Toolkit for Hospitals and Physicians' Offices.* 2009: Available from: http://www2.aap.org/sections/perinatal/PDF/breastfeedingtemplate.pdf (accessed May 20, 2015).
55 Bystrova K, Ivanova V, Edhborg M *et al.* Early contact versus separation: effects on mother-infant interaction one year later. *Birth* 2009;**36**:97–109.
56 Charpak N, Ruiz JG, Zupan J *et al.* Kangaroo Mother Care: 25 years after. *Acta Paediatrica* 2005;**94**:514–522.
57 Moore ER, Anderson GC, and Bergman N. Early skin-to-skin contact for mothers and their healthy newborn infants. *Cochrane Database of Systematic Reviews* 2007;(**3**):CD003519.
58 Ferber SG and Makhoul IR. The effect of skin-to-skin contact (kangaroo care) shortly after birth on the neurobehavioral responses of the term newborn: a randomized, controlled trial. *Pediatrics* 2004;**113**:858–865.
59 Radzyminski S. Neurobehavioral functioning and breastfeeding behavior in the newborn. *Journal of Obstetric, Gynecologic, & Neonatal Nursing* 2005;**34**:335–341.
60 World Health Organization. Breastfeeding Promotion and Support in a Baby-friendly Hospital, a 20-hour course for maternity staff. Baby Friendly Hospital Initiative: Revised, Updated and Expanded for Integrated Care: World Health Organization & UNICEF; 2009. www.who.int
61 Mikiel-Kostyra K, Mazur J, and Wojdan-Godek E. Factors affecting exclusive breastfeeding in Poland: cross-sectional survey of population-based samples. *Soz Praventivmed* 2005;**50**:52–59.

62 Widstrom AM, Lilja G, Aaltomaa-Michalias P *et al.* Newborn behaviour to locate the breast when skin-to-skin: a possible method for enabling early self-regulation. *Acta Paediatrica* 2011;**100**:79–85.
63 Cadwell K. Latching-on and suckling of the healthy term neonate: breastfeeding assessment. *Journal of Midwifery & Womens Health* 2007;**52**:638–642.
64 Ip S, Chung M, Raman G *et al.* A summary of the Agency for Healthcare Research and Quality's evidence report on breastfeeding in developed countries. *Breastfeeding Medicine* 2009;**4**(Suppl. 1):S17–30.
65 Walker M. *Breastfeeding Management for the Clinician: Using the Evidence*. 2nd edn. Sudbury, MA: Jones & Bartlett, 2011.
66 Bartick M and Reinhold A. The burden of suboptimal breastfeeding in the United States: a pediatric cost analysis. *Pediatrics* 2010;**125**:e1048–1056.
67 Geddes DT. Inside the lactating breast: the latest anatomy research. *Journal of Midwifery & Womens Health* 2007;**52**:556–563.
68 Riordan J and Wambach K. *Breastfeeding and Human Lactation*. 4th edn. Sudbury, MA: Jones & Bartlett, 2010.
69 Geddes DT. Ultrasound imaging of the lactating breast: methodology and application. *International Breastfeeding Journal* 2009;**4**:4.
70 Doucet S, Soussignan R, Sagot P *et al.* An overlooked aspect of the human breast: areolar glands in relation with breastfeeding pattern, neonatal weight gain, and the dynamics of lactation. *Early Human Development* 2012;**88**:119–128.
71 Kent JC. How breastfeeding works. *Journal of Midwifery & Womens Health* 2007;**52**:564–570.
72 Colson SD, Meek JH, and Hawdon JM. Optimal positions for the release of primitive neonatal reflexes stimulating breastfeeding. *Early Human Development* 2008;**84**:441–449.
73 Dennis CL and McQueen K. The relationship between infant-feeding outcomes and postpartum depression: a qualitative systematic review. *Pediatrics* 2009;**123**:e736–751.
74 Doan T, Gardiner A, Gay CL *et al.* Breast-feeding increases sleep duration of new parents. *Journal of Perinatal & Neonatal Nursing* 2007;**21**:200–206.
75 Hunter LP, Rychnovsky JD, and Yount SM. A selective review of maternal sleep characteristics in the postpartum period. *Journal of Obstetric, Gynecologic, & Neonatal Nursing* 2009;**38**:60–68.
76 Schytt E, Lindmark G, and Waldenstrom U. Physical symptoms after childbirth: prevalence and associations with self-rated health. *BJOG* 2005;**112**:210–217.
77 Montgomery-Downs HE, Insana SP, Clegg-Kraynok MM *et al.* Normative longitudinal maternal sleep: the first 4 postpartum months. *American Journal of Obstetrics & Gynecology* 2010;**203**:465 e1–7.
78 Blunden SL, Thompson KR, and Dawson D. Behavioural sleep treatments and night time crying in infants: challenging the status quo. *Sleep Medicine Reviews* 2011;**15**:327–334.
79 Hairston IS, Waxler E, Seng JS *et al.* The role of infant sleep in intergenerational transmission of trauma. *Sleep* 2011;**34**:1373–1383.
80 Cook F, Bayer J, Le HN *et al.* Baby Business: a randomised controlled trial of a universal parenting program that aims to prevent early infant sleep and cry problems and associated parental depression. *BMC Pediatrics* 2012;**12**:13.
81 Lee SY, Lee KA, Aycock D *et al.* Circadian activity rhythms for mothers with an infant in ICU. *Frontiers in Neurology* 2010;**1**:155.
82 Tarullo AR, Balsam PD, and Fifer WP. Sleep and Infant Learning. *Infant and Child Development* 2011;**20**:35–46.
83 Henderson JM, France KG, and Blampied NM. The consolidation of infants' nocturnal sleep across the first year of life. *Sleep Medicine Reviews* 2011;**15**:211–220.
84 Horsley T, Clifford T, Barrowman N *et al.* Benefits and harms associated with the practice of bed sharing: a systematic review. *Archives of Pediatrics and Adolescent Medicine* 2007;**161**:237–245.

85 Wong FY, Witcombc NB, Yiallourou SR *et al.* Cerebral oxygenation is depressed during sleep in healthy term infants when they sleep prone. *Pediatrics* 2011;**127**:e558–565.
86 Nelson AM. Transition to motherhood. *Journal of Obstetric, Gynecologic, & Neonatal Nursing* 2003;**32**:465–477.
87 Rubin R. Puerperal change. *Nursing Outlook* 1961;**9**:753–755.
88 Rubin R. Attainment of the maternal role. 2. Models and referrants. *Nursing Research* 1967;**16**:342–346.
89 Attrill B. The assumption of the maternal role: a developmental process. *Australian Journal of Midwifery* 2002;**15**:21–25.
90 Association of Women's Health, Obstetric and Neonatal Nurses. *The Compendium of Postpartum Care*. 2nd edn. Washington, DC: AWHONN, 2006.
91 Mercer RT. The process of maternal role attainment over the first year. *Nursing Research* 1985;**34**:198–204.
92 Martell LK and Mitchell SK. Rubin's "Puerperal Change" reconsidered. *Journal of Obstetric, Gynecologic, & Neonatal Nursing* 1984;**13**:145–149.
93 Parratt JA and Fahy KM. A feminist critique of foundational nursing research and theory on transition to motherhood. *Midwifery* 2011;**27**:445–451.
94 Biehle SN and Mickelson KD. First-time parents' expectations about the division of childcare and play. *Journal of Family Psychology* 2012;**26**:36–45.
95 Yelland J, McLachlan H, Forster D *et al.* How is maternal psychosocial health assessed and promoted in the early postnatal period? Findings from a review of hospital postnatal care in Victoria, Australia. *Midwifery* 2007;**23**:287–297.
96 Mercer RT. Becoming a mother versus maternal role attainment. *Journal of Nursing Scholarship* 2004;**36**:226–232.
97 Ngai FW, Chan SW, and Holroyd E. Chinese primiparous women's experiences of early motherhood: factors affecting maternal role competence. *Journal of Clinical Nursing* 2011;**20**:1481–1489.
98 World Health Organization. *Medical Eligibility Criteria for Contraceptive Use*. 4th edn. Author: Geneva. 2009.
99 Centers for Disease Control. *United States Medical Eligibility Criteria for Contraceptive Use.* Washinton DC: CDC, 2010.
100 Tepper NK, Curtis KM, Jamieson DJ *et al.* Update to CDC's U.S. medical eligibility criteria for contraceptive use, 2010: revised recommendations for the use of contraceptive methods during the postpartum period. *Morbidity and Mortality Weekly Report* 2011;**60**:878–883.
101 Chen BA, Reeves MF, Hayes JL *et al.* Postplacental or delayed insertion of the levonorgestrel intrauterine device after vaginal delivery: a randomized controlled trial. *Obstetrics & Gynecology* 2010;**116**:1079–1087.
102 Kapp N and Curtis KM. Intrauterine device insertion during the postpartum period: a systematic review. *Contraception* 2009;**80**:327–336.
103 Eroglu K, Akkuzu G, Vural G *et al.* Comparison of efficacy and complications of IUD insertion in immediate postplacental/early postpartum period with interval period: 1 year follow-up. *Contraception* 2006;**74**:376–381.
104 Jackson E, Curtis KM, and Gaffield ME. Risk of venous thromboembolism during the postpartum period: a systematic review. *Obstetrics & Gynecology* 2011;**117**:691–703.
105 Pollack A, American College of Obstetrticians & Gynecologists Practice Bulletin No. 46: Benefits and Risks of Sterilization. *Obstetrics & Gynecology* 2003;**102**:647–658.
106 King J. Contraception and lactation. *Journal of Midwifery & Womens Health* 2007;**52**:614–620.
107 Berg CJ, Callaghan WM, Syverson C *et al.* Pregnancy-related mortality in the United States, 1998 to 2005. *Obstetrics & Gynecology* 2010;**116**:1302–1309.

108 Abrams ET and Rutherford JN. Framing postpartum hemorrhage as a consequence of human placental biology: an evolutionary and comparative perspective. *American Anthropologist* 2011;**113**:417–430.
109 Callaghan WM, Kuklina EV, and Berg CJ. Trends in postpartum hemorrhage: United States, 1994–2006. *American Journal of Obstetrics & Gynecology* 2010;**202**:353 e1–6.
110 Haeri S and Dildy GA, III. Maternal mortality from hemorrhage. *Seminars in Perinatology* 2012;**36**:48–55.
111 Lyndon A, Lagrew D, Shields L *et al.* Improving Health Care Response to Obstetric Hemorrhage. 2010; Developed under contract #08-85012 with the California Department of Public Health; Maternal, Child and Adolescent Health Division: http://www.cmqcc.org/ob_hemorrhage (accessed May 20, 2015).
112 Bateman BT, Berman MF, Riley LE *et al.* The epidemiology of postpartum hemorrhage in a large, nationwide sample of deliveries. *Anesthesia & Analgesia* 2010;**110**:1368–1373.
113 Massiah N, Athimulam S, Loo C *et al.* Obstetric care of Jehovah's Witnesses: a 14-year observational study. *Arch Gynecol Obstet* 2007;**276**:339–343.
114 Clark SL and Hankins GD. Preventing maternal death: 10 clinical diamonds. *Obstetrics & Gynecology* 2012;**119**:360–364.
115 American College of Obstetricians and Gynecologists, Clinical Management Guidelines for Obstetrician-Gynecologists, Practice Bulletin No.76: Postpartum Hemorrhage. *Obstetrics & Gynecology* 2006;**108**:1039–1047.
116 Yoong W, Karavolos S, Damodaram M *et al.* Observer accuracy and reproducibility of visual estimation of blood loss in obstetrics: how accurate and consistent are health-care professionals? *Archives of Gynecology and Obstetrics* 2010;**281**:207–213.
117 Al Kadri HM, Al Anazi BK, and Tamim HM. Visual estimation versus gravimetric measurement of postpartum blood loss: a prospective cohort study. *Archives of Gynecology and Obstetrics* 2011;**283**:1207–1213.
118 Dildy GA, III, Paine AR, George NC *et al.* Estimating blood loss: can teaching significantly improve visual estimation? *Obstetrics & Gynecology* 2004;**104**:601–606.
119 Maslovitz S, Barkai G, Lessing JB *et al.* Improved accuracy of postpartum blood loss estimation as assessed by simulation. *Acta Obstetricia et Gynecologica Scandinavica* 2008;**87**:929–934.
120 Bose P, Regan F, and Paterson-Brown S. Improving the accuracy of estimated blood loss at obstetric haemorrhage using clinical reconstructions. *BJOG* 2006;**113**:919–924.
121 Schorn MN. Measurement of blood loss: review of the literature. *Journal of Midwifery & Womens Health* 2010;**55**:20–27.
122 Patel A, Goudar SS, Geller SE *et al.* Drape estimation vs. visual assessment for estimating postpartum hemorrhage. *International Journal of Gynecology & Obstetrics* 2006;**93**:220–224.
123 Toledo P, McCarthy RJ, Hewlett BJ *et al.* The accuracy of blood loss estimation after simulated vaginal delivery. *Anesthesia & Analgesia* 2007;**105**:1736–1740.
124 Singh S, McGlennan A, England A *et al.* A validation study of the CEMACH recommended modified early obstetric warning system (MEOWS). *Anaesthesia* 2012;**67**:12–18.
125 Pacheco LD, Saade GR, Gei AF *et al.* Cutting-edge advances in the medical management of obstetrical hemorrhage. *American Journal of Obstetrics & Gynecology* 2011;**205**:526–532.
126 Bonnet MP, Deneux-Tharaux C, and Bouvier-Colle MH. Critical care and transfusion management in maternal deaths from postpartum haemorrhage. *European Journal of Obstetrics & Gynecology and Reproductive Biology* 2011;**158**:183–188.
127 Saule I and Hawkins N. Transfusion practice in major obstetric haemorrhage: lessons from trauma. *International Journal of Obstetric Anesthesia* 2012;**21**:79–83.
128 Ahonen J. The role of recombinant activated factor VII in obstetric hemorrhage. *Current Opinion in Anaesthesiology* 2012;**25**:309–314.
129 Beringer RM and Patteril M. Puerperal uterine inversion and shock. *British Journal of Anaesthesia* 2004;**92**:439–441.

130 The Joint Commission. Preventing Maternal Death. *Sentinel Event Alert* 2010;**44**. http://www.jointcommission.org/sentinel_event_alert_issue_44_preventing_maternal_death/ (accessed May 20, 2015).

131 Cantwell R, Clutton-Brock T, Cooper G *et al.* Saving Mothers' Lives: Reviewing maternal deaths to make motherhood safer: 2006–2008. The Eighth Report of the Confidential Enquiries into Maternal Deaths in the United Kingdom. *BJOG* 2011;**118**(Suppl. 1):1–203.

132 James AH, Jamison MG, Brancazio LR *et al.* Venous thromboembolism during pregnancy and the postpartum period: incidence, risk factors, and mortality. *American Journal of Obstetrics & Gynecology* 2006;**194**:1311–1315.

133 Heit JA, Kobbervig CE, James AH *et al.* Trends in the incidence of venous thromboembolism during pregnancy or postpartum: a 30-year population-based study. *Annals of Internal Medicine* 2005;**143**:697–706.

134 Pomp ER, Lenselink AM, Rosendaal FR *et al.* Pregnancy, the postpartum period and prothrombotic defects: risk of venous thrombosis in the MEGA study. *Journal of Thrombosis and Haemostasis* 2008;**6**:632–637.

135 Sultan AA, West J, Tata LJ *et al.* Risk of first venous thromboembolism in and around pregnancy: a population-based cohort study. *British Journal of Haematology* 2012;**156**:366–373.

136 Bates SM. Pregnancy-associated venous thromboembolism: prevention and treatment. *Seminars in Hematology* 2011;**48**:271–284.

137 Bremme KA. Haemostatic changes in pregnancy. *Best Practice & Research Clinical Haematology* 2003;**16**:153–168.

138 Brenner B. Haemostatic changes in pregnancy. *Thrombosis Research* 2004;**114**:409–414.

139 Hellgren M. Hemostasis during normal pregnancy and puerperium. *Seminars in Thrombosis and Hemostasis* 2003;**29**:125–130.

140 James AH. Venous thromboembolism in pregnancy. *Arteriosclerosis, Thrombosis, and Vascular Biology* 2009;**29**:326–331.

141 Gherman RB, Goodwin TM, Leung B *et al.* Incidence, clinical characteristics, and timing of objectively diagnosed venous thromboembolism during pregnancy. *Obstetrics & Gynecology* 1999;**94**:730–734.

142 James AH, Tapson VF, and Goldhaber SZ. Thrombosis during pregnancy and the postpartum period. *American Journal of Obstetrics & Gynecology* 2005;**193**:216–219.

143 Sibai BM. Etiology and management of postpartum hypertension-preeclampsia. *American Journal of Obstetrics & Gynecology* 2012;**206**:470–475.

144 Chames MC, Livingston JC, Ivester TS *et al.* Late postpartum eclampsia: a preventable disease? *American Journal of Obstetrics & Gynecology* 2002;**186**:1174–1177.

145 American College of Obstetricians and Gynecologists. Committee Opinion No. 514: emergent therapy for acute-onset, severe hypertension with preeclampsia or eclampsia. *Obstetrics & Gynecology* 2011;**118**:1465–1468.

146 Raheem IA, Saaid R, Omar SZ *et al.* Oral nifedipine versus intravenous labetalol for acute blood pressure control in hypertensive emergencies of pregnancy: a randomised trial. *BJOG* 2012;**119**:78–85.

147 Stella CL, Jodicke CD, How HY *et al.* Postpartum headache: is your work-up complete? *American Journal of Obstetrics & Gynecology* 2007;**196**:318 e1–7.

148 Curry R, Swan L, and Steer PJ. Cardiac disease in pregnancy. *Current Opinion in Obstetrics and Gynecology* 2009;**21**:508–513.

149 Saving Mothers' Lives: Reviewing maternal deaths to make motherhood safer: 2006–2008. *BJOG* 2011;**118**:1–203.

150 Lisonkova S, Liu S, Bartholomew S *et al.* Temporal trends in maternal mortality in Canada II: estimates based on hospitalization data. *Journal of Obstetrics and Gynaecology Canada* 2011;**33**:1020–1030.

151 Callaghan WM. Overview of maternal mortality in the United States. *Seminars in Perinatology* 2012;**36**:2–6.

152 Wolff GA and Weitzel NS. Management of acquired cardiac disease in the obstetric patient. *Seminars in Cardiothoracic and Vascular Anesthesia* 2011;**15**:85–97.

153 Gelson E, Gatzoulis M, and Johnson M. Valvular heart disease. *BMJ* 2007;**335**:1042–1045.

154 Leeman LM and Rogers RG. Sex after childbirth: postpartum sexual function. *Obstetrics & Gynecology* 2012;**119**:647–655.

155 East CE, Begg L, Henshall NE *et al.* Local cooling for relieving pain from perineal trauma sustained during childbirth. *Cochrane Database of Systematic Reviews* 2012;(**5**):CD006304.

156 Hedayati H, Parsons J, and Crowther CA. Topically applied anaesthetics for treating perineal pain after childbirth. *Cochrane Database of Systematic Reviews* 2005;(**2**):CD004223.

157 Lowder JL, Burrows LJ, Krohn MA *et al.* Risk factors for primary and subsequent anal sphincter lacerations: a comparison of cohorts by parity and prior mode of delivery. *American Journal of Obstetrics & Gynecology* 2007;**196**:344 e1–5.

158 Landy HJ, Laughon SK, Bailit JL *et al.* Characteristics associated with severe perineal and cervical lacerations during vaginal delivery. *Obstetrics & Gynecology* **201**;117:627–635.

159 Buppasiri P, Lumbiganon P, Thinkhamrop J *et al.* Antibiotic prophylaxis for third- and fourth-degree perineal tear during vaginal birth. *Cochrane Database of Systematic Reviews* 2010;(**11**):CD005125.

160 Fitzgerald MP, Weber AM, Howden N *et al.* Risk factors for anal sphincter tear during vaginal delivery. *Obstetrics & Gynecology* 2007;**109**:29–34.

161 Hamilton EF, Smith S, Yang L *et al.* Third- and fourth-degree perineal lacerations: defining high-risk clinical clusters. *American Journal of Obstetrics & Gynecology* 2011;**204**:309 e1–6.

162 Williams MK and Chames MC. Risk factors for the breakdown of perineal laceration repair after vaginal delivery. *American Journal of Obstetrics & Gynecology* 2006;**195**:755–759.

163 Payne JL. Antidepressant use in the postpartum period: practical considerations. *American Journal of Psychiatry* 2007;**164**:1329–1332.

164 McGarry J, Kim H, Sheng X *et al.* Postpartum depression and help-seeking behavior. *Journal of Midwifery & Womens Health* 2009;**54**:50–56.

165 Centers for Disease Control. Prevalence of self-reported postpartum depressive symptoms – 17 states, 2004–2005. *Morbidity and Mortality Weekly Report* 2008;**57**:361–366.

166 Kendall-Tackett K. A new paradigm for depression in new mothers: the central role of inflammation and how breastfeeding and anti-inflammatory treatments protect maternal mental health. *International Breastfeeding Journal* 2007;**2**:6.

167 Antoniou E, Vivilaki VG, and Daglas M. Correlation of domestic violence during pregnancy with postnatal depression: systematic review of bibliography. *Health Science Journal* 2008;**2**:15–19.

168 Barr JA and Beck CT. Infanticide secrets: qualitative study on postpartum depression. *Canadian Family Physician* 2008;**54**:1716–1717 e5.

169 Hale TW. *Medications and Mothers' Milk.* 14th edn. Amarillo, TX: Hale Publishing, 2010.

170 Freeman MP. Complementary and alternative medicine for perinatal depression. *Journal of Affective Disorders* 2009;**112**:1–10.

171 Heh SS, Huang LH, Ho SM *et al.* Effectiveness of an exercise support program in reducing the severity of postnatal depression in Taiwanese women. *Birth* 2008;**35**:60–65.

172 Sarris J. Herbal medicines in the treatment of psychiatric disorders: a systematic review. *Phytotherapy Research* 2007;**21**:703–716.

173 Ventura SJ, Abma JC, Mosher WD *et al.* Estimated pregnancy rates by outcome for the United States, 1990–2004 *National Vital Statistics Reports* 2008;**56**:1–25, 8.

174 MacDorman MF and Kirmeyer S. Fetal and perinatal mortality, United States, 2005. *National Vital Statistics Reports* 2009;**57**(8):1–19.

175 VanderWielen B, Zaleski C, Cold C *et al.* Wisconsin stillbirth services program: a multifocal approach to stillbirth analysis. *American Journal of Medical Genetics Part A* 2011;**155A**:1073–1080.

176 Maternal-Fetal Medicine Committee, Clinical Practice Obstetrics Committee, Leduc L, *et al.* Stillbirth and bereavement: guidelines for stillbirth investigation. *Journal of Obstetrics and Gynaecology Canada* 2006;**28**:540–552.

177 Royal College of Obstetricians. Late intrauterine death and stillbirth. Greentop Guideline No. 55. 2010: 1–33.

178 Dudley DJ, Goldenberg R, Conway D *et al.* A new system for determining the causes of stillbirth. *Obstetrics & Gynecology* 2010;**116**:254–260.

179 American College of Obstetricians and Gynecologists Practice Bulletin No. 102: Management of Stillbirth. *Obstetrics & Gynecology* 2009;**113**:748–761.

180 Blackmore ER, Cote-Arsenault D, Tang W *et al.* Previous prenatal loss as a predictor of perinatal depression and anxiety. *British Journal of Psychiatry* 2011;**198**:373–378.

181 Cote-Arsenault D. The influence of perinatal loss on anxiety in multigravidas. *Journal of Obstetric, Gynecologic, & Neonatal Nursing* 2003;**32**:623–629.

182 Armstrong DS, Hutti MH, and Myers J. The influence of prior perinatal loss on parents' psychological distress after the birth of a subsequent healthy infant. *Journal of Obstetric, Gynecologic, & Neonatal Nursing* 2009;**38**:654–666.

183 Rubin R. Maternal tasks in pregnancy. *Journal of Advanced Nursing* 1976;**1**:367–376.

184 Lathrop A and Vandevusse L. Affirming motherhood: validation and invalidation in women's perinatal hospice narratives. *Birth* 2011;**38**:256–265.

185 Geller G, Rushton CH, Francomano C *et al.* Genetics professionals' experiences with grief and loss: implications for support and training. *Clinical Genetics* 2010;**77**:421–429.

186 Swanson KM. Nursing as informed caring for the well-being of others. *Image – The Journal of Nursing Scholarship* 1993;**25**:352–357.

187 Limbo R and Kobler K. The tie that binds: relationships in perinatal bereavement. *American Journal of Maternal/Child Nursing* 2010;**35**:316–321.

188 Capitulo KL. Evidence for healing interventions with perinatal bereavement. *American Journal of Maternal/Child Nursing* 2005;**30**:389–396.

CHAPTER 19

Development of an obstetrical patient safety program

Christian M. Pettker[1] and Edmund F. Funai[2]

[1] Department of Obstetrics, Gynecology, and Reproductive Sciences, Yale University School of Medicine, New Haven, CT, USA

[2] Department of Obstetrics and Gynecology, University of South Florida, Tampa, FL, USA

19.1 Introduction

The Institute of Medicine report from 1999, *To Err is Human: Building a Safer Health System* [1], was the call to arms for the patient safety movement, pointing out that up to 44,000–98,000 hospitalized Americans die annually as a result of medical errors and mishaps. Put into perspective, this is the equivalent of two 747 jets crashing, weekly, or would rank error as the eighth leading cause of death in the United States, ahead of HIV, motor vehicle accidents, and breast cancer. Since then, quality and safety have intercalated into all parts of healthcare delivery, driven by public demand, regulatory oversight, reimbursement incentives, but most of all the desire of healthcare providers to deliver the best and safest care possible.

Obstetrical units have received increased attention in terms of quality and safety. Volume explains much of this: childbirth accounts for over 4 million hospitalizations each year, ranking first for indications for hospitalization in the United States in 2009 [2]. Furthermore, each birth involves *two* patients, mother and child, and injury and an adverse outcome in either case is a significant deviation from the expectation. The liability atmosphere surrounding obstetrics also contributes to the focus on quality and safety. A random sampling of closed-claim cases from five malpractice companies in four regions of the United States demonstrates most cases, 19%, involve obstetrics/gynecology specialists [3]. According to a 2010 Benchmarking Report by CRICO, a medical malpractice company covering the Harvard medical community, the average payment in obstetrics-related malpractice claims ($822,000–1,100,000) is 2–3 times that of other clinical areas ($324,000–389,000) [4].

Management of Labor and Delivery, Second Edition. Edited by George A. Macones.

Liability concerns have affected individual providers in substantial ways. The 2012 American College of Obstetrics and Gynecology (ACOG) Survey on Professional Liability revealed that 77.3% of respondents had experienced at least one professional liability claim in their careers, with an average of 2.64 claims per physician [5]. Notably, 44% of the claims were dropped or settled without any payment on behalf of the obstetrician/gynecologist. The impact of this on practice is also notable: nearly 51% have made changes to practice based on the affordability or availability of professional liability insurance and almost 58% have made changes in clinical practice as a result of the risk or fear of liability claims or litigation.

A proactive and positive approach to quality and safety in obstetrics involves designing a "high reliability" system that attempts to manage a complex and hazardous operation without errors [6]. Such a unit develops purposefully and strategically, with careful attention to implementing programs focusing on standardization, teamwork, professionalism, and self-evaluation. This chapter focuses on the fundamentals and building blocks for transforming a labor and delivery unit into a high reliability operation.

19.2 Background and fundamentals of patient safety

There is no universally accepted definition of patient safety. Precise definitions of patient safety range from simple, like that of the Institute of Medicine ("The prevention of harm caused by errors of commission and omission."), to complex, such as that from Emanuel on behalf of the Agency for Healthcare Research and Quality ("Patient safety is a discipline in the healthcare sector that applies safety science methods toward the goal of achieving a trustworthy system of healthcare delivery. Patient safety is also an attribute of healthcare systems; it minimizes the incidence and impact of, and maximizes recovery from, adverse events.") [7,8]. The term "patient safety," as a result, is likely to evoke many different connotations to patients, nurses, physicians, and administrators.

Much of the work in patient safety is based on advances in safety in aviation and the military. The aviation model of safety begins and builds off four basic assumptions. First, due to the complex systems involved in flying and the basic limitations of human workers, the risk of failure of is inherent. Second, not all risk is foreseeable and the key to safety is recognizing and managing failure. Third, a majority of accidents are based on human error in a team setting, emphasizing the importance of teamwork strategies to mitigate a developing event. Finally, catastrophic events are rarely due to one error, and so maintaining awareness across all activities for potential mishaps or lapses is important. Thus, while error may be inevitable, it may also be prevented or managed; human and technological systems can be built to intercept error before it manifests into injury or to mitigate harm when the error reaches the endpoint.

A patient safety program seeks to change the culture and design of systems that deliver health care, based on the same assumptions. The risks of the complexity of modern medicine are summed up succinctly by Sir Cyril Chantler, Chair of the University College London Partners: "Medicine used to be simple, ineffective, and relatively safe. Now it is complex, effective, and potentially dangerous." Furthermore, this complexity rides on the execution of nearly all tasks by human subjects and human workers. Obstetrics also exemplifies the second point, as most emergencies such as shoulder dystocia and postpartum hemorrhage are unforeseeable but prompt recognition and action can make considerable differences. Third, medicine, as much as any human activity, should be viewed as a team sport, without the benefit of coaches and where the loser, the patient, loses more than the rest of the team [9]. Finally, it is clear from Joint Commission (JCAHO) "sentinel event" and root cause analyses, that a catastrophic injury is typically related to many errors, rather than a singular event, evoking Reason's "Swiss cheese" model of accident causation [10,11].

19.3 Building blocks of an obstetric patient safety program

Beginning a patient safety program requires a commitment for change across all levels of the healthcare team. The change required for a patient safety program should not be underestimated. Importantly, leadership must show a commitment not only by demonstrating willingness to allocate appropriate resources – such as safety nurses and educational/training programs – but also by engaging in the various activities, including teamwork training and promoting a culture of safety, rather than a culture of blame. This improves a transition to a "just culture," which describes a culture that identifies and addresses systems issues that lead individuals to engage in unsafe behaviors while maintaining accountability [12]. This includes promoting transparency and openness in responding to adverse events. In terms of financial commitment, while startup costs are not insignificant, overall payoffs in terms of outcome improvements, workplace satisfaction and worker retention, and liability experience will likely provide significant returns on investment.

1. *Unit audit/assessment*: Knowing where to begin for a patient safety program often requires an unbiased and impartial external assessment of the unit. This begins the culture shift from a culture of fear and blame for errors and adverse events, to one of openness and transparency. To promote a team approach, any combination of nurses, physicians, or administrators can be invited, but the members of this group should be familiar with both obstetrics and safety and quality. Hospital and unit policies and protocols should be reviewed for clarity as well as adherence to national and regulatory standards. A triangulation process, where staff from the various professional domains are interviewed and

differences in perspectives are compared across domains for consistency or variation, can assess the overall culture of safety. The review typically results in a written report offering recommendations for improvement based on local and national standards. The review and report should be transparent, based on local and national standards, informed by the evidence, and focused on core principles of safety.

2. *Safety culture assessment*: A second means for assessing the baseline safety status of a unit is administration of a structured and validated safety culture survey. Two tools, the Safety Attitude Questionnaire (SAQ) and the Hospital Survey on Patient Safety Culture, are available at this time. The SAQ, a tool developed by Sexton and adapted for use in health care, assesses employee perception of safety and teamwork. Respondents are assessed in six domains of safety (teamwork culture, safety culture, job satisfaction, working conditions, stress management, and perceptions of management) and can be used to show differences over time or between employee groups, the latter a product of our being trained and working in silos. Replies are based on a 5-point Likert scale. Differences of 10% or more, over time or between groups, are considered clinically significant and overall scores > 80% are the target for change. To date, the SAQ is the only safety assessment survey validated to correspond improved scores with lower rates of adverse outcomes [13]. Conveniently, an SAQ has been adapted specifically to obstetrics and has been used to demonstrate significant improvements from a comprehensive safety program [14–16]. The Hospital Survey on Patient Safety Culture, developed for the Agency for Healthcare Research and Quality (AHRQ), is a more general assessment tool and is available for free in the public domain [17]. The major advantage of this survey is that results from a particular unit can be compared to a database of national results reported to and accumulated by the AHRQ [18]. Both surveys have similar reliability and predictive validity [19].

3. *Teamwork training*: According to the Joint Commission, communication is the leading root cause of sentinel events [20]. A 2004 JCAHO sentinel event report echoed these findings for obstetrics [21]. Of 47 perinatal deaths, the leading contributor to these adverse events was communication, in over 70% of cases. Medicine is a team sport, as Gawande points out, without the benefit of a coach [9]. However, while we are expected to work in teams, nurses and physicians, for example, are trained in distinct styles and silos. The result is a workforce that works in groups – as individuals working synchronously but independently with distinct goals – rather than in teams.

Crew resource management (CRM) seeks to train workers to develop habits of teams, such as having a clear and valued vision, developing trust and confidence in each other, understanding leadership and following, and adoption of clear communication tools. CRM is currently advocated by the Institute of Medicine, the Institute for Healthcare Improvement, the AHRQ, the Department of Defense, ACOG, and the Joint Commission. In fact, the Joint Commission insists that perinatal units develop CRM programs, as part of their 2004 report on perinatal deaths [21].

MedTeams™ (Should Rhode Island Hospital, Providence, RI) and TeamSTEPPS® (Agency for Healthcare Research and Quality, Rockville, MD) are two examples of teamwork models based on CRM that address four main competencies: leadership, situation monitoring, mutual support, and communication. Specific tools that are often discussed include:

1 Team huddles: Our unit uses multiple huddles throughout the day, including a morning report including midwives and physicians, a post-report labor and delivery "board meeting" of team leadership to assess the team status and resource status, patient bedside huddles or rounds, and a midnight huddle including leadership from all obstetric units to reassess team and resource status.
2 Debriefings: Pre-event debriefings can develop a shared mental model for care and anticipate problems, and a post-event debriefing can develop an appropriate handoff for the next stage of care and educate the team on goals for success for the future.
3 SBAR (situation-background-assessment-recommendation): A handoff tool for precise communication of care pathways.
4 Two-challenge rule: A conflict resolution tool to communicate a staff members' level of concern. If a team member requests clarification or explanation of a treatment, and meets an unsatisfactory result, after two attempts a more assertive strategy or a superior in the chain of command should be invoked.
5 Check-backs: A closed-loop communication tool to verify information exchange where a verbal order or command is written down and read back before it is carried out.
6 Call-outs: Call-outs are communication tools used for emergencies, such as shoulder dystocia, where a designated person identifies and communicates important information (such as who is in charge or who else is being called) to an entire team simultaneously.
7 The "CUS" words of Concerned, Uncomfortable, and Scared used to communicate levels of concern. Using the terms in that order specifies an escalation of concern and should trigger the listener to respect the other team member's discomfort with a particular situation.
8 Chain of command (Figure 19.1): A readily available chain of command demonstrates to workers who is available to manage resolution when team conflict arises. The most effective chains of command include contact information for individuals at each level, to promote a sense of accessibility, and a nursing/provider dyad at each level, to reduce the silos and encourage open discussions between pairs.

While implementation of a team training program is formidable, sustaining the principles in practice is the biggest challenge. Leadership must be committed to asking staff what team training principles they incorporated any time a

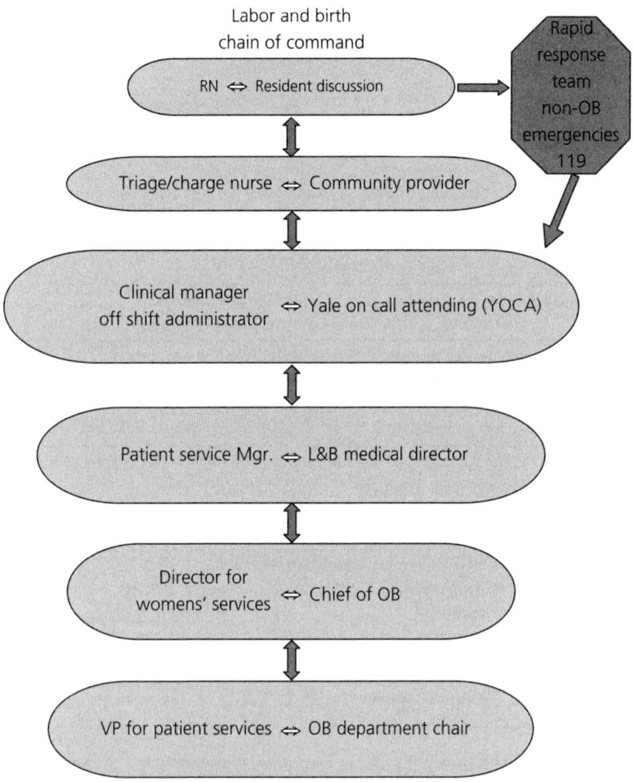

Figure 19.1 Example of a chain of command.

complaint or concern is discussed after an event. We post and supply our staff with laminated cards with the basic principles of CRM (Figure 19.2 and Figure 19.3) for reference and reminding.

The only randomized trial for team-training in obstetrics to date failed to demonstrate improvements in clinical adverse outcomes, though team-trained institutions did see improved cesarean decision-to-incision times (21.2 vs 33.3 minutes; $p = 0.03$) [22]. However, CRM has proven helpful in developing teamwork culture and in improving outcomes in surgical units, demonstrating a 50% improved risk-adjusted mortality rate in CRM-trained programs in the Veterans Health Administration [23].

4. *Standardized protocols, guidelines, checklists*: Protocols, guidelines, and checklists seek to guide decisions and management and standardize care based on best practices and the best available evidence. The best guidelines instruct all levels of caregivers, but in particular both nurses and physicians/midwives. Furthermore, the best guidelines will assert a high level of standardization when the evidence demonstrates superiority of one care pathway or when the concept of using one care pathway, and avoiding variable approaches, reduces exposure to confusion and error.

Team training communication tools	
CUS	Identify level of concern "I'm **c**oncerned" "I'm **u**ncomfortable" } Stop the line "This is a **s**afety concern" "I'm **s**cared"
SBAR	Focus the communication **S**ituation–current clinical situation/what is going on with the patient? **B**ackground–what is the pertinent clinical background or context? **A**ssessment–what do you think is the problem? **R**ecommendation–what would you like done?
Two challenge rule	Refocus the discussion when an initial assertion is ignored Restate and voice concern at least **two times** to ensure it is heard
Call out	Strategy used to communicate important or critical information • Informs all team members simultaneously during emergent situations • Helps team members anticipate next steps • Direct responsibility to a specific individual responsible for the task
Check back	Closing the loop to ensure that information conveyed is understood by the receiver • Sender initiates message • Receiver accepts message and provides feedback–"write it down & read it back" • Sender re-confirms message or clarifies if needed
Chain of command	Escalation of concern until resolution realized • Incorporates nursing and medical representation at all levels • Initiate when: - Above procedures of resolution have not been effective - There is need to proceed to a higher authority for discussions or decisions regarding: ◦ Patient care or safety ◦ Operational issues

Team training key concepts	
Team structure	Team size, membership, leadership, composition, identification and distribution Team includes every staff member that influences patient care; licensed and non-licensed staff have equal responsibility for patient safety
Team leadership	Ability to: • Organize the team • Articulate clear goals • Empower team members to speak up • Make decisions • Role model desired behavior • Skillful at conflict resolution
Team events Brief Huddle Debrief	Planning: session to discuss team formation; assign roles; establish expectations; anticipate outcomes and contingencies Problem solving: ad hoc planning; assessing the need to adjust the plan Process Improvement: after action review; informational exchange to improve Team performance and effectiveness
Situation monitoring **Situation awareness** **Cross monitoring** **Shared mental model**	An individual skill: continual scanning and assessing what's going on around you An individual outcome: knowing what's going on around you A team skill: watching each other's back; provides a team safety net A team outcome: all team members are on the same page
Mutual support **Feedback** **Task assistance**	 Information given for the purpose of improving team performance and patient safety Mutual support; assistance is actively sought and offered
Communication	Process by which information is clearly and accurately exchanged by team members

Figure 19.2 and **Figure 19.3** Examples of a laminated reference card outlining the key principles of team training.

Any program implementing standardized guidelines and protocols will meet resistance from experienced providers who assert the primacy of their experience and knowledge. This resistance is largely based on the fear that standardization will completely dictate all care pathways and will not allow for variation or individualization where it might be necessary. The most effective guidelines create a solid structure for care, but will actually leave room for appropriate variation when reasonable and safe. When developing protocols and guidelines, it is critical to involve an interdisciplinary group of nurses, midwives, physicians, residents, and administrators. Physicians should include both academic and community providers, if relevant. Establishment of consensus and allowing for adequate comment periods prior to implementation will increase the likelihood of success. Over time, as a safety culture develops, even the providers initially most resistant to standardization will begin to ask for protocols that do not yet exist to help guide them in their practice.

Higher risk practices – such as the use of oxytocin, prostaglandins, and magnesium sulfate – and the most common practices – such as cesarean delivery and induction of labor – are particularly aided by standardization. Creation of guidelines in these instances creates a common knowledge structure, or shared mental model, for performing well during times strained by pressure or uncertainty. The practices can also be aided by the institution of checklists, which insist on real-time implementation of the important events and activities required to perform a successful task. In other areas of medicine, checklists have proven in clinical trials to reduce central-line associated bloodstream infections and surgical complications [24,25]. Implementation of an oxytocin checklist has been shown to reduce maximum infusion rates without affecting the length of labor and coinciding with a lower cesarean rate [26].

Standardization is also enhanced through electronic medical records (EMR). Guidelines and protocols may be incorporated into the EMR for quick access. Computerized order entry can reduce the rates of medication errors, particularly when standardized order sets (such as for oxytocin administration or for preeclampsia or preterm premature rupture of membranes) are used. Interactive decision support tools can also be engaged to assist providers in ordering the correct supplemental treatments for certain clinical scenarios. These systems can reduce the possibilities of human error.

ACOG Practice Bulletins, Committee Opinions, and Policies are helpful sources for outlining a clinical protocol. The National Institute for Health and Clinical Excellence (NICE) (http://www.nice.org.uk) in the United Kingdom provides guidelines with special attention given to high-quality evidence and cost effectiveness. For instance, the website offers clinical pathways for cesarean delivery, intrapartum care, induction of labor, and smoking cessation during pregnancy, and includes implementation tools and resources. The National Guideline Clearinghouse (http://www.guideline.gov) gathers guidelines from diverse national, state, local, and hospital organizations on a website; guidelines may be accessed here and adapted to particular local customs or needs.

5. *Perinatal patient safety nurse*: Initiation and maintenance of a comprehensive safety program requires a designated practitioner to oversee daily operations. The responsibilities for patient-care oversight, development and implementation of initiatives, oversight and maintenance of quality metrics, and championing the transformation to a culture of safety should not be underestimated and cannot be administrated piecemeal. A perinatal patient safety nurse can serve as the organizing element of a patient safety program [27]. A nurse with both clinical and administrative experience, with a background in obstetrics, is ideal. Project management will require good organization and skills in directing people and meetings. Many nurses may not have particular backgrounds in quality and safety before beginning in a role such as this, though an interest in developing this expertise is essential. Good communication skills and ability to work with and lead teams is critical, as this person will be an example that clinical teams will look to. The keys to success for this role are to be "available, affable, and able."

The Yale-New Haven obstetric patient safety nurse has diverse responsibilities, including oversight of the anonymous event reporting system, the safety attitude questionnaire, and quality assurance reviews. The latter is part of her role in providing a continuous quantitative and qualitative assessment of the clinical care and outcomes of our service. Cases complicated by adverse outcomes or near-misses are collected through the anonymous event reporting system, attendance at daily rounds, daily review of the services with charge nurses, and review of labor and neonatal logs. Each case complicated by a defined adverse outcome – within the Adverse Outcome Index – gets a formal written assessment for review by leaders and, if appropriate, the obstetrics Patient Safety Committee. Occasionally, the perinatal patient safety nurse will lead a root cause analysis related to an adverse event. Educational programs under her supervision include electronic fetal monitoring education and testing and CRM training. Our patient safety nurse is also involved with preparations and responses to reviews from the various regulatory bodies visiting our hospital.

6. *Safety reporting structure*: Discovering system flaws and adverse events can be assisted with a computerized, ideally web-based, event reporting tool. An anonymous and easily accessible system allows for discreet and real-time reporting of adverse events, near-misses, and unsafe conditions. It is important that reported events be responded to with transparent explanations or corrective action. Over time, as a reporting culture develops, staff are empowered to participate in change and will less frequently see the need to report anonymously. The patient safety nurse can be responsible for investigations and tracking trends. An important caveat is that a patient safety team should not rely on an event reporting system to capture all of the adverse events in a unit or hospital. In fact, a Department of Health and Human Services report from 2012 revealed that

hospital incident reporting systems only captured 14% of important events and that most hospitals rely too much on these systems for data collection [28].

7. *Obstetrics Patient Safety Committee*: Departmental leadership, in conjunction with the patient safety nurse, can be an effective leadership team for a perinatal patient safety initiative. A multidisciplinary committee can provide support for administrative responsibilities by reviewing important adverse event cases, evaluating current practices, and organizing prospective initiatives, and has shown great success in prioritizing the safety culture [29,30]. Regular and structured meetings can be led by the patient safety nurse and another patient safety champion. A multidisciplinary committee comprised of nurses, midwives, obstetricians, residents, pediatricians, anesthesiologists, and administrators is important for representing the interests of all stakeholders and can be an important advocate and example for culture change.

8. *Simulation training*: Simulation can be an important education and training tool for medical teams, particularly as part of a quality improvement effort. The aviation industry developed simulation to recreate workplace conditions to facilitate teaching of new skills and for practice in managing rare scenarios. Labor and delivery is an ideal setting for simulation training because the field, as in aviation, is characterized by long periods of routine activities interrupted by infrequent but high-stakes events like shoulder dystocia, hemorrhage, and eclampsia. Typically, a simulation effort should focus on either knowledge/skills training or teamwork training, rather than both, in order to focus teams on the intended goals. Simulations can occur *in situ*, on a labor and delivery unit, such as during a time of low workload. Surprise *in situ* simulation events, however, can test a unit's preparedness and provide important feedback to a team for troubleshooting or systems improvement. Off-site simulation centers allow for a more controlled atmosphere for practice and learning and often incorporate high-fidelity simulation technologies, but require substantial preparation and resources. Mannequins and simulation monitoring equipment can provide a realistic experience.

Simulation training has proven an important educational intervention in obstetrics, demonstrating improvements in some clinical outcomes (e.g. Apgar scores, hypoxic-ischemic encephalopathy, shoulder dystocia) as well as improved team performance and knowledge/skills [31–34]. Demonstrating its perceived importance for education and improvement, ACOG and the Society for Maternal-Fetal Medicine are developing programs to assist units in implementing simulation programs [35].

9. *Electronic fetal monitoring training*: Historically, fetal monitoring interpretation was considered an art as much as a science. Subjective, but unscientific, descriptions of fetal tracings – using terms such as "ominous," "fetal distress," "reassuring," and "non-reassuring" – were, and still are, common. The 2004 Joint Commission sentinel event review into perinatal deaths demonstrated that 34% involved inadequate fetal monitoring. Included in the Joint Commission's

recommendations was for units to "develop clear guidelines for fetal monitoring of potential high-risk patients, including nursing protocols for the interpretation of fetal heart rate tracings" and to "educate nurses, residents, nurse midwives, and physicians to use standardized terminology to communicate abnormal fetal heart rate tracings" [21]. The next year, ACOG and the Association of Women's Health, Obstetric and Neonatal Nurses advocated universal implementation of the National Institute of Health / National Institute of Child Health and Human Development (NICHD) Workshop guidelines on electronic fetal monitoring [36]. These were subsequently revised, with the addition of a three-tiered classification system, in 2008 [37]. Adoption of such guidelines by a unit is important, and usually relies on formalized programs for training and testing. One example of this is offered by National Certification Corporation (NCC; http://www.nccnet.org), a nonprofit group that offers training and testing of fetal monitoring standards based on the NICHD criteria. We have additionally provided our teams with laminated reference cards to assist in better incorporating standardized terminology into their practices (Figure 19.4 and Figure 19.5).

10. *Obstetrical hospitalist*: Hospitalist coverage of inpatient general medical units has increased in popularity across the country. A dedicated inpatient caregiver who oversees the hospital care of patients from various primary outpatient providers, the hospitalist has primary skillsets related to inpatient care and as such can improve clinical efficiency. Data suggests that clinical outcomes may be better in hospitals that employ hospitalists [38]. In 2003, Weinstein proposed the concept of a laborist, an obstetrician, physically available 24 hours a day, on labor and delivery, with the sole responsibility of managing patients who present to the unit [39]. ACOG now supports the concept of an obstetrics/gynecology hospitalist "as one potential solution to achieving increased professional and patient satisfaction while maintaining safe and effective care across delivery settings" [40].

A variety of laborist models have been proposed. Weinstein's original model proposed that the laborists be employed by the hospital, with their salaries covered by billings for fees and services. This would fit particularly well with a teaching hospital, where a supervising physician is required to be present for oversight of resident activities. This model would allow for a consistent laborist group, a specialized set of individuals with improved familiarity (for the labor unit teams and processes) and efficiency. Not all practices or units can support this type of structure, and other adaptations are possible for private practice and community hospital models [41].

A major criticism of this practice is the loss of continuity between a patient's outpatient and inpatient experiences. It also may not be readily apparent to some units, especially low-volume ones, how to cover the costs of a laborist program. Furthermore, agreement on standardized approaches to particular practices must be obtained for the model to function well. No data exist at this time for whether any type of laborist model improves clinical outcomes or is cost-effective.

2008 NICHD definitions for EFM assessment and documentation		
Baseline		Rounded to increments of 5 bpm (e.g. 140, 145) need baseline duration of ≥ 2 min. during a 10 min segment, between periodic or episodic changes, to determine baseline
	Bradycardia	< 110 bpm for > 10 min.
	Tachycardia	> 160 bpm for > 10 min.
Variability	Absent	Undetectable
	Minimal	> Undetectable- ≤ 5bpm
	Moderate	6–25 bpm
	Marked	>25bpm
Acceleration		**Abrupt** increase ≥ 15 bpm, lasts ≥ 15 sec.
	Prolonged	≥2 min. and < 10 min. (≥ 10 min = a baseline change)
Decelerations	Variable	**Abrupt** decrease onset to nadir <30 sec. decrease ≥ 15 bpm lasting ≥ 15 sec. < 2 min.
	Early	**Gradual** decrease onset to nadir ≥ 30 sec. with contraction
	Late	**Gradual** decrease onset to nadir ≥ 30 sec. nadir of deceleration occurring after peak of contraction
	Prolonged	Decrease ≥ 15 bpm lasting ≥ 2 min. but < 10 min. (≥ 10 min = a baseline change)
	Recurrent	Occur with ≥ 50% of uterine contractions in any 20 min window
	Intermittent	Occur with < 50% of uterine contractions in any 20 min window
Contractions		Consider: frequency, duration, intensity and relaxation
	Normal	≤5 contractions / 10 minutes averaged over a 30 min window
	Tachysystole†	>5 contractions/10 minutes averaged over a 30 min window should always be qualified as to the presence or absence of associated FHR decels. DO NOT USE HYPERSTIMULATION.

Three–tier EFM interpretation system	
Category I *(Must include **all** of these characteristics)*	**Rate**: 110–160 beats per minute (bpm) **Variability**: moderate **Late or variable decelerations**: absent **Early decelerations**: presentor absent **Accelerations**: present or absent
Category II *(All FHR tracings not categorized as Cat. I or Cat. III, including all of these listed)*	**Baseline rate** • Bradycardia not accompanied by absent variability • Tachycardia **Baseline FHR variability** • Minimal variability • Absent variability not accompanied by recurrent decelerations • Marked baseline variability **Accelerations** • Absence of induced accelerations after fetal stimulation **Periodic or episodic decelerations** • Recurrent variable decelerations accompanied by minimal or moderate baseline variability • Prolonged deceleration ≥ 2 minutes but < 10 minutes • Recurrent late decelerations with moderate baseline variability • Variable decelerations with other characteristics, such as slow return to baseline, "overshoots", or "shoulders'
Category III *(Includes either of these listed)*	***Absent* baseline FHR variability *and* any of the following** • Recurrent late decelerations • Recurrent variable decelerations • Bradycardia **Sinusoidal pattern**

Figure 19.4 and **Figure 19.5** Examples of a laminated reference card outlining the key principles of electronic fetal monitoring interpretation.

11. *Medical documentation standardization*: Most, if not all, of the preceding initiatives involved some sort of standardization of processes. EMR provides an additional manner of standardization to support these other processes. Paper medical records rely on handwritten descriptions and facilitate subjective and less rigorous interpretations. Errors of omission are more possible if a provider is not prompted to document every component of the assessment. An electronic intrapartum documentation template can force the use of uniform electronic fetal monitoring nomenclature, based on NICHD criteria, and can prompt a more complete evaluation. Computerized order entry can allow for the integration of bundles and checklists as well as standardized order sets to better guide a provider through the preferred management strategies for various clinical scenarios.

19.4 Measuring patient safety

The science of measuring safety and quality begins with the Donabedian model of patient safety. Beginning with work in the 1960s and developing further in the 1980s, Avedis Donabedian proposed a model for examining healthcare quality based on three domains: structure, process, and outcome [42,43]. Structure is defined as the setting and organization of healthcare delivery, including the building, the staff, and the physical resources necessary. It may also include certain nonphysical qualities, such as the safety culture or climate, of a healthcare institution. Process consists of the actions performed to give care to that patient. Finally, the outcome is the result of the patient's involvement in the healthcare system. In this model, each component directly influences the next. Measuring healthcare quality is often grouped into these domains:

Outcome measures: While outcome measures are typically the *result* of the healthcare process, in terms of assessment, they are the most logical *beginning* for measuring quality. Outcome measures can track how often patients are harmed or how well the organization is providing favorable (expected) outcomes, though most patient safety initiatives focus on adverse outcome measures, as this is often the primary goal of such efforts. In obstetrics, the Adverse Outcome Index (AOI) (Table 19.1) is one such set of measures based on specific outcomes set forth by the Joint Commission, ACOG, and the National Perinatal Information Center [44]. The AOI is calculated as the percentage of mothers with at least one adverse outcome indicator. Thus, a mother with two or more outcomes would only count once in the numerator, with the total number of mothers over the specific period of time making up the denominator. While individual indicators can be tracked on their own, the rate can be calculated on a monthly or quarterly basis to evaluate progress of an initiative. Many quality improvement programs have used the AOI [22,44–46].

Table 19.1 Obstetric Adverse Outcome Index (AOI) indicators [44].

Apgar < 7 at 5 minutes
Blood transfusion
Fetal traumatic birth injury
Intrapartum or neonatal death > 2500 g
Maternal death
Maternal ICU admission
Maternal return to OR or labor and delivery
Unexpected admission to neonatal ICU > 2500 g and for > 24 hours
Uterine rupture

Structure measures: It is easily possible to measure changes in the physical structure of an organization in response to a patient safety effort. A reduction in nurse:patient ratios, for instance, is a change that is easily measured and on its own probably demonstrates an inherent quality improvement. Yet, its association with an outcome measure is sometimes necessary to justify its utility. For instance, Needleman has demonstrated that staffing levels below target (structure measure) are associated with increased mortality (outcome measure) in a large tertiary medical center [47]. The structure of the organization, however, can also be viewed as an intangible element, as in culture. Safety culture is defined as how safety thinking and practices have integrated into clinical activities. Safety climate is the quantitative description of the safety culture and can be measured by calibrating a healthcare team's perceptions about issues related to safety through surveys [14]. Two important safety climate surveys are currently available, and are described previously.

Process measures: Process measures analyze the adherence to common or evidence-based standards and practices, with the assumption that adherence to these performance measures improves outcomes [48]. The Surgical Care Improvement Project (SCIP), which proposes to measure processes like appropriate antibiotic administration and thromboembolism prophylaxis, is one example of a set of process measures. Many quality measures proposed by regulatory bodies such as the Joint Commission and the National Quality Forum consist of process measures (see below). ACOG, in many Practice Bulletins, suggests "Proposed Performance Measures" that may be relevant for a labor unit. Adherence to good practices in one process of care likely produces better compliance across the spectrum of a healthcare encounter, but it remains to be seen if improvements in particular process outcomes actually translate to reduced adverse outcomes or improvements in clinical outcomes [49]. An example of this sort of analysis is provided by a randomized trial of a multifaceted behavioral intervention – which included training, workshops, and guidelines – in South America that tracked the use of episiotomy and of prophylactic postpartum oxytocin [50]. Both of these process measures improved, as did the rate of postpartum hemorrhage.

The science of measuring safety in obstetrics is still evolving. Whether the obstetric AOI is the most appropriate way of tracking a safety program has not been established. A major limitation of the AOI is that while it may have strong internal validity, it is not as good at comparing different units with different levels of acuity, different patient mixes, and varying provider types.

Independent of the scientific utility of such mandates, regulatory bodies will certainly provide some guidance on what should and will be required for tracking by hospitals. The Joint Commission, in the "Perinatal Care Core Measure Set," requires reporting of elective deliveries < 39 weeks of gestation, primary cesarean rates in low-risk women, appropriate use of antenatal steroids, newborn nosocomial bloodstream infections, and rates of exclusive breastfeeding at discharge [51]. The National Quality Forum has endorsed, in addition to those five, additional quality measures for obstetrics, including appropriate use of prophylactic antibiotics prior to cesarean, appropriate use of thromboprophylaxis at the time of cesarean, episiotomy rate, birth trauma rate, and birth of babies under 1500 g at sites with appropriate levels of care [52].

19.5 The evidence on quality improvement in obstetrics

The Yale-New Haven comprehensive obstetric safety program incorporated many, if not most, of the improvement strategies in this chapter [45]. Significant improvements, as measured by the AOI, were seen: over a 3-year period, comprising over 13,000 deliveries, the AOI declined significantly ($p = 0.01$) (Figure 19.6). The mean quarterly AOI for the *second* half of the initiative (2.09 ± 0.57%) was significantly lower than that for the first half (2.90 ± 0.64%) ($p = 0.04$). Further improvements were seen in safety climate, as well, with favorable impressions of teamwork culture and safety culture improving from 39 to 63% and 33 to 63%, respectively [16].

A group from the Hospital Corporation of America healthcare system, which involves more than 200 hospitals across the United States, implemented a comprehensive effort that included a protocol for oxytocin administration, checklist-based protocols for misoprostol and magnesium, and a standardized shoulder dystocia delivery note [53]. Over time they witnessed a reduction in annual malpractice claims from 10–13/ 100,000 deliveries to 6–7.5/ 100,000 births ($p < 0.001$).

Some research is demonstrating that improvements in outcomes may translate to improved liability experiences, as relates to claims and expenditures, in obstetrics. A Rand study has demonstrated that a reduction of 10 adverse events in a given year may lead to a decrease of 3.7 malpractice claims, with approximately one-third of the variance in malpractice claims attributable to patient safety indicators [54]. Smaller studies – limited by local legal climates, claims that remain open or unresolved, and long statutes of limitations – have also reported favorable experiences [55,56].

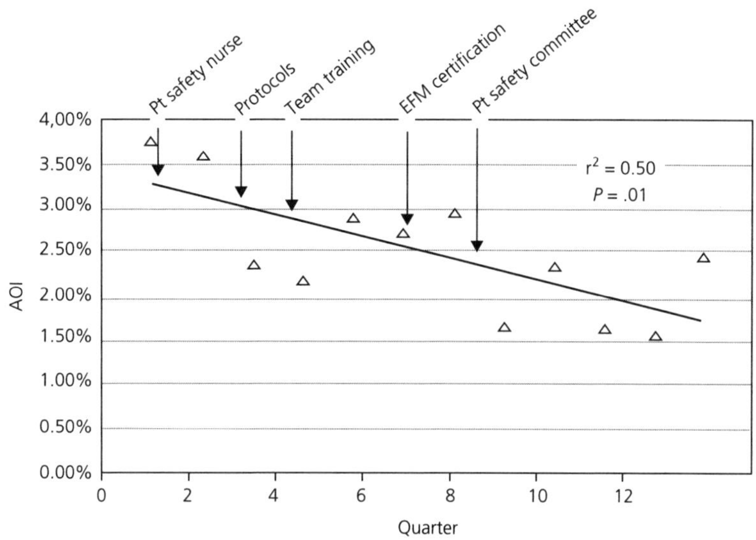

Figure 19.6 The Yale-New Haven Hospital obstetric Adverse Outcomes Index from September 2004 to August 2007. *Source*: Pettker *et al.*, 2009 [44]. Reproduced with permission of Elsevier.

19.6 Conclusion

The science of patient safety is young and evolving. Truthfully, little evidence exists at this time to validate many safety practices, though most appeal for their common sense and practicality. Justification of such efforts by studying outcomes and costs will prove vital in the coming years. Even in the absence of strong, favorable evidence, government and regulatory bodies, in addition to third-party payers, will require adoption of many of these practices. Knowledge of the essential practices of patient safety is essential to keep up with the changes in modern health care. Engaging in these processes can evolve a unit into a "high reliability" organization, where safety is a paramount end, teams are valued over the individual, effective and transparent communication is constantly reinforced, and the unexpected becomes expected.

References

1 Kohn, LT, Corrigan, JM., and Donaldson, Molla S. (eds) *To Err Is Human: Building a Safer Health System*. Washington, DC: Institute of Medicine, National Academy Press, 1999.

2 National Hospital Discharge Survey, 2009. 2009 [cited May 1, 2012]; Available from: http://www.cdc.gov/nchs/data/nhds/2average/2009ave2_firstlist.pdf (accessed 20 May 2015).

3 Studdert DM, Mello MM, Gawande AA, Gandhi TK, Kachalia A, Yoon C *et al.* Claims, errors, and compensation payments in medical malpractice litigation. *New England Journal of Medicine* 2006;**354**(19):2024–2033.

4 CRICO. Malpractice Risks in Obstetrics (2010 Annual Benchmarking Report). Cambridge, MA: CRICO, 2011.
5 American College of Obstetricians and Gynecologists. 2009 ACOG survey on professional liability results. 2009 [cited 2009 February 1, 2012]; Available from: http://www.acog.org/About-ACOG/ACOG-Departments/Professional-Liability/2012-Survey-Results
6 Knox GE and Simpson KR. Perinatal high reliability. *American Journal of Obstetrics & Gynecology* 2011;**204**(5):373–377.
7 Aspden P, Institute of Medicine (U.S.). Committee on Data Standards for Patient Safety. *Patient Safety: Achieving a New Standard for Care*. Washington, DC: National Academies Press, 2004.
8 Emanuel L, Berwick D, Conway J, Combes J, Hatlie M, Leape L *et al.* What exactly is patient safety? In: Henricksen K, Battles J, Keyes M, Grady M (eds) *Advances in Patient Safety: New Directions and Alternative Approaches*. Rockville, MD: Agency for Healthcare Research and Quality, 2008.
9 Gawande A. *Better: A Surgeon's Notes on Performance*. 1st edn. New York: Metropolitan, 2007.
10 Joint Commission on Accreditation of Healthcare Organizations. *Root Cause Analysis in Health Care: Tools and Techniques*. 4th edn. Oakbrook Terrace, IL: Joint Commission Resources, 2009.
11 Reason JT. *Human Error*. Cambridge & New York: Cambridge University Press, 1990.
12 Marx D. *Patient Safety and the "Just Culture": A Primer for Health Care Executives*. New York: Columbia University, 2001.
13 Colla JB, Bracken AC, Kinney LM, and Weeks WB. Measuring patient safety climate: a review of surveys. *Quality & Safety in Health Care* 2005;**14**(5):364–366.
14 Sexton JB, Helmreich RL, Neilands TB, Rowan K, Vella K, Boyden J *et al.* The Safety Attitudes Questionnaire: psychometric properties, benchmarking data, and emerging research. *BMC Health Services Research*. 2006;**6**:44.
15 Sexton JB, Holzmueller CG, Pronovost PJ, Thomas EJ, McFerran S, Nunes J *et al.* Variation in caregiver perceptions of teamwork climate in labor and delivery units. *Journal of Perinatology* 2006;**26**(8):463–470.
16 Pettker CM, Thung SF, Raab CA, Donohue KP, Copel JA, Lockwood CJ *et al.* A comprehensive obstetrics patient safety program improves safety climate and culture. *American Journal of Obstetrics & Gynecology* 2011;**204**(3):216 e1–6.
17 Sorra J and Nieva V. *Hospital Survey on Patient Safety Culture*. Rockville, MD: Agency for Healthcare Research and Quality, 2004.
18 Sorra J. *Hospital Survey on Patient Safety Culture: 2009 Comparative Database Report*. Rockville, MD: Agency for Healthcare Research and Quality, U.S. Department of Health and Human Services, 2009.
19 Etchegaray JM and Thomas EJ. Comparing two safety culture surveys: Safety Attitudes Questionnaire and Hospital Survey on Patient Safety. *BMJ Quality & Safety* 2012;**21**(6):490–498.
20 Joint Commission on Accreditation of Healthcare Organizations. *Sentinel Event Statistics*. 2011 [cited February 1, 2012]; Available from: http://www.jointcommission.org/SentinelEvents/Statistics/ (accessed May 20, 2015).
21 Joint Commission on Accreditation of Healthcare Organizations. *Sentinel Event Alert 30*. 2004 [cited February 1, 2012]; Available from: http://www.jointcommission.org/sentinel_event_alert_issue_30_preventing_infant_death_and_injury_during_delivery/ (accessed May 20, 2015).
22 Nielsen PE, Goldman MB, Mann S, Shapiro DE, Marcus RG, Pratt SD *et al.* Effects of teamwork training on adverse outcomes and process of care in labor and delivery: a randomized controlled trial. *Obstetrics & Gynecology* 2007;**109**(1):48–55.
23 Neily J, Mills PD, Young-Xu Y, Carney BT, West P, Berger DH *et al.* Association between implementation of a medical team training program and surgical mortality. *Journal of the American Medical Association* 2010;**304**(15):1693–1700.

24 Haynes AB, Weiser TG, Berry WR, Lipsitz SR, Breizat AH, Dellinger EP *et al.* A surgical safety checklist to reduce morbidity and mortality in a global population. *New England Journal of Medicine* 2009;**360**(5):491–499.

25 Pronovost P, Needham D, Berenholtz S, Sinopoli D, Chu H, Cosgrove S *et al.* An intervention to decrease catheter-related bloodstream infections in the ICU. *New England Journal of Medicine* 2006;**355**(26):2725–2732.

26 Clark S, Belfort M, Saade G, Hankins G, Miller D, Frye D *et al.* Implementation of a conservative checklist-based protocol for oxytocin administration: maternal and newborn outcomes. *American Journal of Obstetrics & Gynecology* 2007;**197**(5):480 e1–5.

27 Will SB, Hennicke KP, Jacobs LS, O'Neill LM, and Raab CA. The perinatal patient safety nurse: a new role to promote safe care for mothers and babies. *Journal of Obstetric, Gynecologic, & Neonatal Nursing* 2006;**35**(3):417–423.

28 Levinson DR. *Hospital Incident Reporting Systems Do Not Capture Most Patient Harm.* Department of Health and Human Services. January 2012. Available from: https://oig.hhs.gov/oei/reports/oei-06-09-00091.pdf (accessed May 20, 2015).

29 Odwazny R, Hasler S, Abrams R, and McNutt R. Organizational and cultural changes for providing safe patient care. *Quality Management in Health Care* 2005;**14**(3):132–143.

30 Piotrowski MM, Saint S, and Hinshaw DB. The Safety Case Management Committee: expanding the avenues for addressing patient safety. *Joint Commission Journal on Quality Improvement* 2002;**28**(6):296–305.

31 Merien AE, van de Ven J, Mol BW, Houterman S, and Oei SG. Multidisciplinary team training in a simulation setting for acute obstetric emergencies: a systematic review. *Obstetrics & Gynecology* 2010;**115**(5):1021–1031.

32 Deering S, Poggi S, Macedonia C, Gherman R, and Satin AJ. Improving resident competency in the management of shoulder dystocia with simulation training. *Obstetrics & Gynecology* 2004;**103**(6):1224–1228.

33 Draycott T, Sibanda T, Owen L, Akande V, Winter C, Reading S *et al.* Does training in obstetric emergencies improve neonatal outcome? *BJOG* 2006;**113**(2):177–182.

34 Draycott TJ, Crofts JF, Ash JP, Wilson LV, Yard E, Sibanda T *et al.* Improving neonatal outcome through practical shoulder dystocia training. *Obstetrics & Gynecology* 2008;**112**(1):14–20.

35 Argani CH, Eichelberger M, Deering S, and Satin AJ. The case for simulation as part of a comprehensive patient safety program. *American Journal of Obstetrics & Gynecology* 2012;**206**(6):451–455. Epub 2011/921.

36 National Institute of Child Health and Human Development Research Planning Workshop. Electronic fetal heart rate monitoring: research guidelines for interpretation. *American Journal of Obstetrics & Gynecology* 1997;**177**(6):1385–1390.

37 Macones GA, Odibo A, Gross G, Stamilio D, Rampersad R, Ebinger R *et al.* Standardized multidisciplinary EFM training for the entire obstetrical team. *American Journal of Obstetrics & Gynecology* 2009;**199**(6):S211.

38 Lopez L, Hicks LS, Cohen AP, McKean S, and Weissman JS. Hospitalists and the quality of care in hospitals. *Archives of Internal Medicine* 2009;**169**(15):1389–1394.

39 Weinstein L. The laborist: a new focus of practice for the obstetrician. *American Journal of Obstetrics & Gynecology.* 2003;**188**(2):310–312.

40 American College of Obstetricians and Gynecologists. Committee Opinion No. 459: the obstetric-gynecologic hospitalist. *Obstetrics & Gynecology* 2010;**116**(1):237–239.

41 Gussman D and Mann W. The laborist: a flexible concept. 2007 [cited May 20, 2012]; Available from: http://www.acog.org/About-ACOG/ACOG-Departments/Practice-Management-and-Managed-Care/The-Laborist---A-Flexible-Concept

42 Donabedian A. Evaluating the quality of medical care. *The Milbank Memorial Fund Quarterly* 1966;**44**(3):(Suppl.):166–206.

43 Donabedian A. *Explorations in Quality Assessment and Monitoring*. Ann Arbor, MI: Health Administration Press, 1980.
44 Mann S, Pratt S, Gluck P, Nielsen P, Risser D, Greenberg P *et al.* Assessing quality in obstetrical care: development of standardized measures. *Joint Commission Journal on Quality and Patient Safety / Joint Commission Resources* 2006;**32**:497–505.
45 Pettker CM, Thung SF, Norwitz ER, Buhimschi CS, Raab CA, Copel JA *et al.* Impact of a comprehensive patient safety strategy on obstetric adverse events. *American Journal of Obstetrics & Gynecology* 2009;**200**(5):492 e1–8.
46 Walker S, Strandjord TP, and Benedetti TJ. In search of perinatal quality outcome measures: 1 hospital's in-depth analysis of the Adverse Outcomes Index. *American Journal of Obstetrics & Gynecology* 2010;**203**(4):336 e1–7.
47 Needleman J, Buerhaus P, Pankratz VS, Leibson CL, Stevens SR, and Harris M. Nurse staffing and inpatient hospital mortality. *New England Journal of Medicine* 2011;**364**(11):1037–1045.
48 Williams SC, Schmaltz SP, Morton DJ, Koss RG, and Loeb JM. Quality of care in U.S. hospitals as reflected by standardized measures, 2002–2004. *New England Journal of Medicine* 2005;**353**(3):255–264.
49 Hawn MT. Surgical care improvement: should performance measures have performance measures. *Journal of the American Medical Association* 2010;**303**(24):2527–2528.
50 Althabe F, Buekens P, Bergel E, Belizan JM, Campbell MK, Moss N *et al.* A behavioral intervention to improve obstetrical care. *New England Journal of Medicine* 2008;**358**(18):1929–1940.
51 Joint Commission on Accreditation of Healthcare Organizations. *Perinatal Care*. 2010 [cited February 1, 2011]; Available from: http://www.jointcommission.org/perinatal_care/ (accessed 20 May 2015).
52 Forum NQ. *National Quality Forum Endorses National Consensus Standards for Perinatal Care*. 2008 [cited February 1, 2012]; Available from: http://www.qualityforum.org/news_and_resources/press_releases/2012/nqf_endorses_perinatal_measures.aspx.
53 Clark SL, Belfort MA, Byrum SL, Meyers JA, and Perlin JB. Improved outcomes, fewer cesarean deliveries, and reduced litigation: results of a new paradigm in patient safety. *American Journal of Obstetrics & Gynecology* 2008;**199**(2):105 e1–7.
54 Greenberg MD, Haviland AM, Ashwood JS, and Main R. *Is Better Patient Safety Associated with Less Malpractice Activity?* Santa Monica, CA: RAND Institute for Civil Justice, 2010.
55 Grunebaum A, Chervenak F, and Skupski D. Effect of a comprehensive obstetric patient safety program on compensation payments and sentinel events. *American Journal of Obstetrics & Gynecology* 2011;**204**(2):97–105.
56 Iverson RE Jr and Heffner LJ. Obstetric safety improvement and its reflection in reserved claims. *American Journal of Obstetrics & Gynecology* 2011;**205**(5):398–401.

Index

Management of Labor and Delivery, Second Edition. Edited by George A. Macones.